Neuroimmune Interactions

Neuroimmune Interactions

Edited by Chester Robinson

STATES
ACADEMIC PRESS
www.statesacademicpress.com

States Academic Press,
109 South 5th Street,
Brooklyn, NY 11249, USA

Visit us on the World Wide Web at:
www.statesacademicpress.com

ISBN: 978-1-63989-372-0

Cataloging-in-Publication Data

Neuroimmune interactions / edited by Chester Robinson.
p. cm.
Includes bibliographical references and index.
ISBN 978-1-63989-372-0
1. Neuroimmunology. 2. Nervous system--Diseases--Immunological aspects. 3. Immunology.
4. Neurosciences. I. Robinson, Chester.
QP356.47 .N48 2022
616.079--dc23

Table of Contents

Preface VII

Chapter 1 **Inflammatory macrophage phenotype in BTBR T+tf/J mice** 1
Charity E. Onore, Milo Careaga, Brooke A. Babineau, Jared J. Schwartzer, Robert F. Berman and Paul Ashwood

Chapter 2 **Hyperleptinemia is associated with parameters of low-grade systemic inflammation and metabolic dysfunction in obese human beings** 10
Sonia Leon-Cabrera, Lourdes Solís-Lozano, Karina Suárez-Álvarez, Antonio González-Chávez, Yadira L. Béjar, Guillermo Robles-Díaz and Galileo Escobedo

Chapter 3 **Treating depression and depression-like behavior with physical activity: an immune perspective** 16
Harris A. Eyre, Evan Papps and Bernhard T. Baune

Chapter 4 **Hypothalamic neurohormones and immune responses** 42
J. Luis Quintanar and Irene Guzmán-Soto

Chapter 5 **Neuro-immune abnormalities in autism and their relationship with the environment: a variable insult model for autism** 58
Daniel K. Goyal and Jaleel A. Miyan

Chapter 6 **Stress modulates intestinal secretory immunoglobulin A** 67
Rafael Campos-Rodríguez, Marycarmen Godínez-Victoria, Edgar Abarca-Rojano, Judith Pacheco-Yépez, Humberto Reyna-Gar ias, Reyna Elizabeth Barbosa-Cabrera and Maria Elisa Drago-Serrano

Chapter 7 **Immune mechanisms in cerebral ischemic tolerance** 77
Lidia Garcia-Bonilla, Corinne Benakis, Jamie Moore, Costantino Iadecola and Josef Anrather

Chapter 8 **Immune responses at brain barriers and implications for brain development and neurological function in later life** 96
Helen B. Stolp, Shane A. Liddelow, Inês Sá-Pereira, Katarzyna M. Dziegielewska and Norman R. Saunders

Chapter 9 **Calcitonin gene-related peptide is a key neurotransmitter in the neuro-immune axis** 110
Bakri M. Assas, Joanne I. Pennock and Jaleel A. Miyan

Chapter 10 **Hormonal influences on neuroimmune responses in the CNS of females** 119
Nela Monasterio, Edgar Vergara and Teresa Morales

Chapter 11 **Kynurenines in CNS disease: regulation by inflammatory cytokines** 127
Brian M. Campbell, Erik Charych, Anna W. Lee and Thomas Möller

Chapter 12 **The microbiota-gut-brain axis: neurobehavioral correlates, health and sociality** ... 149
Augusto J. Montiel-Castro, Rina M. González-Cervantes, Gabriela Bravo-Ruiseco and Gustavo Pacheco-López

Chapter 13 **Surgical manipulation compromises leukocyte mobilization responses and inflammation after experimental cerebral ischemia in mice** ... 164
Adam Denes, Jesus M. Pradillo, Caroline Drake, Hannah Buggey, Nancy J. Rothwell and Stuart M. Allan

Chapter 14 **Inflammatory process in Alzheimer's Disease** ... 173
Marco A. Meraz-Ríos, Danira Toral-Rios, Diana Franco-Bocanegra, Juana Villeda-Hernández and Victoria Campos-Peña

Chapter 15 **The gateway theory: bridging neural and immune interactions in the CNS** ... 188
Daisuke Kamimura, Moe Yamada, Masaya Harada, Lavannya Sabharwal, Jie Meng, Hidenori Bando, Hideki Ogura, Toru Atsumi, Yasunobu Arima and Masaaki Murakami

Chapter 16 **Fetal cholinergic anti-inflammatory pathway and necrotizing enterocolitis: the brain-gut connection begins *in utero*** ... 193
L. Garzoni, C. Faure and M.G. Frasch

Chapter 17 **Programming of neuroendocrine self in the thymus and its defect in the development of neuroendocrine autoimmunity** ... 202
Vincent Geenen, Gwennaëlle Bodart, Séverine Henry, Hélène Michaux, Olivier Dardenne, Chantal Charlet-Renard, Henri Martens and Didier Hober

Chapter 18 **Pericytes: brain-immune interface modulators** ... 212
Gabriela Hurtado-Alvarado, Adrian M. Cabañas-Morales and Beatriz Gómez-Gónzalez

Chapter 19 **Brain immune interactions and air pollution: macrophage inhibitory factor (MIF), prion cellular protein (PrP^C), interleukin-6 (IL-6), interleukin 1 receptor antagonist (IL-1Ra), and interleukin-2 (IL-2) in cerebrospinal fluid and MIF in serum differentiate urban children exposed to severe vs. low air pollution** ... 222
Lilian Calderón-Garcidueñas, Janet V. Cross, Maricela Franco-Lira, Mariana Aragón-Flores, Michael Kavanaugh, Ricardo Torres-Jardón, Chih-kai Chao, Charles Thompson, Jing Chang, Hongtu Zhu and Amedeo D'Angiulli

Permissions

List of Contributors

Index

Preface

The system of processes and structures which consists of interactions between the nervous system and the immune system is termed as the neuroimmune system. It involves electrophysiological and biochemical processes, and is integral in protecting the neurons from pathogens. Sensory neurons and immune cells are used by the neuroimmune system for the detection and management of harmful stimuli. The neuroimmune system is primarily comprised of glial cells. Neurons and glial cells work together to deal with attacking pathogens. Both glial cells and neurons express chemokine receptors, thus chemokines act as mediators in neuron-glial cell interaction. Different approaches, evaluations, methodologies and advanced studies on neuroimmune interactions and their clinical aspects have been included in this book. It presents this complex subject in the most comprehensible and easy to understand language. This book will serve as a valuable source of reference for graduate and post graduate students.

This book is the end result of constructive efforts and intensive research done by experts in this field. The aim of this book is to enlighten the readers with recent information in this area of research. The information provided in this profound book would serve as a valuable reference to students and researchers in this field.

At the end, I would like to thank all the authors for devoting their precious time and providing their valuable contribution to this book. I would also like to express my gratitude to my fellow colleagues who encouraged me throughout the process.

Editor

1

Inflammatory macrophage phenotype in BTBR T+tf/J mice

Charity E. Onore[1,2], Milo Careaga[1,2], Brooke A. Babineau[3,4], Jared J. Schwartzer[1,5], Robert F. Berman[1,5] and Paul Ashwood[1,2]*

[1] The MIND Institute, University of California, Davis, CA, USA
[2] Department of Medical Microbiology and Immunology, University of California, Davis, CA, USA
[3] Department of Pediatrics, University of California, San Francisco, CA, USA
[4] Institute for Human Genetics, University of California, San Francisco, CA, USA
[5] Department of Neurological Surgery, University of California, Davis, CA, USA

Edited by:
Adam Denes, University of Manchester, UK

Reviewed by:
Jaleel A. Miyan, The University of Manchester, UK
Sylvie Girard, University of Manchester, UK

***Correspondence:**
Paul Ashwood, The MIND Institute, University of California, 2825 50th Street, Sacramento, CA 95817, USA
e-mail: pashwood@ucdavis.edu

Although autism is a behaviorally defined disorder, many studies report an association with increased pro-inflammatory cytokine production. Recent characterization of the BTBR T+tf/J (BTBR) inbred mouse strain has revealed several behavioral characteristics including social deficits, repetitive behavior, and atypical vocalizations which may be relevant to autism. We therefore hypothesized that, asocial BTBR mice, which exhibit autism-like behaviors, may have an inflammatory immune profile similar to that observed in children with autism. The objectives of this study were to characterize the myeloid immune profile of BTBR mice and to explore their associations with autism-relevant behaviors. C57BL/6J (C57) mice and BTBR mice were tested for social interest and repetitive self-grooming behavior. Cytokine production was measured in bone-marrow derived macrophages incubated for 24 h in either growth media alone, LPS, IL-4/LPS, or IFNγ/LPS to ascertain any M1/M2 skewing. After LPS stimulation, BTBR macrophages produced higher levels of IL-6, MCP-1, and MIP-1α and lower IL-10 ($p < 0.01$) than C57 mice, suggesting an exaggerated inflammatory profile. After exposure to IL-4/LPS BTBR macrophages produced less IL-10 ($p < 0.01$) than C57 macrophages and more IL-12p40 ($p < 0.01$) suggesting poor M2 polarization. Levels of IL-12(p70) ($p < 0.05$) were higher in BTBR macrophages after IFNγ/LPS stimulation, suggesting enhanced M1 polarization. We further observed a positive correlation between grooming frequency, and production of IL-12(p40), IL-12p70, IL-6, and TNFα ($p < 0.05$) after treatment with IFNγ/LPS across both strains. Collectively, these data suggest that the asocial BTBR mouse strain exhibits a more inflammatory, or M1, macrophage profile in comparison to the social C57 strain. We have further demonstrated a relationship between this relative increase in inflammation and repetitive grooming behavior, which may have relevance to repetitive and stereotyped behavior of autism.

Keywords: autism, BTBR, behavior, immune system, inflammation, macrophage, M1, M2

BACKGROUND

Autism is a behaviorally defined disorder without a known physiological cause. This disorder is characterized by social deficits, communication deficits, and the presence of repetitive or stereotyped behaviors (APA, 2000). Several studies have attempted to identify a genetic cause for autism (Yrigollen et al., 2008; Voineagu et al., 2011; Lintas et al., 2012); however, the majority of autism cases remain idiopathic in nature (Abrahams and Geschwind, 2008). Although the genetic cause for autism remains undetermined, there is increasing evidence that immune function may play a role in the disorder. A number of studies have identified trends in abnormal immune function in individuals with autism including a trend toward high cytokine production and atypical immune cell function (Ashwood et al., 2006, 2011a,b,c; Enstrom et al., 2010). There is further evidence suggesting that many of these atypical immune profiles are associated with worsening autism-associated behaviors (Onore et al., 2012).

Immune abnormalities in autism spectrum disorders have been characterized in a number of studies, including evidence of increased microglia and astroglia activation in the brain, as well as increased levels of interferon (IFN)γ, interleukin (IL)-1β, IL-6, IL-12, tumor necrosis factor (TNF)-α, and macrophage chemotactic protein (MCP)-1 in brain tissue and cerebral spinal fluid (Vargas et al., 2005; Li et al., 2009; Morgan et al., 2010). In parallel with findings within the central nervous system (CNS), increased plasma levels of these cytokines including IL-1β, IL-6, IL-12p40, and MCP-1 have been reported as well (Ashwood et al., 2011b). Of note, peripheral plasma levels of these cytokines were associated with worsening autism-associated behaviors in the areas of communication and social interaction, suggesting a relationship between peripheral immune activity and behavioral symptoms of the disorder (Ashwood et al., 2011b,c).

Given the unknown pathophysiology of autism and highly variable genetics of the disorder, an animal model that exhibits behavioral characteristics with relevance to autism-features rather than a direct genetic link may be useful for examining potential relationship between physiology and behavior. The BTBR T+tf/J mouse (referred to as BTBR here-in) is an inbred strain that has recently been described to exhibit behaviors relevant to autism, including asocial behavior, repetitive behavior, and atypical vocalizations (Moy et al., 2007; McFarlane et al., 2008; Scattoni et al., 2008, 2011). There is also evidence to suggest that the BTBR mouse exhibits increased ERK signaling (Zou et al., 2011), a common finding in individuals with Fragile X Syndrome, one of the leading known genetic risk factors for autism. However, little is currently known about the relationship between BTBR associated behavior and immunity in the BTBR mouse. Recent research has outlined differences in immune function including increased titers of immunoglobulin (Ig) and inflammatory cytokine levels in brain tissue, and greater susceptibility to listeriosis than C57Bl/6J mice (referred to as C57 here-in) (Heo et al., 2011). Immunity against listeriosis is largely based on the ability of macrophages to polarize to an inflammatory (M1) profile (Pfeffer et al., 1993; Jouanguy et al., 1999; Benoit et al., 2008). This data suggests immunological differences between the two strains and may implicate aberrant macrophage function, but there is as yet no direct evidence of a relationship between the function of the immune cells and behavioral symptoms in the BTBR mouse.

We hypothesized that there are associations between myeloid inflammation and autism relevant behaviors in the BTBR mouse. To further elucidate the relationship between inflammation and behavior, and to examine the role of M1/M2 polarization in BTBR, we analyzed individual mice for social interaction and repetitive grooming behavior and measured macrophage cytokine production *in vitro*. Bone marrow-derived macrophages were generated for each mouse and tested for inflammatory and anti-inflammatory cytokine responses. In addition, we further characterized immune function by testing the ability of BTBR macrophages to polarize to pro-inflammatory IL-12 high (M1) and anti-inflammatory IL-10 high (M2) macrophage subtypes *in vitro* (Mantovani et al., 2005).

METHODS

MICE

C57Bl/6J (C57) mice (Jackson Laboratory-West, Sacramento, CA), BTBR T^{+}tf/J (BTBR) mice (Jackson Laboratory, Bar Harbor, ME), and 129/SvImJ (129) mice (Jackson Laboratory) were maintained by the Campus Laboratory Animal Services, at University of California, Davis at ambient room temperature on a 12 h light/dark cycle. Food and water were provided *ad libitum*. All procedures were performed with approval by the University of California, Davis Institutional Animal Care and Use Committee and in accordance with the guidelines provided by the National Institutes of Health for the humane treatment of animals. Social approach and self-grooming assays were conducted in dedicated behavioral testing rooms during the standard light phase, usually between 1000 and 1500 h. Mice of the 129 strain were used as novel mouse controls in the social approach testing paradigm. Mice were deeply anesthetized with isofluorane and euthanized by decapitation. Femurs and tibia were aseptically removed and stored in RPMI 1640 (Life Technologies) media supplemented with 10% FBS, 100 IU/ml penicillin, 100 IU/ml streptomycin, 25 μg/ml gentimycin (Sigma) prior to processing. For this study, nine C57 mice (male, age 10–12 weeks) and seven BTBR mice (male, age 10–12 weeks), were utilized.

SOCIAL APPROACH

Social approach was assayed in an automated three-chambered apparatus (NIMH Research Services Branch, Bethesda, MD) using methods previously described (Crawley, 2007; Yang et al., 2007, 2009, 2011a,b; Chadman et al., 2008; McFarlane et al., 2008; Moy et al., 2008; Silverman et al., 2010, 2011). Briefly, the apparatus was a rectangular, three-chambered box made of clear polycarbonate. Photocells embedded in the doorways automatically detected entries between chambers and the amount of time spent in each chamber by the subject mouse. The test session began with a 10 min habituation session in the center chamber only, followed by a 10 min habituation to all three empty chambers. At the completion of the second habituation phase, the subject mouse was returned to the center chamber and a clean novel object (wire cup) was placed in one of the side chambers and a novel 129 mouse of similar age and weight was placed in an identical wire cup located in the other side chamber. After both stimuli were positioned, the subject mouse was allowed access to all three chambers for 10 min. Trials were video recorded and time spent sniffing the novel object and time spent sniffing the novel mouse were later scored by a trained observer using a handheld stopwatch. Performance on social approach was plotted as a "social score," which is equal to the amount of time (in seconds) the experimental animal spent sniffing the novel mouse minus the time spent sniffing the novel object. Therefore, high positive scores indicate high sociability, and low or negative scores indicate low sociability.

SPONTANEOUS SELF GROOMING

Mice were scored for spontaneous self-grooming behaviors as described previously (Yang et al., 2007, 2009; McFarlane et al., 2008; Silverman et al., 2010). Briefly, each mouse was given a 10 min habituation in a clean, empty mouse cage and then video recorded for 10 min. The video recorded session was scored for cumulative time spent grooming all body regions by a trained observer using a stopwatch. Differences in color and markings between the inbred strains prevented fully blind ratings. However, the distinguishing features of the strain were less visible in the video recordings, which is why this method was chosen over live scoring. The animals' behavior in the spontaneous self-grooming tasks was plotted as "grooming" which indicates the amount of time (in seconds) the experimental animal spent grooming itself during the 10-min observation phase.

GENERATION OF MACROPHAGE MEDIA

Confluent L929 Cells (ATCC, Manassas, VA) were cultured for 7 days in complete Dubelcco's modified Eagles media (DMEM) F-12 (Life Technologies, Carlsbad, CA) supplemented with 10% low endotoxin, heat inactivated fetal bovine serum (FBS) (Life technologies), 100 IU/ml penicillin, and 100 IU/ml streptomycin (Sigma, St Louis, MO). The resulting L929 conditioned media was passed through a 2 μm filter (Millipore, Billerica, MA) to remove cellular debris and ensure sterility. To create macrophage media, complete DMEM was supplemented 10% with filtered L929 conditioned media. L929 conditioned media was stored at −20°C for less than 60 days before single thaw and use.

BONE MARROW-DERIVED MACROPHAGE GENERATION

Legs with fur and skin removed, including femur and tibia from each mouse, were washed twice in sterile cold (4°C) Hanks buffered saline solution (HBSS) (Mediatech, Herndon, VA). Tissue was removed from the bones with sterile scissors and forceps, and bones were washed in 10 mls cold HBSS. The proximal and distal ends of both the femur and tibia were removed, and the lumens of the femurs and tibia were flushed with 10 mls of cold HBSS using a 25 gauge needle (BD Medical, Franklin Lakes, NJ). Dislodged bone marrow was agitated by aspiration and ejected with a 22 gauge needle (BD Medical). The resulting cell suspension was filtered through a 100 μm nylon mesh (BD Biosciences, Carlsbad, CA). Cells were pelleted by centrifugation at 500 g for 5 min and resuspended in macrophage media to a concentration of 1×10^5 cells/ml, plated in sterile non-cell culture treated petri dishes (BD Biosciences) at a volume of 10 mls per dish and incubated for 3 days at 37°C, 5% CO_2. Five mls of macrophage media was then added to each dish and cells were incubated for a further 4 days at 37°C, 5% CO_2 for a total incubation time of 7 days. Petri dishes containing adherent, mature bone marrow-derived macrophages were washed with 10 mls cold HBSS, and incubated with 3 mls Cell Stripper™ buffer (Mediatech) per plate, for 5 min at 37°C, 5% CO_2. Following incubation, cells were dislodged from the petri dishes by gentle pipetting, diluted in an equal amount of complete DMEM, and pelleted by centrifugation at 400 g for 5 min. Cells were resuspended at 1×10^6 cell/ml in complete DMEM, and 1 ml was plated in 12-well sterile tissue culture plate (Greiner Bio-One, Monroe, NC) and allowed to adhere overnight at 37°C, 5% CO_2. Following adhesion of bone marrow-derived macrophages, complete DMEM was aspirated and replaced with 1 ml/well of 1×10^6 cells with the following eight conditions: media alone, 2 ng/ml recombinant mouse IL-4 (R&D, Minneapolis, MN), 150 ng/ml recombinant mouse IFNγ (R&D), 10 ng/ml lipopolysaccharide (LPS) (Sigma), 2 ng/ml recombinant mouse IL-4 with 10 ng/ml LPS, or 150 ng/ml recombinant mouse IFNγ with 10 ng/ml LPS. Cells were incubated under these conditions for 24 h, at which point supernatants were collected and stored at −80°C until assayed.

CYTOKINE MEASUREMENT

The quantification of the cytokines Granulocyte Macrophage-Colony Stimulating Factor (GM-CSF), IFNγ, IL-1β, IL-6, IL-10, IL-13, IFNγ induced protein (IP)-10 (CXCL10), MCP-1 (CCL2), TNFα, macrophage inflammatory protein (MIP)-1α (CCL3), and MIP-1β (CCL4) in supernatants was determined using mouse specific Milliplex™ multiplexing bead immunoassays (Millipore, Billerica, MA). The cytokines IL-12p40 and IL-12p70 were measured using Bioplex™ multiplexing bead immunoassays (Bio-Rad Laboratories, Hercules, CA). Samples were run in accordance with the instructions of the manufactures protocol. In brief, 25 μL of supernatant was incubated with antibody-coupled beads. After a series of washes, a biotinylated detection antibody was added to the beads, and the reaction mixture was detected by the addition of streptavidin conjugated to phycoerythrin. The bead sets were analyzed using a flow-based Luminex™ 100 suspension array system (Bio-Plex 200; Bio-Rad Laboratories). Unknown sample cytokine concentrations were calculated by Bio-Plex Manager software using a standard curve derived from the known reference cytokine concentrations supplied by the manufacturer. A five-parameter model was used to calculate final concentrations and values are expressed in pg/ml. The sensitivity of this multiplex immunoassay allowed the detection of cytokine concentrations with the following minimal detectable limits: IL-1β (2 pg/ml), IL-6 (1.8 pg/ml), IL-10 (3.3 pg/ml), IL-12(p40) (1.53 pg/ml), IL-12(p70) (1.62 pg/ml), IFNγ (0.9 pg/ml), IP-10 (0.6 pg/ml), MCP-1 (5.3 pg/ml), MIP-1α (8.7 pg/ml), MIP-1β (10.1 pg/ml), and TNFα (1 pg/ml).

STATISTICAL ANALYSIS

Statistical analysis to compare cytokine levels between BTBR and C57 groups was conducted with Mann–Whitney test. Correlation analysis was performed with Spearman correlation analysis. All analyses were two-tailed, and values of $p < 0.05$ were considered statistically significant. Unadjusted p-values are presented for multiplex cytokine data (Rothman, 1990). Medians and interquartile ranges (IQR) are reported for all measured cytokines and chemokines. All analyses were conducted with GraphPad Prism statistical software (GraphPad Software Inc., San Diego, CA).

RESULTS

CYTOKINE RESPONSES

To determine the cytokine response to LPS (a gram negative bacterial endotoxin) with and without polarization, bone marrow macrophages were incubated in media alone, IL-4 (a M2 polarizing cytokine), or IFNγ (a M1 polarizing cytokine) with LPS. Even without presence of polarizing cytokine or LPS stimulus, BTBR macrophages exhibit a trend toward higher inflammatory cytokine production, with significantly higher production of IL-12(p40) [C57 median ± IQR: 15.30 ± 7.56; median ± IQR: 20.58 ± 7.56; $p = 0.0485$] (**Table 1**). Following stimulation with LPS, BTBR macrophages produce significantly higher levels of inflammatory cytokines IL-6 [C57 median ± IQR: 1254 ± 760.2; BTBR median ± IQR: 3112 ± 1189; $p = 0.0003$], IL-12(p40) [C57 median ± IQR: 446.4 ± 322.5; BTBR median ± IQR: 2779 ± 1652; $p = 0.0002$], MCP-1 [C57 median ± IQR: 750.4 ± 442.6; BTBR median ± IQR: 3117 ± 1036; $p = 0.0002$], IP-10 [C57 median ± IQR: 8875 ± 2859; BTBR median ± IQR: 14535 ± 1294; $p = 0.0007$], and MIP-1α [C57 median ± IQR: 1945 ± 713; BTBR median ± IQR: 4342 ± 2828; $p = 0.0002$] and lower levels of anti-inflammatory cytokine IL-10 [C57 median ± IQR: 448.4 ± 307.6; BTBR median ± IQR: 284.2 ± 195.2; $p = 0.0229$] (**Table 1**).

To determine whether BTBR macrophages are more inclined toward a pro-inflammatory M1 phenotype, we measured the levels of M1 and M2 associated cytokines following polarization with IL-4 and LPS to induce a M2 phenotype or IFNγ and LPS to induce a M1 phenotype. Our initial experiments revealed treatment with IL-4 alone was not sufficient to induce a cytokine

Table 1 | Macrophage cytokine levels in unstimulated and LPS stimulated culture conditions.

Cytokines pg/ml	Unstimulated: Median (IQR)			LPS: Median (IQR)		
	C57	BTBR	*p*-value	C57	BTBR	*p*-value
IL-1β	3.9 (14.39)	BLD	N/A	BLD	16.56 (38.26)	0.351
IL-6	0.23 (2.22)	BLD	N/A	1254 (760.2)	3112 (1189)	0.0003*
IL-10	BLD	BLD	N/A	448.4 (307.6)	284.2 (195.2)	0.023*
IL-12p40	15.3 (7.56)	20.58 (7.56)	0.049*	446.4 (322.5)	2779 (1652)	0.0002*
IL-12p70	BLD	BLD	N/A	BLD	56.81 (56.81)	N/A
IP-10	65.45 (30.94)	70.17 (93.81)	0.142	8875 (2859)	14535 (1294)	0.0007*
MCP-1	BLD	15.63 (32.74)	N/A	750.4 (442.6)	3117 (1036)	0.0002*
TNF-α	BLD	0.13 (5.1)	N/A	448.3 (407.5)	595.2 (217.2)	0.408
MIP-1α	39.27 (22.41)	BLD	N/A	1945 (713)	4342 (2828)	0.0002*
MIP-1β	63.35 (36.58)	56.76 (83.06)	0.671	10214 (2530)	23060 (9262)	0.0003*

Median cytokine measurements and interquartile ranges (IQR) in pg/ml. All p-values were calculated by two-tailed Mann Whitney U-test.
**Significant p-values; BLD: Below level of detection; N/A: Not applicable, p-values could not be calculated.*

response distinguishable from that of media alone. Following stimulation with IL-4 and LPS, BTBR macrophages produce significantly lower levels of IL-10 [C57 median ± IQR: 641.9 ± 164.2; BTBR median ± IQR: 222.6 ± 83.4; $p = 0.0.0003$], a M2 cytokine, and higher IL-12p40 [C57 median ± IQR: 182.3 ± 102.6; BTBR median ± IQR: 613.8 ± 359.4; $p = 0.001$], IL-6 [C57 median ± IQR: 558.6 ± 288.1; BTBR median ± IQR: 1264 ± 330; $p = 0.0052$], and MIP-1α [C57 median ± IQR: 2551 ± 1150; BTBR median ± IQR: 4179 ± 4467; $p = 0.0021$]. Following stimulation with IFNγ and LPS, BTBR macrophages produce significantly higher levels of IL-12(p40) [C57 median ± IQR: 12496 ± 5494; BTBR median ± IQR: 18607 ± 326.6; $p = 0.0401$], IL-12(p70) [C57 median ± IQR: 251.9 ± 302.17; BTBR median ± IQR: 625.5 ± 477.1; $p = 0.0108$], and IP-10 [C57 median ± IQR: 3464 ± 1953; BTBR median ± IQR: 7497 ± 3553; $p = 0.0002$] but also more IL-10 [C57 median ± IQR: 35.24 ± 15.36; BTBR median ± IQR: 74.8 ± 30.9; $p = 0.0115$] and MCP-1 [C57 median ± IQR: 1238 ± 802; BTBR median ± IQR: 1954 ± 752; $p = 0.0012$] (**Table 2**). BTBR macrophages appeared to exhibit an overall trend toward increased M1 polarization (**Figure 1**).

BEHAVIORAL AND IMMUNE CORRELATIONS

To examine a potential relationship between the immune profile observed in BTBR macrophages, and the impaired social interaction and repetitive grooming associated with the BTBR strain, we tested for associations by Spearman analysis. There was very little association between cytokine profiles and social behavior in the BTBR mouse; however, for macrophage cell cultures, IL-1β demonstrated a negative association with sociability after IFNγ/LPS incubation [$r = -0.56$; $p = 0.023$] such that as IL-1β levels increased social approach decreased (**Figure 2**). In contrast, grooming behavior was associated with a large number of cytokines including associations with IL-12(p40) [$r = 0.58$; $p = 0.033$] and IP-10 [$r = 0.55$; $p = 0.032$] in unstimulated macrophages (**Figure 3**) suggesting that as cytokine levels increased there was an increase in repetitive behaviors. Following stimulation with LPS, inflammatory cytokines IL-6 [$r = 0.77$; $p = 0.001$] and MIP-1β [$r = 0.67$; $p = 0.006$] were positively associated with grooming behavior, while the anti-inflammatory M2 associated cytokine IL-10 demonstrated a negative association with grooming [$r = -0.63$; $p = 0.012$] (**Figure 4**). This data suggests that inflammatory cytokines are associated with more impaired repetitive behavior whereas anti-inflammatory cytokines are associated with improvement in behaviors. In polarization conditions such as IL-4/LPS incubation, IL-10 again was negatively associated with grooming [$r = -0.86$; $p = 0.0001$], while IL-6 [$r = -0.63$; $p = 0.012$], IP-10 [$r = 0.775$, $p = 0.0007$], and MIP-1β [$r = 0.5286$, $p = 0.0428$] were positively associated with grooming time (**Figure 5**). Macrophage cytokines produced following incubation with the M1 polarizing IFNγ/LPS condition including IL-12(p40) [$r = 0.72$; $p = 0.004$], IL-12(p70) [$r = 0.77$; $p = 0.001$], and TNF-α [$r = 0.63$; $p = 0.011$] also positively associated with increased grooming behavior following incubation with the M1 polarizing IFNγ/LPS condition, such that M1 macrophage cytokine production was associated with more impaired behavior. Interestingly, within the BTBR strain alone, IL-12(p70) [$r = 0.87$; $p = 0.03$] and TNF-α [$r = 0.94$; $p = 0.005$] levels were also positively correlated with grooming (**Figure 6**).

DISCUSSION

In this study we describe several immune features in the asocial BTBR mouse that differ from social C57 mice including higher production of inflammatory cytokines and chemokines in bone-marrow derived macrophages. BTBR macrophages produced increased levels of IL-6 after LPS stimulation. Even without stimulation, BTBR macrophages produced higher levels of IL-12(p40) and IP-10, suggesting a possible M1 polarization even without the presence of M1 polarizing exposure to IFNγ or LPS. After stimulation with LPS, IL-12(p40) remained higher in BTBR mice, while IL-10 was lower, again suggesting M1 polarization even in the absence of IFNγ. Levels of IL-12(p70) were undetectable in C57 mice, but were detectable in the majority of BTBR samples, suggesting IL-12(p70) levels may also be higher in BTBR mice. However, given that IL-12(p70) were below levels of detection in the C57, statistical analysis was limited and p-values could not be calculated. In addition to evidence of M1

Table 2 | Macrophage cytokine levels in IL-4/LPS and IFNγ/LPS stimulated culture conditions.

Cytokines pg/ml	IL-4/LPS: Median (IQR)			IFNγ/LPS: Median (IQR)		
	C57	BTBR	*p*-value	C57	BTBR	*p*-value
IL-1β	20.04 (32.39)	BLD	0.252	BLD	46.36 (28.18)	N/A
IL-6	558.6 (288.1)	1264 (330)	0.005*	10680 (8041)	10667 (5695)	0.919
IL-10	641.9 (164.2)	222.6 (83.4)	0.0003*	35.24 (15.36)	74.8 (30.9)	0.012*
IL-12p40	182.3 (102.6)	613.8 (359.4)	0.001*	12496 (5494)	18607(326.6)	0.040*
IL-12p70	BLD	BLD	N/A	251.9 (302.17)	625.5 (477.1)	0.011*
IP-10	3464 (1953)	7497 (3553)	0.0002*	18319 (7141)	16726 (10137)	0.351
MCP-1	2692 (682)	3373 (1065)	0.351	1238 (802)	1954 (752)	0.001*
TNF-α	418.2 (292.6)	498.5 (282)	0.351	975.2 (451.8)	1393 (974)	0.071
MIP-1α	2551 (1150)	4179 (4467)	0.002*	872.3 (321.6)	1134 (330.2)	0.091
MIP-1β	4264 (2097)	6136 (17675)	0.055	4019 (1492)	5791 (3024)	0.071

Median cytokine measurements and interquartile ranges (IQR) in pg/ml. All p-values were calculated by two-tailed Mann Whitney U-test.
**Significant p-values; BLD: Below level of detection; N/A: Not applicable, p-values could not be calculated.*

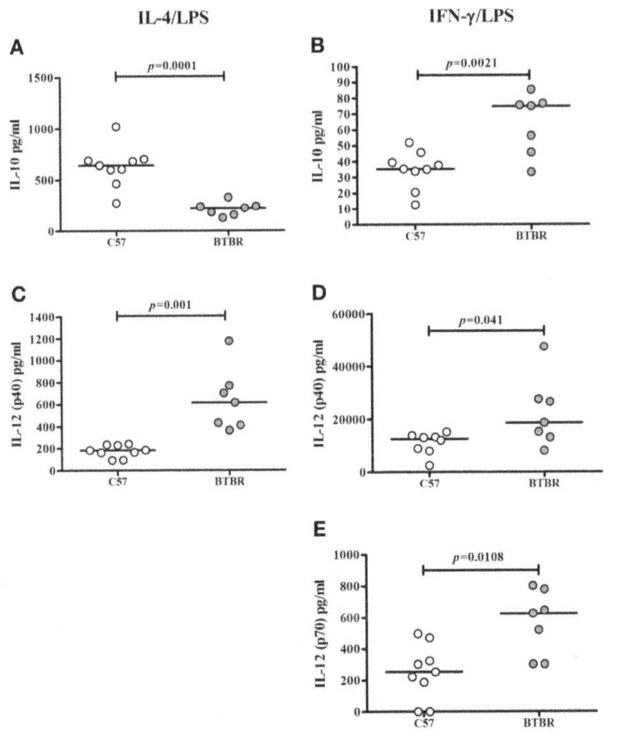

FIGURE 1 | M1 and M2 cytokine polarization in BTBR and C57 macrophages. Scatter graphs and median values of IL-10 **(A,B)**, IL-12p40 **(C,D)** and IL-12p70 **(E)** after IL-4/LPS incubation **(A,C)** and IFNγ/LPS incubation **(B,D,E)**. IL-12(p70) values were below observable levels in IL-4/LPS stimulated samples. *p*-values were calculated with Mann–Whitney test.

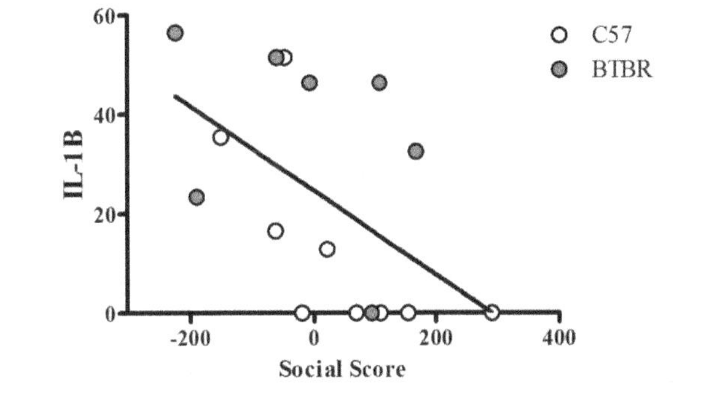

FIGURE 2 | Social correlation in IFNγ/LPS stimulated macrophages. Scatter graphs and linear regression of IL-1β in IFNγ stimulated macrophages. Correlation coefficients (*r*-values) and *p*-values were calculated with Spearman's correlation analysis. C57 *r*-value: −0.80, *p*-value: 0.009*; BTBR *r*-value: −0.43, *p*-value: 0.333; Across strains *r*-value: −0.56, *p*-value: 0.023*; *significant *p*-values.

polarization, levels of chemokines MIP-1α and MCP-1 were also higher in BTBR macrophages after LPS stimulation suggesting chemotactic responses may also be enhanced in this asocial mouse strain.

Macrophage polarization has many similarities to T helper (T_H) cell subtypes and can be divided into two major groups, denoted M1 and M2 (Mantovani et al., 2005; Mosser and Edwards, 2008). M1 macrophages are IL-12^{high}, IL-10^{low}, they are higher inflammatory cytokine producers than their M2 counterparts, and promote a T_H1 response in part through production of IL-12(p70). IL-12(p40) is a subunit of both IL-12(p70) and IL-23, which are both produced in significant quantities by M1 macrophages (Oppmann et al., 2000). While M2 cells can also produce inflammatory cytokines, they tend to produce far less than M1 macrophages, and have an IL-12^{low}, IL-10^{high} phenotype, and promote T_H2 responses. M1 polarization has been implicated in a number of neurological disease including multiple sclerosis and Alzheimer's disease (Mikita et al., 2011), and recent literature suggests that promoting an M2 phenotype may be beneficial to cognitive function (Derecki et al., 2010a). Transplant of wild-type IL-4 competent T cells in to IL-$4^{-/-}$ mice results in improved cognition (Derecki et al., 2010b), and transplant of M2 polarized macrophages results in improved cognitive performance in immune deficient mice (Derecki et al., 2011). Together, this data suggests that M1 macrophage polarization may have

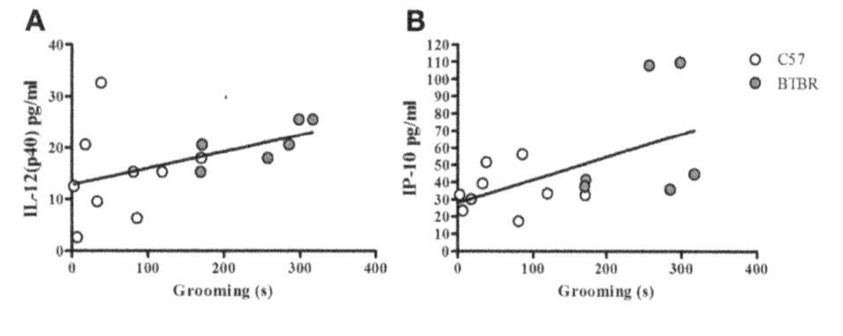

FIGURE 3 | Grooming correlation in unstimulated macrophages. Scatter graphs and linear regression of IL-12(p40) **(A)** and IP-10 **(B)** in unstimulated macrophages. Correlation coefficients (*r*-value) and *p*-values were calculated with Spearman's correlation analysis. **(A)** C57 *r*-value: 0.27, *p*-value: 0.493; BTBR *r*-value: 0.88, *p*-value: 0.033*; Across strains *r*-value; 0.58, *p*-value: 0.024* **(B)** C57 *r*-value: 0.23, *p*-value: 0.546; BTBR *r*-value: 0.43, *p*-value: 0.397; Across strains *r*-value: 0.55, *p*-value: 0.032*; *significant *p*-values.

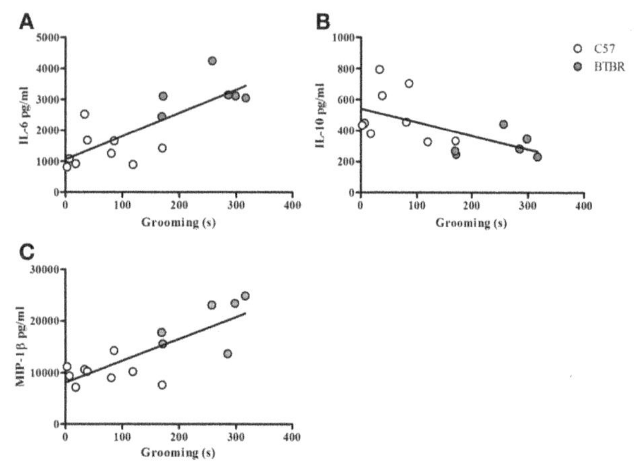

FIGURE 4 | Grooming correlation in LPS stimulated macrophages. Scatter graphs and linear regression of IL-6 **(A)**, IL-10 **(B)**, and **(C)** MIP-1β in LPS stimulated macrophages. Correlation coefficients (*r*-values) and *p*-values were calculated with Spearman's correlation analysis. **(A)** C57 *r*-value: 0.30, *p*-value: 0.433; BTBR *r*-value: 0.20, *p*-value: 0.704; Across strains *r*-value: 0.77, *p*-value: 0.001* **(B)** C57 *r*-value: −0.22, *p*-value: 0.576; BTBR *r*-value: −0.09, *p*-value: 0.872; Across strains *r*-value: −0.63, *p*-value: 0.012* **(C)** C57 *r*-value: −0.15, *p*-value: 0.708; BTBR *r*-value: 0.60, *p*-value: 0.241; Across strains *r*- value: 0.67, *p*-value: 0.006; *significant *p*-values.

detrimental effects on normal brain function whilst M2 can ameliorate some of these effects.

To further examine the proclivity of BTBR macrophages to polarize to an M1 phenotype, C57 and BTBR macrophages were stimulated with LPS in the presence of IFNγ (M1) or IL-4 (M2) (Zhang et al., 2008). Under M1 polarizing conditions, BTBR macrophages produced significantly higher IL-12(p40) and IL-12(p70), mirroring the enhanced M1 polarization. In addition under M2 polarizing conditions, BTBR macrophages produced significantly less IL-10, and significantly more IL-12(p40) suggesting poor relative M2 polarization compared to C57 mice (**Figure 1**). Collectively, these data suggest that BTBR macrophages are innately M1 skewed, and more inclined to produce M1 associated cytokines such as IL-12(p70).

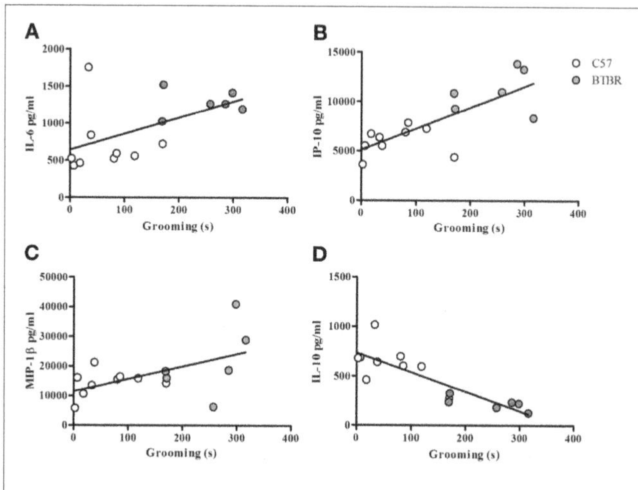

FIGURE 5 | Grooming correlation in IL-4/LPS stimulated macrophages. Scatter graphs and linear regression of IL-6 **(A)**, IP-10 **(B)**, MIP-1β **(C)**, and IL-10 **(D)** in IL-4/LPS stimulated macrophages. Correlation coefficients (*r*-value) and *p*-values were calculated with Spearman's correlation analysis. **(A)** C57 *r*-value: 0.43, *p*-value: 0.244; BTBR *r*-value: 0.09, *p*-value: 0.872; Across strains *r*-value: 0.63, *p*-value: 0.012* **(B)** C57 *r*-value: 0.40, *p*-value: 0.291; BTBR *r*-value: 0.02, *p*-value: 1; Across strains *r*-value: 0.78, *p*-value: 0.0007* **(C)** C57 *r*-value: 0.38, *p*-value: 0.312; BTBR *r*-value: 0.71, *p*-value: 0.136; Across strains *r*-value: 0.53, *p*-value: 0.042* **(D)** C57 *r*-value: −0.48, *p*-value: 0.188; BTBR *r*-value: −0.77, *p*-value: 0.072; Across strains *r*-value: −0.86, *p*-value: 0.0001*; *significant *p*-values.

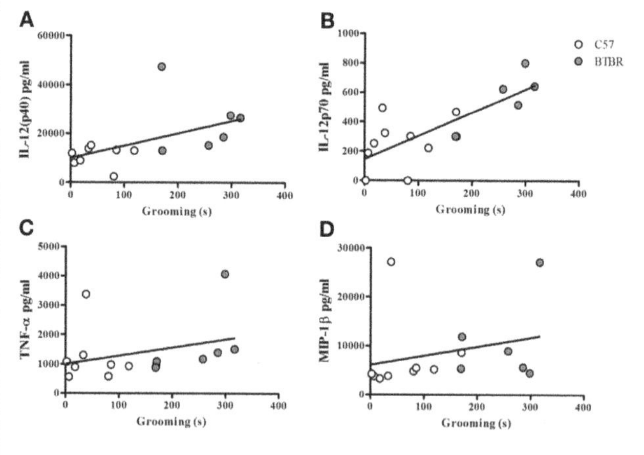

FIGURE 6 | Grooming correlation in IFNγ/LPS stimulated macrophages. Scatter graphs and linear regression of IL-12(p40) **(A)**, IL-12(p70) **(B)**, TNFα **(C)**, and MIP-1β **(D)** in IFNγ/LPS stimulated macrophages. Correlation coefficients (*r*-values) and *p*-values were calculated with Spearman's correlation analysis. **(A)** C57 *r*-value: 0.26, *p*-value: 0.536; BTBR *r*-value: 0.09, *p*-value: 0.919; Across strains *r*-value: 0.72, *p*-value: 0.004* **(B)** C57 *r*-value: 0.39, *p*-value: 0.291; BTBR *r*-value: 0.87, *p*-value: 0.033*; Across strains *r*-value: 0.77, *p*-value: 0.001* **(C)** C57 *r*-value: 0.02, *p*-value: 0.966; BTBR *r*-value: 0.94, *p*-value: 0.005*; Across strains *r*-value 0.51, *p*-value: 0.005* **(D)** C57 *r*-value: 0.70, *p*-value: 0.036*; BTBR *r*-value: 0.20, *p*-value: 0.704; Across strains *r*- value: 0.63, *p*-value: 0.011*; *significant *p*-values.

In this study, we have compared two inbred strains, which were selected for their possession of autism-relevant features or lack thereof (BTBR and C57, respectively) (McFarlane et al., 2008). Given the potential genetic differences between these two inbred strains, it would be possible that these observed immunological differences are circumstantial and unrelated to behavior. To better understand the relationship between autism-like behavior and immune phenotype, we measured social and repetitive behavior in each mouse, and analyzed the correlation between these behavioral measurements and cytokine profiles. We observed only one cytokine correlation with social behavior (**Figure 2**), which may suggest that social behavior is not heavily affected by immune function within BTBR mice as a group.

Although we did not see strong correlations between social behavior and immune measures in these experiments, the inflammation in BTBR mice may have an impact on fetal development *in-utero*. Maternal immune activation (MIA) in C57 mice results in elevated expression of IL-6, IL-12(p40), IL-12(p70), IL-13, IL-15, IFNγ, TNFα, and IL-10 in pregnant dams (Arrode-Bruses and Bruses, 2012), and leads to deficits in sociability in their offspring (Malkova et al., 2012). The data here-in suggest that BTBR mice innately produce higher levels of many of these cytokines, which may suggest that the maternal environment in which BTBR embryos are exposed to naturally resembles that of the MIA C57 model in terms of increased inflammatory cytokine exposure *in-utero*. Potentially, social impairment is more closely associated with prenatal exposures, while repetitive grooming seems to be related to ongoing elevated inflammation. Additional research, such as prenatal cross-fostering, may help differentiate the roles of the maternal BTBR environment and adult immune profiles in the development of autism-like symptoms in the BTBR mice.

Unlike the social behavior, repetitive grooming behavior correlated with a number of cytokine profiles under all tested culture conditions. IL-12(p40) correlated with increasing grooming behavior of BTBR mice in unstimulated macrophages, and this correlation was also observed across the two strains (**Figure 3**). Contrary to the positive correlation between IL-12(p40) and repetitive behavior, macrophage derived IL-10 was negatively associated with repetitive grooming across strains in both LPS stimulated and IL-4/LPS stimulated conditions (**Figures 4**, **5**), suggesting a relationship between M1/M2 polarization and repetitive behavior such that M1 was associated with more impairment and M2 with less grooming behaviors. Moreover, both IL-12(p40) and IL-12(p70) showed positive correlations with repetitive grooming post IFNγ/LPS exposure, further supporting a relationship between M1 macrophage cytokines and repetitive grooming.

Of note, a difference in IL-12(p40) was observed between BTBR and C57 strains. We initially measured IL-12(p40) using an allele specific capture antibody, which recognizes several common strains such as C57, BALB/c, and CH3 mice, but does not recognize IL-12(p40) in autoimmune prone strains such as NOD or SJL strains of mice (Ymer et al., 2002). IL-12(p40) from BTBR was also undetectable with this antibody, but was detectable with a non-allele specific anti-IL-12(p40) capture antibody (data not shown). Although we did not test for IL-12(p40) allelic differences between these two strains, an allelic difference may indicate a functional difference for IL-12(p40) *in-vivo*. Interestingly, IL-10 production is also higher in BTBR mice. The synergistic effect of functionally abnormal IL-12p40 allele and high levels of IL-10 production in response to IFNγ may help explain how BTBR mice can both express higher IL-12(p40) and IL-12(p70) than their C57 counterparts, but also be more susceptible to Listeriosis (Heo et al., 2011).

The relationship between repetitive grooming and immune function, particularly in myeloid cells, has been recently illustrated by research in the Hoxb8 deficient mice. Hoxb8 is a myeloid expressed gene associated with repetitive pathological grooming in mice deficient for the gene and excessive grooming is reduced with wild-type bone marrow transplant (Chen et al., 2010). Given this data suggesting that peripherally derived immune cells can have a profound effect on normal grooming behavior, it is possible that ongoing myeloid inflammation may be related to repetitive grooming behavior in animal models. Further evidence that peripherally derived hematopoietic cells can improve behavior was illustrated in a recent paper demonstrating that bone marrow transplant arrested disease development in MeCP2$^{+/-}$ mouse models of Rett's syndrome (Derecki et al., 2012).

Research in children with autism also implicates the role of myeloid cells in the pathology of the disorder. Immunohistochemistry of postmortem brain samples have revealed elevated numbers of microglia in brain parenchyma, and increased perivascular macrophages as well as elevated microglial and perivascular macrophage activation in the brains of children with autism, and increased levels of MCP-1 (Vargas et al., 2005; Morgan et al., 2010). Consistent with findings in the brain, studies examining peripheral myeloid function have revealed increased numbers of circulatory monocytes in the blood and increased cytokine production following TLR4 stimulation in monocytes of children with autism including increased levels of IL-1β, IL-6, and IL-23 and associations with behavioral assessment scores (Sweeten et al., 2003; Jyonouchi et al., 2008; Enstrom et al., 2010). Similar to findings in microglia and monocytes, there is also evidence of atypical distribution of dendritic cell populations in children with autism (Breece et al., 2013), suggesting that many branches of the myeloid system are affected in the disorder. The data described here-in draws many parallels between previously recorded immune phenomena in humans, and the immune profile of the BTBR mouse and warrants a closer examination of neuro-immune interactions in the development of autism spectrum disorders.

In this study, we have demonstrated an inflammatory immune profile is displayed in the asocial BTBR mouse strain as well as associations between inflammation and M1 associated cytokines with repetitive grooming behavior. The immune phenotype of BTBR mice draws several parallels to observation in children with autism particularly high IL-12, IL-6, and MCP-1 production observed in both children with autism and BTBR mice. Although there are caveats in comparing the immunophenotype of two different strains based on behavior, the observed correlations between autism-relevant behaviors and immunological measures suggest the inflammatory phenotype of the BTBR mouse is more than circumstantial. Together these data suggests that the BTBR mouse may possess more than a behavioral similarity to autism in humans, but may also share some physiological symptoms associated with the disorder as well. Although it may not be possible to find a true animal model for autism, the BTBR mouse may prove to be a useful model to study the relationship between inflammation and behavior, the fruits of which may one day be applied to autism and other inflammatory disorders that manifest in behavioral deficits.

ACKNOWLEDGMENTS

This work was supported by NIH T32MH073124, Jane Botsford Johnson Foundation, Peter Emch Foundation, Barbara and Michael Bass Foundation, and the Brain & Behavior Research Foundation (formerly known as National Alliance for Research on Schizophrenia and Depression). The authors would like to thank Duy Pham for his technical support.

REFERENCES

Abrahams, B. S., and Geschwind, D. H. (2008). Advances in autism genetics: on the threshold of a new neurobi- ology. *Nat. Rev. Genet.* 9, 341–355. doi: 10.1038/nrg2346

APA. (2000). *Diagnostic and Statistical Manual of Mental Disorders.* Arlington, VA: American Psychiatric Publishing Inc.

Arrode-Bruses, G., and Bruses, J. L. (2012). Maternal immune activa- tion by poly(I:C) induces expression of cytokines IL-1beta and IL-13, chemokine MCP-1 and colony stim- ulating factor VEGF in fetal mouse brain. *J. Neuroinflammation* 9, 83. doi:10.1186/1742-2094-9-83

Ashwood, P., Krakowiak, P., Hertz Picciotto, I., Hansen, R., Pessah, I. N., and Van de Water, J. (2011a). Altered T cell responses in children with autism. *Brain Behav. Immun.* 25, 840–849. doi: 10.1016/ j.bbi.2010.09.002

Ashwood, P., Krakowiak, P., Hertz Picciotto, I., Hansen, R., Pessah, I., and Van de Water, J. (2011b). Elevated plasma cytokines in autism spectrum disorders provide evidence of immune dysfunc- tion and are associated with impaired behavioral outcome. *Brain Behav. Immun.* 25, 40–45. doi: 10.1016/j. bbi.2010.08.003

Ashwood, P., Krakowiak, P., Hertz- Picciotto, I., Hansen, R., Pessah, I. N., and Van de Water, J. (2011c). Associations of impaired behaviors with elevated plasma chemokines in autism spectrum disorders. *J. Neuroimmunol.* 232, 196–199. doi: 10.1016/j.jneuroim. 2010.10.025

Ashwood, P., Wills, S., and Van de Water, J. (2006). The immune response in autism: a new frontier for autism research. *J. Leukoc. Biol.* 80, 1–15. doi: 10.1189/jlb.1205707

Benoit, M., Desnues, B., and Mege, J. L. (2008). Macrophage polarization in bacterial infections. *J. Immunol.* 181, 3733–3739.

Breece, E., Paciotti, B., Nordahl, C. W., Ozonoff, S., Van de Water, J. A., Rogers, S. J., et al. (2013). Myeloid dendritic cells frequen- cies are increased in children with autism spectrum disorder and asso- ciated with amygdala volume and repetitive behaviors. *Brain Behav. Immun.* 31, 69–75. doi: 10.1016/j. bbi.2012.10.006

Chadman, K. K., Gong, S., Scattoni, M. L., Boltuck, S. E., Gandhy, S. U., Heintz, N., et al. (2008). Minimal aberrant behavioral phenotypes of neuroligin-3 R451C knockin mice. *Autism Res.* 1, 147–158. doi: 10.1002/aur.22

Chen, S. K., Tvrdik, P., Peden, E., Cho, S., Wu, S., Spangrude, G., et al. (2010). Hematopoietic origin of pathological grooming in Hoxb8 mutant mice. *Cell* 141, 775–785. doi: 10.1016/j.cell.2010.03.055

Crawley, J. N. (2007). Mouse behavioral assays relevant to the symp- toms of autism. *Brain Pathol.* 17, 448–459. doi: 10.1111/j.1750-3639. 2007.00096.x

Derecki, N. C., Cronk, J. C., Lu, Z., Xu, E., Abbott, S. B., Guyenet, P. G., et al. (2012). Wild-type microglia arrest pathology in a mouse model of Rett syndrome. *Nature* 484, 105–109. doi: 10.1038/nature10907

Derecki, N. C., Privman, E., and Kipnis, J. (2010a). Rett syn- drome and other autism spectrum disorders-brain diseases of immune malfunction? *Mol. Psychiatry* 15, 355–363. doi: 10.1038/mp.2010.21

Derecki, N. C., Cardani, A. N., Yang, C. H., Quinnies, K. M., Crihfield, A., Lynch, K. R., et al. (2010b). Regulation of learn- ing and memory by meningeal immunity: a key role for IL-4. *J. Exp. Med.* 207, 1067–1080. doi: 10.1084/jem.20091419

Derecki, N. C., Quinnies, K. M., and Kipnis, J. (2011). Alternatively activated myeloid (M2) cells enhance cognitive function in immune compromised mice. *Brain Behav. Immun.* 25, 379–385. doi: 10.1016/j.bbi.2010.11.009

Enstrom, A. M., Onore, C. E., Van de Water, J. A., and Ashwood, P. (2010). Differential monocyte responses to TLR ligands in children with autism spectrum disorders. *Brain Behav. Immun.* 24, 64–71. doi: 10.1016/j. bbi.2009.08.001

Heo, Y., Zhang, Y., Gao, D., Miller, V. M., and Lawrence, D. A. (2011). Aberrant immune responses in a mouse with behavioral disorders. *PLoS ONE* 6:e20912. doi: 10.1371/journal.pone.0020912

Jouanguy, E., Doffinger, R., Dupuis, S., Pallier, A., Altare, F., and Casanova, J. L. (1999). IL-12 and IFN-gamma in host defense against mycobacteria and salmonella in mice and men. *Curr. Opin. Immunol.* 11, 346–351. doi: 10.1016/S0952-7915(99)80055-7

Jyonouchi, H., Geng, L., Cushing- Ruby, A., and Quraishi, H. (2008). Impact of innate immunity in a sub- set of children with autism spec- trum disorders: a case control study. *J. Neuroinflammation* 5, 52. doi: 10.1186/1742-2094-5-52

Li, X., Chauhan, A., Sheikh, A. M., Patil, S., Chauhan, V., Li, X. M., et al. (2009). Elevated immune response in the brain of autis- tic patients. *J. Neuroimmunol.* 207, 111–116. doi: 10.1016/j.jneuroim. 2008.12.002

Lintas, C., Sacco, R., and Persico, A. M. (2012). Genome-wide expression studies in autism spectrum disor- der, Rett syndrome, and Down syndrome. *Neurobiol. Dis.* 45, 57–68. doi:10.1016/j.nbd.2010.11.010

Malkova, N. V., Yu, C. Z., Hsiao, E. Y., Moore, M. J., and Patterson, P. H. (2012). Maternal immune activation yields offspring display- ing mouse versions of the three core symptoms of autism. *Brain Behav. Immun.* 26, 607–616. doi: 10.1016/j.bbi.2012.01.011

Mantovani, A., Sica, A., and Locati, M. (2005). Macrophage polariza- tion comes of age. *Immunity* 23, 344–346. doi: 10.1016/j.immuni. 2005.10.001

McFarlane, H. G., Kusek, G. K., Yang, M., Phoenix, J. L., Bolivar, V. J., and Crawley, J. N. (2008). Autism- like behavioral phenotypes in BTBR T+tf/J mice. *Genes Brain Behav.* 7, 152–163. doi: 10.1111/j.1601- 183X.2007.00330.x

Mikita, J., Dubourdieu-Cassagno, N., Deloire, M. S., Vekris, A., Biran, M., Raffard, G., et al. (2011). Altered M1/M2 activation patterns of monocytes in severe relaps- ing experimental rat model of multiple sclerosis. Amelioration of clinical status by M2 acti- vated monocyte administration. *Mult. Scler.* 17, 2–15. doi: 10.1177/1352458510379243

Morgan, J. T., Chana, G., Pardo, C. A., Achim, C., Semendeferi, K., Buckwalter, J., et al. (2010). Microglial activation and increased microglial density observed in the dorsolateral prefrontal cortex in autism. *Biol. Psychiatry* 68, 368–376. doi: 10.1016/j.biopsych. 2010.05.024

Mosser, D. M., and Edwards, J. P. (2008). Exploring the full spec- trum of macrophage activation. *Nat. Rev. Immunol.* 8, 958–969. doi: 10.1038/nri2448

Moy, S. S., Nadler, J. J., Young, N. B., Nonneman, R. J., Segall, S. K., Andrade, G. M., et al. (2008). Social approach and repetitive behavior in eleven inbred mouse strains. *Behav. Brain Res.* 191, 118–129. doi: 10.1016/j.bbr.2008.03.015

Moy, S. S., Nadler, J. J., Young, N. B., Perez, A., Holloway, L. P., Barbaro, R. P., et al. (2007). Mouse behavioral tasks relevant to autism: phenotypes of 10 inbred strains. *Behav. Brain Res.* 176, 4–20. doi: 10.1016/j.bbr.2006.07.030

Onore, C., Careaga, M., and Ashwood, P. (2012). The role of immune dys- function in the pathophysiology of autism. *Brain Behav. Immun.* 26, 383–392. doi: 10.1016/j.bbi.2011. 08.007

Oppmann, B., Lesley, R., Blom, B., Timans, J. C., Xu, Y., Hunte, B., et al. (2000). Novel p19 protein engages IL-12p40 to form a cytokine, IL- 23, with biological activities sim- ilar as well as distinct from IL- 12. *Immunity* 13, 715–725. doi: 10.1016/S1074-7613(00)00070-4

Pfeffer, K., Matsuyama, T., Kundig, T. M., Wakeham, A., Kishihara, K., Shahinian, A., et al. (1993). Mice deficient for the 55 kd tumor necrosis factor receptor are resis- tant to endotoxic shock, yet suc- cumbto *L. monocytogenes* infection. *Cell* 73, 457–467. doi: 10.1016/0092- 8674(93)90134-C

Rothman, K. J. (1990). No adjust- ments are needed for multiple com- parisons. *Epidemiology* 1, 43–46. doi: 10.1097/00001648-199001000- 00010 Scattoni, M. L., Gandhy, S. U., Ricceri, ., and Crawley, J. N. (2008). Unusual repertoire of vocaliza- tions in the BTBR T+tf/J mouse model of autism. *PLoS ONE* 3:e3067. doi: 10.1371/journal.pone. 0003067

Scattoni, M. L., Ricceri, L., and Crawley, J. N. (2011). Unusual repertoire of vocalizations in adult BTBR T+tf/J mice during three types of social encounters. *Genes Brain Behav.* 10, 44–56. doi: 10.1111/j.1601-183X.2010.00623.x

Silverman, J. L., Tolu, S. S., Barkan, C. L., and Crawley, J. N. (2010). Repetitive self-grooming behav- ior in the BTBR mouse model of autism is blocked by the mGluR5 antagonist MPEP. *Neuro- psychopharmacology* 35, 976–989. doi: 10.1038/npp.2009.201

Silverman, J. L., Turner, S. M., Barkan, C. L., Tolu, S. S., Saxena, R., Hung, A. Y., et al. (2011). Sociability and motor functions in Shankl mutant mice. *Brain Res.* 1380, 120–137. doi: 10.1016/j.brainres. 2010.09.026

Sweeten, T. L., Posey, D. J., and McDougle, C. J. (2003). High blood monocyte counts and neopterin levels in children with autistic disorder. *Am. J. Psychiatry* 160, 1691–1693. doi: 10.1176/appi.ajp.160.9.1691

Vargas, D. L., Nascimbene, C., Krishnan, C., Zimmerman, A. W., and Pardo, C. A. (2005). Neuroglial activation and neu- roinflammation in the brain of patients with autism. *Ann. Neurol.* 57, 67–81. doi: 10.1002/ana.20315

Voineagu, I., Wang, X., Johnston, P., Lowe, J. K., Tian, Y., Horvath, S., et al. (2011). Transcriptomic analysis of autistic brain reveals convergent molecular pathol- ogy. *Nature* 474, 380–384. doi: 10.1038/nature10110

Yang, M., Clarke, A. M., and Crawley, J. N. (2009). Postnatal lesion evi- dence against a primary role for the corpus callosum in mouse sociability. *Eur. J. Neurosci.* 29, 1663–1677. doi: 10.1111/j.1460- 9568.2009.06714.x

Yang, M., Perry, K., Weber, M. D., Katz, A. M., and Crawley, J. N. (2011a). Social peers rescue autism- relevant sociability deficits in ado- lescent mice. *Autism Res.* 4, 17–27. doi: 10.1002/aur.163

Yang, M., Silverman, J. L., and Crawley, J. N. (2011b). Automated three-chambered social approach task for mice. *Curr. Protoc. Neurosci.* Chapter 8, Unit 8.26. doi: 10.1002/0471142301.ns0826s56

Yang, M., Zhodzishsky, V., and Crawley, J. N. (2007). Social deficits in BTBR T+tf/J mice are unchanged by cross-fostering with C57BL/6J mothers. *Int. J. Dev. Neurosci.* 25, 515–521. doi: 10.1016/j.ijdevneu.2007.09.008

Ymer, S. I., Huang, D., Penna, G., Gregori, S., Branson, K., Adorini, L., et al. (2002). Polymorphisms in the Il12b gene affect structure and expression of IL-12 in NOD and other autoimmune-prone mouse strains. *Genes Immun.* 3, 151–157. doi: 10.1038/sj.gene.6363849

Yrigollen, C. M., Han, S. S., Kochetkova, A., Babitz, T., Chang, J. T., Volkmar, F. R., et al. (2008). Genes controlling affiliative behav- ior as candidate genes for autism. *Biol. Psychiatry* 63, 911–916. doi: 10.1016/j.biopsych.2007.11.015

Zhang, X., Goncalves, R., and Mosser, D. M. (2008). The isolation and characterization of murine macrophages. *Curr. Protoc. Immunol.* Chapter 14, Unit 14.1. doi: 10.1002/0471142735. im1401s83

Zou, H., Yu, Y., Sheikh, A. M., Malik, ., Yang, K., Wen, G., et al. (2011). Association of upregu- lated Ras/Raf/ERK1/2 signaling with autism. *Genes Brain Behav.* 10, 615–624. doi: 10.1111/j.1601- 183X.2011.00702.x

2

Hyperleptinemia is associated with parameters of low-grade systemic inflammation and metabolic dysfunction in obese human beings

Sonia Leon-Cabrera[1], Lourdes Solís-Lozano[2,3], Karina Suárez-Álvarez[2,3], Antonio González-Chávez[4], Yadira L. Béjar[5], Guillermo Robles-Díaz[2] and Galileo Escobedo[2,3]*

[1] Departamento de Biología de la Reproducción y Clínica de Desórdenes de Sueño, Universidad Autónoma Metropolitana-Iztapalapa, D.F., México
[2] Laboratorio de Hígado, Páncreas y Motilidad, Unidad de Medicina Experimental, Hospital General de México, D.F., México
[3] Facultad de Medicina, Departamento de Medicina Experimental, Hospital General de México, Universidad Nacional Autónoma de México, D.F., México
[4] Servicio de Medicina Interna, Hospital General de México, D.F., México
[5] Servicio de Banco de Sangre, Hospital General de México, D.F., México

Edited by:
Beatriz Gomez-Gonzalez, Universidad Autonoma Metropolitana, Unidad Iztapalapa, Mexico

Reviewed by:
Undurti N. Das, UND LIfe Sciences, USA
Martin (Marco) Harmsen, University Medical Center Groningen, Netherlands

***Correspondence:**
Galileo Escobedo, Unidad de Medicina Experimental, Hospital General de México "Dr. Eduardo Liceaga," Dr. Balmis #148, Col. Doctores, C.P. 06726, México D.F., México
e-mail: gescobedo@unam.mx; gescobedog@msn.com

Leptin is an adipose tissue-derived hormone that has been involved in hypothalamic and systemic inflammation, altered food-intake patterns, and metabolic dysfunction in obese mice. However, it remains unclear whether leptin has a relationship with parameters of systemic inflammation and metabolic dysfunction in humans. We thus evaluated in a cross-sectional study the circulating levels of leptin in 40 non-obese and 41 obese Mexican individuals, examining their relationship with tumor necrosis factor alpha (TNF-α), interleukin (IL) 12, IL-10, central obesity, serum glucose and insulin levels, and serum triglyceride and cholesterol concentrations. Circulating levels of leptin, TNF-α, IL-12, IL-10, and insulin were measured by ELISA, while concentrations of glucose, triglyceride, and cholesterol were determined by enzymatic assays. As expected, serum levels of leptin exhibited a significant elevation in obese individuals as compared to non-obese subjects, showing a clear association with increased body mass index ($r = 0.4173$), central obesity ($r = 0.4678$), and body fat percentage ($r = 0.3583$). Furthermore, leptin also showed a strong relationship with serum TNF-α ($r = 0.6989$), IL-12 ($r = 0.3093$), and IL-10 ($r = -0.5691$). Interestingly, leptin was also significantly related with high concentrations of fasting glucose ($r = 0.5227$) and insulin ($r = 0.2229$), as well as elevated levels of insulin resistance ($r = 0.3611$) and circulating triglyceride ($r = 0.4135$). These results suggest that hyperleptinemia is strongly associated with the occurrence of low-grade systemic inflammation and metabolic alteration in obese subjects. Further clinical research is still needed to determine whether hyperleptinemia may be a potential marker for recognizing the advent of obesity-related metabolic disorders in human beings.

Keywords: leptin, hyperleptinemia, obesity, low-grade inflammation, metabolic disease, type 2 diabetes, human

INTRODUCTION

Obesity is now considered a major health problem worldwide, with a growing prevalence in the Mexican population (Olaiz-Fernández et al., 2006; Popkin, 2011). Obese people show a higher risk to develop type 2 diabetes (T2D), coronary heart disease, stroke, arterial hypertension, non-alcoholic steatohepatitis (NASH), and other obesity-related metabolic disorders (Ritchie and Connell, 2007). These pathologies have been recently associated with a low-grade systemic inflammatory state (Odegaard and Chawla, 2008), characterized by altered circulating levels of inflammatory mediators in the obese subject, including tumor necrosis factor alpha (TNF-α), interleukin (IL-) 12, C-reactive protein (CRP), and IL-10 (Rush et al., 2007; Bremer et al., 2011). TNF-α has been shown to increase with adiposity in mice and human beings (Steinberg et al., 2006). Circulating concentrations of IL-12 and CRP are elevated in overweight and obese individuals, exhibiting a significant association with increased body mass index (BMI) and waist circumference, as well high glucose and triglyceride levels (Visser et al., 1999; Suarez-Alvarez et al., 2013). On the contrary, serum IL-10 levels have been shown to decrease in high-fat diet fed-mice (Gotoh et al., 2012). As it can be seen, circulating proinflammatory factors have received growing attention since they could play a major role in mediating the low-grade inflammatory state, which seems to decisively contribute to the advent of obesity-related metabolic disorders (Ritchie and Connell, 2007; Bertola et al., 2010).

Leptin is an adipose tissue-derived hormone belonging to the class-I helical cytokine family (Trinchieri, 2003). Leptin has been shown to regulate food-intake and energy expenditure in both rodents and humans (Houseknecht et al., 1998). Interestingly, circulating levels of leptin have been shown to increase in high-fat diet fed-mice and obese subjects, leading to a state of hyperleptinemia (Maffei et al., 1995; Lin et al., 2000). However, although hyperleptinemia strongly correlates with parameters of low-grade systemic inflammation and metabolic dysfunction in animal models of obesity (Munzberg, 2008; Arruda et al., 2011; Stienstra et al., 2011), they show controversial results in human beings. For instance, it has been reported that serum leptin is augmented in obese individuals with metabolic syndrome (MetS) that also show an elevation in the plasma levels of CRP (Kim et al., 2006). In contrast, obese non-diabetic women subjected to a caloric restriction diet show decreased values in plasma leptin without exhibiting a significant diminution in the circulating levels of TNF-α (Agueda et al., 2012). In the same sense, in obese adolescents leptin has been shown to rise independently of the levels of insulin resistance and TNF-α (Aguilar et al., 2012; Cohen et al., 2012). As it can be seen, it is still unclear whether hyperleptinemia has an association with the occurrence of low-grade systemic inflammation and metabolic dysfunction in humans.

We thus studied the serum levels of leptin in non-obese and obese Mexican individuals, examining their possible relationship with parameters of low-grade systemic inflammation (TNF-α, IL-12, and IL-10) and metabolic alteration (elevated serum glucose and insulin, increased level of insulin resistance, high triglyceride and cholesterol concentrations, as well as increasing waist circumference and body fat percentage).

MATERIALS AND METHODS

SUBJECTS

A total of 81 apparently healthy Mexican adult volunteers from the south-central region of Mexico were included in the study. All of the participants provided written informed consent, previously approved by an institutional review board of the General Hospital of Mexico "Dr. Eduardo Liceaga," which guaranteed that the study was conducted in accordance with the principles described at the Helsinki Declaration. Subjects were excluded from the study if they had previous or recent diagnosis of diabetes mellitus, cardiovascular diseases, chronic hepatic or renal disease, blood pressure higher than 140/90 mm Hg, inflammatory or autoimmune disorders, acute or chronic infectious diseases, cancer, and endocrine disorders. We additionally excluded pregnant or lactating women, subjects under any kind of cardiometabolic medication including anti-inflammatory, anti-aggregant, and anti-hypertensive drugs, and subjects without having an 8–12 h overnight fasting. All of the individuals enrolled into the study received full medical evaluation, including the achievement of clinic history and physical examination by a physician.

MEASUREMENT OF ANTHROPOMETRIC PARAMETERS

According to the World Health Organization criteria for BMI, all of the participants were divided into two groups: control non-obese subjects (BMI 18.5–24.9 kg/m^2) and obese subjects (BMI $\geq$ 30 kg/m^2), where BMI resulted of dividing weight by height squared (kg/m^2). Waist circumference was obtained from each study subject, considering the midpoint between the lower rib margin and the iliac crest, using a conventional tape in centimeters (cm). For women, abdominal obesity was considered when their waist circumference were 80 cm or higher, whereas for men it was considered when their waist circumference were 94 cm or higher. Percentage of body fat was individually recorded by using a body composition analyzer (TANITA®, Body Composition Analyzer, Model TBF-300A, Tokyo, Japan).

MEASUREMENT OF METABOLIC PARAMETERS

Blood samples were individually taken after overnight fasting, and collected into pyrogen-free tubes (VacutainerTM, BD Diagnostics, NJ, USA) at room temperature. Collection tubes were then centrifuged at 1000 g/4°C for 30 min, and serum samples obtained and stored at −80°C in numerous aliquots until use. Total cholesterol and triglyceride were individually measured in triplicate by an enzymatic assay according to manufacturer's instructions (Roche Diagnostics, Mannhein, Germany). Serum insulin levels were individually determined in triplicate by means of the enzyme-linked immunosorbent assay (ELISA), following the manufacturer's instructions (Abnova Corporation, Taiwan). Serum glucose levels were individually determined in triplicate by the glucose oxidase assay, following the manufacturer's instructions (Megazyme International, Ireland). The estimate of insulin resistance was individually determined by means of the HOMA-IR, as follows: fasting insulin concentration (mU/L) × fasting glucose concentration (mmol/L) divided by 22.5.

MEASUREMENT OF LEPTIN AND LOW-GRADE SYSTEMIC INFLAMMATION PARAMETERS

Blood samples were individually taken after overnight fasting, and collected into pyrogen-free tubes (VacutainerTM, BD Diagnostics, NJ, USA) at room temperature. Collection tubes were then centrifuged at 1000 g/4°C for 30 min, and serum samples obtained and stored at −80°C in numerous aliquots until use. Serum levels of leptin, TNF-α, IL-10, and IL-12 were determined in triplicate by ELISA, following the manufacturer's instructions (Peprotech, Mexico).

STATISTICAL ANALYSIS

Data from anthropometric and metabolic parameters were analyzed by using the Student's t-test for determining significant differences. Data from leptin, TNF-α, IL-10, and IL-12 were analyzed by means of using the Mann-Whitney U-test for determining significant differences. The Spearman's correlation coefficient was performed for examining the relationship of leptin with anthropometric, metabolic, and inflammatory parameters. All of the studied groups were matched by gender and age. Statistical analysis was performed using the GraphPad Prism 5 software. Differences were considered significant when $p < 0.05$.

RESULTS

A total of 40 non-obese controls and 41 obese subjects were included in the study. No significant differences were observed in age (for non-obese controls mean age 29.9 ± 10.35 years, whereas for obese subjects mean age 34.9 ± 10.24 years), and women/men proportion (22 women and 18 men in the non-obese control group, and 20 women and 21 men in the obesity group) in the studied groups (**Table 1**). In contrast, BMI, waist circumference, body fat percentage, fasting blood glucose and insulin, circulating levels of triglyceride and cholesterol, and

Table 1 | Anthropometric, metabolic, and inflammatory characteristics of the study subjects.

	Non-obese	Obese	*P*-value
Gender (W/M)	22/18	20/21	N.S.
Age (years)	29.9 ± 10.3	34.9 ± 10.2	N.S.
BMI (kg/m^2)	22.6 ± 1.8	33.7 ± 3.4	$p < 0.0001$
Waist circumference (cm)	79.6 ± 6.5	107.4 ± 9.9	$p < 0.0001$
Body fat percentage	24.6 ± 8.2	37.6 ± 6.9	$p < 0.05$
Fasting blood glucose (mmol/L)	4.3 ± 0.1	5.89 ± 0.3	$p < 0.0001$
Fasting blood insulin (mU/L)	12.6 ± 1.4	15.5 ± 6.7	$p = 0.0088$
HOMA-IR	2.4 ± 0.3	4.08 ± 1.8	$p < 0.0001$
Total cholesterol (mg/dL)	192.8 ± 10.1	198.1 ± 10.3	$p = 0.0219$
Total triglyceride (mg/dL)	137.5 ± 9.1	251.9 ± 14.4	$p < 0.0001$
TNF-α (pg/mL)	271.8 ± 28.05	322.9 ± 58.5	$p < 0.05$
IL-12 (pg/mL)	272.9 ± 13.6	381.5 ± 59.8	$p < 0.0001$
IL-10 (pg/mL)	1145.2 ± 214.6	840.8 ± 96.5	$p < 0.0001$

Abbreviations: W, women; M, men; BMI, body mass index; HOMA-IR, homeostatic model assessment-insulin resistance; TNF-α, tumor necrosis factor alpha; IL, interleukin; N.S., non-significant differences.
Data are presented as mean ± standard deviation.
Differences were considered significant when p < 0.05.

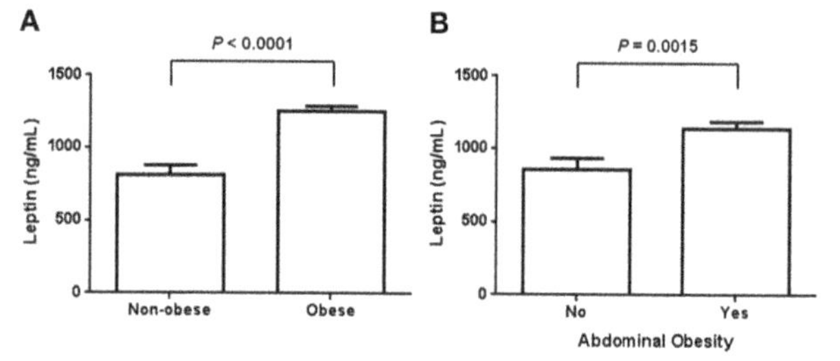

FIGURE 1 | Serum levels of leptin in obese and non-obese individuals. **(A)** Circulating leptin levels were assessed in normal weight and obese subjects, defining obesity according to the World Health Organization criteria for body mass index. In our study population, serum leptin was also evaluated in terms of abdominal obesity **(B)**. For women, abdominal obesity was considered when the waist circumference was 80 cm or higher, whereas for men, it was considered when the waist circumference was 94 cm or higher. Data are expressed as mean ± S. E. Differences were considered significant when $p < 0.05$.

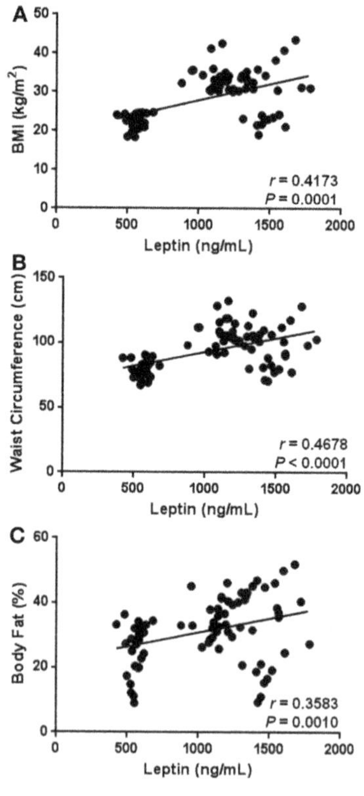

FIGURE 2 | Statistical correlation between serum levels of leptin and anthropometric parameters of obesity. Serum levels of leptin were positively associated with body mass index (BMI) **(A)**, waist circumference **(B)**, and body fat percentage **(C)**. Coefficients (*r*) and *P*-values were calculated by using the Spearman's correlation model. The correlation level was considered significant when $p < 0.05$.

serum concentrations of TNF-α and IL-12 were clearly increased in obese individuals as comparing with non-obese control subjects (**Table 1**). Concomitantly, serum levels of IL-10 were significantly lower in obese individuals than in non-obese subjects (**Table 1**). It merits to mention that BMI was clearly correlated with waist circumference ($r = 0.9297$, $p < 0.0001$) and body fat percentage ($r = 0.7655$, $p < 0.0001$) in our study population. In a similar way, there was also a significant association between waist circumference and body fat percentage ($r = 0.7655$, $p < 0.0001$).

In accordance with previous reports, circulating levels of leptin were significantly increased in obese subjects when comparing to non-obese control individuals. In terms of BMI, leptin exhibited a significant 1.5-fold increase in obese subjects as comparing with normal weight controls (**Figure 1A**). In obese individuals, the mean value of leptin was 1256.1 ± 207.7 ng/mL, whereas in the non-obese group it was around 812.1 ± 417.8 ng/mL (**Figure 1A**). Interestingly, serum values of leptin still showed a significant elevation when examining in subjects with abdominal obesity (**Figure 1B**). For this case, the mean value of leptin in subjects with abdominal obesity was 1141.8 ± 343.6 ng/mL, while it decreased to 858.3 ± 419.6 ng/mL in individuals exhibiting a normal waist perimeter (**Figure 1B**).

As expected, our results show that circulating levels of leptin increase with obesity-related anthropometric parameters. Indeed, leptin was significantly correlated with increased BMI ($r = 0.4173$, $p = 0.0001$), central obesity ($r = 0.4678$, $p < 0.0001$), and body fat percentage ($r = 0.3583$, $p = 0.0010$) (**Figures 2A–C**, respectively). Furthermore, leptin also exhibited a clear association with parameters of metabolic alteration. In this sense, serum leptin was significantly related with increased levels of blood glucose ($r = 0.5227$, $p < 0.0001$) and insulin ($r = 0.2229$, $p = 0.0455$) (**Figures 3A,B**, respectively). There was also a significant relationship between leptin and the level of insulin resistance,

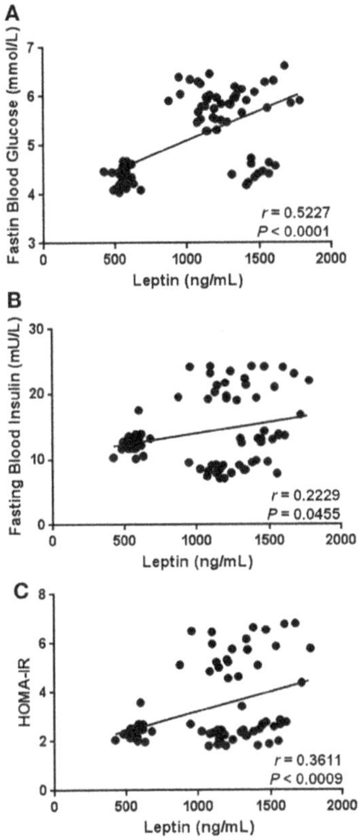

FIGURE 3 | Statistical correlation of the serum levels of leptin with fasting blood glucose, fasting blood insulin, and insulin resistance. Serum concentrations of leptin exhibited a positive significant relationship with high levels of glucose **(A)** and insulin **(B)**, as well increased insulin resistance **(C)**. The level of insulin resistance was estimated using the HOMA-IR index, which results of multiplying fasting insulin concentration (mU/L) by fasting glucose concentration (mmol/L), then divided by the constant 22.5. Coefficients (*r*) and *P*-values were calculated by the Spearman's correlation model. The correlation level was considered significant when $p < 0.05$.

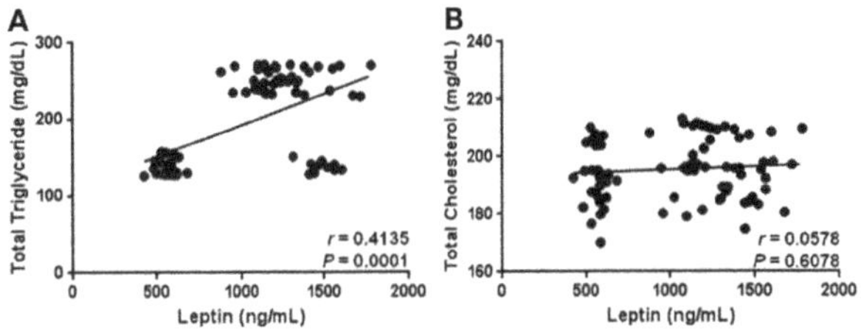

FIGURE 4 | Statistical correlation of the serum levels of leptin with total triglyceride and cholesterol levels. Serum concentrations of leptin showed a positive significant relationship with high levels of triglycerides **(A)**, but not with total cholesterol **(B)**. Coefficients (*r*) and *P*-values were calculated by the Spearman's correlation model. The correlation level was considered significant when $p < 0.05$.

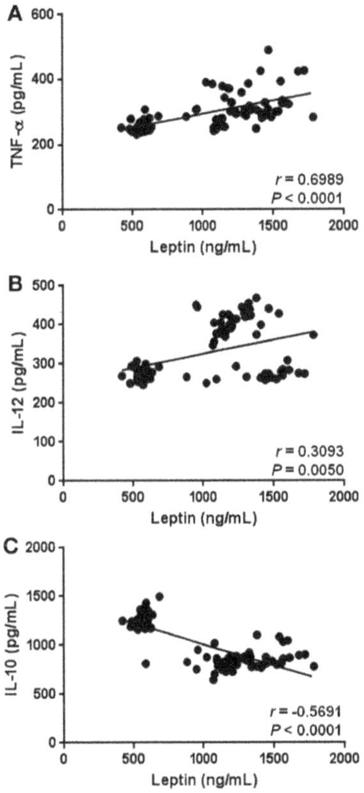

FIGURE 5 | Statistical correlation of the serum levels of leptin with parameters of low-grade systemic inflammation. Serum concentrations of leptin showed a positive significant relationship with increased serum levels of TNF-α **(A)**, and IL-12 **(B)**. At the same time, hyperleptinemia exhibited a significant inverse association with circulating concentrations of IL-10 **(C)**. Coefficients (*r*) and *P*-values were calculated by the Spearman's correlation model. The correlation level was considered significant when $p < 0.05$.

estimated by means of the HOMA-IR ($r = 0.3611$, $p < 0.0009$) (**Figure 3C**). Interestingly, leptin had a positive association with increased triglyceride levels ($r = 0.4135$, $p = 0.0001$), but not with total cholesterol (**Figures 4A,B**, respectively).

Besides having significant relationships with anthropometric and biochemical parameters associated with obesity-related metabolic alterations, hyperleptinemia also showed a strong relation with markers of low-grade systemic inflammation in the study subjects. In fact, circulating leptin was positively correlated with serum levels of TNF-α ($r = 0.6989$, $p < 0.0001$) and IL-12 ($r = 0.3093$, $p = 0.0050$) (**Figures 5A,B**), whereas a significant negative relationship between leptin and IL-10 was observed in the study population ($r = -0.5691$, $p < 0.0001$) (**Figure 5C**).

DISCUSSION

As mentioned, it has been consistently shown that serum concentrations of leptin increase in high-fat diet fed-mice and obese humans. In mice, hyperleptinemia is related to hyperphagia and fat depot augmentation, while it is associated with increased white adipose tissue (WAT) mass and body weight gain in human beings (Stanley et al., 2005). However, recent experimental evidence from animal models of obesity suggests that leptin is not only a marker of weight gain but also seems to have a relationship with developing a systemic state of low-grade inflammation and metabolic disturbance. In fact, obese mice exhibiting hyperleptinemia show increased plasma levels of inflammatory cytokines (Dube et al., 2008; Yang et al., 2010; Enos et al., 2013), accompanied by numerous metabolic disorders including hyperglycemia (Yang et al., 2010), hyperinsulinemia (Stienstra et al., 2011), hyperlipidemia (Kang et al., 2011), liver steatosis (Shih et al., 2010), and insulin resistance (Yang et al., 2010). Taking this experimental evidence into account, it is important to evaluate whether hyperleptinemia could also be associated to the establishment of systemic inflammation and metabolic dysfunction in human beings with high metabolic risk, such as obese individuals.

In humans, the relationship of leptin with a state of metabolic dysfunction has been barely studied, showing inconclusive results to date. Indeed, a study conducted in a group of obese adolescents revealed that high serum levels of leptin correlate with increased BMI and waist circumference, without having a significant relation with the insulin resistance level (Aguilar et al., 2012). In contrast, recent data from a cross-sectional survey conducted in obese adults demonstrated that hyperleptinemia is clearly associated with BMI, hyperinsulinemia, and insulin resistance (Martins Mdo et al., 2012). Our results are consistent with the last study, since high levels of leptin were significantly correlated with hyperglycemia, hyperinsulinemia, increased HOMA-IR, and hypertriglyceridemia in our study population. A possible explanation to understand this apparently controversial finding may involve the age of the subjects included in each study. As it is widely known, the level of sex-steroid hormones reaches a plateau during maturity, in comparison to both childhood and adolescence where numerous hormonal variations are normally observed (Stanhope and Brook, 1988; Rogol, 2004). Interestingly, it has been recently reported that sex-steroid hormones are able to upregulate the leptin expression in human and rat cells (Feng et al., 2011; Gambino et al., 2012). Therefore, it is feasible to expect that synthesis of leptin may be enhanced during adulthood, which may contribute to decrease the leptin levels in children/adolescents in comparison with adults. However, additional clinical studies considering the influence of sex-steroid hormones upon the systemic levels of leptin are necessary in order to address major conclusions.

An interesting finding in this cross-sectional study involves the relationship of hyperleptinemia with a systemic state of low-grade inflammation in obese human beings. A recent study demonstrated that leptin is overexpressed in the subcutaneous adipose tissue (SAT) of obese individuals with MetS, as comparing with SAT from healthy obese subjects and non-obese individuals (Farb et al., 2011). Furthermore, increasing in the leptin expression is accompanied by macrophage infiltration and overexpression of proinflammatory cytokines such as IL-1β, IL-6, and IL-8 in the SAT of those same patients (Bremer et al., 2011; Farb et al., 2011). Consistent with this previous study, our results show that hyperleptinemia is significantly associated with high serum levels of TNF-α and IL-12, as well as reduced concentrations of IL-10 in subjects with central obesity, hyperglycemia, increased insulin resistance, and hypertriglyceridemia. IL-12 is a cytokine with the ability to induce synthesis of interferon-gamma (IFN-γ) in T cells and natural killer cells (Trinchieri, 2003). IFN-γ is a key mediator in releasing of TNF-α by classically activated macrophages (Odegaard and Chawla, 2008). Taking into consideration that serum IFN-γ has been shown to increase during obesity (Azar Sharabiani et al., 2011), it is conceivable to expect a positive relationship among TNF-α, IL-12, and leptin in our study population. Another intriguing issue concerning the positive association among leptin, TNF-α, and IL-12, involves the ability of leptin to regulate the expression of inflammatory cytokines. It has been recently reported that leptin is able to stimulate the *in vitro* production of TNF-α and IL-1β in human mononuclear cells (Tsiotra et al., 2013). Thus, it is now proposed that high levels of leptin may induce the production of proinflammatory cytokines in obese people, contributing in this way to the systemic inflammation observed in these subjects. Nevertheless, before establishing a possible cause-and-effect relation among leptin, TNF-α, and IL-12 in the scenario of obesity, additional prospective clinical research is required. Moreover, consistent with the installation of a systemic state of low-grade inflammation, we observed a significant reduction in the circulating levels of IL-10 in obese individuals as comparing with non-obese subjects. IL-10 is a cytokine with potent anti-inflammatory properties in mice and humans (Saraiva and O'garra, 2010). However, the role of IL-10 during systemic inflammation and metabolic dysfunction is still poorly understood (Formoso et al., 2012; Tajik et al., 2012). For this reason, it is important to mention that the present work is one of the first contributions showing a significant inverse correlation between serum IL-10 and hyperleptinemia in obese individuals. Collectively, these findings suggest that obesity-related hyperleptinemia is accompanied by a low-grade inflammatory profile, characterized by increased circulating levels of TNF-α and IL-12, and reduced concentrations of IL-10. Whether hyperleptinemia is cause or consequence of the systemic inflammatory milieu in humans, is a matter worthy of being considered in further basic and clinical studies.

Present results demonstrate that high circulating levels of leptin are significantly associated with a systemic state of low-grade inflammation and metabolic dysfunction in obese subjects. Additional prospective clinical studies are still required to evaluate whether hyperleptinemia may be used as a marker for recognizing the advent of obesity-related metabolic disorders in human beings.

ACKNOWLEDGMENTS

We thank Jose Alejandro Perez Gonzalez, Guadalupe Gonzalez Galicia, Maria de Jesus Mata Rivera, Alejandra Lopez, Maria Esther Ruiz Escalera, Yazmin Saldaña Arenas, Patricia Enriquez Lemus, and Yolanda Camarillo Ornelas for their technical assistance in the enrollment of the study subjects. This work was supported by grant no. CB-2009-01-129316 from Consejo Nacional de Ciencia y Tecnologia (CONACYT) to Galileo Escobedo. S. Leon-Cabrera thanks the support from the Programa del Mejoramiento del Profesorado (PROMEP)-Mexico. Dr. L. Graue corrected the English version of this manuscript.

REFERENCES

Agueda, M., Lasa, A., Simon, E., Ares, R., Larrarte, E., and Labayen, I. (2012). Association of circulating visfatin concen- trations with insulin resistance and low-grade inflammation after dietary energy restriction in Spanish obese non-diabetic women: role of body composition changes. *Nutr. Metab. Cardiovasc. Dis.* 22, 208–214. doi: 10.1016/j.numecd. 2010.06.010

Aguilar, M. J., Gonzalez-Jimenez, E., Antelo, A., and Perona, J. S. (2012). Insulin resistance and inflammation markers: correla- tions in obese adolescents. *J. Clin. Nurs.* 22, 2002–2010. doi: 10.1111/ jocn.12034

Arruda, A. P., Milanski, M., Coope, A., Torsoni, A. S., Ropelle, E., Carvalho, D. P., et al. (2011). Low- grade hypothalamic inflammation leads to defective thermogenesis, insulin resistance, and impaired insulin secretion. *Endocrinology* 152, 1314–1326. doi: 10.1210/en. 2010-0659

Azar Sharabiani, M. T., Vermeulen, R., Scoccianti, C., Hosnijeh, F. S., Minelli, L., Sacerdote, C., et al. (2011). Immunologic pro- file of excessive body weight. *Biomarkers* 16, 243–251. doi: 10.3109/1354750X.2010.547948

Bertola, A., Bonnafous, S., Anty, R., Patouraux, S., Saint-Paul, M. C., Iannelli, A., et al. (2010). Hepatic expression patterns of inflamma- tory and immune response genes associated with obesity and NASH in morbidly obese patients. *PLoS ONE* 5:e13577. doi: 10.1371/jour- nal.pone.0013577

Bremer, A. A., Devaraj, S., Afify, A., and Jialal, I. (2011). Adipose tissue dysregulation in patients with metabolic syn- drome. *J. Clin. Endocrinol. Metab.* 96, E1782–E1788. doi: 10.1210/jc.2011-1577

Cohen, J. I., Maayan, L., and Convit, A. (2012). Preliminary evidence for obesity-associated insulin resis- tance in adolescents without ele- vations of inflammatory cytokines. *Diabetol. Metab. Syndr.* 4, 26. doi: 10.1186/1758-5996-4-26

Dube, M. G., Torto, R., and Kalra, S. P. (2008). Increased leptin expression selectively in the hypothalamus suppresses inflammatory markers CRP and IL-6 in leptin-deficient diabetic obese mice. *Peptides* 29, 593–598. doi: 10.1016/j.peptides. 2008.01.001

Enos, R. T., Davis, J. M., Velazquez, K. T., Mcclellan, J. L., Day, S. D., Carnevale, K. A., et al. (2013). Influence of dietary saturated fat content on adiposity, macrophage behavior, inflammation, and metabolism: composition matters. *J. Lipid Res.* 54, 152–163. doi: 10.1194/jlr.M030700

Farb, M. G., Bigornia, S., Mott, M., Tanriverdi, K., Morin, K. M., Freedman, J. E., et al. (2011). Reduced adipose tis- sue inflammation represents an intermediate cardiometabolic phenotype in obesity. *J. Am. Coll. Cardiol.* 58, 232–237. doi: 10.1016/j.jacc.2011.01.051

Feng, Y., Shao, R., Weijdegard, B., Wang, T., Johansson, J., Sun, S., et al. (2011). Effects of andro- gen and leptin on behavioral and cellular responses in female rats. *Horm. Behav.* 60, 427–438. doi: 10.1016/j.yhbeh.2011.07.012

Formoso, G., Taraborrelli, M., Guagnano, M. T., D'adamo, M., Di Pietro, N., Tartaro, A., et al. (2012). Magnetic resonance imaging determined visceral fat reduction associates with enhanced IL-10 plasma levels in calorie restricted obese subjects. *PLoS ONE* 7:e52774. doi: 10.1371/journal. pone.0052774

Gambino, Y. P., Perez Perez, A., Duenas, J. L., Calvo, J. C., Sanchez-Margalet, V., and Varone, C.L. (2012). Regulation of leptin expression by 17beta-estradiol in human placental cells involves membrane associated estrogen receptor alpha. *Biochim. Biophys. Acta* 1823, 900–910. doi: 10.1016/j.bbamcr. 2012.01.015

Gotoh, K., Inoue, M., Masaki, T., Chiba, S., Shimasaki, T., Ando, H., et al. (2012). A novel anti-inflammatory role for spleen-derived interleukin-10 in obesity-induced hypothalamic inflammation. *J. Neurochem.* 120, 752–764. doi: 10.1111/j.1471-4159. 2011.07617.x

Houseknecht, K. L., Baile, C. A., Matteri, R. L., and Spurlock, M. E. (1998). The biology of lep- tin: a review. *J. Anim. Sci.* 76, 1405–1420.

Kang, J. S., Lee, W. K., Yoon, W. K., Kim, N., Park, S. K., Park, H. K., et al. (2011). A combination of grape extract, green tea extract and L-carnitine improves high-fat diet-induced obesity, hyperlipi- demia and non-alcoholic fatty liver disease in mice. *Phytother. Res.* 25, 1789–1795. doi: 10.1002/ ptr.3476

Kim, C. S., Park, H. S., Kawada, T., Kim, J. H., Lim, D., Hubbard, N. E., et al. (2006). Circulating levels of MCP-1 and IL-8 are elevated in human obese subjects and associ- ated with obesity-related parame- ters. *Int. J. Obes.* 30, 1347–1355.doi: 10.1038/sj.ijo.0803259

Lin, S., Thomas, T. C., Storlien, L. H., and Huang, X. F. (2000). Development of high fat diet- induced obesity and leptin resistance in C57Bl/6J mice. *Int. J. Obes. Relat. Metab. Disord.* 24, 639–646. doi: 10.1038/sj.ijo.0801209

Maffei, M., Halaas, J., Ravussin, E., Pratley, R. E., Lee, G. H., Zhang, Y., et al. (1995). Leptin levels in human and rodent: measurement of plasma leptin and ob RNA in obese and weight-reduced sub- jects. *Nat. Med.* 1, 1155–1161. doi: 10.1038/nm1195-1155

Martins Mdo, C., Lima Faleiro, L., and Fonseca, A. (2012). [Relationship between leptin and body mass and metabolic syndrome in an adult population]. *Rev. Port. Cardiol.* 31, 711–719.

Munzberg, H. (2008). Differential leptin access into the brain— a hierarchical organization of hypothalamic leptin target sites? *Physiol. Behav.* 94, 664–669. doi: 10.1016/j.physbeh.2008.04.020

Odegaard, J. I., and Chawla, A. (2008). Mechanisms of macrophage activation in obesity-induced insulin resistance. *Nat. Clin. Pract. Endocrinol. Metab.* 4, 619–626. doi: 10.1038/ncpendmet0976

Olaiz-Fernández, G., Rivera- Dommarco, J., Shamah-Levy, T., Rojas, R., Villalpando-Hernández, S., Hernández-Avila, M., et al. (2006). *Encuesta Nacional de Salud y Nutrición 2006*. Cuernavaca: Instituto Nacional de Salud Pública.

Popkin, B. M. (2011). Does global obesity represent a global pub- lic health challenge? *Am. J. Clin. Nutr.* 93, 232–233. doi: 10.3945/ajcn.110.008458

Ritchie, S. A., and Connell, J. M. (2007). The link between abdominal obesity, metabolic syn- drome and cardiovascular disease. *Nutr. Metab. Cardiovasc. Dis.* 17, 319–326. doi: 10.1016/j.numecd. 2006.07.005

Rogol, A. D. (2004). Gender and hormonal regulation of growth. *J. Pediatr. Endocrinol. Metab.* 17(Suppl 4), 1259–1265.

Rush, E. C., Plank, L. D., and Yajnik, C. S. (2007). Interleukin-6, tumour necrosis factor-alpha and insulin relationships to body compo- sition, metabolism and resting energy expenditure in a migrant Asian Indian population. *Clin. Endocrinol. (Oxf)* 66, 684–690. doi: 10.1111/j.1365-2265.2007.02801.x

Saraiva, M., and O'garra, A. (2010). The regulation of IL-10 production by immune cells. *Nat. Rev. Immunol.* 10, 170–181. doi: 10.1038/nri2711

Shih, C. C., Lin, C. H., and Wu, J. B. (2010). Eriobotrya japon- ica improves hyperlipidemia and reverses insulin resistance in high- fat-fed mice. *Phytother. Res.* 24, 1769–1780. doi: 10.1002/ptr.3143

Stanhope, R., and Brook, C. G. (1988). An evaluation of hor- monal changes at puberty in man. *J. Endocrinol.* 116, 301–305. doi: 10.1677/joe.0.1160301

Stanley, S., Wynne, K., Mcgowan, B., and Bloom, S. (2005). Hormonal regulation of food intake. *Physiol. Rev.* 85, 1131–1158. doi: 10.1152/physrev.00015.2004

Steinberg, G. R., Michell, B. J., Van Denderen, B. J., Watt, M. J., Carey, A. L., Fam, B. C., et al. (2006).

Tumor necrosis factor alpha- induced skeletal muscle insulin resistance involves suppression of AMP-kinase signaling. *Cell Metab.* 4, 465–474. doi: 10.1016/j. cmet. 2006.11.005

Stienstra, R., Van Diepen, J. A., Tack, C. J., Zaki, M. H., Van De Veerdonk, F. L., Perera, D., et al. (2011). Inflammasome is a central player in the induction of obesity and insulin resistance. *Proc. Natl. Acad. Sci. U.S.A.* 108, 15324–15329. doi: 10.1073/pnas.1100255108

Suarez-Alvarez, K., Solis-Lozano, L., Leon-Cabrera, S., Gonzalez- Chavez, A., Gomez-Hernandez, G., Quinones-Alvarez, M. S., et al. (2013). Serum IL-12 Is increased in Mexican obese subjects and associ- ated with low-grade inflammation and obesity-related parameters. *Mediators Inflamm.* 2013:967067. doi: 10.1155/2013/967067

Tajik, N., Keshavarz, S. A., Masoudkabir, F., Djalali, M., Sadrzadeh-Yeganeh, H. H., Eshraghian, M. R., et al. (2012). Effect of diet-induced weight loss on inflammatory cytokines in obese women. *J. Endocrinol. Invest.* 36, 211–215. doi: 10.3275/8465

Trinchieri, G. (2003). Interleukin-12 and the regulation of innate resis- tance and adaptive immunity. *Nat. Rev. Immunol.* 3, 133–146. doi: 10.1038/ nri1001

Tsiotra, P. C., Boutati, E., Dimitriadis, G., and Raptis, S. A. (2013). High insulin and leptin increase resistin and inflammatory cytokine production from human mononuclear cells. *Biomed Res. Int.* 2013:487081. doi: 10.1155/ 2013/487081

Visser, M., Bouter, L. M., Mcquillan, G. M., Wener, M. H., and Harris, T. B. (1999). Elevated C-reactive pro- tein levels in overweight and obese adults. *JAMA* 282, 2131–2135. doi: 10.1001/jama.282.22.2131

Yang, J. H., Lim, H. S., and Heo, Y. R. (2010). Sasa borealis leaves extract improves insulin resistance by modulating inflammatory cytokine secretion in high fat dietinduced obese C57/BL6J mice. *Nutr. Res. Pract.* 4, 99–105. doi: 10.4162/ nrp.2010.4.2.99

3

Treating depression and depression-like behavior with physical activity: an immune perspective

Harris A. Eyre[1,2], Evan Papps[1] and Bernhard T. Baune[1]*

[1] Discipline of Psychiatry, School of Medicine, University of Adelaide, Adelaide, SA, Australia
[2] School of Medicine and Dentistry, James Cook University, Townsville, QLD, Australia

Edited by:
Felipe Schuch, Hospital de Clínicas de Porto Alegre, Brazil

Reviewed by:
Oliver Grimm, Central Institute of Mental Health, Germany
Mark Horowitz, King's College London, UK
Bianca W. De Aguiar, Universidade Federal do Rio Grande do Sul, Brazil

***Correspondence:**
Bernhard T. Baune, Discipline of Psychiatry, School of Medicine, University of Adelaide, Adelaide, SA 5005, Australia.
e-mail: bernhard.baune@adelaide.edu.au

The increasing burden of major depressive disorder makes the search for an extended understanding of etiology, and for the development of additional treatments highly significant. Biological factors may be useful biomarkers for treatment with physical activity (PA), and neurobiological effects of PA may herald new therapeutic development in the future. This paper provides a thorough and up-to-date review of studies examining the neuroimmunomodulatory effects of PA on the brain in depression and depression-like behaviors. From a neuroimmune perspective, evidence suggests PA does enhance the beneficial and reduce the detrimental effects of the neuroimmune system. PA appears to increase the following factors: interleukin (IL)-10, IL-6 (acutely), macrophage migration inhibitory factor, central nervous system-specific autoreactive CD4+T cells, M2 microglia, quiescent astrocytes, CX3CL1, and insulin-like growth factor-1. On the other hand, PA appears to reduce detrimental neuroimmune factors such as: Th1/Th2 balance, pro-inflammatory cytokines, C-reactive protein, M1 microglia, and reactive astrocytes. The effect of other mechanisms is unknown, such as: CD4+CD25+T regulatory cells (T regs), CD200, chemokines, miRNA, M2-type blood-derived macrophages, and tumor necrosis factor (TNF)-α [via receptor 2 (R2)]. The beneficial effects of PA are likely to occur centrally and peripherally (e.g., in visceral fat reduction). The investigation of the neuroimmune effects of PA on depression and depression-like behavior is a rapidly developing and important field.

Keywords: physical activity, exercise, depression, psychiatry, immune, neurobiology

The increasing burden of major depressive disorder (MDD; WHO, 2008) makes the search for an extended understanding of etiology, and for the development of additional treatments highly significant. The global "pandemic" of physical inactivity (Lee et al., 2012) – a significant etiological factor for many non-communicable diseases, including depression (Garber et al., 2011; Kohl et al., 2012; Lee et al., 2012) – as well as the growing evidence supporting the clinical utility of physical activity (PA) in many psychiatric disorders, make the biological effects of PA highly relevant (Knochel et al., 2012; Lautenschlager et al., 2012; Rimer et al., 2012). Biological factors may be useful biomarkers for treatment with PA, and neurobiological effects of PA may herald new therapeutic developments in the future.

The neuroimmune system is important in the pathogenesis and pathophysiology of depression-like behaviors (Eyre and Baune, 2012c). Elevations in pro-inflammatory cytokines (PICs), causing neuroinflammation, are well known to be involved in the development of depression-like behaviors – e.g., sickness-like behavior, cognitive dysfunction, and anhedonia – in pre-clinical and clinical populations (Dantzer et al., 2008; McAfoose and Baune, 2009; Miller et al., 2009). The involvement of PICs in the development of depression-like behavior is often referred to as the cytokine model of depression (Dantzer et al., 2008; McAfoose and Baune, 2009; Miller et al., 2009).The neuroinflammatory state is associated with neurotransmitter dysfunction [e.g., reductions in serotonin (5-HT), as well as neurotoxic levels of glutamate (GLU) and tryptophan catabolites], reduced hippocampal (HC) neuroplasticity [e.g., neurogenesis, synaptic plasticity, and long-term potentiation (LTP)], oxidative stress, and glucocorticoid insensitivity (Dantzer et al., 2008; Miller et al., 2009; Eyre and Baune, 2012c; Leonard and Maes, 2012; Moylan et al., 2012).

A variety of novel neuroimmune mechanisms may also be involved in the development of depression-like behaviors (Eyre and Baune, 2012c; Littrell, 2012). Cellular immune factors include various T cells [e.g., CD4+CD25+ T regulatory cells (T regs), CNS-specific autoreactive CD4+ T cells] and macrophages (e.g., M2-type blood-derived macrophages) involved in the model of protective immunosurveillance (Schwartz and Shechter, 2010a,b; Martino et al., 2011; Ron-Harel et al., 2011). These neuroprotective immune cells – found to release neurotrophic factors and anti-inflammatory cytokines (AICs; Schwartz and Shechter, 2010a,b; Martino et al., 2011; Ron-Harel et al., 2011) – may be dysfunctional in the disease state (Schwartz and Shechter, 2010b). Moreover, the function of immunomodulatory proteins such as CX3CL1 (aka fractalkine; Rogers et al., 2011; Corona et al., 2012; Giunti et al., 2012), insulin-like growth factor-1 (IGF-1; Park et al., 2011a), and CD 200 (Lyons et al., 2007; Ojo et al., 2012) may be reduced.

In clinical studies, PA has shown efficacy in the treatment of MDD (Rimer et al., 2012), schizophrenia (SCZ; Knochel et al., 2012), anxiety-based disorders (Asmundson et al., 2013), and in enhancing cognitive function in disorders of cognitive function (i.e., Alzheimer's disease, AD and mild cognitive impairment, MCI; Foster et al., 2011; Knochel et al., 2012; Lautenschlager et al., 2012). There are many reasons why PA is an attractive therapeutic option in psychiatry. It has a low side-effect profile and can be adapted according to a patient's medical co-morbidities and functional status (Garber et al., 2011; Knochel et al., 2012; Rimer et al., 2012). PA also enhances self-esteem (Salmon, 2001), has less stigmatization than psychotherapy, may reduce the use of pharmacotherapies in MDD (Deslandes et al., 2010) and has a positive effect on cardiometabolic risk factors relevant to many psychiatric diseases (e.g., chronic inflammation, visceral fat mass, glucocorticoid sensitivity, glucose control, and insulin sensitivity; Gleeson et al., 2011; Baune et al., 2012c; Hamer et al., 2012; Knochel et al., 2012; Stuart and Baune, 2012).

Physical activity has beneficial effects on depressive symptomatology in a variety of clinical contexts. It is found to have robust effects on the depressive phenotype found in MDD (Rimer et al., 2012), as well as beneficial effects on the depressive symptomatology involved in the negative symptoms of SCZ (Knochel et al., 2012). PA has also been shown to be effective in treating cognitive dysfunction-related depression (Knochel et al., 2012; i.e., in MCI and AD where a significant proportion of patients with AD suffer from co-morbid depression; Lee and Lyketsos, 2003). The clinical utility of PA in MDD is promising given most patients on antidepressants will not achieve remission following initial treatment (Trivedi et al., 2006), and nearly one-third will not achieve remission even following several treatment steps (Rush et al., 2006a,b). Encouragingly, a recent Cochrane meta-analysis of 28 trials (1101 participants) by Rimer et al. (2012) – comparing exercise with no treatment or control intervention – found a moderate clinical effect in MDD. Studies have found that whilst PA has an initial treatment effect equal to that of antidepressants (Rimer et al., 2012), its effects are slower (Blumenthal et al., 1999) with greater relapse prevention (Babyak et al., 2000). PA interventions have been shown to be efficacious as a stand-alone (Rethorst et al., 2009) and as an augmentation treatment for MDD (Trivedi et al., 2011). Adequate levels of PA are also found to have a role in the prevention of MDD (Pasco et al., 2011b).

Physical activity interventions are found to have a multitude of effects on neuroimmune processes (Eyre and Baune, 2012a). Most notably PA interventions are found to reduce PIC levels in the brain of rodents (Eyre and Baune, 2012a) and in the periphery in clinical studies (Beavers et al., 2010a; Rethorst et al., 2012). The anti-inflammatory effects of PA may be related to acute elevations in neuroprotective interleukin-6 (IL-6; Funk et al., 2011), and resultant downstream changes, e.g., increased IL-1ra and reduced neuronal death in the HC (Funk et al., 2011). Reductions in pro-inflammatory visceral fat mass may also play a role in the anti-inflammatory effect of PA (Gleeson et al., 2011).

The neuroimmune effects of PA were recently outlined in our review (Eyre and Baune, 2012a), however, there have been a large number of studies published in 2012 investigating other neuroimmune-related factors (Moon et al., 2012; Rethorst et al., 2012). Novel factors investigated include macrophage migration inhibitor factor (MIF; Moon et al., 2012), CX3CL1 (Vukovic et al., 2012), and IGF-1 (Duman et al., 2009). Taken together, there is a need for a review outlining and summarizing these recent studies in light of pre-existing literature with the intention of better understanding the neuroimmunological effects of PA. From this literature important questions arise: *Are there PA types which are more effective than others? Are there subpopulations of patients with MDD who would benefit more from PA than antidepressants or psychotherapy? Can the neuroimmune effects of PA inform therapeutic development in the future? Are immune biomarkers potentially useful in measuring a treatment effect for PA in depression?*

This paper provides a thorough and up-to-date review of studies examining the neuroimmunomodulatory effects of PA on the brain in depression and depression-like behaviors.

METHODS

This review utilized an electronic search of databases such as PubMed, PsychInfo, OvidSP, and Science Direct. An initial search was conducted using the following keywords: (PA OR exercise) AND (immune OR inflammation OR cytokine OR anti-inflammatory OR immune cell OR glia OR neuroplasticity) AND/OR depression. Abstracts were selected based on the year of publication (between 1995 and December 2012), publication in the English language and of peer-reviewed type. They were excluded if they included anecdotal evidence. A total of 16,000 studies were found using these search terms. A total of 1000 articles remained after assessment of abstracts for relevance to the aims of this review. Of these, 770 studies were excluded after review of the full text if they did not examine the effect of the PA or depression on the immune system. A proportion of papers were found via the reference lists of the 1000 full text articles. Finally, 230 articles were utilized in this review.

CLINICAL EFFICACY OF PHYSICAL ACTIVITY IN DEPRESSION

Evidence supporting the clinical efficacy of PA interventions with depression – and depression co-morbid with other diseases [MCI, coronary heart disease (CHD)] – is growing (Blumenthal et al., 2012a,b; Rimer et al., 2012). In the clinical setting, exercise interventions are defined as "planned, structured, and repetitive bodily movements done to improve or maintain one or more components of physical fitness" (Garber et al., 2011). Exercise types can include aerobic, resistance, neuromotor (involving balance, agility, and co-ordination), and flexibility types (Garber et al., 2011). The following section will outline clinical evidence supporting the use of exercise in depression.

A 2012 re-analysis of available clinical trials by the Cochrane Group (Rimer et al., 2012; 2009 version; Mead et al., 2008) revealed 28 trials (1101 participants) comparing exercise with no treatment or control intervention finding a moderate clinical effect in MDD (standardized mean difference, SMD; −0.67 95% CI −0.90 to −0.43). However, when the meta-analysis was conducted with more strict criteria – i.e., studies with adequate allocation concealment, intention-to-treat analysis, and blinded outcome assessment – there were only four trials (326 participants), the SMD indicated a small clinical effect (SMD −0.31 95% CI −0.63 to 0.01). Moreover, data from the seven trials (373 participants) that provided long-term follow-up also found a small effect for exercise interventions (SMD −0.39, 95% CI −0.69 to −0.09).

In comparison to cognitive behavioral therapy, six trials (152 participants) found no significant difference with exercise.

Further investigating the individual clinical trials analyzed in this field yields interesting information on the clinical effect of exercise regimens. A 16-week randomized controlled trial (RCT) study by Blumenthal et al. (1999) found aerobic exercise and antidepressant (sertraline) treatment were equally effective in reducing depressive symptom severity [as per both Hamilton Depression Rating Scale (HAM-D) and Beck Depression Inventory (BDI)], however, sertaline had a faster initial response (in the first 3 weeks). Shortly after, a paper by Babyak et al. (2000) was published on the same study participants showing – at 6 months follow-up – patients assigned to the exercise program were less likely to relapse (no longer diagnostic for MDD or HAM-D < 8) than patients assigned to antidepressant treatment. Self-initiated exercise after the study intervention was associated with a reduced probability of depression at the end of the follow-up period (OR = 0.49).

Treatment of depression in older people is often hampered by poor recognition and increased prevalence of medication side-effects, polypharmacy, and poor adherence to treatment; therefore, exercise is increasingly being evaluated as a possible treatment. A recent meta-analysis (Bridle et al., 2012) of seven trials of subjects ≥60 years found exercise was associated with significantly lower depression severity (SMD −0.34; 95% CI −0.52 to −0.17). These findings were irrespective of whether participant eligibility was determined by clinical diagnosis or symptom checklist. An RCT in elderly patients (>60 years) with MDD – non-responders to escitalopram – found a 10-week Tai Chi Chih (TCC) exercise intervention augmented antidepressant treatment (Lavretsky et al., 2011). TCC exercise was chosen given it can be readily implemented among older adults with physical limitations (due to chronic medical illnesses or poor balance) and its added stress reduction and mindful cognitive properties. Multiple studies have shown regular, moderate PA can have a positive influence on depressive symptomatology in subjects with AD (Knochel et al., 2012), however Mahendra and Arkin (2003) found this beneficial effect was only significant after >1 year of PA. Deslandes et al. (2010) reported patients with co-morbid MCI and MDD could significantly reduce their antidepressant dose when they underwent a PA program.

Exercise is shown to have some modest beneficial effects on certain aspects of neurocognitive disturbance in depression. An RCT study with patients who met MDD criteria found exercise (both supervised and home-based) performed better with exercise than sertraline on tests of executive functioning, but not on tests of verbal and working memory (Hoffman et al., 2008). A recent meta-analysis (Smith et al., 2010) examining the effects of aerobic exercise on neurocognitive performance found 29 studies (2049 participants) showing modest improvements in attention and processing speed ($g = 0.158$; 95% CI, 0.055–0.260), executive function ($g = 0.123$; 95% CI, 0.021–0.225), and memory ($g = 0.128$; 95% CI, 0.015–0.241).

Depression is a common co-morbidity with a variety of cardiac conditions. Depression affects as many as 40% of patients with heart failure (HF), with up to 75% of patients reporting elevated depressive symptoms (Blumenthal et al., 2012a). For CHD, MDD affects 15–20% of cardiac patients and an additional 20% report elevated depressive symptoms (Blumenthal et al., 2012b). Blumenthal et al. (2012a) recently published an RCT of 2322 stable HF patients who underwent an aerobic exercise program (supervised for 1–3 months followed by home exercise for 9 months) or education and usual guideline-based HF care. Compared with usual care, aerobic exercise resulted in lower mean BDI-II scores at 3 and 12 months (differences of −0.76 and −0.68, respectively). Another study by Blumenthal et al. (2012b) assessed efficacy of 4 months of aerobic exercise and antidepressant treatments (sertraline) in reducing depressive symptoms and improving cardiovascular biomarkers in depressed patients with CHD. At 4 months, exercise and sertraline were equally as effective at reducing depressive symptoms (HRSD) vs. placebo. Exercise tended to result in greater reductions in heart rate variability vs. sertraline.

When considering the anti-depressive effects of exercise – in addition to biological effects – we must consider psychosocial aspects. Studies have shown exercise regimens have a distraction effect (from negative thoughts and ruminations), provide a sense of mastery via the learning of new skills (Lepore, 1997), and hence enhance self-efficacy (Craft, 2005) and self-esteem (Salmon, 2001). A study by Craft (2005) found that those who experienced an increase in mood following exercise showed higher self-efficacy levels at 3 and 9 weeks post-exercise. Self-esteem is considered to be one of the strongest predictors of overall (Diener, 1984), subjective well-being and low self-esteem is considered to be closely related with mental illness (Fox, 2000). The abovementioned beneficial psychological effects may lead to the stress reducing and stress-resilience enhancing effects of exercise (Salmon, 2001). Additionally, exercise regimens in a group setting may have a beneficial effect via training social skill deficits (Rimer et al., 2012).Therefore, considering the immunomodulatory effects of social support, i.e., social isolation stress is repeatedly shown to enhance inflammation in clinical and pre-clinical models (Hafner et al., 2011), the social interaction effects of PA interventions must be considered as a confounder.

Whilst the vast majority of research using PA in psychiatry is positive and encouraging, it is important to also consider potential pre-cautions during PA interventions. Some studies report no effect for PA in depression (Rimer et al., 2012). This may be explained by inappropriate intensity of PA, or a too short duration of PA as a treatment (Rimer et al., 2012). In order to enhance the potential for antidepressant effects, multiple authors now recommend exercise of moderate-intensity and of at least 8 weeks duration (Mead et al., 2008; Trivedi et al., 2011; Rimer et al., 2012). PA regimens must be tailored according to the individual patient's functional status and other co-morbidities. Failing to do so can lead to further morbidity and/or mortality. In patients with social phobia-related symptoms, the approach to PA interventions should be tailored appropriately.

NEUROIMMUNOLOGICAL EFFECTS OF PHYSICAL ACTIVITY IN DEPRESSION

When considering the neuroimmunological effects of PA in depression, it is important to first outline the current understanding on neuroimmunological mechanisms of the depression-like disease states. Therefore, the following section will outline these neuroimmunological mechanisms in detail; following, the neuroimmunological effects of PA will be examined.

NEUROIMMUNOLOGICAL CHANGES IN DEPRESSION

The neuroimmunological changes found in depression involve humoral and cellular factors from both the innate and adaptive immune systems (Eyre and Baune, 2012c; Littrell, 2012). Humoral factors include PICs, AICs, C-reactive protein (CRP) as well as other immunomodulatory factors like CX3CL1, CD200, and IGF-1 (Eyre and Baune, 2012b). Cellular factors include resident glia (e.g., astrocytes, microglia) and centrally migrating immune cells involved in protective immunosurveillance (e.g., CD4+ T cells and macrophages; Eyre and Baune, 2012b).

Neuroinflammation and depression: a well recognized relationship

The neuroinflammatory state is well known to be associated with the depressive phenotype (Dantzer et al., 2008; Dowlati et al., 2010). For example, a recent meta-analysis found a significant correlation between tumor necrosis factor (TNF-α), IL-6, and CRP with depression in humans (Dowlati et al., 2010). Neuroinflammation is characterized by elevations in PICs and reductions in AICs and can arise within the CNS itself, or peripheral inflammatory signals can be transferred into the CNS (Dantzer et al., 2008; see Quan and Banks, 2007; for a review of peripheral-CNS pathways, including: the neural route, circumventricular organs, BBB transport of cytokines, and secretions from BBB cells). The neuroinflammatory state is known to cause neurovegetative or sickness-like symptoms, depression- and anxiety-like behaviors, as well as cognitive dysfunction and symptoms of Chronic Fatigue Syndrome (Dantzer et al., 2008; McAfoose and Baune, 2009; Dowlati et al., 2010; Miller, 2010; Yirmiya and Goshen, 2011; Bansal et al., 2012), and the causation of these phenotypic states by PICs has been modeled in both rodent and human models and extensively reviewed (Dantzer et al., 2008; Miller, 2010).

Neuroinflammation-based models of depression have shown PICs to impact on other major neurobiological systems involved in depression. Neuroinflammation affects the neurotransmitter systems by activation if the tryphophan degrading enzyme, indoleamine 2,3 dioxygenase (IDO), altering metabolism of tryptophan into neurotoxic metabolites (3-hydroxykyurenin, 3-HK and quinolinic acid, QA) and depleting its availability for serotonin (5-HT) synthesis (Miller, 2010; Dantzer et al., 2011; Moylan et al., 2012). Inflammation also stimulates the reuptake of monoamines from the synapse by increasing the activity and the density of 5-HT, noradrenaline, and dopamine transporters (Moron et al., 2003; Nakajima et al., 2004; Zhu et al., 2006). Evidence suggests these immune mechanisms adversely affected glutamatergic neurotransmission causing GLU to rise to neurotoxic levels (McNally et al., 2008; Hashimoto, 2009; Popoli et al., 2012). In the neuroinflammatory state PICs may disrupt the capacity of the glucocorticoid receptor to translocate to the nucleus where it normally acts to suppress the activity of pro-inflammatory transcription factors such as nuclear factor-kappa B (NF-κB) – this is termed glucocorticoid resistance (Dantzer et al., 2008; Miller, 2010; Muller et al., 2011). High levels of PICs impair processes of neuroplasticity in the HC, such as neurogenesis, LTP, neurotrophin production (e.g., brain-derived neurotrophic factor, BDNF), and synaptic plasticity (Miller, 2010; Eyre and Baune, 2012c). In the context of reduced neuroplasticity, elevations in neurotoxic oxidative stress products and markers of apoptosis are found in the HC (Moylan et al., 2012). An in-depth assessment on the effects of inflammation on these systems is outside the scope of this review and have been outlined recently (see Dantzer et al., 2008, 2011; McAfoose and Baune, 2009; Muller et al., 2011; Moylan et al., 2012).

Rationale for examining immune mechanisms in addition to inflammation

Whilst the cytokine and neuroinflammatory models of depression have been helpful in understanding the neurobiology behind the depressive phenotype, there are a number of clinical and biological reasons for investigating neuroimmune mechanisms in addition to inflammation. These factors include:

- A recent meta-analysis by Hannestad et al. (2011) found results arguing against the notion that resolution of a depressive episode is associated with normalization of levels of circulating PICs. This analysis of 22 studies (603 subjects) found – when all antidepressants were grouped – these medications reduced levels if IL-1β with a marginal effect on IL-6 (using less stringent fixed-effects models); there was no effect on TNF-α. However, a sub-group analysis of selective serotonin regulate inhibitors (SSRI) medication found a reduction in IL-6 and TNF-α. Other antidepressants did not reduce PIC levels.
- Recent evidence has emerged to suggest no effect or even an antagonistic effect for anti-inflammatory medications in depression. A large-scale prospective cohort study of treatment-resistant depression, the "sequenced treatment alternatives to relieve depression" (STAR*D), found an antagonistic effect for anti-inflammatory compounds on ADs (Warner-Schmidt et al., 2011). Patients reporting concomitant non-steroidal anti-inflammatory drug (NSAID) or other analgesic treatment showed a reduced therapeutic response to citalopram, hence, the authors suggest concomitant use of NSAIDs may be an important reason for high SSRI treatment resistance rates (Warner-Schmidt et al., 2011). A recent re-analysis reached a similar conclusion, with more modest effects persisting after adjustment for potential confounding variables (Gallagher et al., 2012). Another recently published study shows no difference between infliximab, a TNF-α antagonist, and placebo in a recent 12-week double-blind, placebo-controlled RCT for treatment-resistant depression (Raison et al., 2012). There was a significant effect for infliximab in individuals who had a high baseline hs-CRP (>5 mg/L) and a significant effect for placebo-treated patients at a baseline hs-CRP of <5-mg/L. Schwartz and Shechter hypothesize anti-inflammatory drug compounds may block the production of brain-derived cytokines and chemokines which promote the migration of neuroprotective immune cells involved in protective immunosurveillance toward the CNS (Schwartz and Shechter, 2010b; Warner-Schmidt et al., 2011). Importantly, however, the use of NSAIDs may be most useful when used in the correct stage of neuroinflammatory diseases, i.e., administered early in the neuroinflammatory disease course when transmigratory immune cells have not come into effect (Schwartz and Shechter, 2010b).
- Evidence is emerging to suggest a neuroprotective and physiological role for "PICs." TNF-α and IL-6 have been shown to play an integral roles in processes of memory and learning in

both human and rodent studies, as well as having a physiological role in HC neuroplasticity (Carlson et al., 1999; Eyre and Baune, 2012c). The *TNF-α* gene (*rs1800629*) is correlated with enhanced cognitive processing speed in a healthy human population (Baune et al., 2008a). The *IL-6* gene (*rs1800795*) has been correlated with increased to HC volume in a healthy human population (Baune et al., 2012a). There are other studies outlining a neuroprotective effect of PICs in the brain (see below).

- From a clinical disease course perspective, there are other mechanisms in depression – in addition to inflammation – which may have a role in explaining the absence of correlation between the increase in neuroinflammation in aging and rates of depression. Since aging itself is related to higher levels of systemic inflammation and neuroinflammation (Hein and O'Banion, 2012), this should lead to higher rates of depression in old age, however, rates are highest in those aged 25–45 years, not in old age (Kessler et al., 2005). Other neuroimmune factors which may explain this scenario will be outlined below.

DYSFUNCTION OF NEUROPROTECTIVE IMMUNE FACTORS IN DEPRESSION

When considering neuroimmunological factors in depression, historically the focus has mainly been on high levels of PICs and their detrimental effects on the brain. However, research is beginning to suggest a significant role for neuroprotective neuroimmune factors in depression and other neurobiological disorders (e.g., multiple sclerosis and AD; Martino et al., 2011; Kokaia et al., 2012). When considering these neuroprotective factors in depression, their loss of function may exacerbate the depression-like behaviors (Schwartz and Shechter, 2010b). The following section will outline evidence suggesting a possible beneficial role for a variety of neuroimmune factors.

Neuroprotective and physiological effects of cytokines

There are a number of cytokines are found to have neuroprotective and physiological effects.

Interleukin-6 has been found to have neuroprotective effects via gp130 signaling and related pathways [i.e., Janus Kinase (JAK)/Signal Transducer and Activator of Transcription (STAT), Mitogen-activated Protein Kinase (MAPK)/cAMP Response Element-binding (CREB), Ras-MAPK, Phosphatidylinositol 3-kinases (PI3K); Baune et al., 2012a]. These mechanisms affect the production of neurotrophic factors, cellular survival, and apoptosis (Baune et al., 2012a). A recent imaging genetics study investigated the association between the *IL-6* gene and brain morphology in a large cohort of healthy adult participants in a whole-brain analysis approach (Baune et al., 2012a). Carriers of the G-allele of the *IL-6* genetic variant *rs1800795 (-174 C/G)* showed a significant association with larger HC volumes on the right side in healthy subjects. This genotype effect was remarkably specific to the HC, with no other structure surviving statistical threshold for the entire brain. The findings are suggestive of a neuroprotective role of the *IL-6* gene [*rs1800795 (-174 C/G)*] on HC morphology. Supporting a role of IL-6 in neuroproliferation is an *in vivo* study showing that IL-6 knockout mice have reduced proliferating NSCs specifically in the HC, hence underlining the importance of IL-6 in cell proliferation and cell survival (Bowen et al., 2011). However, other similar studies have shown no effect or a negative effect for IL-6 in neurogenesis processes (Eyre and Baune, 2012c). The difference between the pro- and anti-neurogenic effects of IL-6 may reflect differences in amounts and conditions used experimentally (Eyre and Baune, 2012c).

Tumor necrosis factor-α is thought to exert its protective and restorative effects primarily via TNFR2 (p75; primarily neuroprotective and neuroregenerative pathway) and related signaling pathways [i.e., IκB kinase (IKK)/Nuclear Factor κB (NF-kB), Transforming Growth factor β-activated Kinase 1 (TAK-1), PI3K-PKB-Akt, c-Jun N-terminal kinases (JNK), and IL-6), as opposed to the TNFR1 (p55; primarily neurodegenerative; Eyre and Baune, 2012a; Santello and Volterra, 2012). Importantly, whether the outcome of TNF-α signaling is protective or damaging may depend upon duration of NF-κB activation (Santello and Volterra, 2012). TNF-α has been found to exert beneficial effects in depression-related processes, e.g., cognitive function and HC neurogenesis (Eyre and Baune, 2012a; Santello and Volterra, 2012). During relatively health aging processes, it has been shown that the *TNF-α* gene (*rs1800629*) has protective effects on cognitive processing speed (Baune et al., 2008a) and has been associated with cognitive processes (e.g., response inhibition, error processing, attentional processes, and mental rotation) in young health individuals (Eyre and Baune, 2012a). In behavioral studies, TNF-α deficient mice exhibit impaired HC-dependent memory function in the Morris Water Maze suggesting that during early stages of brain development basal levels of TNF is required for memory and learning (Baune et al., 2008b).

Interleukin-4 has been found to have a beneficial role in depression-like behaviors and a neuroprotective effect. The release of IL-4 from CNS-specific autoreactive CD4+ T cells involved in protective immunosurveillance – in response to increased neurotoxicity (Ron-Harel et al., 2011) – binds to IL-4 receptor on the cytotoxic microglia (Kipnis et al., 2008) causing downregulation of PIC production, induction of BDNF and IGF-1, and an elevation in neurogenesis (Butovsky et al., 2005, 2006b; Lyons et al., 2009; Martino et al., 2011). Microglia under quiescent conditions, after exposure to IL-4 or low levels of IFN-γ (Butovsky et al., 2006b), have been shown to support neurogenesis and NSC differentiation and migration *in vitro* (Aarum et al., 2003; Butovsky et al., 2006b; Walton et al., 2006). IL-4 is also shown to promote the creation of neuroprotective M2-type microglial phenotype (Godbout et al., 2012). A recent study found central IL-4 administration increased microglial-specific M2a-type genes including *Arginase*, *IL-1Rα*, and *BDNF* (Godbout et al., 2012). Microglia activated by IL-4 remain committed to their protective phenotype (M2-type) even when exposed to a threatening environment in the form of LPS, and, exposure of microglia, pre-activated to a cytotoxic phenotype, to IL-4 induces a phenotype switch toward neuroprotection (Butovsky et al., 2005; Schwartz et al., 2006). A study rodent by Derecki et al. (2010) shows T cell-derived IL-4 to have beneficial effects on the regulation of cognitive function in rodents via meningeal myeloid cell phenotypes producing BDNF. IL-4 knockout mice show greater sickness behavior (measured by exploratory behavior) than wildtype mice exposed to LPS (Lyons et al., 2009). Interestingly, Kim et al. (2011) proposes T-bet deficient mice may have a neuroprotective effect by creating a predominance of Th2-derived IL-4, which may in turn stimulate meningeal myeloid cell BDNF production. T-bet is a Th1-specific T-box transcription factor which regulates CD4+ Th1 development by inducing endogenous Th1 cytokines, while simultaneously repressing Th2 development (Wong et al., 2008).

A role for IL-10 in neuroprotection and the prevention of depression-like behavior has been suggested. Central administration of IL-10 prevents the emergence of behavioral signs of depression in an LPS model of sickness behavior (Bluthe et al., 1999). IL-10 over-expression mice display less anxiety-like behaviors, while IL-10 knock-out rodents display greater anxiety and depression-like behavior (forced-swim test) with these effects more pronounced in females (Mesquita et al., 2008). In human studies, IL-10 is found to be reduced in the depressed state (Himmerich et al., 2010). Further papers examining the neuroprotective effects of IL-10 can be found in Raison and Miller (2011).

Immunomodulatory factors

Insulin-like growth factor-1 is a major neurotrophic factor involved in neuroplastic functions such as neurogenesis and is critical in normal memory and LTP functions (Trejo et al., 2007). Recent evidence suggests IGF-1 also has added immunomodulatory effects (Park et al., 2011a,b). In an LPS model of depression, central administration of IGF-1 is shown to prevent LPS-induced sickness- and depression-like behavior (Park et al., 2011a,b) in association with an induction of BDNF and a reduction of TNF-α, IL-1β, and iNOS in the pre-frontal cortex (PFC; Park et al., 2011b). Given the levels of IGF-1 have been found to be low in rodent models of depression (Mitschelen et al., 2011), the absence of this anti-inflammatory factor may exacerbate the neuroinflammatory and anti-neuroplastic state in depression.

CX3CL1 is a chemokine expressed by healthy neurons which has its receptor, CX3CR1, in membrane bound form or as soluble ligand (Rogers et al., 2011). It has an important role in inhibiting the activation of microglia (Rogers et al., 2011). A recent study with CX3CR1 knock-out mice and the LPS model of sickness behavior found a deficiency in the action of CX3CL1 resulted in protracted microglial activation, as measured by IL-1β and CD14 (Corona et al., 2010). These mice have extended LPS-induced depression-like behavior in association with the activated microglial phenotype described (Corona et al., 2010). In another study with CX3CR1 knock-out mice, a lack of the CX3CR1 receptor resulted in contextual fear conditioning (associative memory) and Morris Water Maze deficits (spatial memory), as well as impairment in LTP (Rogers et al., 2011). Disruption of the CX3CL1/CX3CR1-pathway in young rodents decreases both survival and proliferation of HC neural progenitor cells (Bachstetter et al., 2011).

CD200 is a membrane glycoprotein which has been identified as an immune-suppressive molecule (Cox et al., 2012). It is expressed in neurons and oligodendrocytes, but not on microglia (Cox et al., 2012). The receptor for CD200, CD200R, is also a membrane glycoprotein and is primarily restricted to cells of the myeloid lineage, hence being found on microglia, but not neurons or astrocytes (Cox et al., 2012). The interaction between CD200 and its receptor play a significant role in maintaining microglia in a quiescent state, therefore, a decrease in CD200 expression is associated with evidence of microglia activation (Cox et al., 2012). A rodent study by Frank et al. (2007) shows an inescapable shock model of stress over 24 h resulted in a downregulation of HC CD200 in association with enhanced LPS-induced cytokine production in HC microglia. This suggests stress can activate microglia via downregulation of CD200, enhancing the PIC production of microglia (Frank et al., 2007). A study by Cox et al. (2012) found a CD200 fusion protein (CD200Fc), activator of CD200R, attenuated age-related microglial immunoreactivity in the HC (indicated by MHCII, CD40, and iNOS). CD200Fc also attenuated LPS-induced microglial activation (indicated by elevated MHCII, CD40, CD11b, and CD68) and LTP deficits (Cox et al., 2012). Using CD200 knock-out mice and LPS-induced sickness behavior, Costello et al. (2011) found the neuroinflammatory changes resulting from CD200 deficiency have a negative impact on LTP in the CA1 region of the dentate gyrus. Interestingly, a study by Lyons et al. (2009) has shown IL-4 as a key inducer of CD200 expression.

Dysfunction of protective immunosurveillance

Emerging data suggests a role for CNS-specific autoreactive CD4+ T cells, blood-derived macrophages (in the form of M2 alternatively activated macrophages) in physiological, protective immunosurveillance functions of the brain (Derecki et al., 2010, 2011; Martino et al., 2011; Ron-Harel et al., 2011). Evidence suggests these cell types may have established a physiological connection between the immune system and the brain, and have assisted in explaining processes of HC-dependent neurogenesis and cognitive dysfunction (Kipnis et al., 2004b; Butovsky et al., 2006b, 2007; Ziv et al., 2006; Brynskikh et al., 2008; Derecki et al., 2010, 2011), anxiety- and depression-like behavior (Cohen et al., 2006; Lewitus et al., 2008; Cardon et al., 2010) due to an insufficient immune response (Derecki et al., 2010, 2011; Schwartz and Shechter, 2010a,b; Ron-Harel et al., 2011). The role of these cells in neuroprotection and higher neurocognitive functions has been reviewed in detail elsewhere (Martino et al., 2011; Yirmiya and Goshen, 2011); however, a brief summary will be given, below.

Immune cells involved in protective immunosurveillance can populate meningeal areas of the choroid plexus and the cerebrospinal fluid, hence gaining access to the healthy brain without entering the parenchyma (Ransohoff et al., 2003; Derecki et al., 2010, 2011; Schwartz and Shechter, 2010a). CNS-specific autoreactive CD4+ T cells are suggested to react to three signals, (1) T-cell receptor (TCR; Ron-Harel et al., 2011), (2) co-stimulatory signals (CD28/CD80,86; Jenkins and Johnson, 1993), and (3) PICs and reactive oxygen species (ROS; Curtsinger et al., 1999; Tse et al., 2007; Ron-Harel et al., 2011). The T cells in question, activated in response to increased neurotoxicity (Ron-Harel et al., 2011), are thought to secrete increased levels of IL-4 (Ron-Harel et al., 2011), where IL-4 penetrates the brain parenchyma and binds to IL-4R on the cytotoxic microglia (Kipnis et al., 2008). Exposure of cytotoxic microglia to IL-4 causes downregulation of PIC secretion, induction of BDNF and IGF-1 secretion, and an elevation in neurogenesis (Butovsky et al., 2005, 2006b; Martino et al., 2011). All of these signals support the restoration of brain homeostasis (Ron-Harel et al., 2011). Furthermore, the T cells boost infiltration of neuroprotective blood-borne monocytes upon need (Shechter et al., 2009). A recent commentary by Ron-Harel et al. (2011) suggests any destabilization in brain homeostasis that cannot be locally contained by microglia and/or astrocytes will increase T cell recruitment as well as subsequent IL-4 release and recruitment of blood-derived macrophages.

According to the "protective immunosurveillance" model, increased susceptibility to mental illness may result from a deficiency in circulating T cells and the IL-4 they can produce, as the IL-4 mediates processes which are able to counteract neuroinflammation and restore brain homeostasis (Ron-Harel et al., 2011). Indeed, the brains of immune-deficient mice show accumulation of toxicity (i.e., increased glyoxalase-1, a compensatory mechanism against free radical and carbonyl levels; Ron-Harel et al., 2011).

According to the protective immunosurveillance model, activation of CNS-specific autoreactive CD4+ T cells (mentioned above) support the infiltration of neuroprotective, alternatively activated M2 macrophages to the sub-arachnoid meningeal spaces and choroid plexus, via IL-4 and IFN-γ secretion (Derecki et al., 2010, 2011; Ron-Harel et al., 2011). These infiltrating macrophages, together with the microglia they regulate, remove dead cells and cellular debris, buffer toxic compounds (such as GLU and ROS), and produce growth factors (i.e., BDNF and IGF-1), while down-regulating inflammation-associated compounds such as IL-1β, TNF-α, iNOS, and COX-2 (Hauben et al., 2000; Butovsky et al., 2005, 2006a,b, 2007; Shaked et al., 2005; Beers et al., 2008; Chiu et al., 2008; Rolls et al., 2008; Shimizu et al., 2008; Koronyo-Hamaoui et al., 2009; Shechter et al., 2009; Derecki et al., 2010, 2011; Prinz et al., 2011). These neurobiological functions are thought to contribute to blood-derived macrophages support of learning and memory (as determined via the Morris Water Maze and Barnes Maze; Derecki et al., 2010, 2011). Importantly, intravenous injection of M2 cells into immune-deficient mice can circumvent the need for CNS-specific autoreactive CD4+ T cells (Derecki et al., 2011). For a review of the role of blood-derived macrophages see recent papers (Derecki et al., 2010; Martino et al., 2011; Yirmiya and Goshen, 2011).

The type of macrophage – classical (M1), alternatively activated (M2), and deactivated types – determines the role in sickness behavior (for thorough review see Moon et al., 2011). Classical macrophages produce PICs and, hence, induce sickness behaviors (Dantzer et al., 2008; Moon et al., 2011). M2 macrophages which reduce PIC production, as outlined above, are associated with a reduction in sickness behavior (Derecki et al., 2010, 2011; Sherry et al., 2010). Deactivated macrophages which inhibit PIC production via IL-10 secretion are also thought to have beneficial effects of sickness behaviors, however, this finding has not been replicated (Moon et al., 2011).

It is important to mention a recent critique of the protective immunosurveillance concept recently produced by Rook et al. (2011). One important issue raised is that the phenotype of the neuroprotective, CNS-specific autoreactive CD4+ T cells is poorly understood (Rook et al., 2011). The authors suggest immune cells involved with the function of protective autoimmunity is likely from a regulatory cell – not always CD25+ – given the involvement of IL-4 and IL-10. Suggestions for potential cell types include Th3, Tr1, Th2, IL-10^{+}TH1, CD8+ reg cells, regulatory Foxp3+ NKT, IL-10^{+}CD56^{bright}NK, or various other IL-10-secreting cell types (Fujio et al., 2010; Rook et al., 2011). Another important consideration raised is the effect of T cell produced IL-4 on T reg differentiation. T cell differentiation into the T reg cell type can be enhanced or opposed by IL-4 depending on the context (Chapoval et al., 2010; Rook et al., 2011). Further, one study shows IL-4 increased certain chemokines (CCL1, CCL17, and CCL22) in an experimental autoimmune encephalitis (EAE) model capable of recruiting T regs (Butti et al., 2008). The above mentioned issues are relevant to the neuroimmune model of depression considering the dynamic relationship between T regs and effector T cells.

Glial cells

The role of the immunocompetent glia, astrocytes, and microglia, in depression is complex and poorly understood (Beumer et al., 2012); importantly, however, there is a developing literature supporting a neuroprotective effect of these cells under certain conditions (Schwarz and Bilbo, 2011, 2012; Ekdahl, 2012). The follow section will summarize most recent evidence available in this field.

Microglia

The function of microglia is dynamic even in the resting state whereby they continually survey their microenvironments by extending and contracting processes into nearly synapses (Bilbo et al., 2012). Microglia are the resident macrophages of the CNS and are recognized as the primary component of the neuroimmune system (Ekdahl, 2012). Once activated – by chronic stress conditions, or immune challenge with LPS or PICs – microglia are capable of producing PICs and neurotoxic mediators such as nitric oxide, PGE2, and superoxide anions (Liu et al., 2011; Bilbo et al., 2012; Ekdahl, 2012). A recent study by Walker and colleagues has shown a role for microglia in mediating the effects of stress on PFC neuronal function and PFC-regulated behavior (Hinwood et al., 2012). This study found restraint stress conditions caused a decline in working memory performance associated with increased microglial activity (measured by a 25% increase in Iba-1 labeling, ΔFosB, and a hyper-ramified state) in the medial PFC and no association was found with increased antigen presentation (MHCII) or apoptosis (caspase-3; Walker et al., 2011).

Given the pre-existing association with the inflammatory hypothesis of depression much research centers on reducing the PIC production of microglia (Liu et al., 2011). Recent evidence suggests a neuroprotective function of microglia under certain circumstances (Yirmiya and Goshen, 2011; Ekdahl, 2012). For example, microglia under quiescent conditions, after exposure to IL-4 or low levels of IFN-γ (Butovsky et al., 2006b), have been shown to support neurogenesis and NSC differentiation and migration *in vitro* (Aarum et al., 2003; Butovsky et al., 2006b; Walton et al., 2006). Microglia activated by IL-4 remain committed to their protective phenotype even when exposed to a threatening environment in the form of LPS, and, exposure of microglia pre-activated to a cytotoxic phenotype to IL-4 induces a phenotype switch toward neuroprotection (Butovsky et al., 2005; Schwartz et al., 2006). Exposure of rats to environmental enrichment (EE) increases neurogenesis alongside increased HC microglia proliferation (microglia assumed a neuroprotective phenotype expressing

MHC II and IGF-1; Ziv et al., 2006). As mentioned previously, the pro-neurogenic effects of microglia may be related to their interactions with CNS-specific autoreactive CD4+ T cells, this was further confirmed by a study showing transgenic mice with an excess of these T cells – and associated increases in neurogenesis – showed attenuated neurogenesis by chronic treatment with the microglial inhibitor, minocycline (Ziv et al., 2006). Furthermore, a rodent model of amyotrophic lateral sclerosis (ALS) illustrates the interaction between T cells and microglia whereby Th1 cytokines promote M1 microglia and Th2 or Treg cytokines promote M2 microglia (Chiu et al., 2008). Microglia were also shown to support neurogenesis in adrenalectomized rodents via TGF-β (Battista et al., 2006; Mathieu et al., 2010). Opposing the above neuroprotective findings is a rodent study demonstrating that PA-induced neurogenesis was not associated with microglial proliferation or activation, and no indication of T-cell-microglial interactions (i.e., no MHC II expression or T cells in the HC; Olah et al., 2009).

In summary, microglial function is closely intertwined with the immune system and neurogenesis (Ekdahl, 2012), with the cross-talk between these systems requiring further investigation. For instance, a recent review by Ekdahl (2012) suggests microglial activation patterns may by region-specific. Moreover, there appears to be a primarily beneficial interaction between microglia and new neurons in the intact brain, however, the cross-talk is complex and probably double-edged in pathological conditions, especially following long-term microglial activation (Ekdahl, 2012).

Astrocytes

Astrocytes are physically and functionally appositioned with most synapses, known as the "tripartite synapse" (Araque et al., 1999). They possess immune-like properties whereby they have an ability to respond to inflammatory cytokines (particularly IL-1β), to secrete PICs (i.e., TNF-α and IL-6) and to phagocytose cellular processes and debris (Yirmiya and Goshen, 2011). These cells play an important role in neural and synaptic functioning. For example, a rodent study by Bracchi-Ricard et al. (2008) shows female mice where the transcription factor NF-κB was inhibited specifically in astrocytes displayed deficits in learning, memory, and LTP. These cells were also found to mediate homeostatic synaptic scaling following prolonged inhibition of neuronal activity via TNF-α secretion, a known synaptic strength enhancer (Stellwagen and Malenka, 2006; Kaneko et al., 2008). The role of astrocytic IL-1 signaling in memory functioning and LTP was recently demonstrated by Ben Menachem-Zidon et al. (2011). In this study neural precursor cells (NPCs) derived from either WT or IL-1rKO neonatal mice were labeled with BrdU and transplanted into the HC of either IL-1rKO or WT adult host mice. Transplanted NPCs showed long-term survival and differentiated into astrocytes (expressing GFAP and S100β), but did not differentiate into neurons. Several weeks post-transplantation, IL-1rKO mice transplanted with IL-1rKO cells, or sham operated, displayed severe memory disturbances and a marked impairment in LTP. However, IL-1rKO mice transplanted with WT NPCs (expressing IL-1R) displayed complete rescue of the impaired memory functioning, as well as partial restoration of LTP. IL-4 is also found to be important in astrocyte functioning with the secretion of BDNF by *in vitro* astrocytes being markedly enhanced by this cytokine (Martino et al., 2011). Furthermore – and in fitting with the abovementioned model of protective immunosurveillance by Schwartz et al. – astrocytes also acquire a neuroprotective phenotype following their co-culture with T cells (Garg et al., 2008).

There is a paucity of evidence correlating the role of the abovementioned glial cells in models and tests of depression-like behavior. This is an important area for future research as these cells appear to be involved in depression-related pathophysiological processes.

Additional cellular immune factors

The role of T regs in depression is uncertain, and may be both positive and negative in depression pathophysiology depending on the surrounding environment (Cohen et al., 2006; Himmerich et al., 2010). In relation to the positive effects of T regs, some authors propose these cells may function to inhibit inappropriate or excessive immune responses, i.e., PIC production (Dantzer et al., 2008; Miller, 2010). Some human studies have found reduced IL-10 and TGF-β have been found in depressed patients, and are thought to be consistent with reduced T reg expression and/or function (Myint et al., 2005; Sutcigil et al., 2007; Dhabhar et al., 2009; Musil et al., 2011). One study found decreased T regs, alongside intracellular Foxp3, in association with IL-10 and TGF-β in depressed patients vs. controls (Li et al., 2010). A second study found 6 weeks of AD treatment led to increased T reg (CD4+CD25^{hi}) percentage in association with decreased IL-1β (Himmerich et al., 2010). A recent rodent study shows T reg cell depleted mice undergoing chronic immobilization stress displayed markedly increased anxiety in the Elevated Plus Maze and increased depression-like behavior in the Forced-Swim Test (Kim et al., 2012). These finds were found in correlation with elevated serum cytokines (i.e., IL-6, TNF-α, IL-2, IFN-γ, and IL-4) and reduced levels of HC 5-HT. In addition, a rodent model of cholestatic liver disease due to bile duct ligation found T regs suppress sickness-like behavior alongside inhibiting monocyte and hepatic IL-6 production, and subsequent signaling via circulating IL-6 acting (via p-STAT3 at the level of the cerebral endothelium; Nguyen et al., 2012). However, T regs have also been found to inhibit the beneficial effects of CNS-specific autoreactive CD4+ T cells on mitigating stress-induced anxiety-like behaviors in rodents (Cohen et al., 2006). This suggests T regs may inhibit the neuroprotective functions of these autoreactive T cells, a counterproductive effect. Interestingly, other studies with an optic nerve injury model have shown both Treg-free CD4+ T cells and T regs, respectively, can exhibit neuroprotective functions via preventing neuronal cell loss (Kipnis et al., 2004a). T regs exhibit significant plasticity and can lose regulatory activity, expressing effector cell function under certain circumstances (Zhou et al., 2009). Therefore, the balance of these two cells types may play a role in neuroprotective functions. Interestingly, T regs constitutively express CD25, a high affinity IL-2 receptor. The expression of CD25 is thought to be one of the ways by which T regs suppress proliferation of T effector cells, that is, by acting as a sink for IL-2 which is needed for T effector cell proliferation (Walsh and Kipnis, 2011). Interestingly, IL-2 is known to increase the suppressive abilities of T regs (Kohm et al., 2006), hence, the reduction of IL-2 which is seen in some studies of depression may reduce the anti-inflammatory effects of T regs (Anisman et al., 1999; Blume et al., 2011). A recent review paper summarizes literature suggesting T reg phenotypes are flexible depending on background chemokine and cytokine levels (Rook et al., 2011). Flexibility of phenotype means these cells can change from anti- to pro-inflammatory functions (Rook et al., 2011); indeed, authors remark that T-cell phenotype may change from the start to the end of studies (Rook et al., 2011). Furthermore, gut microbiota may affect the immunosuppressive function of T regs as well as their effects on higher neurocognitive behaviors of the brain (Rook et al., 2011). Clearly, the effect of T regs in depression requires further research.

Other T-cell subtypes in depression – Th1, Th2 cells, and T-bet

The balance of Th1 vs. Th2 cytokines in depression is currently debated by prominent authors in the field (Capuron and Miller, 2011; Rook et al., 2011). The majority of evidence suggests a net Th1 production as a key feature of immune dysfunction in depression, however, some studies suggest increased Th2 production (Myint et al., 2005; Capuron and Miller, 2011; Rook et al., 2011; Leonard and Maes, 2012). Th1 cells can produce IFN-γ, IL-2, and TNF-α; Th2 cells can produce IL-4, IL-6, and IL-10. Recent evidence suggests T-bet is associated with depression-like behaviors (Wong et al., 2008; Kim et al., 2011). T-bet deficient mice, Th1/IFN-γ depleted, are shown to be resistant to stress-induced depression-like behavior and stress-induced neuroinflammation (i.e., IL-6 and TNF-α; Kim et al., 2011). A clinical study by Wong et al. (2008) in a sample of Mexican Americans with major depression, shows evidence that single nucleotide polymorphisms (SNPs) in the *T-bet* (*Tbx21*) gene, which is critical for helper T (Th) 1-cell function, are associated with susceptibility to major depression. Moreover, the same study showed T-cell involvement in AD treatment response of genes associated with T-cell development (T-cell antigen receptor-ε subunit of T3, CD3E; Wong et al., 2008).

BALANCING BENEFICIAL AND DETRIMENTAL EFFECTS OF THE NEUROIMMUNE SYSTEM IN DEPRESSION

In the sections above we have outlined both the beneficial and detrimental effects of the neuroimmune system in depression. From this information, we suggest that depression-related pathophysiology and depression-like behaviors may be dictated by the balance between the beneficial and detrimental effects of neuroimmune factors. See **Figure 1** for a graphical representation of this balance. It is possible that when the balance is skewed toward the detrimental effects of the neuroimmune system, this leads to the development of depression-like behaviors, may prolong depressive episodes and lead to more severe symptomatology and behaviors. Alternatively, if the balance becomes skewed toward the beneficial effects of the neuroimmune system, this would reduce symptomatology and behavior and may drive the end of depressive episodes and prolong relapse remission.

NEUROBIOLOGICAL EFFECTS OF PHYSICAL ACTIVITY IN DEPRESSION

The neurobiological effects of PA in depression include effects on neurotransmitter, neuroendocrine systems, effects on neuroplasticity, and effects on neuroimmunological factors. The following section will outline the effects of PA on these systems, below, with a focus on neuroimmunological factors.

Neurobiological effects

Physical activity has been shown to upregulate monoamine neurotransmitters in the brain (e.g., 5-HT, dopamine, and noradrenaline) as well as endorphins (Knochel et al., 2012; Lautenschlager et al., 2012; Sarris et al., 2012). Reductions in glucocorticoid stress hormones are also found alter PA interventions whereby PA appears to re-regulate the HPA axis (Eyre and Baune, 2012c). Oxidative stress is reduced in the hippocampus in pre-clinical populations (Marosi et al., 2012).

Hippocampal neuroplasticity (e.g., neurogenesis, HC volume, and neurotrophin production) is increased with PA interventions in both clinical and pre-clinical populations (Erickson et al., 2012; Knochel et al., 2012; Lautenschlager et al., 2012). Pereira et al. (2007) reported that aerobic exercise resulted in increased HC blood volume which correlated with improved aerobic capacity and neurogenesis in the dentate gyrus. A recent RCT by Erickson et al. (2011) found that an aerobic exercise program in older adults, for 3 days a week over 1 year, increased HC volume by 2%. This was associated with increased serum BDNF and improvements in spatial memory. Further work is required to investigate the effects of PA on neuroplasticity in the PFC and amygdala.

Neuroimmunological effects in clinical populations

A recent study by Rethorst et al. (2012) aimed to determine the extent to which inflammatory markers can be used to predict treatment response to exercise treatment, and if this effect was dependent upon the dose of exercise. This prospective study used participants who were incomplete responders to an SSRI and randomized them to two doses of aerobic exercise for 12 weeks [4 or 16 kilocalories per kilogram of body weight per week (KKW))] 16 KKW was designed to meet or exceed current PA guidelines for public health from professional associations. The study found participants with a high baseline TNF-α (>5.493 pg/ml) had a greater reduction in depressive symptoms (measured by IDS-C) than those with a low TNF-α level. Interestingly, this finding may suggest TNF-α as a moderator between SSRI and exercise treatment, and TNF-α levels could be used to recommend exercise rather than medication as part of a personalized treatment algorithm (Rethorst et al., 2012). This is given Eller et al. (2008) found high baseline TNF-α associated with non-response to an SSRI, and the Hannestad et al. (2011) meta-analysis also supports this association. There was a significant correlation between change in IL-1β and depression symptoms for the 16 KKW group, but not the 4 KKW group. The meta-analysis by Hannestad et al. (2011) also found a reduction in IL-1β correlated with better outcomes with SSRIs. Interestingly there was no change in cytokines levels following either exercise dosage. The authors suggest this may have occurred due to pre-treatment with SSRIs – a well known anti-inflammatory agent (Hannestad et al., 2011) – which obscured the ability to detect changes in cytokine levels. Indeed, many past studies have shown exercise to have a robust anti-inflammatory effect in both human and rodent studies (Rethorst et al., 2011; Eyre and Baune, 2012a).

Another recent study by Irwin and Olmstead (2012) utilized a 9-week TCC program in a healthy older adult population to investigate the effect of exercise on depression symptoms. This study

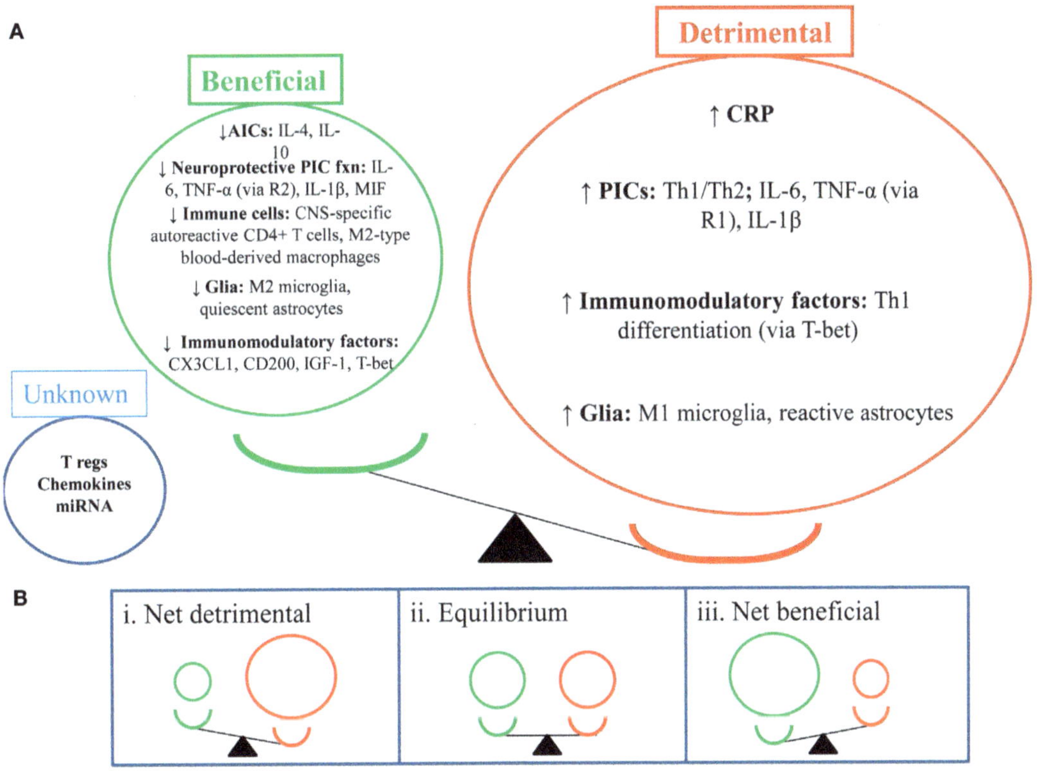

FIGURE 1 | Depression-like behavior: balancing the beneficial and detrimental effects of the neuroimmune system. (A) This section shows the balance of the detrimental (red) and beneficial (green) effects of neuroimmune factors in the depressed state (i.e., detrimental factors out way beneficial factors). NB: depression-like behavior includes sickness-like behavior, anhedonia, anxiety-, and cognition-like behaviors. **(B)** This section shows a number of potential outcomes for the balance between the abovementioned neuroimmune factors. (i) Shows a net detrimental effect which would lead to depression-like behaviors; clinically this could mean a depressive episode and could also increase relapse rates. (ii) Shows an equilibrium position which may suggest a stable/steady state in behavior; clinically this could mean a euthymic state. (iii) Shows a net beneficial effect which may attenuate depression-like behavior; clinically this could mean reduction or resolution of depressive symptoms and reduced relapse rates.

found TCC reduced depressive symptoms (BDI) in correlation with a reduction in IL-6 levels. TCC, however, had no effect on cellular markers of inflammation (i.e., sIL-1ra, sIL-6, sICAM, and IL-18). The authors suggest PA treatments may modulate IL-6 via decreasing sympathetic outflow. Aging and stress are associated with increases in circulating catecholamine levels, which are known to increase IL-6.

A study by Kohut et al. (2006) found aerobic exercise reduced pro-inflammatory factors (i.e., CRP, IL-5, TNF-α, and IL-18) more than a combination of flexibility and strength exercise over a 10-month period. These exercise types both reduced depressive symptoms in the Geriatric Depression Scale (GDS).

The robust lipolytic effects of PA are suggested to play a role in the antidepressant effects of PA in depression, via reducing the systemic pro-inflammatory state seen in obesity (Gleeson et al., 2011). A high visceral fat mass has been shown to cause a chronic inflammatory state, and this chronic inflammatory state may link depression and obesity (Stuart and Baune, 2012). Gleeson et al. (2011) also suggests physical inactivity is a risk factor for the accumulation of visceral fat which may predispose individuals to chronic illness like depression and heart disease via systemic PIC production by visceral fat mass.

See **Tables 1** and **2** for clinical studies examining the effects of exercise on neuroimmunological factors with and without depressive symptom correlations, respectively.

Neuroimmunological effects in pre-clinical populations

As seen in **Tables 3** and **4**, there are a large number of studies investigating the neuroimmunological effects of PA. Studies have been variously conducted with and without behavioral correlates. The following section will summarize the salient studies in this field.

A recent study found a voluntary exercise regimen to be associated with increased HC MIF, as well as *Bdnf* and *Tph2* (tryphophan hydroxylase, involved in the synthesis of 5-HT) gene expression (Moon et al., 2012). These changes occurred in the context of reduced depression-like behavior (FST), and the effect of PA on these factors was mediated by the CD74-GTPase (MIF receptor) and RhoA-ERK1/2 pathway. MIF is a PIC expressed in the CNS whose deletion is associated with increased anxiety- and depression-like behaviors, as well as of impaired HC-dependent memory and HC neurogenesis (Conboy et al., 2011). Taken together, this information suggests a role of MIF in mediating the antidepressant action of exercise, probably by enhancing 5-HT neurotransmission and neurogenesis.

Table 1 | Neuroimmune effects of physical activity in human populations with depressive symptom correlation.

Study	Study objective	Study details	Exercise details	Neuropsychological testing	Immune testing	Results
Rethorst et al. (2012)	To examine the extent to which inflammatory markers can be used to predict response to exercise treatment after an incomplete response to an SSRI To examine how the inflammatory markers change with exercise and if those changes are associated with dose of exercise or changes in symptom severity	Prospective. Randomized. TREAD study Participants had MDD and were partial responders to an SSRI (i.e., ≥14 HRSD-17 following >6 weeks but <6 months of treatment) Excluded if regularly engaging in PA Age 18–70 years 73 participants 12-week	Randomized to either 16 or 4 KWW Aerobic EXC (treadmill or cycle ergometers) Combination of supervised and home-based sessions	Clinician: IDS-C30 Self-rated: IDS-SR30 and HRSD-17	ELISA of serum at baseline and 12 weeks. IFN-γ, IL-1β, IL-6, and TNF-α	High baseline TNF-α (>5.493 pg/ml) α greater ↓ in depression sxs (IDS-C) over 12 weeks ($p < 0.0001$) Sig pos α between Δ IL-1β and Δ depression sxs ($p = 0.04$). For 16KKW not 4 KKW NS change in cytokine levels following 12 weeks of EXC. NS relationship between EXC dose and change in cytokine levels High TNF-α may predict better outcomes with EXC vs. ADs ↓ IL-1β α positive depression treatment outcomes
Rethorst et al. (2011)	To determine whether the relationship between IL-6 and depressive symptoms is moderated by participation in moderate-intensity physical activity in a sample of primary care patients	Cross-sectional 97 participants. Family medicine clinic ≥40 years CES-D > 15	Moderate-intensity PA. Measured using modified Community Health Activities Model program for Seniors Activity Questionnaire for older adults	CES-D	ELISA of serum IL-6	Correlation between IL-6 and depressive sxs NS ($r = 0.086$, $p = 0.40$) Association between IL-6 and depressive symptoms was moderated by PA ($p = 0.02$) Among those who did not engage in mod PA, higher depressive sxs α ↑ IL-6 ($r = 0.28$, $p = 0.05$) Association was NS for moderate PA ($r = -0.13$, $p = 0.38$)
Irwin and Olmstead (2012)	To evaluate the effects of a behavioral intervention, TCC on circulating markers of inflammation in older adults	83 healthy older adults (59–86 years) RCT. Two arms – TCC, HE 16 weeks intervention + 9 weeks follow-up	TCC and HE Groups of 7–10 TCC 20 min, 3/week	BDI PSQI	ELISA of plasma for IL-6, CRP, sIL-1ra, sIL-6, sICAM, IL-18 [NB] *High IL-6 > 2.46 pg/ml*	High IL-6 at entry: TCC ↓ IL-6 comparable to those in TCC and HE who had low IL-6 at entry IL-6 in HE remained higher than TCC and HE with low entry IL-6 TCC ns Δ cellular markers of inflammation TCC = ↓ depressive sxs α ↓ IL-6

(Continued)

Table 1 | Continued

Study	Study objective	Study details	Exercise details	Neuropsychological testing	Immune testing	Results
Kohut et al. (2006)	To determine if a long-term exercise intervention among older adults would reduce serum inflammatory cytokines, and if this reduction would be mediated, in part, by improvements in psychosocial factors and/or by β-adrenergic receptor mechanisms	Adults ≥ 64 years. Community-based Randomized to aerobic or flexibility/strength EXC. 10 months A sub-group of patients on non-selective β1β2-adrenergic antagonists were included	Aerobic (CARDIO) or flexibility/strength EXC (FLEX) 3 days/week, 45 min/day, 10 months	GDS, PSS, CS, SPS, and LOT	ELISA of plasma: CRP, IL-6, TNF-α, and IL-18	EXC = ↓ depressive symptoms, ↑ optimism CARDIO EXC = ↓ IL-6, IL-18, CRP, TNF-α vs. FLEX FLEX EXC = ↓ TNF-α, no change in IL-6, IL-18, CRP ↓ CRP α ↓ depressive symptoms No effect for non-selective β1β2-adrenergic antagonists

TREAD, treatment with exercise augmentation for depression; KKW, kilocalories per kilogram of body weight per weeks; HE, health education; PSQI, Pittsburgh Sleep Quality Index; GDS, Geriatric Depression Scale; PSS, Perceived Stress Scale; CS, Coherence Scale; SPS, Social Previsions Scale; LOT, Life Orientation Test; α, association with or correlation with; EXC, exercise; IDS-C30, Inventory of Depressive Symptomatology; IL, interleukin; TNF, tumor necrosis factor; IFN, interferon; ELISA, enzyme-linked immunosorbent assay; CRP, C-reactive protein; CES-D. Center for Epidemiologic Studies Depression Scale; NS, non-significant; TCC, Tai Chi Chih.

Other studies found investigating the effects of PA on neuroimmune-related factors suggest PA increases anti-inflammatory or immunomodulatory factors, e.g., IL-10, IGF-1, and CX3CL1. Sigwalt et al. (2011) shows that in a rat model of depression induced by repeated dexamethasone administration, swimming exercise reduces depression-like behavior in correlation with increased HC IL-10, BDNF, and DNA oxidation. Duman et al. (2009) and Kohman et al. (2012) show voluntary wheel running associated with increased IGF-1, a factor recently shown to have anti-inflammatory effects.

Physical activity has been found to have beneficial effects on immunocompetent glial cells. A study by Latimer et al. (2011) has shown PA to revise age-related astrocyte hypertrophic/reactivity and myelin dysregulation – changes associated with neuroinflammation, cognitive decline, and reduced vascular function. Kohman et al. (2012) recently published a study showing PA attenuates aging associated increases in the proportion of new microglia within the HC (Iba-1 labeled). Furthermore, they show PA increases the pro-neurogenic phenotype of microglia (i.e., IGF-1-releasing microglia) which may contribute to increased HC neurogenesis. Given the robust anti-inflammatory effect of PA, the authors suggest PA may reduce PIC protein production leading to impaired microglial proliferation. A recent study by Barrientos et al. (2011) shows access to a running wheel reduced PIC expression from cultured microglia of aged rats. A recent study by Vukovic et al. (2012) suggests PA enhances the immunomodulatory factor CX3CL1 in the HC, with this associated with enhanced microglia-dependent neural precursor activity, as per the *ex vivo* neurosphere assay.

A study by Funk et al. (2011) demonstrates that PA can offer significant protection to the HC in a chemical-induced injury model [via trimethyltin (TMT)] that involves TNF receptor signaling. PA attenuated TMT-induced changes such as loss of DG neurons and microglial activation. Furthermore, PA was accompanied by a significant elevation in IL-6 and IL-1ra mRNA levels and repressed elevations in PICs and chemokines (CCL2 and CCL3). Interestingly, the investigators identified a functional role for IL-6 in neuroprotection given mice deficient in IL-6 (IL-6 knock-out) were not responsive to the neuroprotective effects of PA on the HC. The effects of PA and TMT on IL-6 downstream signal events differed at the level of STAT3 activation. The beneficial effects of acute spikes in IL-6 with PA is clearly a significant factor in the anti-inflammatory effect of PA. In a human study by Starkie et al. (2003), 3 h of cycling blunted the endotoxin-induced increase in circulating TNF-α levels, and this effect was mimicked by an IL-6 infusion. Further, this regulatory role of IL-6 on TNF-α levels was demonstrated in anti-IL-6 treated mice and IL-6 knock-out mice (Mizuhara et al., 1994; Matthys et al., 1995). Whilst acute elevations in IL-6 are found throughout the body (Funk et al., 2011), a recent study shows a selective increase in IL-6 localized to the HC (Rasmussen et al., 2011).

Neuroimmune cells may also have a role in the beneficial effects of PA. A study by Ziv et al. (2006) found PA, a component of the EE protocol, was associated with enhanced HC neurogenesis alongside a neuroprotective microglia phenotype and in the presence of a T-cell population. The role of CNS-specific T cells in the neuroprotective effects of PA is suggested given severe combined

Table 2 | Neuroimmune effects of physical activity in human populations without depressive symptom correlation.

Study	Study objective	Study details	Exercise details	Immune testing	Results
Nicklas et al. (2008)	To determine the effects of a long-term exercise intervention on two prominent biomarkers of Inflammation, CRP and IL-6, in elderly men and women	Single-blind, randomized, controlled trial 424 elderly (70–89 years), non-disabled, and community-dwelling men and women 12 months of moderate-intensity PA vs. successful aging (SA) health education intervention	Moderate-intensity PA. Combined aerobic, strength, balance, and flexibility exercise Approx 1 h sessions, 3/week. Starting in center and transition to home-based exercise	ELISA of plasma: CRP and IL-6	PA = ↓ IL-6 vs. SA. No ΔCRP
Donges et al. (2010)	To determine the effects of 10 weeks of resistance or aerobic exercise training on IL-6 and CRP. Further, to determine pre-training and post-training associations between alterations of IL-6 and CRP and alterations of total body fat mass (TB-FM), intra-abdominal fat mass (IA-FM), and total body lean mass (TB-LM)	102 sedentary subjects Resistance group (RG), aerobic group (AG), or control. 10 weeks Subjects were involved in DEXA, muscle strength, aerobic fitness measures, and lipid profiling	Supervised exercise Control group maintained sedentary lifestyle and dietary patterns	IL-6, CRP	RG and AG = ↓ CRP, no effect on IL-6
Martins et al. (2010)	Effect of exercise on metabolic profile in a healthy elderly sample	RCT $N = 63$ 16 weeks	Aerobic: 40–80% HR max Resistance: 8 exercises – 1 set/8reps to 3sets/15reps	Total cholesterol, triglycerides – colorimetric end-point assay HDL, LDL – two-point kinetic assay Hs-CRP – immunoturbidometry [@ baseline, 16 weeks]	Aerobic and resistance exercise = improvement in all measures
Stewart et al. (2007)	The purpose of this study was to examine the influence of a 12-week exercise training program on inflammatory cytokine and CRP concentrations. A secondary purpose was to determine whether training-induced changes in cytokines and CRP were influenced by age	29 younger (18–35 years) and 31 old (65–85 years) subjects Assigned to young physically active, young physically inactive, older physically active, older physically inactive groups	Inactive groups complete 12 weeks (3 days/week) of aerobic and resistance exc Physically active control groups continue their normal exc programs	ELISA of serum: CRP ELISA of plasma: IL-6, TNF-α, and IL-1β	Prescribed EXC = ↓ CRP, no change for IL-6, IL-1β, TNF-α for both young and older subjects

(Continued)

Table 2 | Continued

Study	Study objective	Study details	Exercise details	Immune testing	Results
Black et al. (2012)	To examine if a yogic meditation might alter the activity of inflammatory and antiviral transcription control pathways that shape immune cell gene expression	45 family dementia caregivers Randomized to either Kirtan Kriya Meditation (KKM) or Relaxing Music (RM)	8 weeks of KKM or RM. Both 12-min/day	Genome-wide transcriptional profiles collected from PBMC at baseline and 8 weeks follow-up. RNA extraction ◇ cRNA Transcript Origin Analysis	KKM = ↑ 19 gene's expression (immunoglobulin-related transcripts) KKM = ↓ 49 gene's expression (PIC, activation-related immediate-early genes). From plasmacytoid dendritic cells and B lymphocytes Effects may be due to ↓ NF-κB and IRF-1
Santos et al. (2012)	To assess the effects of moderate exercise training on sleep in elderly people as well as their cytokine profiles	22 male, sed, health, elderly Polysomnography collected week – 1 and 6 Total body mass and% fat. Whole-body plethysmography	Mod training for 24 weeks. 60 min/day, 3 days/week Work rate equiv to ventilator aerobic threshold (VO_{2max}, VATI)	ELISA plasma: TNF-α, IL-6, IL-1, and IL-10	EXC = ↑ aerobic fitness, ↓ REM latency, ↓ time awake EXC = ↓ IL-6, TNF-α, TNF-α/IL-10 EXC = ↑ IL-10
Cordova et al. (2011)	To investigate the association between long-term RT and circulating levels of the pro-inflammatory mediators IL-6, TNF-α, and IFN-γ in elderly women	Cross-sectional 54 years. Women RT – $N = 28$ Sed – $N = 26$	In RT group women underwent 8.6 ± 0.3 months of EXC. Mod-intensity (70% 1RM) 50 min, 3/week, 3 sets of 12 reps per exercise	ELISA plasma: TNF-α, IL-6, and IFN-γ	RT = ↓ IFN-γ, ↓ IL-6, ↓ TNF-α vs. sed RT = ↓ caloric intake, sBP FFM 1/α IL-6
Libardi et al. (2012)	The aim of the present study was to evaluate the effects of 16 weeks of RT, ET, and CT on inflammatory markers, CRP, and functional capacity in sedentary middle-age men	Healthy inactive subjects. ~ 49.5 years ± 5 Randomized to RT ($N = 11$), ET ($N = 12$), CT ($N = 11$), or ctrl ($N = 13$) BMI, waist-to-hip ration, DEXA for FFM Diet contents recorded	3 weekly sessions for 60 min for 16 weeks Max strength (1RM) tested in bench press and leg press VO_{2peak} measured in incremental exc test	ELISA plasma: TNF-α, IL-6, and CRP	RT and CT = ↑ max strength ET and CT = ↑ VO_{2peak} Ns Δ TNF-α, IL-6, CRP
Beavers et al. (2010b)	Effect of chronic exercise on inflammation in the elderly	RCT $N = 424$	12 months combined aerobics, strength, flexibility/balance training	CRP, IL-6, IL-6sR, IL-8, and IL-15, Adiponectin, Il-1rα, IL-2sRα, TNF-α, and sTNFRI and II ELISA	Exercise = ↓ IL-8, no Δ in others

(Continued)

Table 2 | Continued

Study	Study objective	Study details	Exercise details	Immune testing	Results
Colbert et al. (2004)	Effect of exercise on inflammation in the elderly	Cross-sectional $N = 3075$	Questionnaire	CRP, IL-6, and TNF-α (blood/serum) – ELISA	↑ Exercise α ↓ CRP ($p < 0.01$), ↓ IL-6 ($p < 0.001$), ↓ TNF-α ($p = 0.02$)
Geffken et al. (2001)	Effect of physical activity on inflammation in healthy elderly	Cross-sectional $N = 5201$	Questionnaire	Blood: CRP, fibrinogen, Factor VIII activity, and WCC	↑ Physical activity α ↓ Inflammatory markers
Nybo et al. (2002)	Is prolonged exercise associated with an altered cerebral IL-6 response?	Quasi-experimental $N = 8$, young men Injected with radiotracer (133-Xe)	2 min × 60 min bouts of cycle ergometer at 50% VO_{2max} at different temperatures	Blood: IL-6 – ELISA	Prolonged exercise = ↑ IL-6 release
Kohut et al. (2006)	Effect of different exercise types on inflammation in the elderly	RCT $N = 87$ M34/F53 Subset administered non-selective β-adrenergic antagonists	10 months: 45 min 3×/week Cardio: 65–80% VO_{2max} Strength/flexibility: 10–15 reps (moderate-intensity)	Blood: CRP, IL-6, TNF-α, and IL-18	Cardio = ↓ all markers ($p < 0.05$) Strength/flex = ↓ TNF-α ($p = 0.001$) β-inhibitors made no effect
Reuben et al. (2003)	Effect of physical activity on inflammation in elderly	Cross-sectional $N = 877$	Sef-reported: Yale Physical activity survey	Blood: IL-6, CRP – ELISA	↑ Physical activity α ↓ IL-6 and CRP

RT, resistance training; ET, endurance training; CT, concurrent training; FFM, free fat mass; VATI, ventilator anaerobic threshold; TCC, Tai Chi Chih; RCT, randomized controlled trial; IL, interleukin; TNF, tumor necrosis factor; IFN, interferon; ELISA, enzyme-linked immunosorbent assay; CRP, C-reactive protein.

Table 3 | Neuroimmunological effects of physical activity in rodent populations: with behavioral correlates.

Study	Study objective	Animal	Exercise type	Behavioral assessment	Immune measures	Results: behavioral	Results: neuroimmune
Moon et al. (2012)	To determine the underlying mechanism of MIF in HC neurogenesis and its role in exercise-induced antidepressant therapy	Rat MIF−/− and WT	Voluntary EXC vs. ECT	FST	*In vivo*: HC, RT-PCR, IB, IHC	*MIF−/−* = depression-like behavior	EXC = ↑ *Tph2 in vitro* and *in vivo* (*in vitro* α ↑ 5-HT)
		In vivo component	28 days of EXC or 10 days of ECT		*In vitro*: PCR, RT-PCR	*MIF−/−* = blunted antidepressant effect of EXC in FST	EXC = ↑ *Bdnf in vitro* and *in vivo*
			ICV injection with MIF *In vitro*: neuronal cell lines treated with MIF. Neuro 2A			Administration of MIF protein = antidepressant effect in FST	CD 74-GPTase (MIF receptor) and RhoA-ERK1/2 pathway mediated MIF-induced Tph2 and Bdnf gene expression and 5-HT content
			MIF −/− = ↓ *Dcx* and *Pax6* siRNAs, GTPase RhoA inhibitor CT04, MEK inhibitor U0126				EXC = ↑ MIF (HC) (IHC and IB)
Sigwalt et al. (2011)	The aim of the present study was to investigate the influence of swimming exercise training on behavior and neurochemical parameters in a rat model of depression induced by repeated dexamethasone administration	Adult Wistar rats. 60 days Daily s.c. dex (1.5 mg/kg) or saline administration	4 groups: CTRL, EXC, DEX, and DEX + EXC	SPT	RIA blood corticosterone	DEX: ↓ sucrose consumption, ↑ immob time	DEX: ↑ HC DNA oxidation, ↑ IL-10, ↑ BDNF, ↓ blood corticosterone levels, ↓ adrenal weight, ↓ body mass
			EXC: swimming/aerobic. 1 h/day, 5 days/week for 3 weeks. Overload of 5% of rat body weight	FST	IHC HC: BDNF 8OHdG	EXC: ↑ sucrose consumption	EXC: normalization of BDNF and IL-10, ↑ blood testosterone, ↓ HC DNA oxidation
			CTRL: fluoxetine 10 mg/kg		RT-PCR HC: BDNF, IL-10		
Duman et al. (2009)	To assess the role of peripheral IGF-I in mediating antidepressant-like behavior under resting physiological conditions	Mice. C57Bl/6	Voluntary wheel running for 4 weeks	FST	PFC and HC	IGF-1 = ↓ immob time, ↑ sucrose consumption	Anti-IGF-1 blocked the BDNF producing effect of EXC
	To investigate the extent to which IGF-I might contribute to antidepressant-like behavior in exercising mice	uCMS		NIH	ELISA for IGF-1	Anti-IGF-1 blocked the antidepressant effect of EXC (FST)	EXC = ↑ IGF-1 mRNA
		IGF-1 and anti-IGF-1 was administered s.c.		SCT	ISH for IGF-1 and BDNF		EXC ≠ PFC IGF-1 mRNA, nor HC and PFC BDNF

IHC, immunohistochemistry; IB, immunoblot; HC, hippocampus; PFC, pre-frontal cortex; SPT, sucrose preference test; dex, dexamethasone; FST, forced-swim test; MIF, macrophage migration inhibitory factor; RT-PCR, reverse transcription polymerase chain reaction; IB, immunoblot; ELISA, enzyme-linked immunosorbent assay; CTRL, control; BDNF, brain-derived neurotrophic factor; ISH, in situ hybridization.

Table 4 | Neuroimmune effects of physical activity in rodent populations: without behavioral correlates.

Study	Study objective	Animal	Exercise Type	Neuroimmune measures	Results: immune
Funk et al. (2011)	To examine the impact of voluntary exercise on a model of TNF receptor activation dependent neuronal apoptosis	Mice. Pathogen-free CD-1	Voluntary running wheel access for 2 weeks	Flow cytometry of CD11b, CD4, and GFP	EXC = ↓ neuronal death, TNF-α, TNFr1, *MyD88*, TGF-β, CCL2, CCL3
		WT and IL-6−/−		IHC HC GFP+, Iba-1 cells; IL-6, IL-6 Rα, gp130, pAkt, p-STAT3	EXC = ↑ IL-1α mRNA, IL-1RA mRNA, IL-6 (mRNA and protein), neuronal IL-6-Rα
		IP injection of TMT (2.4 mg/kg) or saline		Mass spect: Tin (sn)	TMT = ↑ IL-1α mRNA, IL-1RA mRNA, IL-6 (mRNA and protein), neuronal IL-6-Rα
		Bone-marrow chimera mice used to confirm lack of infiltrating monocytes with TMT injury		Fluorescent microscopy HC for cell death and microglia phenotyping	EXC = ↓ TNF-α cell death signaling pathways with TMT. IL-6 pathway recruitment occurred in both EXC and TMT conditions – IL-6 downstream signal events differed in the level of STAT3 activation
				qPCR	EXC ≠ BDNF mRNA, NGF mRNA, GDNF mRNA
				Microarray analysis: cell death and IL-6 pathways	IL-6−/− mice: EXC showed ↓ neuroprotection against TMT-induced injury
Kohman et al. (2012)	To evaluate whether exercise modulates division and/or activation state of microglia in the dentate gyrus of the hippocampus	Adult (3.5 months) and aged (18 months) BALB/c mice	Vol running wheel for 8 weeks	IHC: BrdU HC IF (confocal microscopy): HC: microglia (Iba-1 +), microglial division (Iba-1+ and BrdU +), co-expression of IGF-1, new neuron survival (BrdU × fraction displaying NeuN)	Aged mice = ↑ new microglia EXC = ↓ new microglia in aged mice, ↑ microglial IGF-1 expression, ↑ survival of new neurons + proliferation EXC ≠ microglial survival or proliferation in adult mice [NB] *IGF-1-releasing microglia considered pro-neurogenic*
Yi et al. (2012)	To determine if regular treadmill running may blunt the effect of western diet on hypothalamic inflammation	Ldlr−/− (low-density lipoprotein receptor deficiency) and WT mice	Moderate, regular treadmill running exercise. Involuntary. 30 min/day, 5 days/week, 26 weeks	IP glucose tolerance test performed	EXC = ↓ hypothalamic inflammation, ↓ microglial activation
		High-fat diet exposure Indirect calorimetry performed	Exhaustion tests at weeks 0 and 25	Blood glucose levels measured Plasma insulin via ELISA Blood markers: TNF-α, IL-6, INF-g, IL-1α, PAI-1, and MCP-1 IHC: hypothalamus for iba-1	EXC = ↑ glucose tolerance EXC ≠ circulating cytokines
Ehninger et al. (2011)	Effect of exercise on cell genesis in the adult amygdala	Female C57BL6/J mice, 2 mo	Exercise vs. 2 sedentary controls (environmental enrichment, standard housing) 10 days, voluntary wheel running	Iba-1, S100β, BrdU, NeuN, NG2, CNPase, GFAP, and ki67 (hippocampus) – immunofluorescence	Exercise and environmental enrichment = ↑ oligodendroglial precursor proliferation, ↓ microgliogenesis, ↑ neuroplasticity

(Continued)

Table 4 | Continued

Study	Study objective	Animal	Exercise Type	Neuroimmune measures	Results: immune
Latimer et al. (2011)	To test the hypothesis that exercise initiated at mid-age can slow the development of hippocampal glial and vascular biomarkers of early aging	C57BL/6 mice: young, middle and aged	Voluntary exercise for 6 weeks	BP monitoring IHC HC: astrocyte (GFAP) and myelin staining (MBP) ELISA HC: VEGF (angiogenesis marker) Vascular casting: scanning electron micrographs of MCA were utilized	EXC = ↓ HC GFAP and MBP which were associated with aging EXC = astrocytic changes, i.e., fewer branches, finer processes, less hypertrophied EXC = ↑ VEGF which was associated with aging EXC = improved endothelial functioning (less ragged and irregular, ↑ ECN) and ↓ BP
Jeon et al. (2012)	To examine the effects of aging vs. exercise on serum profiles of cytokines and chemokines in mice models	C57BL/6 mice. Young (2 months) and old (20 months)	Forced treadmill exc for 4 weeks. 30 min/day, 5 days/week	Multiplexed bead-based sandwich immunoassay of 50 serum cytokines/chemokines	Treadmill EXC ≠ Δ serum cytokines/chemokines significantly Older mice = ↑ eotaxin, IL-9, TARC vs. young mice
Wu et al. (2012)	Effect of exercise on hippocampal neurogenesis in infection	Male/female IL-1β^{XAT} (IL-1β over-expression) C57BL/6 mice, 8–12 months vs. WT	Exercise vs. sedentary control Intra-hippocampal FIV (feline immunodeficiency virus) injection vs. vehicle 2 weeks, voluntary wheel running	MHCII DCX, BrdU, Iba-1 (HC) – immunohistochemistry	EXC ≠ normalized neurogenesis in presence of centrally mediated infection in IL-1β over-expression
Nichol et al. (2008)	Effect of exercise on amyloid load and neuroinflammation in AD mice	Male/female Tg2576 C57B16/SJL mice, 16–18 months vs. WT	Exercise vs. sedentary control 3 weeks, voluntary wheel running	HC and cortex Pro-inflammatory: IL-1β, TNF-α – ELISA Adaptive/alternate immune markers: IFN-γ, CD40, MHCII – Western blot CD11c, MIP-1α – Immunohistochemistry Aβ – ELISA, Dot-blot analysis CD68, mannose receptor – Immunohistochemistry Iba-1 – Western blot	EXC = ↓ TNF-α, IL-1β EXC = ↑ IFN-γ, CD11c, MHCII, CD40, MIP-1α EXC = ↑ CD68, mannose receptor (↑ Perivascular MΦ infiltrate)

(Continued)

Table 4 | Continued

Study	Study objective	Animal	Exercise Type	Neuroimmune measures	Results: immune
Vukovic et al. (2012)	Effect of exercise on microglial-dependent hippocampal neurogenesis	Female TG-Csf1r-GFP C57BL/6J mice, 6–8-week old	Exercise vs. sedentary control *Ex vivo* neurosphere culture with/without microglia 2 weeks, voluntary wheel running	HC BrdU, DCX, Iba-1 – immunostaining CX3CL1 – ELISA MHCII – FACS	EXC = microglial-dependent ↑ neural precursor activity EXC = ↓ MHCII+ve microglia, EXC = ↑ CX3CL1 (neuroprotective phenotype)
Ziv et al. (2006)	Role of immune cells in neurogenesis	Male Sprague Dawley rats, 12-week old	EE vs. standard lab control Healthy rats vs. immune-deficient (SCID mice)	From HC: IHC: BrdU, MHCII, IB-4, IGF-1, NeuN, BDNF, and TCR	EE = ↑ neurogenesis and adaptive microglial profile in presence of function T-cell population
Leem et al. (2011)	Effect of exercise in neuroinflammation in AD mice	Male/Female Tg-Ad (NSE/htau23) C57BL/6 mice 16 months vs. WT	EXC vs. sedentary control Intermediate (12 m/min) vs. high intensity exercise (19 m/min)	From HC RT-PCR: TNF-α, IL-6, and IL-1β WB: iNOS, ERK, COX-2, p38 IHC: phosphoTau, GFAP, MAC-1, and p65	High intensity EXC = ↓ phosphoTau ($p < 0.05$) High intensity EXC = ↓ gliosis [MAC-1, GFAP] ($p < 005$) High intensity EXC = ↓ μAPK-dependent signaling pathway [↓ iNOS, TNF-α, IL-6, IL-1β] ($p < 0.05$)
Herring et al. (2012)	Effect of exercise in pregnancy on AD pathology in offspring	Female Tg-AD APP695 CRND8 x C57BL/6-C3H-HeJ vs. WT	Exercise vs. sedentary control Duration of pregnancy, voluntary wheel running	From entire brain, except, cerebellum, brainstem IHC: Aβ, A1F1, laminin, RELN RT-PCR: Gapdh, APP, Lpap1, ApoE1, Clu, A2m, Mmp9, Mme DC protein assay: $A\beta_{40}$, $A\beta_{42}$, sAPPα WB: APP, CTFβ, RELn, APOER2, VLDR, ADC, CYP, IDE, IBA-1, PTGER2, SOD1, SOD2	EXC = ↓ Aβ in offspring via altered APP processing ($p < 0.022$) EXC = ↑ angiogenesis ($p < 0.022$) EXC = ↑ neuroplasticity EXC = ↓ microgliosis ($p = 0.002$), pro-inflammatory mediators, oxidative stress mediators ($p = 0.029$)
Carmichael et al. (2010)	Role of brain MΦ on central cytokines and fatigue post-exercise	Male C57Bl/6 mice, 8-week old	Exercise vs. sedentary control MΦ depletion with clodronate injection or saline Single bout of exercise, 22 m/min for 150 m	IL-1β (cerebrum) – ELISA	EXC = ↑ IL-1β from MΦs

ECN, endothelial cell nuclei; EE, environmental enrichment; IHC, immunohistochemistry; WB, western blot; TCR, T-cell receptor; IL, interleukin; TNF, tumor necrosis factor; IFN, interferon; ELISA, enzyme-linked immunosorbent assay; CRP, C-reactive protein; EXC, exercise; APP, amyloid precursor protein; TMT, trimethyltin; NGF, nerve growth factor, BDNF, brain-derived neurotrophic factor; VEGF, vascular endothelial growth factor.

immunodeficiency (SCID) mice exposed to EE did not show an increase in neurogenesis.

MODEL OF NEUROIMMUNOLOGICAL EFFECTS OF PA IN DEPRESSION

Emerging evidence suggests the neuroimmune system is critical in both the development of depression-related pathophysiology and in the treatment of depression. From the evidence available in this field, PA has a multitude of beneficial neuroimmune effects which may lead to the improvement of depression-related neurobiological processes, hence leading to reduced depression-like behaviors.

From a neuroimmune perspective, evidence suggests PA does enhance the beneficial and reduce the detrimental effects of the neuroimmune system. **Figure 2** outlines these effects. PA appears to increase the following factors: IL-10, IL-6 (acutely), MIF, CNS-specific autoreactive CD4+ T cells, M2 microglia, quiescent astrocytes, CX3CL1, and IGF-1. On the other hand, PA appears to reduce detrimental neuroimmune factors such as: Th1/Th2 balance, PICs, CRP, M1 microglia, and reactive astrocytes. The effect of other factors is unknown, such as: T regs, CD200, chemokines, miRNA, M2-type blood-derived macrophages, and TNF-α (via R2). The beneficial effects of PA are likely to occur centrally and peripherally (e.g., in visceral fat reduction).

Based on the strong relationship between the neuroimmune system and other neurobiological systems (i.e., neuroplasticity, neuroendocrine function, and neurotransmission), we believe PA may exert beneficial behavioral effects via these neurobiological systems. PA's neuroimmune effects are likely involved in enhanced neuroplasticity, reduced oxidative stress, increases in 5-HT, dopamine, and noradrenaline, and enhanced glucocorticoid sensitivity.

The neurobiological effects of PA – mediated largely via the neuroimmune system – are likely involved with reduced depression-like behaviors in rodents (i.e., sickness-like behavior, anhedonia, anxiety-, and cognition-like behaviors) and positive clinical effects (i.e., reduced depressive symptoms, enhanced cognitive function, relapse reduction, and early intervention).

DISCUSSION

Physical activity is increasingly investigated as a preventative, early intervention, and treatment option in depression. The interest in investigation of PA may have arisen for a number of reasons: the burden of depression is rising so novel therapeutic and preventative options are required (WHO, 2008; Berk and Jacka, 2012; Cuijpers et al., 2012; Southwick and Charney, 2012). Rates of physical inactivity are high and rising in modern society (Lee et al., 2012) with early evidence suggesting a link to the development of depression (Pasco et al., 2011a,b). Pharmacotherapy in depression is hampered by relatively high rates of resistance (Rush et al., 2006a,b) and considerable side-effects. Evidence is emerging to suggest co-morbid links between obesity, diabetes,

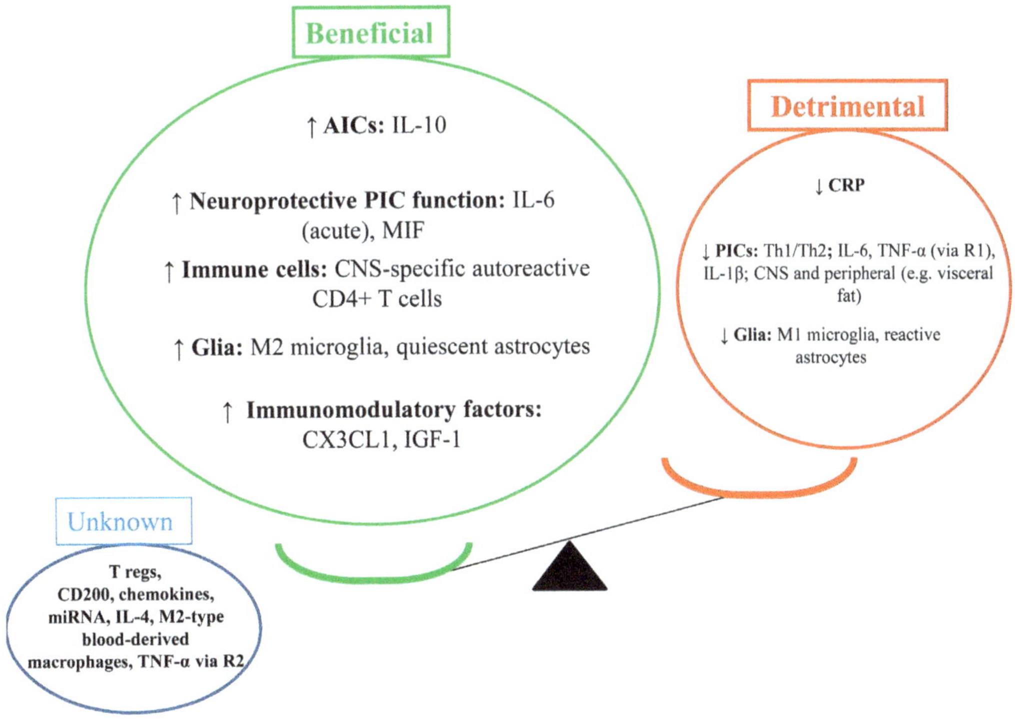

FIGURE 2 | Physical activity in depression: antidepressant via enhancing the beneficial effects of the neuroimmune system. This figure illustrates the effects of PA on the brain as per the balance between beneficial and detrimental effects of neuroimmune factors. PA appears to enhance the beneficial effects of the neuroimmune system and reduce the detrimental effects. From a behavioral perspective, this may lead to reduced depression-like behaviors. From a clinical perspective, this may lead to reduced depressive symptoms, depressive episode resolution, and reduced relapse rates (disease prevention).

heart disease, and depression (Baune and Thome, 2011; Stuart and Baune, 2012), and PA is a therapeutic option with beneficial cardio-metabolic effects (Gleeson et al., 2011; Baune et al., 2012c; Hamer et al., 2012; Knochel et al., 2012; Stuart and Baune, 2012).

Based on the abovementioned factors, research has been reviewed to better understand the clinical efficacy of different types of PA, to understand the mechanism of action of PA and to investigate for suitable biomarkers to measure the treatment effect of PA in depression. Further, a model has been suggested in order to assist in understanding the neuroimmune effects of PA in depression.

An important consideration in the field of exercise immunology includes understanding the mechanisms of treatment response in depression vs. other psychiatric disorders. At present the authors feel there is no enough data to address this issue systematically, with research evidence. Whilst it would appear that the effects of PA on the immune system in various disorders – in both clinical and pre-clinical studies – is quite similar, i.e., PICs are reduced (particularly in anxiety disorders and depression; Gleeson et al., 2011; Eyre and Baune, 2012a), this considers only a narrow range of neuroimmune factors. The authors speculate that the therapeutic difference in PA may occur due to subtle variations in the neuroimmune and neurobiological effect, dependent upon the CNS environment with each pathophysiological state. Studies investigating the effects of a standardized exposure to PA, in various psychiatric disorders in parallel, may assist in unraveling this complex issue.

When considering the balance between the beneficial and detrimental effects of immune system and the effect of PA tipping this balance toward beneficial effects, it is important to consider: *Is it possible to restore the balance of the immune system and still suffer from a low mood?* This is an interesting question and open to debate. It would seem that the majority of evidence suggests that as inflammation increases, mood worsens, and as inflammation reduces, mood appears to return to normal. For example, this is shown in meta-analysis by Dowlati et al. (2010) and a review by Maes (2011) whereby depressive symptoms are associated with elevations in PIC levels. Another meta-analysis shows inflammation reduces with the use of SSRIs in the treatment of depression (Hannestad et al., 2011). However, there are other therapies such as SNRIs which appear to improve mood, yet have no effect on levels of inflammation (Hannestad et al., 2011). Therefore, more work is required to understand the effect of various therapies (pharmacological and non-pharmacological) on a wider variety of immune-related factors such as cytokines (anti- and pro-inflammatory), anti-inflammatory factors like IGF-1, CD200, CX3CL1, MIF, neuroprotective systemic immune cells, etc. Interestingly, Walker (2012) suggests the concentration of antidepressant drug molecules in the CNS also alters the immunomodulatory effects.

FUTURE DIRECTIONS

From current evidence, it is not possible to ascertain the type of PA which is most efficacious in the treatment of depression. Although, most evidence surrounds aerobic exercise. We suggest the need for head-to-head clinical trials comparing different types and intensities of PA to assist in making this issue clearer. Moreover, when considering the effects of distinct types of PA on neuroimmune factors, we also suggest the need for more head-to-head clinical trials (Baune and Eyre, 2012).

The most recent study examining the effects of PA on depressive symptoms was conducted by Rethorst et al. This study suggests that a high baseline TNF-α level was associated with a greater reduction in depressive symptomatology as opposed a high baseline TNF-α level being a negative factor for SSRI efficacy (Hannestad et al., 2011; Rethorst et al., 2012). The authors suggest TNF-α levels may be a moderator between SSRI and exercise treatment, and may have a role in personalized treatment algorithms. Whilst this is a promising suggestion, further research is needed to replicate these findings.

Our understanding of the neuroimmune effects of PA in depression will continue to develop as the understanding of the neuroimmune effects of PA develop. It is important to consider the use of multi-biomarker methods within this area in order to better understand potential biomarkers. For example, the use of neuroimaging, serum protein and genetic markers, and behavioral analysis. This type of methodology is increasingly employed in biological psychiatry (Baune et al., 2010, 2012a,b).

There are a number of neuroimmune-related factors which are yet to be considered in the effect of PA in depression. These factors include micro ribonucleic acid (miRNA), neuroimmune-related Positron Emission Tomography (PET) ligands, the neuroprotective effects of neuroimmune factors, and immune cells. Evidence is emerging to suggest a role for miRNAs, factors involved in regulating gene expression at the post-translational level, in modulating the effects of the immune system (Ponomarev et al., 2012). For example, various miRNAs such as miR-155 and miR-124 may have a role in polarizing microglia toward pro- or anti-inflammatory phenotypes, respectively (Ponomarev et al., 2012). The PET ligand, Translocator Protein (TPSO) ligand [(11)C]PBR28, a marker of microglial activation, was recently found to be elevated by LPS-induced systemic inflammation in non-human primates (Hannestad et al., 2012). This ligand has the potential to be utilized as a biomarker to investigate if activation of microglia may be a mechanism through which systemic inflammatory processes influence the disease course of depression. The biology of centrally migrating immune cells and CNS immune cells in depression is complex and far from understood. Regarding the debated issue of blood-derived macrophages can enter the brain parenchyma: research and development into novel methods for permanent differential labeling of circulating monocytes, as contrasted with resident microglia, is underway (Prinz et al., 2011). Studies are required to better understand the role of protective immunosurveillance in clinical and rodent models of depression.

CONCLUSION

The investigation of the neuroimmune effects of PA on depression and depression-like behavior is a rapidly developing and important field. This paper summarizes the most recent findings in the area and proposes a model whereby PA enhances the beneficial effects of the neuroimmune system and reduces the detrimental effects of the neuroimmune system.

REFERENCES

Aarum, J., Sandberg, K., Haeberlein, S. L., and Persson, M. A. (2003). Migration and differentiation of neural precursor cells can be directed by microglia. *Proc. Natl. Acad. Sci. U.S.A.* 100,15983–15988.

Anisman, H., Ravindran, A. V., Griffiths, J., and Merali, Z. (1999). Endocrine and cytokine correlates of major depression and dysthymia with typ- ical or atypical features. *Mol. Psychi- atry* 4,182–188.

Araque, A., Parpura, V., Sanzgiri, R. P., and Haydon, P. G. (1999). Tripartite synapses: glia, the unacknowl- edged partner. *Trends Neurosci.* 22, 208–215.

Asmundson, G. J. G., Fetzner, M. G., DeBoer, L. B., Powers, M. B., Otto, M. W., and Smits, J. A. J. (2013). Let's get physical: a con- temporary review of the anxiolytic effects of exercise for anxiety and its disorders. *Depress. Anxiety.* doi: 10.1002/da.22043. [Epub ahead of print].

Babyak, M., Blumenthal, J. A., Herman, S., Khatri, P., Doraiswamy, M., Moore, K., et al. (2000). Exer- cise treatment for major depression: maintenance of therapeutic benefit at 10 months. *Psychosom. Med.* 62, 633–638.

Bachstetter, A. D., Morganti, J. M., Jern- berg, J., Schlunk, A., Mitchell, S. H., Brewster, K. W., et al. (2011). Fractalkine and CX3CR1 regulate hippocampal neurogenesis in adult and aged rats. *Neurobiol. Aging* 32, 2030–2044.

Bansal, A. S., Bradley, A. S., Bishop, K. N., Kiani-Alikhan, S., and Ford, B. (2012). Chronic fatigue syndrome, the immune system and viral infec- tion. *Brain Behav. Immun.* 26, 24–31. Barrientos, R. M., Frank, M. G., Crys- dale, N. Y., Chapman, T. R., Ahrend- sen, J. T., Day, H. E., et al. (2011). Little exercise, big effects: revers- ing aging and infection-induced memory deficits, and underly- ing processes. *J. Neurosci.* 31, 11578–11586.

Battista, D., Ferrari, C. C., Gage, F. H., and Pitossi, F. J. (2006). Neuro- genic niche modulation by activated microglia: transforming growth fac- tor beta increases neurogenesis in the adult dentate gyrus. *Eur. J. Neurosci.* 23, 83–93.

Baune, B. T., Dannlowski, U., Dom- schke, K., Janssen, D. G., Jordan, M. A., Ohrmann, P., et al. (2010). The interleukin 1 beta (IL1B) gene is associated with failure to achieve remission and impaired emotion processing in major depression. *Biol. Psychiatry* 67, 543–549.

Baune, B. T., and Eyre, H. (2012). Novel perspectives on the role of immune biomarkers in exercise and depression. *Brain Behav. Immun.* 26,512.

Baune, B. T., Konrad, C., Grotegerd, D., Suslow, T., Birosova, E., Ohrmann, P., et al. (2012a). Interleukin-6 gene (IL-6): a possible role in brain mor- phology in the healthy adult brain. *J. Neuroinflammation* 9,125.

Baune, B. T., Konrad, C., Grotegerd, D., Suslow, T., Ohrmann, P., Bauer, J., et al. (2012b). Tumor necrosis factor gene variation predicts hippocam- pus volume in healthy individuals. *Biol. Psychiatry* 72,655–662.

Baune, B. T., Stuart, M., Gilmour, A., Wersching, H., Heindel, W., Arolt, V., et al. (2012c). The relationship between subtypes of depression and cardiovascular disease: a systematic review of biological models. *Transl. Psychiatry* 2, e92.

Baune, B. T., Ponath, G., Rothermundt, M., Riess, O., Funke, H., and Berger, K. (2008a). Association between genetic variants of IL-1beta, IL-6 and TNF-alpha cytokines and cog- nitive performance in the elderly general population of the MEMO- study. *Psychoneuroendocrinology* 33, 68–76.

Baune, B. T., Wiede, F., Braun, A., Golledge, J., Arolt, V., and Koerner, H. (2008b). Cognitive dysfunction in mice deficient for TNF and its receptors. *Am. J. Med. Genet. B Neu- ropsychiatr. Genet.* 147B, 1056–1064. Baune, B. T., and Thome, J. (2011). Translational research approach to biological and modifiable risk fac- tors of psychosis and affective dis- orders. *World J. Biol. Psychiatry* 12(Suppl 1),28–34.

Beavers, K. M., Brinkley, T. E., and Nick- las, B. J. (2010a). Effect of exercise training on chronic inflammation. *Clin. Chim. Acta* 411,785–793.

Beavers, K. M., Hsu, F. C., Isom, S., Kritchevsky, S. B., Church, T., Good- paster, B., et al. (2010b). Long-term physical activity and inflammatory biomarkers in older adults. *Med. Sci. Sports Exerc.* 42,2189–2196.

Beers, D. R., Henkel, J. S., Zhao, W., Wang, J., and Appel, S. H. (2008). CD4+ T cells support glial neu- roprotection, slow disease progres- sion, and modify glial morphology in an animal model of inherited ALS. *Proc. Natl. Acad. Sci. U.S.A.* 105, 15558–15563.

Ben Menachem-Zidon, O., Avital, A., Ben-Menahem, Y., Goshen, I., Kreisel, T., Shmueli, E. M., et al. (2011). Astrocytes support hippocampal-dependent memory and long-term potentiation via interleukin-1 signaling. *Brain Behav. Immun.* 25, 1008–1016.

Berk, M., and Jacka, F. (2012). Preven- tive strategies in depression: gath- ering evidence for risk factors and potential interventions. *Br. J. Psychi- atry* 201, 339–341.

Beumer, W., Gibney, S. M., Drex- hage, R. C., Pont-Lezica, L., Door- duin, J., Klein, H. C., et al. (2012). The immune theory of psychiatric diseases: a key role for activated microglia and circulating mono- cytes. *J. Leukoc. Biol.* 92,959–975.

Bilbo, S. D., Smith, S. H., and Schwarz, J. M. (2012). A lifespan approach to neuroinflammatory and cognitive disorders: a critical role for glia. *J. Neuroimmune Pharmacol.* 7, 24–41. Black, D. S., Cole, S. W., Irwin, M. R., Breen, E., St Cyr, N. M., Nazarian, N., et al. (2012). Yogic meditation reverses NF-kappaB and IRF-related transcriptome dynamics in leuko cytes of family dementia caregivers in a randomized controlled trial. *Psychoneuroendocrinology.* doi: 10.1016/j.psyneuen.2012.06.011. [Epub ahead of print].

Blume, J., Douglas, S. D., and Evans, D. L. (2011). Immune suppression and immune activation in depression. *Brain Behav. Immun.* 25, 221–229.

Blumenthal, J. A., Babyak, M. A., Moore, K. A., Craighead, W. E., Herman, S., Khatri, P., et al. (1999). Effects of exercise training on older patients with major depression. *Arch. Intern. Med.* 159,2349–2356.

Blumenthal, J. A., Babyak, M. A., O'Connor, C., Keteyian, S., Landzberg, J., Howlett, J., et al. (2012a). Effects of exercise training on depressive symptoms in patients with chronic heart failure: the HF-action randomized trial. *JAMA* 308, 465–474.

Blumenthal, J. A., Sherwood, A., Babyak, M. A., Watkins, L. L., Smith, P. J., Hoffman, B. M., et al. (2012b). Exercise and pharmacological treatment of depressive symptoms in patients with coronary heart disease: results from the UPBEAT (understanding the prognostic benefits of exercise and antidepressant therapy) Study. *J. Am. Coll. Cardiol.* 60,1053–1063.

Bluthe, R. M., Castanon, N., Pousset, F., Bristow, A., Ball, C., Lestage, J., et al. (1999). Central injection of IL-10 antagonizes the behavioural effects of lipopolysaccharide in rats. *Psy- choneuroendocrinology* 24,301–311.

Bowen, K. K., Dempsey, R. J., and Vemuganti, R. (2011). Adult interleukin-6 knockout mice show compromised neurogenesis. *Neuroreport* 22, 126–130.

Bracchi-Ricard, V., Brambilla, R., Levenson, J., Hu, W. H., Bramwell, A., Sweatt, J. D., et al. (2008). Astroglial nuclear factor-kappaB regulates learning and memory and synaptic plasticity in female mice. *J. Neurochem.* 104,611–623.

Bridle, C., Spanjers, K., Patel, S., Ather- ton, N. M., and Lamb, S. E. (2012). Effect of exercise on depression severity in older people: systematic review and meta analysis of ran- domised controlled trials. *Br. J. Psychiatry* 201,180–185.

Brynskikh, A., Warren, T., Zhu, J., and Kipnis, J. (2008). Adaptive immunity affects learning behavior in mice. *Brain Behav. Immun.* 22,861–869.

Butovsky, O., Koronyo-Hamaoui, M., Kunis, G., Ophir, E., Landa, G., Cohen, H., et al. (2006a). Glatiramer acetate fights against Alzheimer's disease by inducing dendritic-like microglia expressing insulin-like growthfactor1. *Proc. Natl. Acad. Sci. U.S.A.* 103,11784–11789.

Butovsky, O., Ziv, Y., Schwartz, A., Landa, G., Talpalar, A. E., Pluchino, S., et al. (2006b). Microglia acti- vated by IL-4 or IFN-gamma differentially induce neurogenesis and oligodendrogenesis from adult stem/progenitor cells. *Mol. Cell. Neurosci.* 31,149–160.

Butovsky, O., Kunis, G., Koronyo Hamaoui, M., and Schwartz, M. (2007). Selective ablation of bone marrow-derived dendritic cells increases amyloid plaques in a mouse Alzheimer's disease model. *Eur. J. Neurosci.* 26,413–416.

Butovsky, O., Talpalar, A. E., Ben- Yaakov, K., and Schwartz, M. (2005). Activation of microglia by aggre- gated beta-amyloid or lipopolysac- charide impairs MHC-II expression and renders them cytotoxic whereas IFN-gamma and IL-4 render them protective. *Mol. Cell. Neurosci.* 29, 381–393.

Butti, E., Bergami, A., Recchia, A., Bram- billa, E., Del Carro, U., Amadio, S., et al. (2008). IL4 gene delivery to the CNS recruits regulatory T cells and induces clinical recovery in mouse models of multiple sclerosis. *Gene Ther.* 15,504–515.

Capuron, L., and Miller, A. H. (2011). Immune system to brain sig- naling: neuropsychopharmacologi- cal implications. *Pharmacol. Ther.* 130, 226–238.

Cardon, M., Ron-Harel, N., Cohen, H., Lewitus, G. M., and Schwartz, M. (2010). Dysregulation of kisspeptin and neurogenesis at adolescence link inborn immune deficits to the late onset of abnormal sensorimo- tor gating in congenital psycholog- ical disorders. *Mol. Psychiatry* 15, 415–425.

Carlson, N. G., Wieggel, W. A., Chen, J., Bacchi, A., Rogers, S. W., and Gahring, L. C. (1999). Inflamma- tory cytokines IL-1 alpha, IL-1 beta, IL-6, and TNF-alpha impart neuro- protection to an excitotoxin through distinct pathways. *J. Immunol.* 163, 3963–3968.

Carmichael, M. D., Davis, J. M., Mur- phy, E. A., Carson, J. A., Van Rooijen, N., Mayer, E., et al. (2010). Role of brain macrophages on IL-1beta and fatigue following eccentric exercise-induced muscle damage. *Brain Behav. Immun.* 24, 564–568.

Chapoval, S., Dasgupta, P., Dorsey, N. J., and Keegan, A. D. (2010). Reg- ulation of the T helper cell type 2 (Th2)/T regulatory cell (Treg) bal- ance by IL-4 and STAT6. *J. Leukoc. Biol.* 87,1011–1018.

Colbert, L. H., Visser, M., Simonsick, E. M., Tracy, R. P., Newman, A. B., Kritchevsky, S. B., et al. (2004). Physical activity, exercise, and inflamma- tory markers in older adults: findings from the Health, Aging and Body Composition Study. *J. Am. Geriatr. Soc.* 52,1098–1104.

Conboy, L., Varea, E., Castro, J. E., Sakouhi-Ouertatani, H., Calandra, T., Lashuel, H. A., et al. (2011). Macrophage migration inhibitory factor is critically involved in basal and fluoxetine-stimulated adult hip- pocampal cell proliferation and in anxiety, depression, and memory related behaviors. *Mol. Psychiatry* 16, 533–547.

Cordova, C., Lopes, E. S. F. Jr., Pires, A. S., Souza, V. C., Brito, C. J., Moraes, C. F., et al. (2011). Long- term resistance training is associated with reduced circulating levels of IL- 6, IFN-gamma and TNF-alpha in elderly women. *Neuroimmunomod- ulation* 18,165–170.

Corona, A. W., Huang, Y., O'Connor, J. C., Dantzer, R., Kelley, K. W., Popovich, P. G., et al. (2010). Fractalkine receptor (CX3CR1) deficiency sensitizes mice to the behavioral changes induced by lipopolysaccharide. *J. Neuroinflammation* 7,93.

Corona, A. W., Norden, D. M., Skendelas, J. P., Huang, Y., O'Connor, J. C., Lawson, M., et al. (2012). Indoleamine 2,3- dioxygenase inhibition attenuates lipopolysaccharide induced per- sistent microglial activation and depressive-like complications in fractalkine receptor (CX(3)CR1)- deficient mice. *Brain Behav Immun.* doi:10.1016/j.bbi.2012.08.008. [Epub ahead of print].

Costello, D. A., Lyons, A., Denieffe, S., Browne, T. C., Cox, F. F., and Lynch, M. A. (2011). Long term potentia- tion is impaired in membrane glycoprotein CD200-deficient mice: a role for Toll-like receptor activation. *J. Biol. Chem.* 286, 34722–34732.

Cox, F. F., Carney, D., Miller, A. M., and Lynch, M. A. (2012). CD200 fusion protein decreases microglial activation in the hippocampus of aged rats. *Brain Behav. Immun.* 26, 789–796.

Craft, L. (2005). Exercise and clinical depression: examining two psycho- logical mechanisms. *Psychol. Sport. Exerc.* 6, 151–171.

Cuijpers, P., Beekman, A. T., and Reynolds, C. F. III. (2012). Prevent- ing depression: a global priority. *JAMA* 307,1033–1034.

Curtsinger, J. M., Schmidt, C. S., Mondino, A., Lins, D. C., Kedl, R. M., Jenkins, M. K., et al. (1999). Inflam- matory cytokines provide a third sig- nal for activation of naive CD4+ and CD8+ T cells. *J. Immunol.* 162, 3256–3262.

Dantzer, R., O'Connor, J. C., Freund, G. G., Johnson, R. W., and Kelley, K. W. (2008). From inflammation to sickness and depression: when the immune system subjugates the brain. *Nat. Rev. Neurosci.* 9,46–56.

Dantzer, R., O'Connor, J. C., Lawson, M. A., and Kelley, K. W. (2011). Inflammation-associated depres- sion: from serotonin to kynurenine. *Psychoneuroendocrinology* 36, 426–436.

Derecki, N. C., Cardani, A. N., Yang, C. H., Quinnies, K. M., Crihfield, A., Lynch, K. R., et al. (2010). Reg- ulation of learning and memory by meningeal immunity: a key role for IL-4. *J. Exp. Med.* 207,1067–1080.

Derecki, N. C., Quinnies, K. M., and Kipnis, J. (2011). Alternatively activated myeloid (M2) cells enhance cognitive function in immune compromised mice. *Brain Behav. Immun.* 25,379–385.

Deslandes, A. C., Moraes, H., Alves, H., Pompeu, F. A., Silveira, H., Mouta, R., et al. (2010). Effect of aero- bic training on EEG alpha asym- metry and depressive symptoms in the elderly: a 1-year follow-up study. *Braz. J. Med. Biol. Res.* 43, 585–592.

Dhabhar, F. S., Burke, H. M., Epel, E. S., Mellon, S. H., Rosser, R., Reus, V. I., et al. (2009). Low serum IL-10 con- centrations and loss of regulatory association between IL-6 and IL-10 in adults with major depression. *J. Psychiatr. Res.* 43,962–969.

Diener, E. (1984). Subjective well being. *Psychol. Bull.* 94,542–575. Donges, C. E., Duffield, R., and Drinkwater, E. J. (2010). Effects of resistance or aerobic exercise train- ing on interleukin-6, C-reactive pro- tein, and body composition. *Med. Sci. Sports Exerc.* 42,304–313.

Dowlati, Y., Herrmann, N., Swardfager, W., Liu, H., Sham, L., Reim, E. K., et al. (2010). A meta-analysis of cytokines in major depression. *Biol. Psychiatry* 67, 446–457.

Duman, C. H., Schlesinger, L., Ter- williger, R., Russell, D. S., Newton, S. S., and Duman, R. S. (2009). Periph- eral insulin-like growth factor-I pro- duces antidepressant-like behavior and contributes to the effect of exer- cise. *Behav. Brain Res.* 198, 366–371.

Ehninger, D., Wang, L. P., Klempin, F., Romer, B., Kettenmann, H., and Kempermann, G. (2011). Enriched environment and physical activity reduce microglia and influence the fate of NG2 cells in the amygdala of adult mice. Cell Tissue Res. 345, 69–86.

Ekdahl, C. T. (2012). Microglial activa- tion – tuning and pruning adult neu- rogenesis. Front. Pharmacol. 3:41. doi:10.3389/fphar.2012.00041

Eller, T., Vasar, V., Shlik, J., and Maron, E. (2008). Pro-inflammatory cytokines and treatment response to escitalopram in major depressive disorder. Prog. Neuropsychopharmacol. Biol. Psychiatry 32, 445–450.

Erickson, K. I., Miller, D. L., and Roecklein, K. A. (2012). The aging hippocampus: interactions between exercise, depression, and BDNF. Neuroscientist 18, 82–97.

Erickson, K. I., Voss, M. W., Prakash, R. S., Basak, C., Szabo, A., Chaddock, L., et al. (2011). Exercise training increases size of hippocampus and improves memory. Proc. Natl. Acad. Sci. U.S.A. 108, 3017–3022.

Eyre, H., and Baune, B. T. (2012a). Neu- roimmunological effects of physical exercise in depression. *Brain Behav. Immun.* 26,251–266.

Eyre, H., and Baune, B. T. (2012b). Neuroimmunomodulation in unipolar depression: a focus on chronobiology and chronotherapeutics. *J. Neural Transm.* 119,1147–1166.

Eyre, H., and Baune, B. T. (2012c). Neuroplastic changes in depression: a role for the immune sys- tem. *Psychoneuroendocrinology* 37, 1397–1416.

Foster, P. P., Rosenblatt, K. P., and Kuljis, R. O. (2011). Exercise-induced cog- nitive plasticity, implications for mild cognitive impairment and Alzheimer's disease. Front. Neurol. 2:28. doi:10.3389/fneur.2011.00028

Fox, K. (2000). "The effects of exercise on self-perceptions and self esteem," in *Physical Activity and Psychological Well-Being*, ed. F. K. Biddle Sjh (London: Routledge), 88–117.

Frank, M. G., Baratta, M. V., Sprunger, D. B., Watkins, L. R., and Maier, S. F. (2007). Microglia serve as a neuroimmune substrate for stress- induced potentiation of CNS proinflammatory cytokine responses. *Brain Behav. Immun.* 21,47–59.

Fujio, K., Okamura, T., and Yamamoto, K. (2010). The Family of IL- 10-secreting CD4+ T cells. *Adv. Immunol.* 105,99–130.

Funk, J. A., Gohlke, J., Kraft, A. D., McPherson, C. A., Collins, J. B., and Jean Harry, G. (2011). Voluntary exercise protects hippocampal neurons from trimethyltin injury: possible role of interleukin-6 to modulate tumor necrosis factor receptor-mediated neurotoxicity. *Brain Behav. Immun.* 25,1063–1077.

Gallagher, P. J., Castro, V., Fava, M., Weilburg, J. B., Murphy, S. N., Gainer, V. S., et al. (2012). Antidepressant response in patients with major depression exposed to NSAIDs: a pharmacovigilancestudy. *Am. J. Psy- chiatry* 169,1065–1072.

Garber, C. E., Blissmer, B., Deschenes, M. R., Franklin, B. A., Lamonte, M. J., Lee, I. M., et al. (2011). American College of Sports Medicine position stand. Quantity and quality of exercise for developing and maintaining cardiorespiratory, musculoskele- tal, and neuromotor fitness in appar- ently healthy adults: guidance for prescribing exercise. *Med. Sci. Sports Exerc.* 43,1334–1359.

Garg, S. K., Banerjee, R., and Kipnis, J. (2008). Neuroprotective immunity: T cell-derived glutamate endows astrocytes with a neuroprotective phenotype. *J. Immunol.* 180, 3866–3873.

Geffken, D. F., Cushman, M., Burke, G. L., Polak, J. F., Sakkinen, P. A., and Tracy, R. P. (2001). Association between physical activity and mark- ers of inflammation in a healthy elderlypopulation. *Am. J. Epidemiol.* 153, 242–250.

Giunti, D., Parodi, B., Usai, C., Ver- gani, L., Casazza, S., Bruzzone, S., et al. (2012). Mesenchymal stem cells shape microglia effector functions through thereleaseofCX3CL1. *Stem Cells* 30,2044–2053.

Gleeson, M., Bishop, N. C., Stensel, D. J., Lindley, M. R., Mastana, S. S., and Nimmo, M. A. (2011). The anti-inflammatory effects of exer- cise: mechanisms and implications for the prevention and treatment of disease. *Nat. Rev. Immunol.* 11, 607–615.

Godbout, K., Fenn, A., Huang, Y., and Gensel, J. (2012). Central interleukin-4 infusion after a peripheral lipopolysaccharide injec- tion promotes a neuroprotective CNS environment with increased M2 microglia. *Brain Behav. Immun.* 26, S29–S30.

Hamer, M., Sabia, S., Batty, G. D., Shipley, M. J., Tabak, A. G., Singh- Manoux, A., et al. (2012). Physi- cal activity and inflammatory mark- ers over 10 years: follow-up in men and women from the Whitehall II Cohort Study. *Circulation* 126, 928–933.

Hannestad, J., Dellagioia, N., and Bloch, M. (2011). The effect of antidepres- sant medication treatment on serum levels of inflammatory cytokines: a meta-analysis. *Neuropsychopharma- cology* 36,2452–2459.

Hannestad, J., Gallezot, J. D., Schaf bauer, T., Lim, K., Kloczynski, T., Morris, E. D., et al. (2012). Endotoxin-induced systemic inflammation activates microglia: [(1)(1)C]PBR28 positron emission tomography in nonhuman primates. *Neuroimage* 63,232–239.

Hashimoto, K. (2009). Emerging role of glutamate in the pathophysiology of major depressive disorder. *Brain Res. Rev.* 61,105–123.

Hauben, E., Butovsky, O., Nevo, U., Yoles, E., Moalem, G., Agranov, E., et al. (2000). Passive or active immunization with myelin basic protein promotes

recovery from spinal cord contusion. *J. Neurosci.* 20, 6421–6430.
Hein, A. M., and O'Banion, M. K. (2012). Neuroinflammation and cognitive dysfunction in chronic dis- ease and aging. *J. Neuroimmune Pharmacol.* 7, 3–6.
Herring, A., Donath, A., Yarmolenko, M., Uslar, E., Conzen, C., Kanakis, D., et al. (2012). Exercise dur- ing pregnancy mitigates Alzheimer- like pathology in mouse offspring. *FASEB J.* 26, 117–128.
Himmerich, H., Milenovic, S., Fulda, S., Plumakers, B., Sheldrick, A. J., Michel, T. M., et al. (2010). Reg- ulatory T cells increased while IL- 1beta decreased during antidepres- sant therapy. *J. Psychiatr. Res.* 44, 1052–1057.
Hinwood, M., Morandini, J., Day, T. A., and Walker, F. R. (2012). Evi- dence that microglia mediate the neurobiological effects of chronic psychological stress on the Medial prefrontal cortex. *Cereb. Cortex* 22, 1442–1454.
Hoffman, B. M., Blumenthal, J. A., Babyak, M. A., Smith, P. J., Rogers, S. D., Doraiswamy, P. M., et al. (2008). Exercise fails to improve neurocog- nition in depressed middle-aged and older adults. *Med. Sci. Sports Exerc.* 40, 1344–1352.
Irwin, M. R., and Olmstead, R. (2012). Mitigating cellular inflammation in older adults: a randomized con- trolled trial of Tai Chi Chih. *Am. J. Geriatr. Psychiatry* 20, 764–772.
Jenkins, M. K., and Johnson, J. G. (1993). Molecules involved in T-cell costimulation. *Curr. Opin. Immunol.* 5, 361–367.
Jeon, H., Mun, G. I., and Boo, Y. C. (2012). Analysis of serum cytokine/ chemokine profiles affected by aging and exercise in mice. *Cytokine* 60, 487–492.
Kaneko, M., Stellwagen, D., Malenka, C., and Stryker, M. P. (2008). Tumor necrosis factor-alpha medi- ates one component of competitive, experience-dependent plasticity in developing visual cortex. *Neuron* 58, 673–680.
Kessler, R. C., Berglund, P., Dem- ler, O., Jin, R., Merikangas, K. R., and Walters, E. E. (2005). Lifetime prevalence and age-of-onset distrib- utions of DSM-IV disorders in the National Comorbidity Survey Repli- cation. *Arch. Gen. Psychiatry* 62, 593–602.
Kim, S. J., Lee, H., Joung, H. Y., Lee, G., Lee, H. J., Shin, M. K., et al. (2011) T-bet deficient mice exhibit resistance to stress-induced develop- ment of depression-like behaviors. *J. Neuroimmunol.* 240–241, 45–51.
Kim, S. J., Lee, H., Lee, G., Oh, J., Shin, M. K., Shim, I., et al. (2012). CD4+CD25+ regula- tory T cell depletion modulates anxiety and depression-like behav- iors in mice. *PLoS ONE* 7:e42054. doi:10.1371/journal.pone.0042054
Kipnis, J., Avidan, H., Caspi, R. R., and Schwartz, M. (2004a). Dual effect of CD4+CD25+ regulatory T cells in neurodegeneration: a dialogue with microglia. *Proc. Natl. Acad. Sci. U.S.A.* 101(Suppl 2), 14663–14669.
Kipnis, J., Cohen, H., Cardon, M., Ziv, Y., and Schwartz, M. (2004b). T cell deficiency leads to cognitive dysfunction: implications for ther- apeutic vaccination for schizophre- nia and other psychiatric conditions. *Proc. Natl. Acad. Sci. U.S.A.* 101, 8180–8185.
Kipnis, J., Derecki, N. C., Yang, C., and Scrable, H. (2008). Immu- nity and cognition: what do age- related dementia, HIV-dementia and 'chemo-brain' have in common? *Trends Immunol.* 29, 455–463.
Knochel, C., Oertel-Knochel, V., O'Dwyer, L., Prvulovic, D., Alves, G., Kollmann, B., et al. (2012). Cognitive and behavioural effects of physical exercise in psychiatric patients. *Prog. Neurobiol.* 96, 46–68.
Kohl, H. W. III, Craig, C. L., Lambert, E. V., Inoue, S., Alkandari, J. R., Lee- tongin, G., et al. (2012). The pan- demic of physical inactivity: global action for public health. *Lancet* 380, 294–305.
Kohm, A. P., McMahon, J. S., Podo- jil, J. R., Begolka, W. S., Degutes, M., Kasprowicz, D. J., et al. (2006). Cutting edge: anti-CD25 mono- clonal antibody injection results in the functional inactivation, not depletion, of CD4+CD25+ T reg- ulatory cells. *J. Immunol.* 176, 3301–3305.
Kohman, R. A., Deyoung, E. K., Bhattacharya, T. K., Peterson, L. N., and Rhodes, J. S. (2012). Wheel run- ning attenuates microglia prolifer- ation and increases expression of a proneurogenic phenotype in the hippocampus of aged mice. *Brain Behav. Immun.* 26, 803–810.
Kohut, M. L., McCann, D. A., Russell, D. W., Konopka, D. N., Cunnick, J. E., Franke, W. D., et al. (2006). Aerobic exercise, but not flexibility/resistance exercise, reduces serum IL-18, CRP, and IL-6 independent of beta- blockers, BMI, and psychosocial fac- tors in older adults. *Brain Behav. Immun.* 20, 201–209.
Kokaia, Z., Martino, G., Schwartz, M., and Lindvall, O. (2012). Cross talk between neural stem cells and immune cells: the key to better brain repair? *Nat. Neurosci.* 15, 1078–1087. Koronyo-Hamaoui, M., Ko, M. K., Koronyo, Y., Azoulay, D., Seksenyan, A., Kunis, G., et al. (2009). Atten- uation of AD-like neuropathology by harnessing peripheral immune cells: local elevation of IL-10 and MMP-9. *J. Neurochem.* 111, 1409–1424.
Latimer, C. S., Searcy, J. L., Bridges, M. T., Brewer, L. D., Popovic, J., Blalock, E. M., et al. (2011). Reversal of glial and neurovas- cular markers of unhealthy brain aging by exercise in middle-aged female mice. PLoS ONE 6:e26812. doi:10.1371/journal.pone.0026812
Lautenschlager, N. T., Cox, K., and Cyarto, E. V. (2012). The influence of exercise on brain aging and demen- tia. *Biochim. Biophys. Acta* 1822, 474–481.
Lavretsky, H., Alstein, L. L., Olmstead, R. E., Ercoli, L. M., Riparetti-Brown, M., Cyr, N. S., et al. (2011). Com- plementary use of Tai Chi Chih augments escitalopram treatment of geriatric depression: a randomized controlled trial. *Am. J. Geriatr. Psy- chiatry* 19, 839–850.
Lee, H. B., and Lyketsos, C. G. (2003). Depression in Alzheimer's disease: heterogeneity and related issues. *Biol. Psychiatry* 54, 353–362.
Lee, I. M., Shiroma, E. J., Lobelo, F., Puska, P., Blair, S. N., and Katz- marzyk, P. T. (2012). Effect of physical inactivity on major non- communicable diseases worldwide: an analysis of burden of disease and life expectancy. *Lancet* 380, 219–229.
Leem, Y. H., Lee, Y. I., Son, H. J., and Lee, S. H. (2011). Chronic exer- cise ameliorates the neuroinflamma- tion in mice carrying NSE/htau23. *Biochem. Biophys. Res. Commun.* 406, 359–365.
Leonard, B., and Maes, M. (2012). Mechanistic explanations how cell-mediated immune activation, inflammation and oxidative and nitrosative stress pathways and their sequels and concomitants play a role in the pathophysiology of unipolar depression. *Neurosci. Biobehav. Rev.* 36, 764–785.
Lepore, S. J. (1997). Expressive writ- ing moderates the relation between intrusive thoughts and depressive symptoms. *J. Pers. Soc. Psychol.* 73, 1030–1037.
Lewitus, G. M., Cohen, H., and Schwartz, M. (2008). Reducing post-traumatic anxiety by immu- nization. *Brain Behav. Immun.* 22, 1108–1114.
Li, Y., Xiao, B., Qiu, W., Yang, L., Hu, B., Tian, X., et al. (2010). Altered expression of CD4+CD25+ regulatory T cells and its 5-HT(1a) recep- tor in patients with major depression disorder. *J. Affect. Disord.* 124, 68–75. Libardi, C. A., De Souza, G. V., Cavaglieri, C. R., Madruga, V. A., and Chacon-Mikahil, M. P. (2012). Effect of resistance, endurance, and con- current training on TNF-alpha, IL-6, and CRP. *Med. Sci. Sports Exerc.* 44, 50–56.
Littrell, J. L. (2012). Taking the perspective that a depressive state reflects inflammation: implications for the use of anti- depressants. Front. Psychol. 3:297. doi:10.3389/fpsyg.2012.00297
Liu, D., Wang, Z., Liu, S., Wang, F., Zhao, S., and Hao, A. (2011). Anti-inflammatory effects of flu- oxetine in lipopolysaccharide(LPS)- stimulated microglial cells. *Neu- ropharmacology* 61, 592–599.
Lyons, A., Downer, E. J., Crotty, S., Nolan, Y. M., Mills, K. H., and Lynch, M. A. (2007). CD200 ligand recep- tor interaction modulates microglial activation *in vivo* and *in vitro*: a role for IL-4. *J. Neurosci.* 27, 8309–8313. Lyons, A., McQuillan, K., Deighan, B. F., O'Reilly, J. A., Downer, E. J., Mur- phy, A. C., et al. (2009). Decreased neuronal CD200 expression in IL-4-deficient mice results in increased neuroinflammation in response to lipopolysaccharide. *Brain Behav. Immun.* 23, 1020–1027.
Maes, M. (2011). Depression is an inflammatory disease, but cell- mediated immune activation is the key component of depression. *Prog. Neuropsychopharmacol. Biol. Psychi- atry* 35, 664–675.
Mahendra, N., and Arkin, S. (2003). Effects of four years of exercise, lan- guage, and social interventions on Alzheimer discourse. *J. Commun. Disord.* 36, 395–422.
Marosi, K., Bori, Z., Hart, N., Sarga, L., Koltai, E., Radak, Z., et al. (2012). Long-term exercise treat- ment reduces oxidative stress in the hippocampus of aging rats. *Neuro- science* 226, 21–28.
Martino, G., Pluchino, S., Bonfanti, L., and Schwartz, M. (2011). Brain regeneration in physiology and pathology: the immune signature driving therapeutic plasticity of neural stem cells. *Physiol. Rev.* 91, 1281–1304.
Martins, R. A., Neves, A. P., Coelho- Silva, M. J., Verissimo, M. T., and Teixeira, A. M. (2010). The effect of aerobic versus strength-based train- ing on high-sensitivity C-reactive protein in older adults. *Eur. J. Appl. Physiol.* 110, 161–169.
Mathieu, P., Piantanida, A. P., and Pitossi, F. (2010). Chronic expres- sion of transforming growth factorbeta enhances adult neurogene- sis. *Neuroimmunomodulation* 17, 200–201.
Matthys, P., Mitera, T., Heremans, H., Van Damme, J., and Billiau, A. (1995). Anti-gamma interferon and anti-interleukin-6 antibodies affect staphylococcal enterotoxin B-induced weight loss, hypoglycemia, and cytokine release in D-galactosamine-sensitized and unsensitized mice. *Infect. Immun.* 63, 1158–1164.
McAfoose, J., and Baune, B. T. (2009). Evidence for a cytokine model of cognitive function. *Neurosci. Biobe- hav. Rev.* 33, 355–366.
McNally, L., Bhagwagar, Z., and Hannes- tad, J. (2008). Inflammation, glu- tamate, and glia in depression: a literature review. *CNS Spectr.* 13, 501–510.

Miller, A. H. (2010). Depression and immunity: a role for T cells? *Brain Behav. Immun.* 24, 1–8.

Miller, A. H., Maletic, V., and Raison, C. L. (2009). Inflammation and its discontents: the role of cytokines in the pathophysiology of major depres- sion. *Biol. Psychiatry* 65, 732–741.

Mitschelen, M., Yan, H., Farley, J. A., Warrington, J. P., Han, S., Herenu, C. B., et al. (2011). Long-term deficiency of circulating and hip- pocampal insulin-like growth fac- tor I induces depressive behavior in adult mice: a potential model of geri- atric depression. *Neuroscience* 185, 50–60.

Mizuhara, H., O'Neill, E., Seki, N., Ogawa, T., Kusunoki, C., Otsuka, K., et al. (1994). T cell activation- associated hepatic injury: mediation by tumor necrosis factors and pro- tection by interleukin 6. *J. Exp. Med.* 179, 1529–1537.

Moon, H. Y., Kim, S. H., Yang, Y. R., Song, P., Yu, H. S., Park, H. G., et al. (2012). Macrophage migration inhibitory factor mediates the anti- depressant actions of voluntary exer- cise. *Proc. Natl. Acad. Sci. U.S.A.* 109, 13094–13099.

Moon, M. L., McNeil, L. K., and Fre- und, G. G. (2011). Macrophages make me sick: how macrophage activation states influence sickness behavior. *Psychoneuroendocrinology* 36, 1431–1440.

Moron, J. A., Zakharova, I., Ferrer, J. V., Merrill, G. A., Hope, B., Lafer, E. M., et al. (2003). Mitogen-activated protein kinase regulates dopamine transporter surface expression and dopamine transport capacity. *J. Neu- rosci.* 23, 8480–8488.

Moylan, S., Maes, M., Wray, N. R., and Berk, M. (2012). The neuroprogres- sive nature of major depressive dis- order: pathways to disease evolu- tion and resistance, and therapeu- tic implications. *Mol. Psychiatry.* doi: 10.1038/mp.2012.33. [Epub ahead of print].

Muller, N., Myint, A. M., and Schwarz, M. J. (2011). Inflammatory bio- markers and depression. *Neurotox. Res.* 19, 308–318.

Musil, R., Schwarz, M. J., Riedel, M., Dehning, S., Cerovecki, A., Spell- mann, I., et al. (2011). Elevated macrophage migration inhibitory factor and decreased transforming growth factor-beta levels in major depression – no influence of cele- coxib treatment. *J. Affect. Disord.* 134, 217–225.

Myint, A. M., Leonard, B. E., Steinbusch, H. W., and Kim, Y. K. (2005). Th1, Th2, and Th3 cytokine alterations in major depression. *J. Affect. Disord.* 88, 167–173.

Nakajima, A., Yamada, K., Nagai, T., Uchiyama, T., Miyamoto, Y., Mamiya, T., et al. (2004). Role of tumor necrosis factor-alpha in methamphetamine-induced drug dependence and neurotoxicity. *J. Neurosci.* 24, 2212–2225.

Nguyen, K., D'Mello, C., Le, T., Urbanski, S., and Swain, M. G. (2012). Regulatory T cells sup- press sickness behaviour develop- ment without altering liver injury in cholestatic mice. *J. Hepatol.* 56, 626–631.

Nichol, K. E., Poon, W. W., Parachikova, A. I., Cribbs, D. H., Glabe, C. G., and Cotman, C. W. (2008). Exercise alters the immune profile in Tg2576 Alzheimer mice toward a response coincident with improved cogni- tive performance and decreased amyloid. *J. Neuroinflammation* 5, 13.

Nicklas, B. J., Hsu, F. C., Brinkley, T. J., Church, T., Goodpaster, B. H., Kritchevsky, S. B., et al. (2008). Exercise training and plasma C- reactive protein and interleukin-6 in elderly people. *J. Am. Geriatr. Soc.* 56, 2045–2052.

Nybo, L., Nielsen, B., Pedersen, B. K., Moller, K., and Secher, N. H. (2002). Interleukin-6 release from the human brain during prolonged exercise. *J. Physiol. (Lond.)* 542, 991–995.

Ojo, B., Rezaie, P., Gabbott, P. L., Davies, H., Colyer, F., Cowley, T. R., et al. (2012). Age-related changes in the hippocampus (loss of synap- tophysin and glial-synaptic interac- tion) are modified by systemic treat- ment with an NCAM-derived pep- tide, FGL. *Brain Behav. Immun.* 26, 778–788.

Olah, M., Ping, G., De Haas, A. H., Brouwer, N., Meerlo, P., Van Der Zee, E. A., et al. (2009). Enhanced hippocampal neurogenesis in the absence of microglia T cell interac- tion and microglia activation in the murine running wheel model. *Glia* 57, 1046–1061.

Park, S. E., Dantzer, R., Kelley, K. W., and McCusker, R. H. (2011a). Central administration of insulin- like growth factor-I decreases depressive-like behavior and brain cytokine expression in mice. *J. Neuroinflammation* 8, 12.

Park, S. E., Lawson, M., Dantzer, R., Kelley, K. W., and McCusker, R. H. (2011b). Insulin-like growth factor-I peptides act centrally to decrease depression-like behavior of mice treated intraperitoneally with lipopolysaccharide. *J. Neuroinflam- mation* 8, 179.

Pasco, J. A., Jacka, F. N., Williams, L. J., Brennan, S. L., Leslie, E., and Berk, M. (2011a). Don't worry, be active: positive affect and habitual physical activity. *Aust. N. Z. J. Psychiatry* 45, 1047–1052.

Pasco, J. A., Williams, L. J., Jacka, F. N., Henry, M. J., Coulson, C. E., Brennan, S. L., et al. (2011b). Habitual physical activity and the risk for depressive and anxiety disorders among older men and women. *Int. Psychogeriatr.* 23, 292–298.

Pereira, A. C., Huddleston, D. E., Brick- man, A. M., Sosunov, A. A., Hen, R., McKhann, G. M., et al. (2007). An *in vivo* correlate of exercise-induced neurogenesis in the adult dentate gyrus. *Proc. Natl. Acad. Sci. U.S.A.* 104, 5638–5643.

Ponomarev, E. D., Veremeyko, T., and Weiner, H. L. (2012). MicroRNAs are universal regulators of differen- tiation, activation, and polarization of microglia and macrophages in normal and diseased CNS. *Glia* 61, 91–103.

Popoli, M., Yan, Z., McEwen, B. S., and Sanacora, G. (2012). The stressed synapse: the impact of stress and glucocorticoids on glutamate transmis- sion. *Nat. Rev. Neurosci.* 13, 22–37.

Prinz, M., Priller, J., Sisodia, S. S., and Ransohoff, R. M. (2011). Hetero- geneity of CNS myeloid cells and their roles in neurodegeneration. *Nat. Neurosci.* 14, 1227–1235.

Quan, N., and Banks, W. A. (2007). Brain-immune communication pathways. *Brain Behav. Immun.* 21, 727–735.

Raison, C. L., and Miller, A. H. (2011). Is depression an inflammatory dis- order? *Curr. Psychiatry Rep.* 13, 467–475.

Raison, C. L., Rutherford, R. E., Wool- wine, B. J., Shuo, C., Schettler, P., Drake, D. F., et al. (2012). A random- ized controlled trial of the tumor necrosis factor antagonist infliximab for treatment-resistant depression: the role of baseline inflammatory biomarkers. *Arch. Gen. Psychiatry.* doi: 10.1001/2013. jamapsychiatry.4. [Epub ahead of print].

Ransohoff, R. M., Kivisakk, P., and Kidd, G. (2003). Three or more routes for leukocyte migration into the central nervous system. *Nat. Rev. Immunol.* 3, 569–581.

Rasmussen, P., Vedel, J. C., Olesen, J., Adser, H., Pedersen, M. V., Hart, E., et al. (2011). In humans IL-6 is released from the brain during and after exer- cise and paralleled by enhanced IL-6 mRNA expression in the hippocam- pus of mice. *Acta Physiol. (Oxf.)* 201, 475–482.

Rethorst, C. D., Moynihan, J., Lyness, J. M., Heffner, K. L., and Chapman, B. P. (2011). Moderating effects of moderate-intensity physical activity in the relationship between depres- sive symptoms and interleukin-6 in primary care patients. *Psychosom. Med.* 73, 265–269.

Rethorst, C. D., Toups, M. S., Greer, T. L., Nakonezny, P. A., Car- mody, T. J., Grannemann, B. D., et al. (2012). Pro-inflammatory cytokines as predictors of antide- pressant effects of exercise in major depressive disorder. *Mol. Psychiatry.* doi: 10.1038/mp.2012.125. [Epub ahead of print].

Rethorst, C. D., Wipfli, B. M., and Landers, D. M. (2009). The antide- pressive effects of exercise: a meta- analysis of randomized trials. *Sports Med.* 39, 491–511.

Reuben, D. B., Judd-Hamilton, L., Har- ris, T. B., and Seeman, T. E. (2003). The associations between physical activity and inflammatory mark- ers in high-functioning older per- sons: MacArthur Studies of Success- ful Aging. *J. Am. Geriatr. Soc.* 51, 1125–1130.

Rimer, J., Dwan, K., Lawlor, D. A., Greig, C. A., McMurdo, M., Morley, W., et al. (2012). Exercise for depres- sion. *Cochrane Database Syst. Rev.* 7, CD004366.

Rogers, J. T., Morganti, J. M., Bach- stetter, A. D., Hudson, C. E., Peters, M. M., Grimmig, B. A., et al. (2011). CX3CR1 deficiency leads to impairment of hippocampal cogni- tive function and synaptic plasticity. *J. Neurosci.* 31, 16241–16250.

Rolls, A., Schori, H., London, A., and Schwartz, M. (2008). Decrease in hippocampal neurogenesis during pregnancy: a link to immunity. *Mol. Psychiatry* 13, 468–469.

Ron-Harel, N., Cardon, M., and Schwartz, M. (2011). Brain home- ostasis is maintained by "danger" signals stimulating a supportive immune response within the brain's borders. *Brain Behav. Immun.* 25, 1036–1043.

Rook, G. A., Lowry, C. A., and Raison, C. L. (2011). Lymphocytes in neu- roprotection, cognition and emo- tion: is intolerance really the answer? *Brain Behav. Immun.* 25, 591–601.

Rush, A. J., Trivedi, M. H., Wisniewski, S. R., Nierenberg, A. A., Stewart, J. W., Warden, D., et al. (2006a). Acute and longer-term outcomes in depressed outpatients requiring one or several treatment steps: a STAR*D report. *Am. J. Psychiatry* 163, 1905–1917.

Rush, A. J., Trivedi, M. H., Wis- niewski, S. R., Stewart, J. W., Nieren- berg, A. A., Thase, M. E., et al. (2006b). Bupropion-SR, sertraline, or venlafaxine-XR after failure of SSRIs for depression. *N. Engl. J. Med.* 354, 1231–1242.

Salmon, P. (2001). Effects of physical exercise on anxiety, depression, and sensitivity to stress: a unify- ing theory. *Clin. Psychol. Rev.* 21, 33–61.

Santello, M., and Volterra, A. (2012). TNFalpha in synaptic function: switching gears. *Trends Neurosci.* 35, 638–647.

Santos, R. V., Viana, V. A., Boscolo, R. A., Marques, V. G., Santana, M. G., Lira, F. S., et al. (2012). Moderate exercise training modulates cytokine profile and sleep in elderly people. *Cytokine* 60, 731–735.

between health and disease. *Mol. Psychiatry* 15, 342–354.

Schwartz, M., and Shechter, R. (2010b). Systemic inflammatory cells fight off neurodegenerativedisease. *Nat. Rev. Neurol.* 6,405–410.

Schwarz, J. M., and Bilbo, S. D. (2011). "The immune system and the devel- oping brain," in *Colloquium Series on the Developing Brain*, Vol. 2, No. 3, ed. M. M. McCarthy (San Rafael: Morgan and Claypool Publishers), 1–128.

Schwarz, J. M., and Bilbo, S. D. (2012). Sex, glia, and development: interac- tions in health and disease. *Horm. Behav.* 62,243–253.

Shaked, I., Tchoresh, D., Gersner, R., Meiri, G., Mordechai, S., Xiao, X., et al. (2005). Protective autoimmunity: interferon-gamma enables microglia to remove glutamate without evok- ing inflammatory mediators. J. Neu- rochem. 92, 997–1009.

Shechter, R., London, A., Varol, C., Raposo, C., Cusimano, M., Yovel, G., et al. (2009). Infiltrating blood- derived macrophages are vital cells playing an anti-inflammatory role in recovery from spinal cord injury in mice. PLoS Med. 6:e1000113. doi:10.1371/journal.pmed.1000113

Sherry, C. L., Kim, S. S., Dilger, R. N., Bauer, L. L., Moon, M. L., Tapping, R. I., et al. (2010). Sickness behavior induced by endotoxin can be mit- igated by the dietary soluble fiber, pectin, through up-regulation of IL- 4 and Th2 polarization. *Brain Behav. Immun.* 24,631–640.

Shimizu, E., Kawahara, K., Kajizono, M., Sawada, M., and Nakayama, H. (2008). IL-4-induced selective clear- ance of oligomeric beta-amyloid peptide(1–42) by rat primary type 2 microglia. *J. Immunol.* 181, 6503–6513.

Sigwalt, A. R., Budde, H., Helmich, I., Glaser, V., Ghisoni, K., Lanza, S., et al. (2011). Molecular aspects involved in swimming exercise train- ing reducing anhedonia in a rat model of depression. *Neuroscience* 192, 661–674.

Smith, P. J., Blumenthal, J. A., Hoff- man, B. M., Cooper, H., Strauman, T. A., Welsh-Bohmer, K., et al. (2010). Aerobic exercise and neurocognitive performance: a meta-analytic review of randomized controlled trials. *Psy- chosom. Med.* 72,239–252.

Southwick, S. M., and Charney, D. S. (2012). The science of resilience: implications for the prevention and treatment of depression. *Science* 338, 79–82.

Starkie, R., Ostrowski, S. R., Jauffred, S., Febbraio, M., and Peder- sen, B. K. (2003). Exercise and IL-6 infusion inhibit endotoxin-induced TNF-alpha production in humans. *FASEB J.* 17,884–886.

Stellwagen, D., and Malenka, R. C. (2006). Synaptic scaling mediated by glial TNF-alpha. *Nature* 440, 1054–1059.

Stewart, L. K., Flynn, M. G., Campbell, W. W., Craig, B. A., Robinson, J. P., Timmerman, K. L., et al. (2007). The influence of exercise training on inflammatory cytokines and C- reactive protein. *Med. Sci. Sports Exerc.* 39, 1714–1719.

Stuart, M. J., and Baune, B. T. (2012). Depression and type 2 diabetes: inflammatory mechanisms of a psychoneuroendocrine comorbidity. *Neurosci. Biobehav. Rev.* 36, 658–676.

Sutcigil, L., Oktenli, C., Musabak, U., Bozkurt, A., Cansever, A., Uzun, O., et al. (2007). Pro- and anti- inflammatory cytokine balance in major depression: effect of sertraline therapy. *Clin. Dev. Immunol.* 2007, 76396.

Trejo, J. L., Piriz, J., Llorens-Martin, M. V., Fernandez, A. M., Bolos, M., Leroith, D., et al. (2007). Central actions of liver-derived insulin-like growth factor I underlying its pro- cognitive effects. *Mol. Psychiatry* 12, 1118–1128.

Trivedi, M. H., Greer, T. L., Church, T. S., Carmody, T. J., Grannemann, B. D., Galper, D. I., et al. (2011). Exercise as an augmentation treatment for nonremitted major depressive dis- order: a randomized, parallel dose comparison. *J. Clin. Psychiatry* 72, 677–684.

Trivedi, M. H., Rush, A. J., Wisniewski, S. R., Nierenberg, A. A., Warden, D., Ritz, L., et al. (2006). Evalua- tion of outcomes with citalopram for depression using measurement- based care in STAR*D: implications for clinical practice. *Am. J. Psychiatry* 163, 28–40.

Tse, H. M., Milton, M. J., Schreiner, S., Profozich, J. L., Trucco, M., and Piganelli, J. D. (2007). Disruption of innate-mediated proinflammatory cytokine and reactive oxygen species third signal leads to antigen-specific hyporesponsiveness. *J. Immunol.* 178, 908–917.

Vukovic, J., Colditz, M. J., Blackmore, D. G., Ruitenberg, M. J., and Bartlett, P. F. (2012). Microglia modulate hip- pocampal neural precursor activity in response to exercise and aging. *J. Neurosci.* 32,6435–6443.

Walker, F. R. (2012). A review of the mechanism of action for selective serotonin reuptake inhibitors: do these drugs possess anti- inflammatory properties and is this relevant in the treatment of depression? *Neuropharmacology* 67C, 304–317.

Walker, P. A., Letourneau, P. A., Bedi, S., Shah, S. K., Jimenez, F., and Cox, C. S. Jr (2011). Progenitor cells as remote "bioreactors": neuroprotection via modulation of the systemic inflam- matory response. *World J. Stem Cells* 3, 9–18.

Walsh, J. T., and Kipnis, J. (2011). Regu- latory T cells in CNS injury: the sim- ple, the complex and the confused. *Trends. Mol. Med.* 17, 541–547.

Walton, N. M., Sutter, B. M., Lay- well, E. D., Levkoff, L. H., Kearns, S. M., Marshall, G. P. II, et al. (2006). Microglia instruct subven- tricular zone neurogenesis. *Glia* 54, 815–825.

Warner-Schmidt, J. L., Vanover, K. E., Chen, E. Y., Marshall, J. J., and Greengard, P. (2011). Antide- pressant effects of selective sero- tonin reuptake inhibitors (SSRIs) are attenuated by antiinflamma- tory drugs in mice and humans. *Proc. Natl. Acad. Sci. U.S.A.* 108, 9262–9267.

WHO. (2008). *Global Burden of Disease: 2004 Update.* Geneva: WHO. Wong, M. L., Dong, C., Maestre-Mesa, J., and Licinio, J. (2008). Poly- morphisms in inflammation-related genes are associated with suscepti- bility to major depression and anti- depressant response. *Mol. Psychiatry* 13, 800–812.

Wu, M. D., Hein, A. M., Moravan, M. J., Shaftel, S. S., Olschowka, J. A., and O'Banion, M. K. (2012). Adult murine hippocampal neuro- genesis is inhibited by sustained IL- 1beta and not rescued by voluntary running. *Brain Behav. Immun.* 26, 292–300.

Yi, C. X., Al-Massadi, O., Donelan, E., Lehti, M., Weber, J., Ress, C., et al. (2012). Exercise protects against high-fat diet-induced hypothalamic inflammation. *Physiol. Behav.* 106, 485–490.

Yirmiya, R., and Goshen, I. (2011). Immune modulation of learn- ing, memory, neural plasticity and neurogenesis. *Brain Behav. Immun.* 25, 181–213.

Zhou, X., Bailey-Bucktrout, S., Jeker, L. T., and Bluestone, J. A. (2009). Plas- ticity of CD4+ FoxP3+ T cells. *Curr. Opin. Immunol.* 21, 281–285.

Zhu, C. B., Blakely, R. D., and Hewlett, W. A. (2006). The proinflamma- tory cytokines interleukin-1beta and tumor necrosis factor-alpha activate serotonin transporters. *Neuropsy- chopharmacology* 31, 2121–2131.

4

Hypothalamic neurohormones and immune responses

J. Luis Quintanar* and Irene Guzmán-Soto

Laboratory of Neurophysiology, Department of Physiology and Pharmacology, Centro de Ciencias Básicas, Universidad Autónoma de Aguascalientes, Aguascalientes, México

Edited by:
Beatriz Gomez-Gonzalez, Universidad Autonoma Metropolitana, México
Reviewed by:
Dumitru A. Iacobas, Albert Einstein College of Medicine of Yeshiva University, USA
Fatih Tanriverdi, Erciyes University Medical School Endocrinology Department, Turkey
****Correspondence:***
J. Luis Quintanar, Department of Physiology and Pharmacology, Centro de Ciencias Básicas, Universidad Autónoma de Aguascalientes, Av. Universidad 940, C.P. 20131, Aguascalientes Ags., México
e-mail: jlquinta@correo.uaa.mx

The aim of this review is to provide a comprehensive examination of the current literature describing the neural-immune interactions, with emphasis on the most recent findings of the effects of neurohormones on immune system. Particularly, the role of hypothalamic hormones such as Thyrotropin-releasing hormone (TRH), Corticotropin-releasing hormone (CRH) and Gonadotropin-releasing hormone (GnRH). In the past few years, interest has been raised in extrapituitary actions of these neurohormones due to their receptors have been found in many non-pituitary tissues. Also, the receptors are present in immune cells, suggesting an autocrine or paracrine role within the immune system. In general, these neurohormones have been reported to exert immunomodulatory effects on cell proliferation, immune mediators release and cell function. The implications of these findings in understanding the network of hypothalamic neuropeptides and immune system are discussed.

Keywords: TRH, CRH, CRF, GnRH, LHRH, immune system, extrapituitary, receptors

INTRODUCTION

The neurosecretion in the hypothalamus can be traced back to the work of Scharrer and Scharrer (1940). Posterior studies by Harris specified that the hypothalamic substances secreted into the portal vessels were pituitary specific and propose the concept of "releasing factors" whose purpose was to initiate a cascade of events resulting in the release of peripherally active hormones (Harris, 1948).

The discovery and chemical characterization of the first identified hypothalamic releasing factor by Burgus et al. (1969) and Boler et al. (1969) provided ultimate confirmation for the founding principles of neuroendocrinology and was followed by the discovery of other peptide-releasing factors (Nillni and Sevarino, 1999).

THYROTROPIN-RELEASING HORMONE (TRH)

TRH, the smallest known peptide hypophyseotropic hormone, is a tripeptide (pGlu-His-Pro-NH_2; where pGlu stands for pyroglutamic acid) that is released from the hypothalamus and transported via the portal vascular system to the anterior pituitary where it stimulates the release of thyroid-stimulating hormone (TSH) and prolactin from the anterior pituitary (Matre et al., 2003).

TRH it is also known as thyrotropin-releasing factor (TRF), thyroliberin or protirelin (Khomane et al., 2011) and was the first chemically defined hypophyseotropic hormone (Bílek et al., 2011).

SYNTHESIS

This small tripeptide (362.42 Da) is indeed processed from a larger precursor protein, prepro-TRH (ppTRH), through now classic cleavage mechanisms, C-terminal amidation, and cyclization of the N-terminal Gln to pGlu (Guillemin, 2005).

The rat ppTRH is a 29 kDa polypeptide composed of 255 amino acids. The rat precursor contains an N-terminal 25-amino-acid leader sequence, five copies of the TRH progenitor sequence Gln-His-Pro-Gly flanked by paired basic amino acids (Lys-Arg or Arg-Arg), four non-TRH peptides lying between the TRH progenitors, an N-terminal flanking peptide, and a C-terminal flanking peptide. Rats and mice have five Gln-His-Pro-Gly TRH progenitor sequences, whereas humans have six TRH sequences (Chiamolera and Wondisford, 2009).

TRH EXPRESSION REGULATION

The maintenance of euthyroidism is dependent on a highly regulated balance of neuropeptides and neurotransmitters, where the dominant positive hypothalamic control for TSH is TRH, and the principal feedback control is through thyroid hormones (THs) (Nillni and Sevarino, 1999).

THs exert powerful feedback inhibition over the TRH response system by inhibiting TRH synthesis and processing in TRH neurons in the paraventricular region of the hypothalamus and decreasing TRH receptors (TRHR) and responses in the pituitary gland (Hinkle et al., 2012).

TRH gene expression is also regulated by temperature, food intake, and stress. Thus the TRH neuron is well positioned to integrate information about the environment as well as circulating TH levels and ultimately affect metabolism in response to these physiological changes (Chiamolera and Wondisford, 2009).

HALF-LIFE

The short half-life (4–5 mins) of TRH is most likely due to rapid degradation of the TRH at both the carboxy (COOH) and amino (NH_2) termini. Cleavage of the pyroglutamyl moiety of TRH by enzymes like aminopeptidases and deamidases causes formation of the metabolite histidyl proline diketopiperazine (ClycoHistine-Proline, CHP) while its deamidation results in the formation of the free acid, that is, TRH-OH (Khomane et al., 2011).

TRHR

The TRHR is a member of a large family of transmembrane proteins (G-protein-coupled receptors, GPCRs) for which an interaction with an intracellular G protein is a critical part of the signal transduction pathway mediated by the receptor. It is thought that all GPCRs have a common tertiary structure composed of seven transmembrane helices. The topology of these membrane-bound proteins is defined by an extracellular amino terminus and an intracellular COOH terminus. Consequently, the helices are connected by intracellular-extracellular loops. Colson et al. (1998) suggested that TRH initially interacts with residues within the extracellular loops and then moves into the transmembrane binding pocket, aided by the motion of the loops.

A single TRHR gene has been found in humans and higher mammals and two genes encoding homologous receptors, TRHR1 and TRHR2, in rodents (Sun et al., 2003). TRHR1 predominates in the anterior pituitary gland while both TRHR1 and TRHR2 are found in rodent central nervous system (CNS) (Hinkle et al., 2012).

EXTRAHYPOTHALAMIC AND EXTRAPITUITARY LOCATION OF TRH AND TRHR RESPECTIVELY

Originally discovered in the hypothalamus, consistent with its classical role as a hypothalamic hypophysiotrophic factor, TRH and TRHR are now known to be distributed throughout the central and peripheral nervous system (PNS) and are found extensively in extrahypothalamic brain structures and in other organs and tissues (Sun et al., 2003; Kamath et al., 2009).

TRH OUTSIDE THE PITUITARY ZONE

TRH has been located in several brain areas other than the paraventricular nucleus as well as in non-CNS tissues:

- Pancreatic β-cells (Engler et al., 1981; Kawano et al., 1983).
- The whole gastrointestinal tract where it may modulate contractions (Morley, 1979; Engler et al., 1981).
- The genitourinary system. TRH is found in rat, canine and human prostate, seminal vesicles, ovary, testis, Leydig cells and epididymis (Pekary et al., 1980, 1983a,b; Feng et al., 1992).
- The presence of TRH in rat, human, porcine and bovine retina has been reported (Schaeffer et al., 1977; Martino et al., 1980a,b).
- Shambaugh et al. (1979) identified TRH activity in placental extracts by specific radioimmunoassay test (RIA).
- TRH has been found as part of immune system tissues and blood elements (Matre et al., 2003). This topic will be discussed in depth in the following sections.

TRHR OUTSIDE THE HYPOTHALAMIC ZONE

Besides the well-known TRHR location in the pituitary zone, TRH binding sites have been described throughout the central and PNS and in non-CNS tissues including:

- Uterus, ovary and testis where TRHR mRNA levels appear to be relatively high (Fukusumi et al., 1995; Montagne et al., 1999).
- Wang et al. (1997) reported that small intestine epithelial cells were found to express receptors for TRH and to be a primary source of intestine-derived TSH.
- TRHR is also found in retina (Satoh et al., 1993) and adrenal gland (Montagne et al., 1999).

Furthermore, TRHR expression in organs and cells of the immune system has been confirmed:

- Expression of TRHR mRNA and TRHR in lymphoid tissues has been found: Thymus, mesenteric lymph nodes and spleen (Raiden et al., 1995; Mellado et al., 1999).
- Thymus expression of the TRHR has been reported by several authors (Fukusumi et al., 1995; Mellado et al., 1999; Montagne et al., 1999; Matre et al., 2003).
- Expression analysis in rat demonstrated the presence of TRHR mRNA in bone marrow (Montagne et al., 1999; Matre et al., 2003) and in the rat natural-killer cell line RNK-16 (Matre et al., 2003). This expression was shown to be functional as evidenced by TRH binding to surface receptors on thymocytes and RNK-16 cells.
- Analysis of human peripheral blood lymphocyte (Raiden et al., 1995; Mellado et al., 1999) and tonsil-derived leukocyte populations showed TRHR expression in non-activated and phytohemagglutinin-activated T and B cells (Mellado et al., 1999).

The widespread distribution of TRH and the TRHR within and outside the CNS supports a diverse range of roles for this molecule, roles likely to involve many functions outside of the traditional hypothalamic-pituitary-thyroid (HPT) axis (Nillni and Sevarino, 1999).

TRH FUNCTIONS

TRH indirectly stimulates TH biosynthesis and release. Thus, TRH is central in regulating the HPT axis. TRH influences the release of other hormones, including prolactin, growth hormone, vasopressin, insulin, and the classic neurotransmitters noradrenaline and adrenaline (Nillni and Sevarino, 1999).

EXTRAHYPOPHYSIOTROPIC FUNCTIONS OF TRH

More than two-thirds of immunoreactive-TRH in the brain is found outside of the traditional "thyrotrophic zone" of the hypothalamus. This extrahypophysiotropic TRH is believed to function as a neuromodulator of known neurotransmitters. Indeed, it might act as a neurotransmitter itself; it is present in secretory granules whose exocytosis is responsive to membrane depolarization, it acts through specific receptors that are widely distributed throughout the CNS, and it is rapidly cleared through specific catabolic pathways. In several areas of the brain, TRH is colocalized with other neurotransmitters and/or neuromodulators (Nillni and Sevarino, 1999).

These effects of TRH have been demonstrated using TRH and/or TRH analogs. Available TRH analogs have higher affinities for the TRHR, longer half-lives, etc. (Engel et al., 2006; Khomane et al., 2011; Monga et al., 2011).

Beside endocrine functions, TRH also possesses several neuropharmacological effects like cerebral nerve activation (stimulation of motor function), effects on sympathetic nervous system (elevation of blood pressure and stimulation of respiratory), effects on spinal function (stimulation of spinal motor neuron), effects on CNS (antidepressant activity) and peripheral actions (suppression of gastric acid secretion, stimulation of glucagon secretion). These CNS-mediated effects provide the rationale for the use of TRH in the treatment of brain/spinal injury and certain CNS disorders, including schizophrenia, Alzheimer's disease, epilepsy, amyotrophic lateral sclerosis, Parkinson's disease and depression (Khomane et al., 2011).

TRH AND IMMUNE SYSTEM

Two-way communication between the immune and neuroendocrine systems is now well recognized. These interactions are mediated by cytokines, neuropeptides, hormones, other soluble factors and their receptors (Grasso et al., 1998).

As mentioned above, cells of the immune system have been found to contain receptors for neuroendocrine hormones and can also be considered a source of pituitary and hypothalamic peptides (Matre et al., 2003).

IMMUNE RESPONSE TO TRH ADMINISTRATION

Proliferation

Induction. Acute and chronic administration of TRH enhances the proliferation of splenic and thymic lymphocytes in rats (Pawlikowski et al., 1992; Raiden et al., 1995; Winczyk and Pawlikowski, 2000). In fact, it has been reported that TRH promotes thymic reconstitution in mice with anterior hypothalamic area lesions (Lesnikov et al., 1991). According with these data, it was also reported that TRH enhances the *in vitro* plaque-forming cell response (Kruger et al., 1989), antagonizes the dexometasone-induced thymocyte and splenocyte suppression (Winczyk and Pawlikowski, 2000) and administration in humans led to increased secretion of IL-2 into the blood (Komorowski et al., 1993).

Suppression. It has also been reported that TRH significantly inhibits monocyte activity (Lersch et al., 1989). The experimental work of Kunert-Radek et al. (1991) addressed the proliferation of murine splenocytes *in vitro* considering the ^{3}H-thymidine incorporation into splenocyte DNA as an index of proliferation. They found that TRH suppressed the proliferation of splenocytes.

TRH has the capability to modulate the natural cell-mediated cytotoxicity. To try it out, TRH was added to the feed of White Leghorn male chicks and peripheral blood lymphocytes were cultured *in vitro* with or without different mitogens (Phytohaemagglutinin-A (PHA), ConA, or Lipopolysaccharide (LPS)), and the culture supernatants were tested for the presence of lymphokines. Results showed that the supernatant from *in vivo* 5 ppm TRH-treated lymphocytes significantly suppressed the natural cell-mediated cytotoxicity (Haddad and Mashaly, 1992).

Recently was published that oral administration of TRH in mice with experimental autoimmune encephalomyelitis (EAE), an animal model of multiple sclerosis, reduces the spinal cord inflammatory foci without increased frequency of regulatory T cells (Treg) in spleen (Brod and Bauer, 2013).

Induces TSH production by immune cells

At very low concentrations, TRH induces splenocyte production of TSH *in vitro* (Kruger et al., 1989).

Peripheral blood mononuclear cells (PBMC), rat splenocytes and transformed T cell lines produce TSH in response to TRH (Harbour et al., 1989; Raiden et al., 1995).

Induces immune mediators production

PBMC, rat splenocytes and transformed T cell lines can enhance or modulate the *in vitro* antibody response in response to TRH (Kruger et al., 1989; Hart et al., 1990).

Koshida and Kotake (1993) investigated the role of TRH on the superoxide anion (O_2^-) production of rabbit peritoneal macrophages. Their results showed that TRH acts on macrophages and suggest that TRH possesses the priming action of O_2^- release in response to the chemotactic peptide N-formyl-methionyl-leucyl-phenylalanine, and opsonized zymosan. Authors suggest that if this type of priming exists *in vivo* there should be a role to play in an inflammation process.

In vitro studies have shown that a TRH fixation occurs at the level of the human polymorphonuclear neutrophil, which suggests putative membrane receptor (s) for the hypothalamic hormone. The correspondent *in vivo* analyses demonstrated that after TRH administration, enzyme modifications (myeloperoxydase, alkaline phosphatase) and metabolism changes (PAS, Sudan black) happen, showing a functional activation of that blood cell (Blum et al., 1976). These *in vivo* effects could be due to TRH is being directly attached to its receptor on neutrophils or an indirect effect is being mediated by TSH or THs.

Intravenous bolus of TRH in normoprolactinemic women increases plasma gamma interferon (IFN-γ) levels 45 mins after administration. In order to investigate a possible direct action of TRH on immune cells, the authors also examined the effects of this hypothalamic peptide on IFN-γ production by PBMCs stimulated *in vitro* with suboptimal concentration of bacterial superantigen staphylococcal enterotoxin A or concanavalin A (ConA), collected before the intravenous administration of TRH. The *in vitro* findings showed a directly enhanced IFN-γ production by activated lymphocytes (Grasso et al., 1998).

Furthermore, splenic and CNS lymphocytes showed significant decrease in levels of profile 17 helper t cells (T_H17) and T_H1 cytokines: Interleukin-17 (IL-17), tumor necrosis factor (TNF-α) and IL-2 respectively, after oral administration of TRH in EAE mice. This treatment also increased CNS lymphocyte production of T_H2 cytokines, in particular IL-13 (Brod and Bauer, 2013). Thus, oral TRH shows a unique pattern of immunomodulation for an ingested neuropeptide although the poor oral bioavailability associated with TRH and some of its analogs (Khomane et al., 2011).

TRH expression response against immune system challenges

It is known that high concentrations of TRH seem to decrease the production of antibodies against sheep red blood cells (SRBC) (Kukain et al., 1982).

Pérez Castro et al. (1999) investigated whether TRH mRNA levels in the hypothalamus are altered after SRBC (a T cell-dependent antigen) immunization. An increased level of TRH mRNA detected by Northern blot autoradiography was observed at 4, 6, and 24 h post immunization in SRBC-injected animals.

The SRBC-induced effects on TRH mRNA levels are opposite to those induced by LPS, a T cell-independent response through macrophage and B lymphocyte activation. LPS induces a decrease in hypothalamic TRH mRNA levels that is observed at 24 h and more pronounced at 4 h (Pérez Castro et al., 1999).

As we can see, TRH effects could seem controversial but is important to consider that interactions between the CNS, the endocrine system and the immune system are mediated at multiple levels. These mediators include secreted chemical messengers such as hormones, cytokines, neurotransmitters and neuropeptides acting directly or via the nervous system.

Evidence indicates interactions at the level of receptors (e.g., the presence of neuroendocrine peptide receptors on immune cells), at the level of secretory function (e.g., the synthesis and secretion of neuroendocrine peptides by immune cells), and at the level of signal transduction (Kamath et al., 2009). Integration of these complex interactions in a single route would be inaccurate, for this reason, the most wise conclusion could be consider the TRH-immune system homeostatic hypothesis proposed by Gary et al. (2003) and Kamath et al. (2009), which states that TRH mediated mechanisms respond to many elements of the immune system and affect them in ways that tend to maintain or restore homeostasis.

The effects of TRH administration on immune system are summarized in **Figure 1**.

CLINICAL RELEVANCE AND FUTURE DIRECTIONS

Studies on the effects of TRH *in vitro* hardly can be extrapolated to *in vivo* conditions. The direct effect of TRH on the immune system provides a modulatory physiological role. However, pharmacological administration in humans and in experimental animals involves two pathways impact (1) through stimulation of TSH secretion and therefore of THs and (2) the direct effect on the immune system. TRH administration may affect these two ways and with addition or synergy effects. One possibility to explore the direct mode might be using hypophysectomized or thyroidectomized animals to avoid endocrine influence. According to the studies described above, it is possible to consider the possibility that clinical treatment with TRH may improve the immune response in patients with immune deficiencies or reduced response in autoimmune diseases such as multiple sclerosis or lupus erythematosus. Such expectations are a challenge to be explored in the future.

CORTICOTROPIN-RELEASING HORMONE (CRH)

CRH or Corticotropin-releasing factor (CRF) was characterized, purified and synthesized in 1981 by Vale. The composition of this 41 amino-acid peptide is different from one species to another. Its principal origin in the brain are the neurons from paraventricular nucleus of the hypothalamus. By the portal hypothalamic-pituitary vessels, it reaches the anterior pituitary lobe where it stimulates the corticotroph cells (Raux-Demay and Girard, 1985; Emeric-Sauval, 1986). The plasma half-life of CRH in humans is 4 mins (Schürmeyer et al., 1984). The action of CRH on adrenocorticotrophic hormone (ACTH) secretion is predominant, but it acts in relation with arginine-vasopressin and potentially with angiotensin and catecholamines. Adrenal steroids (glucocorticoids) act on feedback control of CRH secretion in the hypothalamus and also on pituitary corticotrophs. CRH has shown to be an important regulator of the endocrine stress response, and it is now known to play a role in diverse functions in the homeostatic balance, important in mobilization of resources and behaviors during stress (Bale and Vale, 2004), it is involved in the regulation of food intake and satiety, as well as gastrointestinal tract motility, vascular tone, and development, and also acoustic and cardiac function (Heinrichs et al., 1992; Koob and Heinrichs, 1999; Maillot et al., 2000; Inoue et al., 2003; Janssen and Kozicz, 2013).

CRH RECEPTOR (CRHR)

High-affinity CRHRs which mediate the actions of the hypothalamic peptide on ACTH release, have been principal identified in the anterior pituitary gland. Interaction of the pituitary receptor by CRH agonists stimulates ACTH release. CRH exerts its effects by binding to specific cell surface receptors, of which two receptor subtypes have been reported, CRH-R1 and CRH-R2. These receptors share high sequence homology and belong to the family of seven transmembrane GPCRs (Vaughan et al., 1995; Lewis et al., 2001).

Actions of this peptide are initiated by binding and activating GPCRs and subsequently the activation of adenylate cyclase and cyclic adenosine monophosphate dependent protein kinase (Grammatopoulos and Chrousos, 2002). In the regulation of ACTH secretion, the effects of CRH on the corticotroph are integrated with the stimulatory actions of cyclic adenosine monophosphate and the inhibitory effects of glucocorticoids. Following adrenalectomy, the progressive elevation of plasma ACTH levels is accompanied by a concomitant decrease in pituitary CRHRs (down-regulation) (Wynn et al., 1985; Aguilera et al., 1986).

Extrapituitary expression of CRHR

CRH-R1 is a 415 amino acid peptide and has a widespread expression in stress-related areas located in the CNS (Justice et al., 2008; Kuhne et al., 2012). Outside the CNS, the CRH-R1 is expressed in the adrenal gland, gastrointestinal tissue, ovary, testis, skin, thymus and spleen (Dufau et al., 1993; Nappi and Rivest, 1995; Slominski et al., 1995; Baigent and Lowry, 2000; Müller et al., 2001; Chatzaki et al., 2004). CRH-R2 is a 397–437 amino acid protein and it is abundantly expressed in the CNS (Korosi et al., 2007; Justice et al., 2008; Kuhne et al., 2012). In the periphery, the receptor has been identified in the retina, heart, skeletal muscle, vasculature, adrenal gland, and gastrointestinal tissue (Lovenberg et al., 1995; Müller et al., 2001; Chatzaki et al., 2004).

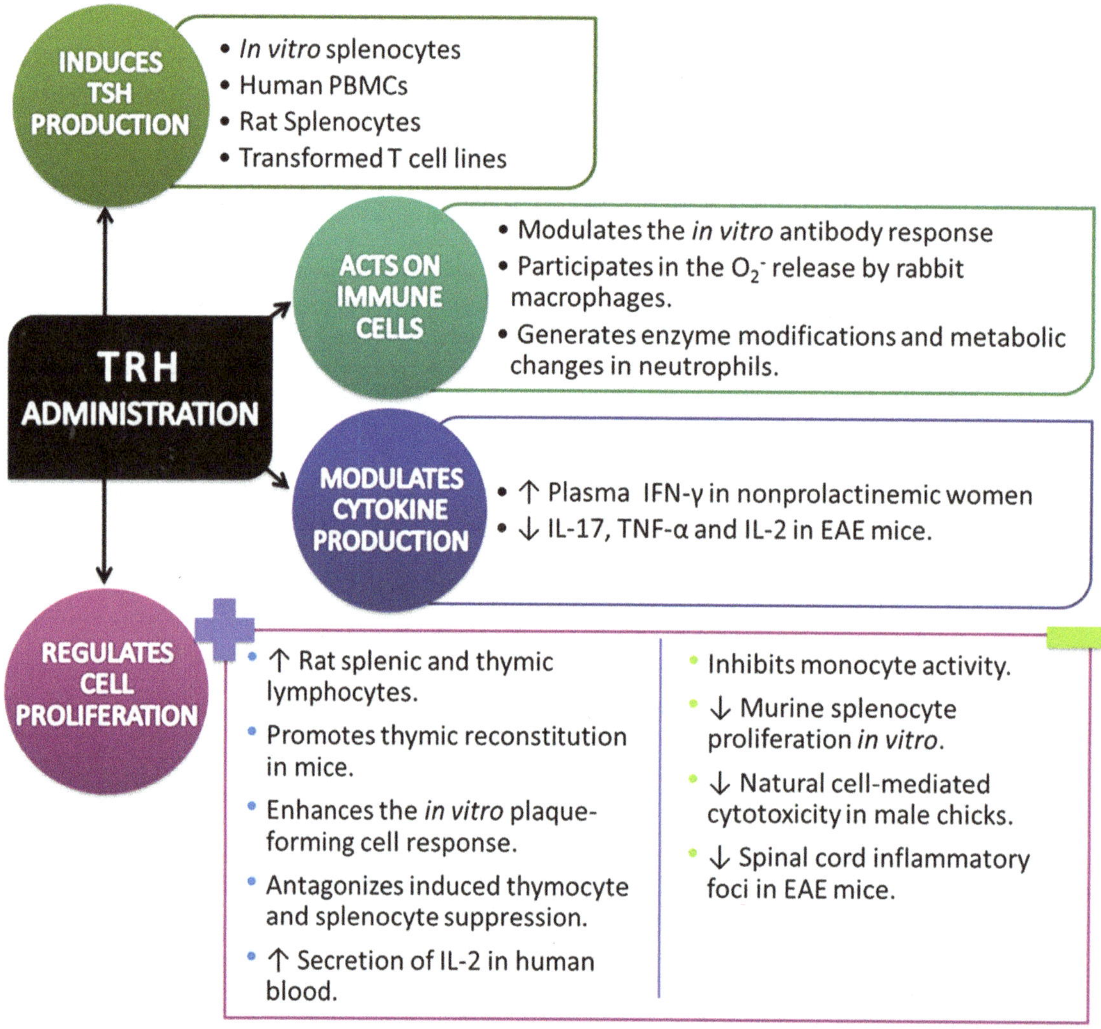

FIGURE 1 | Immune response against Thyrotropin-Releasing Hormone/Thyrotropin-Releasing Hormone agonist administration in a diversity of normal and pathological conditions (↑ = increase, ↓ = decrease).

Binding sites for CRH have been reported on adherent splenocytes (Webster et al., 1990), monocyte-macrophages (Audhya et al., 1991) and T lymphocytes (Singh and Fudenberg, 1988). CRH-R1 and CRH-R2 expression was described in granulocytes and lymphocytes in inflamed tissues (Mousa et al., 2003). CRH-R1 mRNA expression had been reported in the human leukemic mast cell line (Theoharides et al., 1998) and mast cells were reported to express immunoreactive CRH-R1 in inflamed human synovial tissue (McEvoy et al., 2001).

CRH EFFECTS ON CNS AND PNS

Independently of anterior pituitary, CRH has effects within of nervous system. The central administration of CRH produces hypertension, tachycardia and an elevated oxygen consumption. CRF acts within the brain to increase plasma concentrations of noradrenaline and adrenaline resulting in increased plasma concentrations of glucagon and in hyperglycemia. Likewise, also acts increasing the plasma concentrations of vasopressin. CRH induces a reduction in food intake and increases grooming behavior and locomotor activity. The physiological significance of the peripheral actions of CRH on various organ systems is unknown. Intravenous administration of CRH reduces gastric acid secretion, gastric emptying and blood pressure but increases heart rate, venous return to the heart, mesenteric and aortic blood flow and pancreatic bicarbonate and protein secretions (Lenz, 1987; Chen et al., 2007).

CRH AND IMMUNE SYSTEM

The cellular components of the immune-inflammatory response include leukocytes, such as monocytes–macrophages, polymorphonuclear neutrophils, eosinophils and basophils, platelets, dentritic cells, mast cells, epithelial and endothelial cells, and fibroblasts which belong to the innate immune system, as well as lymphocytes T, B and natural killer (NK) which are included in the adaptive immune system. These cells cooperate using molecular signals, including ILs, colony-stimulating factors, TNF, IFNs, transforming growth factor, and chemokines, vasoactive amines (histamine and serotonine), plasma proteases (kinine and complement systems), arachidonic acid metabolites (prostaglandins, leukotrienes, and lipoxins), platelet-activating factor, nitric oxide, and neuropeptides (Mastorakos et al., 2006).

The majority of *in vivo* studies suggest that direct stimulation of hypothalamic CRH by cytokines is the principal route by which immune activation stimulates the hypothalamic–pituitary–adrenal (HPA) axis (Besedovsky et al., 1986; Harbuz et al., 1992) and this process is prostaglandin-dependent. Thus, experimental evidence suggests that CRH may modulate the immune and inflammatory responses via two pathways: an anti-inflammatory one operated by centrally released CRH, most likely through stimulation of glucocorticoid and catecholamine release, and one pro-inflammatory, through direct action of peripherally secreted CRH (Karalis et al., 1997).

CRH in immune cells

Mast cells. Mast cells are critical for allergic reactions due to their secretion of numerous vasoactive molecules and cytokines (Kobayashi et al., 2000). Evidence indicates that mast cells are also involved in innate and acquired immunity (Marone et al., 2002), as well as in neuroinflammatory conditions such as those affected by stress (Theoharides and Cochrane, 2004). Mast cells secrete numerous pro-inflammatory cytokines, such as IL-6, IL-8, and TNF-α (Kobayashi et al., 2000; Marone et al., 2002), and secretion of vascular endothelial growth factor (VEGF) by CRH stimulation (Cao et al., 2005). Interestingly, human mast cells were shown to synthesize and secrete large amounts of CRH, suggesting that this peptide could regulate mast cells through CRH receptor in an autocrine manner. Secretion of CRH from mast cells could also be triggered by pro-inflammatory molecules that are released during the initial phases of inflammation (Kempuraj et al., 2004). CRH causes mast cell degranulation in human skin, releasing great amounts of histamine, which appears to be the principal mediator of the vasodilatory effects of CRH (Wright, 2003).

Mononuclear cells. In mononuclear cells, it has been reported that CRH stimulates immune functions, proliferation of lymphocytes both in the absence and presence of T cell mitogens, and the expression of IL-2R antigen on T cells (Singh, 1989; Singh et al., 1990). It has also been reported the presence of binding sites for CRH on monocytes, T and B lymphocytes and thymus (Singh and Fudenberg, 1988). The CRH is also a stimulator of production of two interleukins, IL-1 and IL-2. IL-1 has been shown to stimulate the secretion of CRH by hypothalamic cells (Sapolsky et al., 1987) and CRH stimulates the production of IL-1 and IL-2, suggesting the presence of a complete network between the neuroendocrine system and the immune system (Singh and Leu, 1990).

The release of CRH plays a role in modulating NK activity following stress also implies that CRH in the brain may be involved in the functional population of lymphocytes. Studies have been conducted to analyze the effect of CRF on the reduction of several cellular immune measures such as splenic and peripheral blood NK activity and lymphocyte responses to mitogenic stimulation (Strausbaug and Irwin, 1992; Boyadjieva et al., 2006). Other observations also indicate that central doses of CRH slow the kinetics and reduce the level of IgG response to a specific T-cell-dependent antigen (Irwin, 1993). The administration of central CRH antagonist induces suppression of NK cytotoxicity. In contrast, peripheral application has no effect on CRH modulation of immunity (Irwin et al., 1987).

Other studies have shown CRH to inhibit IFN-γ secretion (Angioni et al., 1993). IL-2-induced splenocyte proliferation as well as LPS-mediated IL-1 and IL-6 production by peripheral blood monocytes (Hagan et al., 1992).

The effects of CRH were almost exclusively examined in the mononuclear cells, however in other studies has been reported that polymorphonuclear cells (neutrophils), express higher levels of CRH-R1 than mononuclear immune cells in mouse (Radulovic et al., 1999). It has been shown that CRH inhibits the secretion of IL-1β from mature neutrophils purified from spleens of mice injected with LPS (Radulovic and Spiess, 2001).

It has been described the CRH presence in macrophages (Brouxhon et al., 1998). Results showed that CRH could be detected in normal peritoneal macrophages and the levels increased significantly after stimulation with LPS (Wang et al., 2012). The role of CRH may be immunomodulatory, however the effects remains to be studied.

On other hand, studies shown that cluster of differentiation (CD14+) group of cell surface marker proteins, the CRH can activate CD14+ cells to produce TNF-α cells and compromise endothelial barrier function by inducing apoptosis of the endothelial cells (Song et al., 2013).

CRH and its relationship to immune therapies

Drugs have been proposed to either block CRHR-1 and CRHR-2 receptors as CRH inhibitors with therapeutic properties through modifying the immune response as tool for both CNS and inflammatory disorders associated with central and peripheral CRH. CRH-R1 antagonist could be considered for the treatment of allergic conditions, such as urticaria, asthma, eczema, or disorders that increase blood–brain barrier permeability (Theoharides et al., 1998; Esposito et al., 2002), chronic inflammatory bowel syndromes, irritable bowel disease, and ulcerative colitis and other pathologies (Kawahito et al., 1995; Gravanis and Margioris, 2005).

The effects of CRH administration on immune system are summarized in **Figure 2**.

Future directions

There are two major problems associated with the HPA axis. The inflammatory process and the reduction in the immune response. Chronic exposure to antiinflammatory steroids have effects such as immunosuppression which under certain conditions can cause undesired effect. Identifying specific receptor subtypes to CRH, or applying interleukin receptor blockers may provide a viable alternative to maintaining of the homeostatic mechanisms.

Emotional stress causes somatic alterations including the immune response and is perhaps, one of the most pressing problems in global public health that needs to be addressed.

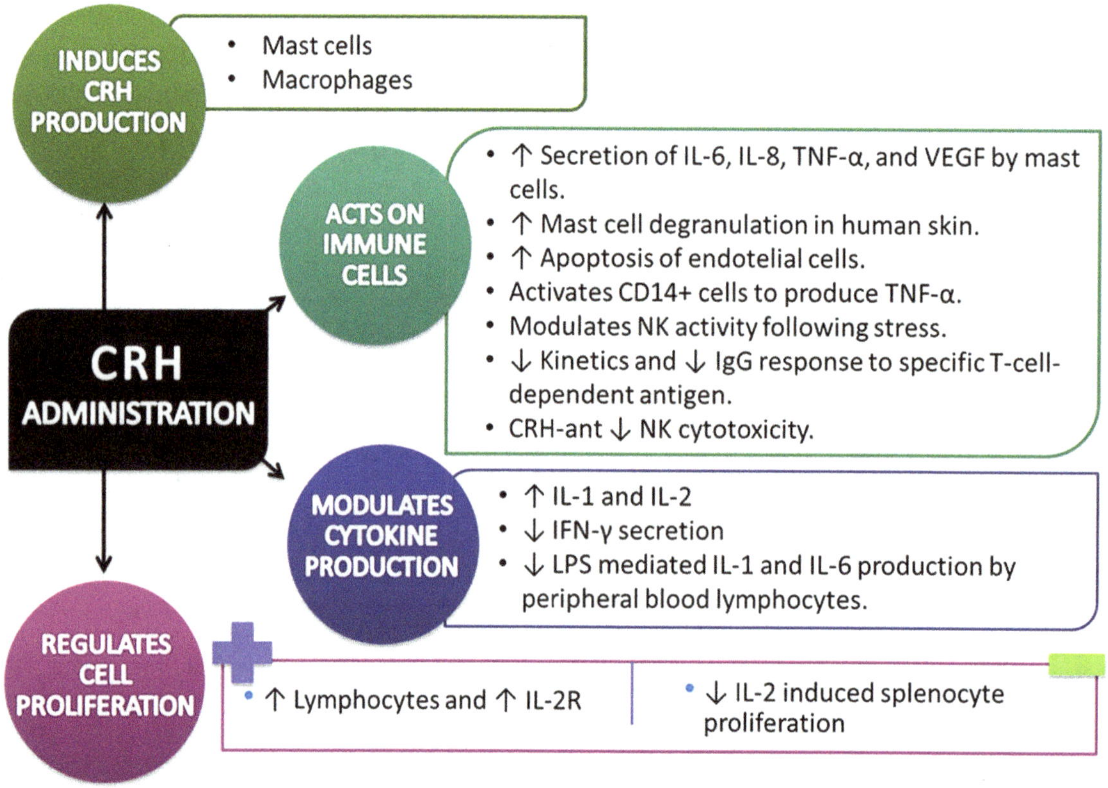

FIGURE 2 | Experimental data of Corticotropin-Releasing Hormone/Corticotropin-Releasing Hormone agonist impact on immune system cells and processes (↑ = increase, ↓ = decrease).

GONADOTROPIN-RELEASING HORMONE (GnRH)

GnRH, also known as luteinizing hormone releasing hormone (LHRH), is a small peptide hormone (pGlu-His-Trp-Ser-Tyr-Gly-Leu-Arg-Pro-Gly-NH_2) of 1.2 kDa, with an established role as central regulator of the neuroendocrine reproductive axis in both males and females (Cheung and Wong, 2008).

This neuropeptide is mainly synthesized in hypothalamic neurons of the medial preoptic area. It is well established that adenohypophysial gonadotropic cells stimulate the synthesis and secretion of gonadotropic hormones such as follicle stimulating hormone (FSH) and luteinizing hormone (LH) (Cheng and Leung, 2005). LH and FSH are released into the systemic circulation in a pulsatile pattern, which is dependent upon the GnRH pulse frequency, and act to affect gonadal steroidogenesis and gametogenesis (Sasaki and Norwitz, 2011).

GnRH ISOFORMS

At the present, it is known that, in addition to the hypothalamic GnRH, several other isoforms of the decapeptide exist in vertebrates. All these isoforms are characterized by the conservation of the length of the peptide as well as by the amino acid sequences of the N-terminal (Glp-His-Trp-Ser) and C-terminal (Pro-Gly-NH_2) domains, indicating that these molecular features are critical for the binding to, and the activation of, the receptor (Limonta and Manea, 2013). The classical hypophysiotropic GnRH located in the anterior hypothalamus/preoptic area is also designed as GnRH-I (Stevenson et al., 2012).

A second isoform of GnRH, originally isolated from the chicken hypothalamus and referred to as chicken GnRH or cGnRH, has been isolated in most vertebrate species—including humans—is now referred to as GnRH-II and is 70% homologous to GnRH-I (Sasaki and Norwitz, 2011). GnRH-II is expressed at a higher level outside of the brain (Tan and Bukulmez, 2011).

A third GnRH isoform, GnRH-III, was isolated from sea lamprey and was also detected in the brain of mammals (Tan and Bukulmez, 2011). This isoform has 60% homology with GnRH-I. In the lamprey, GnRH-III is localized in brain areas involved in the control of reproductive functions and it has been reported to stimulate steroidogenesis and gametogenesis, but it has 500–1000 times less potency in LH and FSH secretion both *in vitro* and *in vivo* (Limonta and Manea, 2013).

GnRH is small and has good thermal and chemical stability and no internal Cys bridges (minimal fixed structure). Its size and stability has led to the availability of thousands of analogs (Conn and Janovick, 2009).

SYNTHESIS AND SECRETION

GnRH is synthesized as a prohormone, human preproGnRH that contains 92 amino acids (Harrison et al., 2004). The gene encoding preproGnRH1 gene has been cloned in number of species and is approximately 4300-bp with four relatively short exons separated by three large introns (Clarke and Pompolo, 2005).

Neurons that synthesize and release GnRH (GnRHergic neurons) have their origin in embryonic olfactory placodes. These embryonic cells, migrate and colonize the basal forebrain, preoptic area around the basal and medium hypothalamus. The median eminence in mammals contains a large amount of GnRH, so is the area in which the peptide is stored in neural terminals before release into the hypothalamus-pituitary portal system (Clarke and Pompolo, 2005).

GnRH is released as synchronized pulses from the nerve endings of about 1000 neurons into the hypophyseal portal system every 30–120 mins to stimulate the biosynthesis and secretion of LH and FSH from gonadotrophs (Millar, 2005). In adult rodents, GnRH is released from the median eminence at a frequency of about one pulse every 30 mins. A slightly slower frequency of release (approximately 50–60 mins intervals) is observed in primates (Yin and Gore, 2006). On the other hand, continuous (non-pulsatile) GnRH administration or long-lasting GnRH-a desensitize GnRHR, thereby decreasing/inhibiting the release of LH and FSH by the pituitary (Wilson et al., 2007).

HALF-LIFE

GnRH half-life normally is about 2–4 mins (Walters et al., 2008). Its short half-life is because of the rapid cleavage of the bonds between amino acids at positions 5–6, 6–7, and 9–10. Substitution at position 6 in GnRH agonists (GnRH-a) yields them resistant to degradation and increases its half-life and the time of receptor occupancy (Magon, 2011).

GnRH RECEPTOR (GnRHR)

The human pituitary GnRHR belongs to the family of GPCRs and is one of the smallest GPCRs (328 amino acid protein in the human); it may contain only the essentials required for ligand binding and signal transduction (Conn and Janovick, 2009).

Distinct forms of the GnRHR can be broadly divided into two groups:

1. The type I GnRH-Rs have greater affinity for GnRH-I than for GnRH-II and lacks a typical intracellular COOH terminus; this group contains all known mammalian GnRH-Rs except for the recently described primate type II GnRH-R (McArdle et al., 2002; Ciechanowska et al., 2010).
2. Type II GnRH-Rs have greater affinity for the GnRH-II and possess C-terminal tails of varying length; this group contains all the known receptors from non-mammalian vertebrates (catfish, goldfish, chicken, goldfish, *Xenopus*, etc.) in addition to the type II primate GnRH-Rs (McArdle et al., 2002).

EXTRAHYPOTHALAMIC AND EXTRAPITUITARY LOCATION OF GnRH AND GnRHR RESPECTIVELY

GnRH outside the pituitary zone

GnRH has been located in several extrahypothalamic cells and tissues: GnRH-like substances have been reported to be secreted from tissues outside the CNS of rats and humans. Particularly, a (GnRH)-like protein has been detected in human ovaries (Aten et al., 1987; Dong et al., 1993; Peng et al., 1994). Also, Oikawa demonstrated by PCR amplification of cDNA from rat hypothalamus, granulosa cells, and whole ovary, a 241-bp product identical to the authentic GnRH sequence based on analysis on both strands (Oikawa et al., 1990).

RT-PCR analysis together with Southern blot analysis demonstrated the presence of GnRH mRNA in human testes and mammary gland (Dong et al., 1993).

Furthermore, the gene coding for GnRH is expressed in immune tissue and immunoreactive GnRH is measurable in immune cells. Analysis of mononuclear cells by RT-PCR coupled to Southern hybridization of total RNA confirmed that GnRH genes are expressed in human peripheral blood lymphocytes. The GnRH transcripts in mononuclear cells were identical to the hypothalamic GnRH and PRL release inhibiting factor cDNA, at least within this 380-bp fragment (Chen et al., 1999).

Rat splenocytes contain an immunoactive and bioactive GnRH (Emanuele et al., 1990; Azad et al., 1991) that has also been found in lymphocytes from rat thymus (Marchetti et al., 1990; Maier et al., 1992). Moreover, it has been reported that normal and leukemic human T cells produce GnRH-II and GnRH-I and that the incubation of those cells with these neuropeptides triggered *de novo* gene transcription and cell-surface expression of a 67-kDa non-integrin laminin receptor that is involved in cellular adhesion and migration and in tumor invasion and metastasis (Chen et al., 2002).

The fact that recent evidence shows the existence of diverse isoforms of GnRH, with high sequence homology and a core variable region raises the issue that previous GnRH distribution studies may have identified a variety of isoforms. To confirm the distribution of GnRH-I only, Khan et al. (2003), reported that intense GnRH-I immunoreactivity was found in Kupffer cells, and less intense in spleen lymphocytes and follicular dendritic cells in rat.

Other cells that have been reported to express GnRH and its mRNA are mast cells from the nervous system and the peritoneal cavity, as detected by immunohistochemistry and RT-PCR, respectively (Silverman et al., 1994; Gill and Rissman, 1998; Khalil et al., 2003).

Extrapituitary GnRHR

GnRH binding sites have been described throughout the CNS and PNS as in several non-CNS cells and tissues:

Human ovarian granulosa-luteal cells also express the GnRHR mRNA (Chen et al., 1999).

GnRHR expression in organs and cells of the immune system has been confirmed: GnRH binding sites have been reported in rat spleen (Batticane et al., 1991) and thymus, thus potentially enabling GnRH-a to have direct stimulatory effects that might contribute to improved T-cell function (Marchetti et al., 1989; Batticane et al., 1991; Morale et al., 1991).

RT-PCR coupled to Southern hybridization of total RNA obtained from mononuclear cells confirmed that the GnRHR is expressed in human peripheral blood lymphocytes (Chen et al., 1999) as in porcine lymphocytes (Standaert et al., 1992).

Chen and colleagues reported that the GnRHR transcript expressed in mononuclear cells has an identical nucleotide sequence as the pituitary GnRHR cDNA. In this work, a time-course study of the effect of GnRH on mononuclear cells was performed and it was found that GnRHR mRNA increased gradually after *in vitro* culture, and this increase was further augmented by treatment with GnRH for up to 24h. In contrast, the expression of GnRH mRNA was decreased by GnRH treatment in a dose-dependent manner and the IL-2Rγ subunit gene was highly expressed in mononuclear cells. At this point we can speculate that these GnRH-binding sites in lymphocytes are probably functional, as many studies have demonstrated that GnRH-a caused a dose-dependent increase in LH production, whereas GnRHR antibodies blocked this action (Chen et al., 1999).

It has also been shown that blockade of central and peripheral GnRHR with a potent GnRH antagonist (GnRH-ant) during a critical period of maturation can impair the morphological development of thymus and the cellular and humoral immune responses in rats (Morale et al., 1991) and monkeys (Mann et al., 1994).

Particularly, neonatal exposure of male primates to a GnRH-ant alters early postnatal programming of immune function by reducing the number of B cells and T cells in the thymic medulla and T cells in the periarterial lymphatic sheaths of the spleen. GnRH-ant treatment increased the frequency of clinical problems, lowered circulating levels of lymphocytes, total T cells, CD8+ T cells and B cells, and altered the proliferative index of lymphocytes to mitogens. As adults, the cell- and humorally-mediated immune responses remained impaired (Mann et al., 2000).

To evaluate regions of GnRH-I binding activity, a biotinylated GnRH-I sequence was used with avidin-labelled HRP, and results showed GnRH-I binding activity present in Kupffer cells, spleen lymphocytes and follicular dendritic cells, as well as in thymocytes and peripheral blood lymphocytes and neutrophils (Khan et al., 2003).

GnRH AND IMMUNE SYSTEM

GnRH and sex steroids seem to be important components of immune system modulation and may play a role in the regulation of immune mediated diseases. A comprehensive description of such interactions has been reviewed by Tanriverdi et al. (2003) and Quintanar (2011).

Immune response to GnRH administration

Proliferation

Induction. When splenocytes and thymocytes are preincubated with GnRH-a or GnRH peptide, an augmentation of the proliferative response is obtained. Marchetti et al. (1989) showed a significant dose-dependent increase on proliferative response to the mitogen ConA in rat thymocytes. This response was abolished with simultaneous addition of a GnRH-ant. Also, splenocytes and thymocytes from proestrus female rats incubated with GnRH or its analogs, significantly increased the basal proliferative activity which was accompanied by a specific increase in IL-2 receptor-positive cells (Batticane et al., 1991).

Furthermore, *in vivo* GnRH-a treatment prevents thymus atrophy and markedly stimulates thymocyte blastogenic activity in hypophysectomized rats, thus suggesting that GnRH and its agonistic analogs are may capable to exert a direct modulation of immune system function (Marchetti et al., 1989).

Injection of GnRH-a increases CD8+ T-cell levels and proliferation to a variety of mitogens (Mann et al., 1994). In another study, it has been reported that GnRH immunization in rats induced the presence of eosinophils in intertubular tissue of testes whereas in unimmunized controls these cells were not present (Duckett et al., 1997).

Moreover, in a rat model of pregnancy-induced thymic involution, GnRH-a infusions markedly attenuated pregnancy-induced thymic involution resulting in significant increases in thymic weight and thymocyte numbers (Dixit et al., 2003a).

In the same way, Sutherland et al. (2008) made a pilot study in patients, where a GnRH-a (goserelin) was given prior to allogeneic or autologous hematopoietic stem cell transplantation. GnRH-a administration significantly increased neutrophil and lymphocyte numbers within the first month of posttransplantation indicating that either directly or indirectly, GnRH induced an increase in circulating neutrophils.

It has been reported that treatment with the GnRH-a, leuprolide acetate (50 μg/mouse, s.c.) prior to restraint stress, significantly prevented its effect on cell-mediated immunity, antibody titer levels, total leukocyte count and relative thymus weight, showing a significant increase of these immunological parameters (Umathe et al., 2008).

Supression. To test whether a GnRH-a could alter *in vivo* human immune cells, Ho et al. (1995) treated a group of infertile patients under a protocol of buserelin acetate administration and peripheral B cells, NK cells, CD4+ and CD8+ T cells, and the expression of CD69, CD25, human leucocyte antigen-DR (HLA-DR), and CD71 antigens on the T cells were serially examined by dual-color flow cytometry. They found that the GnRH-a had a transiently immunosuppressive effect on CD4+ and CD25+ T cells, but CD69+, CD25+, and HLA-DR+ T cells were activated during and after successful implantation. Regarding to the B cells, NK cells, CD8+ T cells, and CD71+ T lymphocyte subpopulations there were no changes throughout the whole course of treatment.

On the other hand, several groups have provided evidence that the *in vitro* proliferation of a variety of human ovarian, endometrial, and breast cancer cell lines can be inhibited by agonistic and/or antagonistic analogs of GnRH in a dose- and time-dependent manner (Eidne et al., 1987; Thompson et al., 1991; Emons et al., 1993a,b; Emons and Schally, 1994).

In ovarian cancer cells, GnRH seems to have two opposite activities:

1. The antimitotic activity through inhibition of signal transduction of mitogens such as epidermal growth factor, and
2. The inhibition of Doxorubicin-induced apoptosis via activation of transcription nuclear factor kappa B (NFkB) as shown by Gründker et al. (2000). In this report is clearly suggested that GnRH-a Triptorelin inhibits Doxorubicin-induced apoptosis via activation of NFkB.

Furthermore, biopsy specimens collected from lesions, myometria and corresponding endometria of women with ovarian endometrioma, adenomyosis and uterine myoma treated with the GnRH-a, leuprolide acetate, for a variable period of 3–6 months before surgery, showed a significantly decrease in the infiltration of CD68-positive Mϕ, micro-vessel density and tissue levels of monocyte chemotactic protein I (MCP-I). Furthermore, when compared with the non-treated group, a significant increase in apoptotic index and quantitative-histogram scores of activated caspase-3 after GnRH-a therapy were observed in the eutopic endometria, lesions and myometria of these diseases (Khan et al., 2010).

Tanriverdi et al. (2005) demonstrated that GnRH-I and GnRH-II have differential modulatory effects on human PBMC proliferation and IL-2Rγ-chain mRNA expression in healthy males. Treatment of *in vitro* PMBCs with GnRH-I and with IL-2 resulted in a significant increase in cell proliferation as well as in an increased expression of IL-2Rγ mRNA in a dose dependent manner compared with the untreated control. In contrast, GnRH-II administration did not affect the proliferation of PMBCs alone, and IL-2Rγ expression was significantly decreased in all concentrations. This study clearly indicates the potential stimulatory effects of GnRH-I in PBMCs and reduction of these effects by GnRH-II.

Induces GnRH production by immune cells. Numerous interesting and solid studies show that T-cells (and other immune cells) can in fact produce and secrete various endogenous neurotransmitters, either spontaneously or after induction by external stimuli. Among neurotransmitters produced by T-cells are GnRH-I and GnRH-II (Levite, 2008).

Immunoactive and bioactive GnRH peptide is present and the GnRH message is expressed in human peripheral blood T-cells. Both $CD4^+$ and $CD8^+$ subsets of T-cells produce GnRH and it is significantly increased when cells are activated by either phytohemagglutinin or anti-CD3 antibody. This GnRH production in activated T-cells is an early activation event that is independent of IL-2 system activation and DNA synthesis (Azad et al., 1993).

Induces immune mediators production. To investigate the role of GnRH in the modulation of T helper cytokines in pregnant rats undergoing termination of pregnancy, Dixit et al. (2003b) administrated a GnRH-a to evaluate effects on Th-1 and Th-2 cytokines. A marked increase in IFN-γ, inhibition of IL-4 production and an IL-2 and IL-10 absent response was observed. It is possible that IL-2 levels are unchanged because it might has been consumed by activated T cells (Quintanar, 2011).

Recently, Goldberg et al. (2009) demonstrated in a clinically relevant model of allogeneic bone marrow transplantation, that after leuprolide acetate treatment, the enhanced peripheral T cell reconstitution is due to both increases in lymphoid-committed precursors as well as enhanced thymic regeneration.

GnRH has also been reported to regulate four angiogenic chemokines expression (CXCL2, CXCL3, CXCL6, and CXCL8) in human placenta, where trophoblasts were subsequently shown to recruit lymphocytes. Additionally, in Jurkat T cells and primary peripheral blood T and uterine NK cells; chemokine release was detected in chemotaxis assays and this was shown to be GnRH dependent (Cavanagh et al., 2009).

There are two works evaluating the efficacy of the GnRH-a, leuprolide acetate, on NK cells activity in endometriosis. Results are contradictory since the first one suggests an increased NK cell activity in peripheral blood samples determined by 51Cr release assay (Umesaki et al., 1999); and the second one reported that NK cell cytotoxicity from control and patients was significantly decreased with leuprolide acetate (Wong and Simon, 2004). These findings suggest a direct immunomodulatory role of GnRH on NK cell activity.

In an attempt to know the possible immunomodulatory effects of GnRH on LPS activated human peripheral blood monocytes cultured *in vitro*, Komorowski and Stepien (1995) found that GnRH did not affect the secretion of the cytokines IL-1β and IL-6.

On the other hand, there is a report where the immunomodulation exerted by GnRH on freshly isolated primary peritoneal macrophages is clearly observed. In this work the authors found that the production of nitric oxide, co-stimulated with LPS and IFNγ, and the activity of NF-kB was suppressed by GnRH exposure. Taken together, these results demonstrate that GnRH participates in macrophage function and indicate that the NF-kB signaling pathway may be responsible for GnRH-mediated immune modulation (Min et al., 2009).

GnRH expression response against immune system challenges

There is a work that reported that when lymphocyte lysates were applied to rat anterior pituitary cells in monolayer culture, significant stimulation of GnRH secretion was seen. This response evoked by lymphocyte lysates was found to be dose dependent and could be significantly inhibited by a GnRH-ant (Emanuele et al., 1990).

Otherwise, TNF has a number of regulatory actions on gonadotrophic functions: TNF and other cytokines, notably IL-1β, have powerful LH suppressing abilities on pituitary activity (Kalra et al., 1998).

GnRH and autoimmunity

Given that GnRH possesses direct immunostimulatory actions, it has been hypothesized that GnRH might play a role in the development of autoimmune disease.

Jacobson et al. (1994) demonstrated that the administration of GnRH antagonists in a mouse model of systemic lupus erythematosus (SLE), led to a reduction in autoantibody levels, total immunoglobulin levels, renal disease, and significantly improved survival, independently of gonadal steroids.

Based on the above mentioned findings and considering that (1) in the nonobese mouse model of autoimmune diabetes (NOD mouse), castration of male NOD mice leads to increased incidence of diabetes, and that (2) castration of male mice leads to an increase in GnRH action, Ansari et al. (2004) determined the effect of GnRH agonists and antagonists on expression of autoimmune diabetes in this mouse model. Their results showed that Antide administration prevented the increased incidence of diabetes, reduced total serum IgG levels, IL-6 cytokine expression in cultured splenocytes, and the lymphocytic infiltration of islets. GnRH administration exerted reciprocal effects, leading to earlier timing of onset of diabetes and increased serum total IgG levels.

In addition, due to that has been reported that motoneurons of spinal cord of rat from embryonic until adult stage, express GnRHRs which respond to GnRH (Quintanar et al., 2009) a possible clinical use in spinal cord injury (Calderón-Vallejo and Quintanar, 2012) and CNS autoimmune diseases has been proposed. Specifically, treatment with GnRH (Quintanar, 2011) or a synthetic analog (Guzmán-Soto et al., 2012) induces an improvement of clinical signs in the EAE model, where they remained significantly lower in EAE rats with GnRH administration compared to animals without treatment. In these experiments, also a significantly increased expression of neurofilaments (NFs) and myelin basic protein as well as more axons of larger areas in the spinal cord of EAE animals were found.

A great advantage of GnRH and its analog leuprolide acetate, is that they are capable to cross the blood brain barrier (Kastin et al., 1980; Barrera et al., 1991) and reach their targets into the CNS. Taking into account this advantage of leuprolide acetate and its effect on recovery in locomotion and increased expression of biological markers, the use of this agonist as a potential therapeutic approach for traumatic or neurodegenerative diseases such as multiple sclerosis should be considered.

The effects of GnRH on immune system are summarized in **Figure 3**.

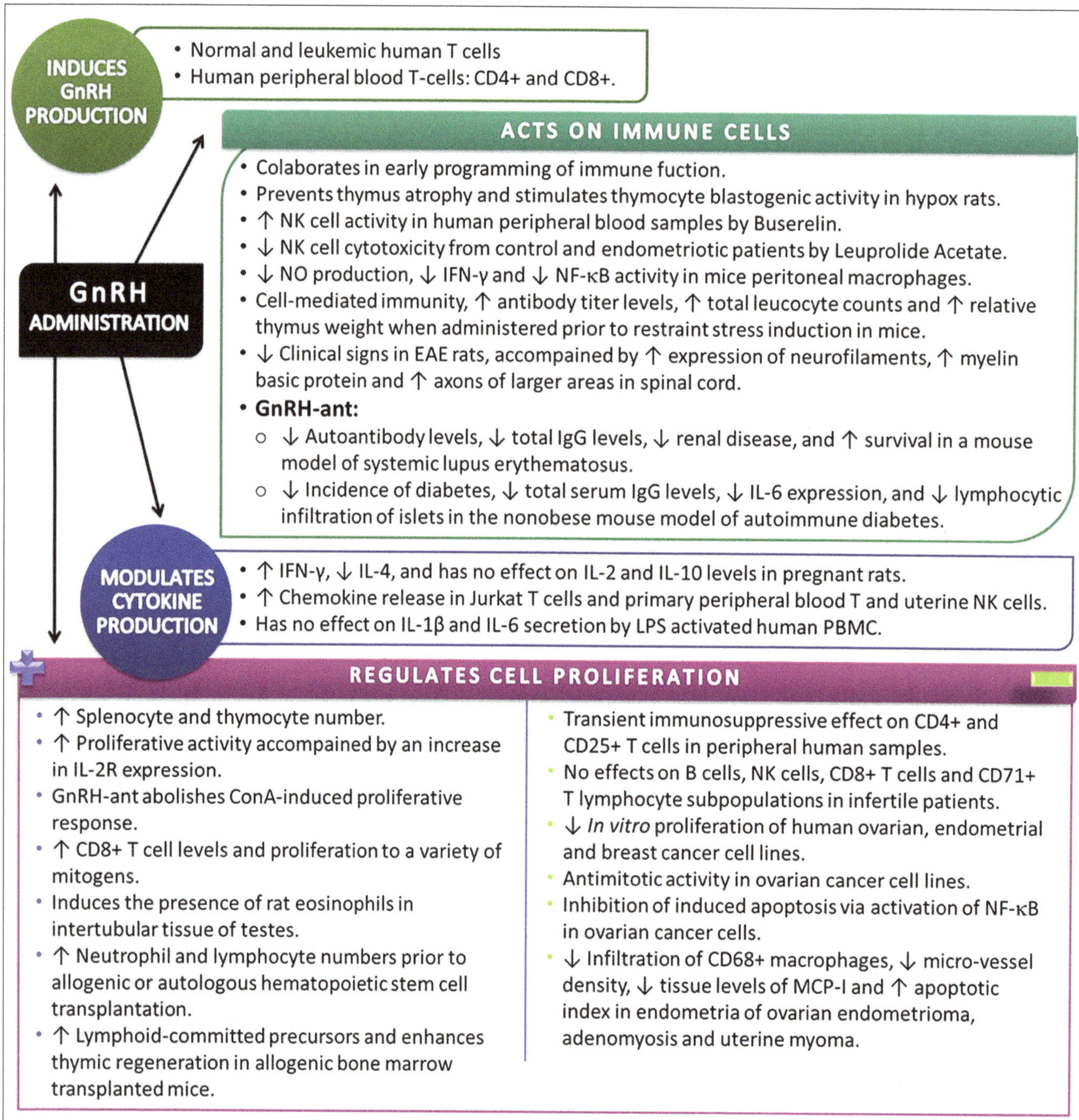

FIGURE 3 | Summary of experimental data showing the effects of Gonadotropin-Releasing Hormone/Gonadotropin-Releasing Hormone agonist on the immune system. Extrapituitary GnRH is implicated in a wide range of immunological processes, including direct cell immunomodulation and proliferative responses (↑ = increase, ↓ = decrease).

Clinical relevance and future directions

GnRH induces the secretion of FSH-LH and consequently of sex hormones, which are involved in the immune response. Controversial is the idea that sex hormones are immunoprotective because depending on the type of hormone and experimental conditions can be obtained opposite effects.

The presence of GnRH receptors and GnRH secretion by cells of the immune system, opening the spectrum of possibilities for interaction of autocrine or paracrine regulation. However, the pharmacological use of GnRH or its analogues, independently of the direct effect of sex hormones, raise the possibility that can be used as a inflammatory regulator in autoimmune diseases. Retrospective studies can be analyzed to establish whether treatment with GnRH analogues have improved immunological conditions of patients with autoimmune pathology. This option can be explored in future works.

CONCLUSION

Hypothalamic hormones are closely related to the immune system. Their direct and indirect effects establish a bidirectional network to establish the required mechanisms to maintain homeostasis.

TRH, CRH and GnRH exhibit common patterns of specific receptors in immune cells and tissues. It is hard to think in the action of a single independent factor within the neuroimmunoendocrine network. When any of these elements destabilize, the system is altered and is difficult to define which factor of all may have been responsible for the alteration. Perhaps because of the complexity of the network, experiments to demonstrate such events become complicated to study. Using *in vitro* models allow clarify in a specific manner some of the elements involved in the homeostasis, however, extrapolate it to *in vivo* models could lead to unreliable interpretations.

In the evolution of the knowledge of the involvement of neurohormones on the immune system, we can find that many of the investigations are related to their pharmacological application, however, few of them concern to the physiological mechanism of its immunomodulation either autocrine or paracrine. If more is known about the physiology of these neurohormones, expectations about their applications at therapeutic level or to the understanding of our complex responses to internal or external challenges to maintain the survival of the individual could be proposed.

REFERENCES

Aguilera, G., Wynn, P. C., Harwood, J. P., Hauger, R. L., Millan, M. A., Grewe, C., et al. (1986). Receptor-mediated actions of corticotropin-releasing factor in pituitary gland and nervous system. *Neuroendocrinology* 43, 79–88. doi: 10.1159/000124513

Angioni, S., Petraglia, F., Gallineli, A., Cosarizza, A., Franceschi, C., Michela, M., et al. (1993). Corti- cotropin releasing hormone modulates cytokines release in cultured human peripheral blood mononuclear cells. *Life Sci.* 53, 1735–1742. doi: 10.1016/0024-3205(93)90160-5

Ansari, M. A., Dhar, M., Spieker, S., Bakht, N., Rahman, A. M.,Moore, W. V., et al. (2004). Modulation of diabetes with gonadotropin-releasing hormone antagonists in the nonobese mouse model of autoimmune diabetes. *Endocrinology* 145, 337–342. doi: 10.1210/en.2003-0512

Aten, R. F., Polan, M. L., Bayless, R., and Behrman, H. R. (1987). A gonadotropin-releasing hormone (GnRH)-like protein in human ovaries: similarity to the GnRH-like ovarian protein of the rat. *J. Clin. Endocrinol. Metab.* 64, 1288–1293. doi:10.1210/jcem-64-6-1288

Audhya, T., Jain, R., and Hollan- der, C. S. (1991). Receptor- mediated immunomodulation by corticotropin-releasing factor. *Cell. Immunol.* 134, 77–84. doi: 10.1016/0008-8749(91)90332-6

Azad, N., Jurgens, J., Young, M., Reda, D., Duffner, L., and Kirsteins, L. (1991). Presence of luteiniz- ing hormone-releasing hormone in rat thymus. *Prog. Neuro. Endocr. Immunol.* 4, 113–120.

Azad, N., La Paglia, N., Jurgens, K. A., Kirsteins, L., Emanuele, N. V., Kelley, M. R., et al. (1993). Immunoactivation enhances the concentration of luteinizing hormone-releasing hormone pep- tide and its gene expression in human peripheral T-lymphocytes. *Endocrinology* 133, 215–223. doi: 10.1210/en.133.1.215

Baigent, S. M., and Lowry, P. J. (2000). mRNA expression pro- files for corticotrophin-releasing factor (CRF), urocortin, CRF receptors and CRF-binding pro- tein in peripheral rat tissues. *J. Mol. Endocrinol.* 25, 43–52. doi: 10.1677/jme.0.0250043

Bale, T. L., and Vale, W. W. (2004). CRF and CRF receptors: role in stress responsivity and other behav- iors. *Annu. Rev. Pharmacol. Toxicol.* 44, 525–557. doi: 10.1146/annurev. pharmtox.44.101802.121410

Barrera, C. M., Kastin, A. J., Fasold, M. B., and Banks, W. A. (1991). Bidirec- tional saturable transport of LHRH across the blood-brain barrier. *Am. J. Physiol.* 261, E312–E318.

Batticane, N., Morale, M. C., Gallo, F., Farinella, Z., and Marchetti, B. (1991). Luteinizing hormone- releasing hormone signaling at the lymphocyte involves stimulation of interleukin-2 receptor expression. *Endocrinology* 129, 277–286. doi: 10.1210/endo-129-1-277

Bílek, R., Bicíková, M., and Šafarík, L. (2011). TRH-Like peptides. *Physiol. Res.* 60, 207–215.

Blum, C., Grozdea, J., and Vergnes, H. (1976). Cytochemical aspects of human polynuclear neutrophils under the *in vitro* and in vivo action of TRH. *C. R. Seances Soc. Biol. Fil.* 170, 666–671.

Boler, J., Enzmann, F., Folkers, K., Bow- ers, C. Y., and Shally, A. V. (1969). The identity of chemical and hor- monal properties of the thyrotropin releasing hormone and pyro- glutamyl-histidil-proline amide. *Biochem. Biophys. Res. Commun.* 37, 705–710. doi: 10.1016/0006-291x(69)90868-7

Boyadjieva, N., Advis, J. P., and Sarkar, D. K. (2006). Role of beta- endorphin, corticotropin-releasing hormone and autonomic nervous system in mediation of the effect of chronic ethanol on natural killer cell cytolytic activity. *Alcohol. Clin. Exp. Res.* 30, 1761–1767. doi: 10.1111/j.1530-0277.2006.00209.x

Brod, S., and Bauer, V. (2013). Ingested (oral) thyrotropin releasing factor (TRH) inhibits EAE. *Citokine* 61, 323–328. doi: 10.1016/j.cyto.2012.10.015

Brouxhon, S. M., Prasad, A. V., Joseph, S. A., Felten, D. L., and Bellinger, D. L. (1998). Localiza- tion of corticotropin releasing factor in primary and secondary lymphoid organs of the rat. *Brain Behav. Immun.* 12, 107–122. doi: 10.1006/brbi.1998.0520

Burgus, R., Dunn, T. F., Desiderio, D., Vale, W., and Guillemin, R. (1969). Derives polypeptidiques de syn- theses doues d'activite hypophys- iotrope TRF. Nouvelles observa- tions. *C. R. Acad. Sci. Hebd. Seances Acad. Sci. D.* 269, 226–228.

Calderón-Vallejo, D., and Quintanar, J. L. (2012). Gonadotropin-releasing hormone treatment improves locomotor activity, urinary func- tion and neurofilament protein expression after spinal cord injury in ovariectomized rats. *Neu- rosci. Lett.* 515, 187–190. doi: 10.1016/j.neulet.2012.03.052

Cao, J., Papadopoulou, N., Kempuraj, D., Boucher, W. S., Sugimoto, K., Cetrulo, C. L., et al. (2005). Human mast cells express corticotropin- releasing hormone (CRH) receptors and CRH leads to selective secretion of vascular endothelial growth fac- tor. *J. Immunol.* 174, 7665–7675.

Cavanagh, P. C., Dunk, C., Pampillo, M., Szereszewski, J. M., Taylor, J. E., Kahiri, C., et al. (2009). Gonadotropin-releasing hormone- regulated chemokine expression in human placentation. *Am. J. Physiol. Cell Physiol.* 297, 17- 27. doi: 10.1152/ajpcell.00013. 2009

Chatzaki, E., Murphy, B. J., Wang, L., Million, M., Ohning, G. V., Crowe, P. D., et al. (2004). Dif- ferential profile of CRF receptor distribution in the rat stomach and duodenum assessed by newly developed CRF receptor antibod- ies. *J. Neurochem.* 88, 1–11. doi: 10.1046/j.1471-4159.2003.02078.x

Chen, A., Ganor, Y., Rahimipour, S., Ben-Aroya, N., Koch, Y., and Levite, M. (2002). The neuropep- tides GnRH-II and GnRH-I are produced by human T cells and trigger laminin receptor gene expression, adhesion, chemotaxis and homing to specific organs. *Nat. Med.* 8, 1421–1426. doi: 10.1038/nm801 messenger ribonucleic acids that are regu- lated by GnRH *in vitro*. *J. Clin. Endocrinol. Metab.* 84, 743–750. doi: 10.1210/jc.84.2.743

Chen, X. Q., Dong, J., Niu, C. Y., Fan, J. M., and Du, J. Z. (2007). Effects of hypoxia on glucose, insulin, glucagon and modula- tion by corticotropin-releasing factor receptor type 1 in the rat. *Endocrinology* 148, 3271–3278. doi: 10.1210/en.2006-1224

Cheng, C. K., and Leung, P. C. K. (2005). Molecular biology of gonadotropin-releasing hormone (GnRH)-I, GnRH-II and their receptors in humans. *Endocr. Rev.* 26, 283–306. doi: 10.1210/er.2003-0039

Cheung, L. W., and Wong, A. S. (2008). Gonadotropin-releasing hormone: GnRH receptor signaling in extra- pituitary tissues. *FEBS J.* 275, 5479–5495. doi: 10.1111/j.1742-4658.2008.06677.x

Chiamolera, M. I., and Wondisford, F.E. (2009). Minireview: thyrotropin-releasing hormone and the thy- roid hormone feedback mechanism. *Endocrinology* 150, 1091–1096. doi: 10.1210/en.2008-1795

Ciechanowska, M., Lapot, M., Mateu- siak, K., and Przekop, F. (2010). Neuroendocrine regulation of GnRH release and expression of GnRH and GnRH receptor genes in the hypothalamus-pituitary unit in different physiological states. *Reprod. Biol.* 10, 85–124. doi: 10.1016/s1642-431x(12)60054-0

Clarke, I. J., and Pompolo, S. (2005). Synthesis and secretion of GnRH. *Anim. Reprod. Sci.* 88, 29–55. doi: 10.1016/j.anireprosci.2005.05.003

Colson, A.-O., Perlman, J. H., Smolyar, A., Gershengorn, M. C., and Osman,R. (1998). Static and dynamic roles of extracellular loops in G-Protein- Coupled receptors: a mechanism for sequential binding of thyrotropin- releasing hormone to its recep- tor. *Biophys. J.* 74, 1087–1100. doi: 10.1016/s0006-3495(98)77827-0

Conn, P. M., and Janovick, J. A. (2009). Trafficking and quality con- trol of the gonadotropin releasing hormone receptor in health and disease. *Mol. Cell. Endocrinol.* 299, 137–145. doi: 10.1016/j.mce.2008.10.051

Dixit, V. D., Sridaran, R., Edmonsond, M. A., Taub, D., and Thompson, W.E. (2003a). Gonadotropin-releasing hormone attenuates pregnancy- associated thymic involution and modulates the expression of antiproliferative gene product pro- hibitin. *Endocrinology* 144, 1496– 1505. doi: 10.1210/en.2002-220955

Dixit, V. D., Yang, H., Udhayaku- mar, V., and Sridaran, R. (2003b). Gonadotropin-releasing hormone alters the T helper cytokine balance in the pregnant rat. *Biol. Reprod.* 68, 2215–2221. doi: 10.1095/biolre- prod.102.012211

Dong, K. W., Yu, K. L., and Roberts, J.L. (1993). Identification of a major up-stream transcription start site for the human progonadotropin- releasing hormone gene used in reproductive tissues and cell lines. *Mol. Endocrinol.* 7, 1654–1666. doi: 10.1210/me.7.12.1654

Duckett, R. J., Hedger, M. P., McLachlan, R. I., and Wreford,N. G. (1997). The effects of gonadotropin-releasing hormone immunization and recombinant follicle-stimulating hormone on the leydig cell and macrophage populations of the adult rat testis. *J. Androl.* 18, 417–423.

Dufau, M. L., Tinajero, J. C., andFabbri, A. (1993). Corticotropin- releasing factor: an antireproductive hormone of the testis. *FASEB J.* 7, 299–307.

Eidne, K. A., Flanagan, C. A., Harris, N. S., and Millar, R. P. (1987). Gonadotropin-releasing hormone (GnRH)-binding sites in human breast cancer cell lines and inhi- bitory effects of GnRH antagonists.*J. Clin. Endocrinol. Metab.* 64, 425– 432. doi: 10.1210/jcem-64-3-425

Emanuele, N. V., Emanuele, M. A., Tentler, J., Kirsteins, L., Azad, N., and Lawrence, A. M. (1990). Rat spleen lymphocytes contain an immunoactive and bioactive luteinizing hormone-releasing hormone. *Endocrinology* 126, 2482–2486. doi: 10.1210/endo-126-5-2482

Emeric-Sauval, E. (1986). Corticotropin-releasing factor (CRF) a review. *Psychoneuroen- docrinology* 11, 277–294. doi: 10.1016/0306-4530(86)90014-4

Emons, G., and Schally, A. V. (1994). The use of luteinizing hormone releasing hormone agonists and antagonists in gynecological can- cers. *Hum. Reprod.* 9, 1362–1379.

Emons, G., Schröder, B., Ortmann, O., Westphalen, S., Schulz, K. D., and Schally, A. V. (1993a). High affinity binding and direct antipro- liferative effects of luteinizing hormone-releasing hormone analogs in human endome- trial cancer cell lines. *J. Clin. Endocrinol. Metab.* 77, 1458–1464. doi: 10.1210/jc.77.6.1458

Emons, G., Ortmann, O., Becker, M., Irmer, G., Springer, B., Laun, R., et al. (1993b). High-affinity bind- ing sites and direct antiprolifera- tive effects of LHRH analogues in human ovarian cancer cell lines. *Cancer Res.* 53, 5439–5446. doi: 10.1210/jc.77.6.1458

Engel, S., Neumann, S., Kaur, N., Monga, V., Jain, R., Northup, J., et al. (2006). Low affinity analogs of thyrotropin-releasing hormone are super-agonists. *J. Biol. Chem.* 281, 3103–13109. doi: 10.1074/jbc.m600440200

Engler, D., Scanlon, M. F., and Jack- son, I. M. D. (1981). Thyrotropin-releasing hormone in the systemic circulation of the neonatal rat is derived from the pancreas and other extraneural tissues. *J. Clin. Invest.* 67, 800–808. doi: 10.1172/jci 110097

Esposito, P., Chandler, N., Kandere, K., Basu, S., Jacobson, S., Conolly, R., et al. (2002). Corticotropin-releasing hormone and brain mast cells reg- ulate BBB permeability induced by acute stress. *J. Pharmacol. Exp. Therapeut.* 303, 1061–1066. doi: 10.1124/jpet.102.038497

Feng, P., Carnell, N. E., Kim, U. J., Jacobs, S., and Wilber, J. F. (1992). The human testis: a novel locus for thyrotropin-releasing hormone (TRH) and TRH mRNA. *Trans. Assoc. Am. Physicians* 105, 222–228.

Fukusumi, S., Ogi, K., Onda, H., and Hinuma, S. (1995). Distribution of thyrotropin-releasing hormone receptor mRNA in rat peripheral tis- sues. *Regul. Pept.* 57, 115–121. doi: 10.1016/0167-0115(95)00026-8

Gary, K. A., Sevarino, K. A., Yarbrough, G. G., Prange, A. J. Jr., and Winokur,A. (2003). The thyrotropin- releasing hormone (TRH) hypoth- esis of homeostatic regulation: implications for TRH-based ther- apeutics. *J. Pharmacol. Exp. Ther.* 305, 410–416. doi: 10.1124/jpet.102. 044040

Gill, C. J., and Rissman, E. F. (1998). Mast cells in the neonate musk shrew brain: implications for neuroendocrine immune interac- tions. *Brain Res. Dev. Brain Res.* 111, 129–136. doi: 10.1016/s0165-3806(98)00121-7

Goldberg, G. L., King, C. G., Nejat,R. A., Suh, D. Y., Smith, O. M., Bretz, J. C., et al. (2009). Luteiniz- ing hormone-releasing hormone enhances T cell recovery following allogeneic bone marrow transplan- tation. *J. Immunol.* 182, 5846–5854. doi: 10.4049/jimmunol.0801458

Grammatopoulos, D. K., and Chrousos, G. P. (2002). Functional characteristics of CRH receptors and potential clinical applications of CRH-receptor antagonists. *Trends Endocrinol. Metab.* 13, 436–444. doi: 10.1016/s1043-2760(02)00670-7

Grasso, G., Massai, L., De Leo, V., and Muscettola, M. (1998). The effect of LHRH and TRH on human Interferon-y production in vivo and *invitro.Life Sci.* 62, 2005–2014. doi: 10.1016/s0024-3205(98)00172-6

Gravanis, A., and Margioris, A. (2005).The corticotropin-releasing factor (CRF) family of neuropeptides in inflammation: potential therapeu- tic applications. Bioactive peptides for immune disease therapy. *Curr. Med. Chem.* 13, 1503–1512. doi: 10.2174/0929867054039008

Gründker, C., Schulz, K., Günthert,A. R., and Emons, G. (2000). Luteinizing hormone-releasing hor- mone induces nuclear factor kappa B-activation and inhibits apopto- sis in ovarian cancer cells. *J. Clin. Endocrinol. Metab.* 85, 3815–3820. doi: 10.1210/jc.85.10.3815

Guillemin, R. (2005). Hypothalamichormones a.k.a. hypothalamic releasing factors. *J. Endocrinol.* 184, 11–28. doi: 10.1677/joe.1.05883

Guzmán-Soto, I., Salinas, E., Hernández-Jasso, I., and Quin- tanar, J. L. (2012). Leupro- lide acetate, a GnRH agonist, improves experimental autoim- mune encephalomyelitis: a possible therapy for multiple sclerosis. *Neu- rochem. Res.* 37, 2190–2197. doi: 10.1007/s11064-012-0842-x

Haddad, E. E., and Mashaly, M. M. (1992). Augmentation of natural cell-mediated cytotoxic activity by supernatant from *in vitro* mitogen-stimulated, in vivo hormone-treated lymphocytes in immature male (K strain) chickens. *Immunol. Invest.* 21, 365–375. doi: 10.3109/08820139209069376

Hagan, P., Poole, S., and Bristow, A. F. (1992). Immunosuppressive activ- ity of corticotropin releasing factor: inhibition of IL-1 and IL-6 produc- tion by human mononuclear cells. *Biochem. J.* 281, 251–254.

Harbour, D. V., Kruger, T. E., Cop- penhaver, D., Smith, E. M., and Meyer, W. J. (1981). Differential expression and regulation of thy- rotropin (TSH) in T cell lines. *Mol. Cell. Endocrinol.* 64, 229–241. doi: 10.1016/0303-7207(89)90150-0

Harbuz, M. S., Stephanou, A., Sarlis, N., and Lightman, S. L. (1992). The effects of recombinant human IL-1-alpha, Il-1-beta or IL-6 on hypothalamic–pituitary–adrenal axis activation. *J. Endocrinol.* 133, 349–355.

Harris, G. W. (1948). Neural control of the pituitary gland. *Physiol. Rev.* 28, 139–179.

Harrison, G. S., Wierman, M. E., Nett, T. M., and Glode, L. M. (2004). Gonadotropin-releasing hormone and its receptor in nor- mal and malignant cells. *Endocr. Relat. Cancer* 11, 725–748. doi: 10.1677/erc.1.00777

Hart, R., Wagner, F., Steffens, W., Lersch, C., Dancygier, H., Dun- tas, L., et al. (1990). Effect of thyrotropin-releasing hormone on immune functions of peripheral blood mononuclear cells. *Regul. Pept.* 27, 335–342. doi: 10.1016/0167-0115(90)90122-d

Heinrichs, S. C., Cole, B. J., Pich, E. M., Menzaghi, F., Koob, G. F., and Hauger, R. L. (1992). Endoge- nous corticotropin-releasing factor modulates feeding induced by neuropeptide Y or a tail-pinch stressor. *Peptides* 13, 879–884. doi: 10.1016/0196-9781(92)90044-4

Hinkle, P. M., Gehret, A. U., and Jones, B. W. (2012). Desensiti- zation, trafficking and resensitiza- tion of the pituitary thyrotropin- releasing hormone receptor. *Front. Neurosci.* 6:180. doi: 10.3389/fnins. 2012.00180

Ho, H. N., Chen, H. F., Chen, S. U., Chao, K. H., Yang, Y. S., Huang, C., et al. (1995). Gonadotropin releasing hormone (GnRH) ago- nist induces down-regulation of the CD3+CD25+ lympho- cyte subpopulation in peripheral blood. *Am. J. Reprod. Immunol.* 33, 243–252. doi: 10.1111/j.1600-0897.1995. tb00891.x

Inoue, K., Valdez, G. R., Reyes, T. M., Reinhardt, L. E., Tabarin, A., Riv- ier, J., et al. (2003). Human uro- cortin II, a selective agonist for the type 2 corticotropin-releasing fac- tor receptor decreases feeding and drinking in the rat. *J. Pharma- col. Exp. Ther.* 305, 385–393. doi: 10.1124/jpet.102.047712

Irwin, M. R. (1993). Brain corti- cotropin releasing hormone and interleukin-1β induced suppression of specific antibody production. *Endocrinology.* 133, 1352–1360. doi: 10.1210/en.133.3.1352

Irwin, M. R., Vale, W., and Britton, K. (1987). Central corticotropin- releasing factor suppresses nat- ural killer cytotoxicity. *Brain Behav. Immun.* 1, 81–87. doi: 10.1016/0889-1591(87)90009-2

Jacobson, J. D., Nisula, B. C., and Steinberg, A. D. (1994). Modulation of the expression of murine lupus by gonadotropin-releasing hor- mone analogs. *Endocrinology* 134, 2516–2523. doi: 10.1210/en.134.6. 2516

Janssen, D., and Kozicz, T. (2013). Is it really a matter of simple dual- ism? Corticotropin-releasing factor receptors in body and mental health. *Front. Endocrinol. (Lausanne)* 4:28. doi: 10.3389/fendo.2013.00028

Justice, N. J., Yuan, Z. F., Sawchenko, P. E., and Vale, W. (2008). Type 1 corticotropin-releasing fac- tor receptor expression reported in BAC transgenic mice: impli- cations for reconciling ligand- receptor mismatch in the central corticotropin-releasing factors sys- tem. *J. Comp. Neurol.* 511, 479–496. doi: 10.1002/cne.21848

Kalra, P. S., Edwards, T. G., Xu, B., Jain, M., and Kalra, S. P. (1998). The anti-gonadotropic effects of cytokines: the role of neuropeptides. *Domest. Anim. Endocrinol.* 15, 321–332. doi: 10.1016/s0739-7240(98)00030-7

Kamath, J., Yarbrough, G. G., Prange, A. J. Jr., and Winokur, A. (2009). The thyrotropin-releasing hor- mone (TRH)–immune system homeostatic hypothesis. *Phar- macol. Ther.* 121, 20–28. doi: 10.1016/j.pharmthera.2008.09.004

Karalis, K., Muglia, L. J., Bae, D., Hilderbrand, H., and Majzoub, J. A. (1997). CRH and the immune sys- tem. *J. Neuroimmunol.* 72, 131–136. Kastin, A. J., Coy, D. H., Schally, A. V., and Zadina, J. E. (1980). Dissociation of effects of LH-RH analogs on pituitary regulation and reproductive behavior. *Pharmacol. Biochem. Behav.* 13, 913–914. doi: 10.1016/0091-3057(80)90228-2

Kawahito, Y., Sano, H., Mukai, S., Asai, K., Kimura, S., Yamamura, Y., et al. (1995). Corticotropin releasing hor- mone in colonic mucosa in patients with ulcerative colitis. *Gut* 37, 544–551. doi: 10.1136/gut.37.4.544

Kawano, H., Daikoku, S., and Saito, S. (1983). Location of thyrotropin-releasing hormone-like immunoreactivity in rat pancreas. *Endocrinology* 112, 951–955. doi: 10.1210/endo-112-3-951

Kempuraj, D., Papadopoulou, N. G., Lytinas, M., Huang, M., Kandere-Grzybowska, K., Madhappan, B., et al. (2004). Corticotropin-releasing hormone and its structurally related urocortin are synthesized and secreted by human mast cells. *Endocrinology* 145, 43–48. doi: 10.1210/en.2003-0805

Khalil, M. H., Silverman, A. J., and Silver, R. (2003). Mast cells in the rat brain synthesize gonadotropin- releasing hormone. *J. Neurobiol.* 56, 113–124. doi: 10.1002/neu. 10220

Khan, K. N., Kitajima, M., Hiraki, K., Fujishita, A., Sekine, I., Ishi- maru, T., et al. (2010). Changes in tissue inflammation, angiogenesis and apoptosis in endometriosis, adenomyosis and uterine myoma after GnRH agonist therapy. *Hum. Reprod.* 25, 642–653. doi: 10.1093/humrep/dep437

Khan, M. A., Ferro, V. A., and Stimson, W. H. (2003). Use of a highly specific monoclonal antibody against the central variable amino acid sequence of mammalian gonadotropin releasing hormone to evaluate GnRH-I tissue distribution compared with GnRH-I binding sites in adult male rats. *Am. J. Reprod. Immunol.* 49, 239–248. doi: 10.1034/j.1600-0897.2003.01202.x

Khomane, K. S., Meena, C. L., Jain, R., and Bansal, A. K. (2011). Novel thyrotropin-releasing hormone analogs: a patent review. *Expert. Opin. Ther. Pat.* 21, 1673–1691. doi: 10.1517/13543776.2011.623127

Kobayashi, H., Ishizuka, T., and Okayama, Y. (2000). Human mast cells and basophils as sources of cytokines. *Clin. Exp. Allergy* 30, 1205–1212. doi: 10.1046/j.1365-2222.2000.00808.x

Komorowski, J., and Stepien, H. (1995). Somatostatin (SRIF) stimulates the release of interleukin-6 (IL-6) from human peripheral blood mono- cytes (PBM) *in vitro*. *Neuropep- tides* 29, 77–81. doi: 10.1016/0143- 4179(95)90087-x

Komorowski, J., Stepled, H., and Paw˜ likowski, M. (1993). The evidence of thyroliberin/triiodothyronin con- trol of TSH secretory response from human peripheral blood mono- cytes cultured *in vitro*. *Neuropep- tides* 25, 31–34. doi: 10.1016/0143- 4179(93)90065-i

Koob, G. F., and Heinrichs, S. C. (1999). A role for corticotrophin-releasing factor and urocortin in behavioral responses to stressors. *Brain Res.* 848, 141–152. doi: 10.1016/s0006-8993(99)01991-5

Korosi, A., Kozicz, T., Richter, J., Veen- ing, J. G., Olivier, B., and Roubos, E.W. (2007). Corticotropin-releasing factor, urocortin 1, and their recep- tors in the mouse spinal cord. *J. Comp. Neurol.* 502, 973–989. doi: 10.1002/cne.21347

Koshida, H., and Kotake, Y. (1993). Thyrotropin-releasing hormone enhances the superoxide anion production of rabbit peritoneal macrophages stimulated with N-Formyl-Methionyl-Leucyl- Phenylalanine and opsonized zymosan. *Life Sci.* 53, 725–731. doi: 10.1016/0024-3205(93)90249-3

Kruger, T. E., Smith, L. R., Harbour, D.V., and Blalock, J. E. (1989). Thy- rotropin: an endogenous regulator of the *in vitro* immune response. *J. Immunol.* 142, 744–747.

Kuhne, C., Puk, O., Graw, J., Hrabe de Angelis, M., Schutz, G., Wurst, W., et al. (2012). Visualizing corticotropin-releasing hormone receptor type 1 expression and neu- ronal connectivities in the mouse using a novel multifunctional allele. *J. Comp. Neurol.* 520, 3150–3180. doi: 10.1002/cne.23082

Kukain, E. M., Mutsenietse, R. K., and Klusha, V. E. (1982). Comparison of the neuro- and immunomodulator properties of low-molecular neu- ropeptides. *Biull. Eksp. Biol. Med.* 94, 79–82. doi: 10.1007/bf00830729

Kunert-Radek, J., Pawlikowski, M., Stepien, H., and Janecka, A. (1991). Inhibitory effect of thyrotropin releasing hormone on spontaneous proliferation of mouse spleen lymphocytes *in vitro*. *Biochem. Biophys. Res. Commun.* 181, 562–565. doi: 10.1016/0006-291x(91) 91226-3

Lenz, H. J. (1987). Extrapituitary effects of corticotropin-releasing factor. *Horm. Metab. Res. Suppl.* 16, 17–23.

Lersch, C., Hammer, C., Krombach, F., and Dancygier, H. (1989). Effect of thyrotropin-releasing hormone (TRH) on the chemiluminescence (CL) activity of human mononu-clear cells. *J. Clin. Lab. Immunol.* 28, 69–71.

Lesnikov, V. A., Korneva, E. A., Dall'ara, A., and Pierpaoli, W. (1991). The involvement of pineal gland and melatonin in immunity and aging: II. Thyrotropin-releasing hormone and melatonin forestall involution and promote reconstitution of the thymus in anterior hypotha- lamic area (AHA)-lesioned mice. *Int. J. Neurosci.* 62, 141–153. doi: 10.3109/00207459108999767

Levite, M. (2008). Neurotransmitters activate T-cells and elicit crucial functions via neurotransmitter receptors. *Curr. Opin. Pharmacol.* 8, 460–471. doi: 10.1016/j.coph.2008. 05.001

Lewis, K., Li, C., Perrin, M. H., Blount, A., Kunitake, K., Donaldson, C., et al. (2001). Identification of uro- cortin III, an additional member of the corticotropin-releasing fac- tor (CRF) family with high affinity for the CRF2 receptor. *Proc. Natl. Acad. Sci. U S A* 98, 7570–7575. doi: 10.1073/ pnas.121165198

Limonta, P., and Manea, M. (2013). Gonadotropin-releasing hormone receptors as molecular therapeutic targets in prostate cancer: current options and emerging strategies. *Cancer Treat. Rev.* 39, 647–663. doi: 10.1016/j. ctrv.2012.12.003

Lovenberg, T. W., Chalmers, D. T., Liu, C., and DeSouza, E. B. (1995). CRF2 alpha and CRF2 beta recep- tor mRNAs are differentially dis- tributed between the rat central ner- vous system and peripheral tissues. *Endocrinology* 136, 4139–4142. doi: 10.1210/en.136.9.4139

Magon, N. (2011). Gonadotropin releasing hormone agonists: expanding vistas. *Indian J. Endocrinol. Metab.* 15, 261–267. doi: 10.4103/2230-8210.85575

Maier, C., Marchetti, B., LeBoeuf, R., and Blalock, J. (1992). Thymocytes express a mRNA that is identical to hypothalamic luteinizing hormone- releasing hormone mRNA. *Cell. Mol. Neurobiol.* 12, 447–454. doi: 10.1007/bf00711545

Maillot, C., Million, M., Wei, J. Y., Gauthier, A., and Tache, Y. (2000). Peripheral corticotropin-releasing factor and stress-stimulated colonic motor activity involve type 1 receptor in rats. *Gastroen- terology* 119, 1569–1579. doi: 10.1053/ gast.2000.20251

Mann, D. R., Akinbami, M. A., Lunn, S. ., Fraser, H. M., Gould, K. G., and Ansari, A. A. (2000). Endocrine- immune interaction: alterations in immune function resulting from neonatal treatment with a GnRH antagonist and seasonality in male primates. *Am. J. Reprod. Immunol.* 44, 30–40.

Mann, D. R., Ansari, A. A., Akinbami, M. A., Wallen, K., Gould, K. G. and McClure, H. M. (1994). Neona- tal treatment with luteinizing hor- mone releasing hormone analogs alters peripheral lymphocyte subsets and cellular and humorally medi- ated immune responses in juvenile and adult male monkeys. *J. Clin. Endocrinol. Metab.* 78, 292–298. doi: 10.1210/jc.78.2.292

Marchetti, B., Guarcello, V., Morale, M. C., Bartoloni, G., Farinella, Z., Cor- daro, S., et al. (1989). Luteinizing hormone-releasing hormone bind- ing sites in the rat thymus: char- acteristics and biological function. *Endocrinology* 125, 1025–1036. doi: 10.1210/endo-125-2-1025

Marchetti, B., Guarcello, V., Morale, M. C., Bartoloni, G., Palumbo, G. Jr., Raiti, F., et al. (1990). A phys- iological role for the neuropeptide luteinizing hormone-releasing hor- mone (LHRH) during the matu- ration of thymus gland function. *Int. J. Neurosci.* 51, 287–289. doi: 10.3109/00207459008999722

Marone, G. S., Galli, J., and Kita- mura, Y. (2002). Probing the roles of mast cells and basophils in nat- ural and acquired immunity, physi- ology and disease. *Trends Immunol.* 23, 425–427. doi: 10.1016/s1471-4906(02)02274-3

Martino, E., Nardi, M., Vaudagna, G., Simonetti, S., Cilotti, A., Pinchera, A., et al. (1980a). Thyrotropin- releasing hormone-like material in human retina. *J. Endocrinol. Invest.* 3, 267–271.

Martino, E., Nardi, M., Vaudagna, ., Simonetti, S., Cilotti, A., and Pinchera, A. (1980b). Presence of thyrotropin-releasing hormone in porcine and bovine retina. *Experientia* 36, 622–623. doi: 10.1007/bf01965840

Mastorakos, G., Karoutsou, E. I., and Mizamtsidi, M. (2006). Corti- cotropin releasing hormone and the immune/ inflammatory response. *Eur. J. Endocrinol.* 155, S77–S84.

Matre, V., Høvring, P. I., Fjeldheim, Å. -K., Helgeland, L., Orvain, C., andersson, K. B., et al. (2003). The human neuroendocrine thyrotropin-releasing hormone receptor promoter is activated by the haematopoietic transcription factor c-Myb. *Biochem. J.* 372, 851–859.doi:10.1042/bj20030057

McArdle, C. A., Franklin, J., Green, L., and Hislop, J. N. (2002). Signalling, cycling and desensitisation of gonadotrophin-releasing hormone receptors. *J. Endocrinol.* 173, 1–11. doi: 10.1677/joe.0.1730001

McEvoy, A. N., Bresnihan, B., FitzGer- ald, O., and Murphy, E. P. (2001). Corticotropin-releasing hormone signaling in synovial tissue from patients with early inflammatory arthritis is mediated by the type 1 corticotropin-releasing hormone receptor. *Arthritis Rheum.* 44, 1761–1767.

Mellado, M., Fernández-Agulló, T., Rodríguez-Frade, J. M., García San Frutos, M., de la Peña, P., Martínez- A, C., et al. (1999). Expression analysis of the thyrotropin-releasing hormone receptor (TRHR) in the immune system using agonist anti-TRHR monoclonal antibod- ies. *FEBS Lett.* 451, 308–314. doi: 10.1016/s0014-5793(99)00607-9

Millar, R. P. (2005). GnRHs and GnRH receptors. *Anim. Reprod. Sci.* 88, 5–28. doi: 10.1016/j.anireprosci.2005.05.032

Min, J. Y., Park, M. H., Lee, J. K., Kim, H. J., and Park, Y. K. (2009). Gonadotropin-releasing hormone modulates immune system func- tion via the nuclear factor-kappa B pathway in murine Raw264.7 macrophages. *Neuroimmunomodu- lation* 16, 177–184.

Monga, V., Meena, C. L., Rajput, S., Pawar, C., Sharma, S. S., Lu, X., et al. (2011). Synthesis, receptor binding and CNS pharmacological studies of new thyrotropin-releasing hormone (TRH) analogues. *Chem. Med. Chem.* 6, 531–543. doi: 10.1002/cmdc.201000481

Montagne, J.-J., Ladram, A., Nicolas, P., and Bulant, M. (1999). Cloning of thyrotropin-releasing hormone precursor and receptor in rat thymus, adrenal gland and testis. *Endocrinology* 140, 1054–1059. doi: 10.1210/en.140.3.1054

Morale, M. C., Batticane, N., Bar- toloni, G., Guarcello, V., Farinella, Z., Galasso, M. G., et al. (1991). Blockade of central and peripheral luteinizing hormone-releasing hormone (LHRH) receptors in neonatal rats with a potent LHRH-antagonist inhibits the morphofunctional development of the thymus and maturation of the cell-mediated and humoral immune responses. *Endocrinology* 128, 1073–1085. doi: 10.1210/endo-128-2-1073

Morley, J. E. (1979). Extrahypothala- mic thyrotropin-releasing hormone (TRH)-its distribution and its functions. *Life Sci.* 25, 1539–1550. doi: 10.1016/0024-3205(79)90435-1

Mousa, S. A., Bopaiah, C. P., Stein, C., and Schafer, M. (2003). Involve- ment of corticotropin-releasing hor- mone receptor subtypes 1 and 2 in peripheral opioid mediated inhi- bition of inflammatory pain. *Pain* 106, 297–307. doi: 10.1016/s0304-3959(03)00302-6

Müller, M. B., Preil, J., Renner, U., Zim- mermann, S., Kresse, A. E., Stalla, G. K., et al. (2001). Expression of CRHR 1 and CRHR 2 in mouse pituitary and adrenal gland: impli- cations for HPA system regulation. *Endocrinology* 142, 4150–4153. doi: 10.1210/en.142.9.4150

Nappi, R. E., and Rivest, S. (1995). Stress-induced genetic expression of a selective corticotropin-releasing factor-receptor subtype within the rat ovaries: an effect dependent on the ovulatory cycle. *Biol. Reprod.* 53, 1417–1428. doi: 10.1095/biolre- prod53.6.1417

Nillni, E. A., and Sevarino, K. A. (1999). The biology of pro-thyrotropin- releasing hormone-derived pep- tides. *Endocr. Rev.* 20, 599–648. doi: 10.1210/er.20.5.599

Oikawa, M., Dargan, C., Ny, T., and Hsueh, A. J. (1990). Expression of gonadotropin releasing hor- mone and prothymosin-messenger ribonucleic acid in the ovary. *Endocrinology* 127, 2350–2356. doi: 10.1210/endo-127-5-2350

Pawlikowski, M., Zerek-Melen, G., and Winczyk, K. (1992). Thyroliberin (TRH) increases thymus cell pro- liferation in rats. *Neuropeptides* 23, 199–202. doi: 10.1016/0143-4179(92)90123-e

Pekary, A. E., Meyera, N. V., Vail- lanta, C., and Hershmana, J. M. (1980). Thyrotropin-releasing hor- mone and a homologous peptide in the male rat reproductive system. *Biochem. Biophys. Res. Commun.* 95, 993–1000. doi: 10.1016/0006-291x(80)91571-5

Pekary, A. E., Ross, R., de Kernion, J., and Hershman, J. M. (1983a). Human reproductive tissues con- tain thyrotropin releasing hormone (TRH) and TRH-homologous pep- tides. *J. Androl.* 4, 408–414.

Pekary, A. E., Richkind, M., andHershman, J. M. (1983b). Thy- rotrophin releasing hormone and related peptides in canine tissues. *J. Endocrinol.* 98, 299–306. doi: 10.1677/joe.0.0980299

Peng, C., Fan, N. C., Ligier, M., Vaananen, J., and Leung, P. C.K. (1994). Expression and regu- lation of gonadotropin-releasing hormone (GnRH) and GnRH receptor messenger ribonucleic acids in human granulosa-luteal cells. *Endocrinology* 135, 1740–1746. doi: 10.1210/en.135.5.1740

Pérez Castro, C., Peñalva, R., Páez Pereda, M., Renner, U., Reul, J. M., Stalla, G. K., et al. (1999). Early activation of Thyrotropin- Releasing-Hormone and prolactin plays a critical role during a T cell-dependent immune response. *Endocrinology* 140, 690–697. doi: 10.1210/en.140.2.690

Quintanar, J. L. (2011). Neuroim- munomodulation by Gonadotropin Releasing Hormone. *Adv. Neuroim- mune Biol.* 1, 125–132.

Quintanar, J. L., Salinas, E. and González, R. (2009). Gonadotropin- releasing hormone receptor in spinal cord neurons of embryos and adult rats. *Neurosci. Lett.* 461, 21–24. doi: 10.1016/j.neulet.2009.06.028

Quintanar, J. L., Salinas, E., and Quintanar-Stephano, A. (2011). Gonadotropin-releasing hormone reduces the severity of experimental autoimmune encephalomyelitis, a model of multiple sclerosis. *Neuropeptides* 45, 43–48. doi: 10.1016/j.npep.2010.10.003

Radulovic, M., and Spiess, J. (2001). Immunomodulatory role of the Corticotropin-Releasing Factor. *Arch. Immunol. Ther. Exp. (Warsz)* 49, 33–38.

Radulovic, M., Dautzenberg, F. M., Shydow, S., Radulovic, J., and Spiess, J. (1999). Corticotropin-releasing factor receptor 1 in a mouse spleen: expression after immune stimula- tion and identification of receptor- bearingcells. *J. Immunol.* 162, 3013– 3021.

Raiden, S., Polack, E., Nahmod, V., Labeur, M., Holsboer, F., and Arzt, E. (1995). TRH receptor on immune cells: *in vitro* and *in vivo* stimula- tion of human lymphocyte and rat splenocyte DNA synthesis by TRH. *J. Clin. Immunol.* 15, 242–249. doi: 10.1007/bf01540881

Raux-Demay, M. C., and Girard, F. (1985). The physiology of corticotropin-releasing factor (CRF). *Reprod. Nutr. Dev.* 25, 931–943.

Sapolsky, R., Rivier, C., Yamamoto, G., Plotsky, P., and Vale, W. (1987). Interleukin-I stimulates the secre- tion of hypothalamic corticotropin-releasing factor. *Science* 238, 522–524. doi: 10.1126/science.2821621

Sasaki, K., and Norwitz, E. R. (2011). Gonadotropin-releasing hormone/ gonadotropin-releasinghormone receptor signaling in the placenta. *Curr. Opin. Endocrinol. Diabetes Obes.* 18, 401–408. doi: 10.1097/MED.0b013e32834cd3b0

Satoh, T., Feng, P., Kim, U. J., and Wilber, J. F. (1993). Identifica- tion of thyrotropin releasing hor- mone receptor messenger RNA in the rat central nervous system and eye. *Brain Res. Mol. Brain Res.* 19, 175–178. doi: 10.1016/0169-328x(93)90165-l

Schaeffer, J. M., Brownstein, M. J., and Axelrod, J. (1977). Thyrotropin- releasing hormone-like material in the rat retina: changes due to envi- ronmental lighting. *Proc. Natl. Acad. Sci. U S A* 74, 3579–3581. doi: 10.1073/pnas.74.8.3579

Scharrer, E., and Scharrer, B. (1940). Secretory cells within the hypotha- lamus. *Res. Publ. Assoc. Res. Nerv. Ment. Dis.* 20, 170–194.

Schürmeyer, T. H., Avgerinos, P.., Gold, P. W., Gallucci, W. T., Tomai, T. P., Cutler, G. B. Jr., et al. (1984). Human corticotropin- releasing factor in man: pharma- cokinetic properties and dose- response of plasma adrenocorti-cotropin and cortisol secretion. *J. Clin. Endocrinol. Metab.* 59, 1103–1108. doi: 10.1210/jcem-59- 6-1103

Shambaugh, G., Kubek, M., and Wilber, J. F. (1979). Thyrotropin-releasing hormone activity in the human pla- centa. *J. Clin. Endocrinol. Metab.* 48, 483–486. doi: 10.1210/jcem-48- 3-483

Silverman, A. J., Millar, R. P., King, J. A., Zhuang, X., and Silver, R. (1994). Mast cells with gonadotropin- releasing hormone-like immunore- activity in the brain of doves. *Proc. Natl. Acad. Sci. U S A* 91, 3695–3699.doi: 10.1073/pnas.91.9.3695

Singh, V. K., and Fudenberg, H. H. (1988). Binding of [125I] corti- cotropin releasing factor to blood immunocytes and its reduction in Alzheimer's disease. *Immunol. Lett.* 18, 5–8. doi: 10.1016/0165-2478(88)90061-2

Singh, V. K., and Leu, S. J. (1990). Enhancing effect of corticotropin- releasing neurohormone on the production of interleukin-1 and interleukin-2. *Neurosci. Lett.* 120, 151–154. doi: 10.1016/0304-3940(90)90025-5

Singh, V. K., Warren, R. P., White, E. D., and Leu, S. J. C. (1990).Corticotropin-releasing factor- induced stimulation of immune functions. *Ann. N Y Acad. Sci.* 594, 416–419. doi: 10.1111/j.1749-6632.1990.tb40514.x

Singh, V.K. (1989). Stimulatory effect of corticotropin-releasing neuro- hormone on human lymphocyte proliferation and interleukin-2 receptor expression. *J. Neu- roimmunol.* 23, 257–262. doi: 10.1016/0165-5728(89)90058-1

Slominski, A., Ermak, G., Hwang, J., Chakraborty, A., Mazurkiewicz, J. E., and Mihm, M. (1995). Proo- piomelanocortin, corticotrophin- releasing hormone and corti- cotrophin releasing hormone receptor genes are expressed in human skin. *FEBS Lett.* 374, 113–116.

Song, J. P., Chen, X., and Hu, S. (2013). Corticotropin releasing hormone activates CD14+ cells to induce endothelial barrier dys- function. *Cell Biol. Int.* 37. doi: 10.1002/cbin.10133. [Epub ahead of print].

Standaert, F. E., Chew, B. P., De Avila, D., and Reeves, J. J. (1992). Presence of luteinizing hormone- releasing hormone binding sites in cultured porcine lymphocytes. *Biol. Reprod.* 46, 997–1000. doi: 10.1095/biolreprod46.6.997

Stevenson, T. J., Hahn, T. P., MacDougall-Shackleton, S. A., and Ball, G. F. (2012). Gonadotropin- releasing hormone plasticity: a comparative perspective. *Front. Neuroendocrinol.* 33, 287–300. doi: 10.1016/j.yfrne.2012.09.001

Strausbaug, H., and Irwin, M. (1992).Central corticotropin releasing hor- mone reduces cellular immunity. *Brain Behav. Immun.* 6, 11–17. doi: 10.1016/0889-1591(92)90055-s

Sun, Y., Lu, X., and Gershengorn, M. C. (2003). Thyrotropin-releasing hor- mone receptors - similarities and differences. *J. Mol. Endocrinol.* 30, 87–97. doi: 10.1677/jme.0.0300087

Sutherland, J. S., Spyroglou, L., Muir- head, J. L., Heng, T. S., Prieto- Hinojosa, A., Prince, H. M., et al. (2008). Enhanced immune system regeneration in humans following allogeneic or autologous hemopoi- etic stem cell transplantation by temporary sex steroid blockade. *Clin. Cancer Res.* 14, 1138–1149. doi: 10.1158/1078-0432.ccr-07-1784

Tan, O., and Bukulmez, O. (2011). Biochemistry, molec- ular biology and cell biology of gonadotropin-releasing hor- mone antagonists. *Curr. Opin. Obstet. Gynecol.* 23, 238–244. doi: 10.1097/gco.0b013e328348a3ce

Tanriverdi, F., Gonzalez-Martinez, D., Hu, Y., Kelestimur, F., and Bouloux, P. M. (2005). GnRH-I and GnRH- II have differential modulatory effects on human peripheral blood mononuclear cell proliferation and interleukin-2 receptor gamma- chain mRNA expression in healthy males. *Clin. Exp. Immunol.* 142, 103–110.

Tanriverdi, F., Silveira, L. F., Mac Coll, G. S., and Bouloux, P. M. (2003). The hypothalamic- pituitary-gonadal axis: immune function and autoimmunity. *J. Endocrinol.* 176, 293–304. doi: 10.1677/joe.0.1760293

Theoharides, T. C., and Cochrane, D. E. (2004). Critical role of mast cells in inflammatory diseases and the effect of acute stress. *J. Neuroimmunol.* 146, 1–12. doi: 10.1016/j.jneuroim.2003.10.041

Theoharides, T. C., Singh, L. K., Boucher, W., Pang, X., Letourneau, R., Webster, E., et al. (1998). Corticotropin-releasing hormone induces skin mast cell degran- ulation and increased vascular permeability, a possible explanation for its proinflammatory effects. *Endocrinology* 139, 403–413. doi: 10.1210/en.139.1.403

Thompson, M. A., Adelson, M. D., and Kaufman, L. M. (1991). Lupron retards proliferation of ovarian epithelial tumour cells cultured in serum-free medium. *J. Clin. Endocrinol. Metab.* 72, 1036–1041. doi: 10.1210/jcem-72-5-1036

Umathe, S. N., Dixit, P. V., Wan- jari, M. M., and Ullewar, M. P. (2008). Leuprolide–a GnRH agonist–prevents restraint stress- induced immunosuppression via sex steroid-independent periph- eral mechanism in mice. *Int. Immunopharmacol.* 8, 71–79. doi: 10.1016/j.intimp.2007.10.011

Umesaki, N., Tanaka, T., Miyama, M., Mizuno, K., Kawamura, N., and Ogita, S. (1999). Increased natural killer cell activities in patients treated with gonadotropin releasing hormone agonist. *Gynecol. Obstet. Invest.* 48, 66–68. doi: 10.1159/000010137

Vaughan, J., Donaldson, C., Bitten-court, J., Perrin, M. H., Lewis, K., Sutton, S., et al. (1995). Uro- cortin, a mammalian neuropeptide related to fish urotensin I and to corticotropin-releasing fac- tor. *Nature* 378, 287–292. doi: 10.1038/378287a0

Walters, K., Wegorzewska, I. N., Chin, Y. P., Parikh, M. G., and Wu, T. J. (2008). Luteinizing hormone- releasing hormone I (LHRH-I) and its metabolite in peripheral tissues. *Exp. Biol. Med.* 233, 123–130. doi: 10.3181/0707-mr-201

Wang, J., Whetsell, M., and Klein, J. R. (1997). Local hormone networks and intestinal T cell homeosta- sis. *Science* 275, 1937–1939. doi: 10.1126/science.275.5308. 1937

Wang, W., Zhang, X., Yang, L., Liu, ., Liu, G., and Zhou, J. (2012). Lipopolysaccharide upregulates the expression of corticotropin- releasing hormone via MAP kinase pathway in rat peritoneal macrophages. *Mol. Cell. Biochem.* 361, 1–7. doi: 10.1007/s11010-011-1080-2

Webster, E. L., Tracey, D. E., Jutila, M. A., Wolfe, S. A. Jr., and de Souza, E. B. (1990). Corticotropin-releasing factor receptors in mouse spleen: identification of receptor-bearing cells as resident macrophages. *Endocrinology* 127, 440–452. doi: 10.1210/endo-127-1-440

Wilson, A. C., Meethal, S. V., Bowen, R. L., and Atwood, C. S. (2007). Leuprolide acetate: a drug of diverse clinical applications. *Expert Opin. Investig. Drugs* 16, 1–13. doi: 10.1517/13543784.16.11.1851

Winczyk, K., and Pawlikowski, M. (2000). Time of day-dependent effects of thyroliberin and thy- rotropin on thymocyte proliferation in rats. *Neuroimmunomodulation* 7, 89–91.doi:10.1159/000026425

Wong, K. H., and Simon, J. A. (2004). *In vitro* effect of gonadotropin- releasing hormone agonist on nat- ural killer cell cytolysis in women with and without endometriosis. *Am. J. Obstet. Gynecol.* 190, 44–49. doi: 10.1016/j.ajog.2003.08.032

Wright, I. M. R. (2003). Corticotropin- releasing hormone causes vasodi- lation in human skin via mast cell-dependent pathways. *J. Clin. Endocrinol. Metab.* 88, 5427–5432. doi: 10.1210/jc.2003-030377

Wynn, P. C., Harwood, J. P., Catt, K. J., and Aguilera, G. (1985). Reg- ulation of corticotrophin releasing factor (CRF) receptors in the rat pituitary gland: effects of adrenalec- tomy on CRF receptors and cor- ticotroph responses. *Endocrinology* 116, 1653–1659. doi: 10.1210/endo-116-4-1653

Yin, W., and Gore, A. C. (2006). Neu- roendocrine control of reproduc- tive aging: roles of GnRH neu- rons. *Reproduction* 131, 403–414. doi: 10.1530/rep.1.00617

5

Neuro-immune abnormalities in autism and their relationship with the environment: a variable insult model for autism

Daniel K. Goyal* and Jaleel A. Miyan

Faculty of Life Sciences, The University of Manchester, Manchester, UK

Edited by:
Adam Denes, The University of Manchester, UK

Reviewed by:
Cynthia L. Bethea, Oregon Health and Science University, USA
Jozsef Halasz, Vadaskert Child Psychiatry Hospital, Hungary

****Correspondence:***
Daniel K. Goyal, Faculty of Life Sciences, The University of Manchester, AV Hill Building, Oxford Road, Manchester M13 9PT, UK
e-mail: danielgoyal@doctors.org.uk

Autism spectrum disorder (ASD) is a heterogeneous condition affecting an individual's ability to communicate and socialize and often presents with repetitive movements or behaviors. It tends to be severe with less than 10% achieving independent living with a marked variation in the progression of the condition. To date, the literature supports a multifactorial model with the largest, most detailed twin study demonstrating strong environmental contribution to the development of the condition. Here, we present a brief review of the neurological, immunological, and autonomic abnormalities in ASD focusing on the causative roles of environmental agents and abnormal gut microbiota. We present a working hypothesis attempting to bring together the influence of environment on the abnormal neurological, immunological, and neuroimmunological functions and we explain in brief how such pathophysiology can lead to, and/or exacerbate ASD symptomatology. At present, there is a lack of consistent findings relating to the neurobiology of autism. Whilst we postulate such variable findings may reflect the marked heterogeneity in clinical presentation and as such the variable findings may be of pathophysiological relevance, more research into the neurobiology of autism is necessary before establishing a working hypothesis. Both the literature review and hypothesis presented here explore possible neurobiological explanations with an emphasis of environmental etiologies and are presented with this bias.

Keywords: autism spectrum disorder, neuro-immune, environment, gut microbiota, neuroinflammation

INTRODUCTION

Autism spectrum disorder (ASD) is a neurodevelopmental disorder of unknown etiology. Recent evidence suggests a strong environmental component (1) and persistent neuroinflammation (2–5). Within the phenology of ASD and associated disorders, the subjectivity involved in attributing an infant or toddler with introversion (or being in one's own world, autism) is fraught with difficulty. The difficulty is not whether such behavioral abnormalities represent a neurobiological illness – consensus is for an organic brain disorder – the challenge stems from the wide-ranging possibilities underlying the visible disease (6, 7). A secondary obstacle to the adequate identification of disease process in ASD patients pertains to scientific disparity. Research efforts have focused more on the genetic aspects of ASD than on environmental factors over the previous 15 years (8). Consequently, several important factors have impinged upon progress for ASD sufferers and those at risk.

The fixation on genetics led to reprioritization by medical staff and displacement of non-genetic scientific researchers. Many clinicians awaited the genetic answer and the promise of targeted, scientifically originated treatment. Conveying the certainty of the scientific consensus at the time, clinicians are now faced with the same patients and a different, almost polar growing certainty: there are likely to be prognostic factors one can mitigate (9, 10).

Previous twin studies suggested a predominant genetic component; however, these studies were poorly designed and had weak power (16, 17). A recent twin study published in July 2011 was well-designed with a substantial statistical power. One hundred ninety-four twin groups were studied and clinically evaluated prior to statistical analysis. Probandwise concordance for monozygotic twins was 77% (95% CI, 65–86%) for 45 male pairs and 50% (95% CI, 16–84%) for 9 female pairs. Concordance rates for dizygotic twins were 31% (95% CI, 16–46%) and 36% (95% CI, 11–60%) for 45 male and 13 female pairs, respectively. The study concluded: autism has substantial environmental factors, and indeed the environmental factors were of more significance than genetic factors (1).

There has been another compounding factor. Diagnostic labeling has changed substantially. Since its discovery in the late 1930s, autism has gradually become the diagnosis of choice. It has replaced and superseded childhood schizophrenia and feeblemindedness and has encompassed within the spectrum, a host of neurodevelopmental disorders [for review see Ref. (11)]. This allowed a rational argument for the increase in prevalence, and as such a tempering of the strict scientific critique required.

Recent advancements in ASD research has led to a surge in research activity, in particular neuro-immune and environmental factors. Here, we present a view of ASD related to neurological, immunological, and neuroimmunological findings from the bias of an environmental etiology standpoint. We briefly discuss the pertinent literature concerning the frequently reported abnormal gut microflora composition in ASD patients. Finally, based on the growing consensus in biological scientific evidence and clinical experience, we present the variable insult model of ASD with the aim of contributing further to a useful research direction for those suffering from ASD and for those faced with managing the condition.

EPIDEMIOLOGY

Autism spectrum disorder was first identified by Kanner in 1938 (12). Over the subsequent 10 years, Kanner discovered 50 further cases (13). Kanner subsequently reviewed the first 11 patients at 30-year follow-up. Only one known patient achieved employment (14). More recent evidence also suggests a high level of disability in affected individuals, with 60–75% achieving poor or very poor outcomes in adulthood (15).

Autism spectrum disorder case detection rates are now substantially higher – from 1 in 3000 reported in 1966 (including both autism and psychosis) (16), 1 in 150 in 8-year-olds in 2007 [Centre for Disease Control (CDC), (17)], and in 2012 a rate of 1 in 88 [CDC, (18)]. In UK, Cohen et al. described a prevalence rate of 1 in 64 (19).

MORBIDITY AND MORTALITY

Shavelle et al. investigated the mortality rate of ASD in over 13,000 patients between 1983 and 1997 (20) and found it to be more than twice that of neurotypical peers. Standardized mortality ratio (SMR) was estimated as 2.4. Certain causes carried significantly higher SMR (see **Table 1**). Similar mortality rates have been reported in other studies (21, 22) with a consistent increased mortality rate for ASD, and a substantially greater risk in female ASD patients. Whilst mental retardation predicted risk of early demise, those without mental retardation also had increased risk.

Table 1 | Causes of death in ASD with moderate to severe retardation or none to mild retardation (in brackets).

Cause of death	Early childhood SMR (5–10 years)	Late childhood SMR (10–20 years)	Adulthood SMR (>20 years)
Drowning	90.6 (14.1)	n/s	n/s
Digestive	n/s	40.8	5.9
Respiratory	n/s	24.5	9.4
Cancer	n/s	12.0 (3.8)	2.4 (1.6)
Nervous and sense	n/s	6.4 (15.9)	4.1
Seizures	n/s	n/s	30.8 (33.1)
Cardiovascular	n/s	n/s	3.7 (2.2)

Adapted from Ref. (20). SMR, standardized mortality ratio; n/s, no significant increase in SMR found in either group.

DISEASE PROGRESSION

There have been several studies evaluating diagnostic stability over time. Turner et al. reassessed 2-year-olds diagnosed with ASD at 4.5 years of age (23) and found no change in their diagnosis of ASD but did find that 20% of children worsened between 2 years of age and 4.5 years of age and 20% improved. Within the parameters addressed, 60% remained relatively stable. No reason was identified for the variation.

Levy et al. have recently reviewed the literature regarding long-term outcome in ASD finding cognitive improvement in 20–55%, cognitive stability in 20–70%, and cognitive loss in 10–15% (24). No reasons were identified for why some ASD patients suffer a progressive illness and others make some recovery. ASDs as a group carry a poorer prognosis than other developmental disorders in almost all domains (24).

SUMMARY OF EPIDEMIOLOGICAL FINDINGS

Even though ASD is associated with high health, social, and financial impacts, investigative epidemiology has been limited. Perhaps the premature acceptance of ASD as a genetic condition limited the power of epidemiological science beyond that of detection of cases [for review see Ref. (25)]. The Interagency Autism Coordinating Committee (IACC) and Centers for Autism and Developmental Disabilities Research and Epidemiology (CADDRE) Network are co-ordinating a large epidemiological study in the US: the study to explore early development (SEED) (26). This is in keeping with the responsibilities set out in the US through "The Combating Autism Act 2006."

IMMUNE ABNORMALITIES AND NEUROINFLAMMATION IN ASD

Perhaps one of the most substantive studies in the last decade was conducted at the John Hopkins Institute, and involved an analysis of autopsy specimens and cerebrospinal fluid (CSF) samples from affected individuals and controls (2). The results indicated a neuroinflammatory response, regardless of age (in patients between 5 and 46 years of age), involving excess microglial activation and increased pro-inflammatory cytokine profiles. The study carries high statistical significance [for review of study, see Ref. (27)] and indicates an inflammatory state probably exists in the brains of these patients. Similar findings were found in a more recent autopsy study of microglia densities in fronto-insular and visual cortices of patients with ASD versus controls, and found a statistically significant ($p \leq 0.0002$) increase in microglial density in both regions (4). Other immune abnormalities have also been found indicating an inflammatory state. Transforming growth factor beta 1 (TGF-β1) is reduced in ASD cohorts versus controls and individuals with other developmental disorders and was found to be inversely proportional to behavior outcomes (irritability, lethargy, stereotypy, and hyperactivity) as well as with levels of social adaptability (28).

Natural killer cells (NK cells) are abnormal in sub-groups of ASD. NK cells respond to macrophage-derived cytokines and are essential in tumor prevention and host anti-viral activity. Enstrom et al. (29) found a significant reduction in NK cell cytotoxicity and a 2.5-fold increase in KSP-37, an NK gene normally induced during active viral infection. They concluded that ASD patients have activated but resting NK cells with increased levels of cytolytic proteins and an altered response to stimulation with changes in gene expression (29). Supporting these findings, cancer mortality rates are higher in ASD (20), and the only identified risk factor for mortality associated with the recent H1N1 outbreak was developmental delay (30). Both of these findings suggest immune dysfunction in

ASD, and either or both of these findings could be linked with the NK cell abnormalities identified by Enstrom et al. (29).

There have been studies making correlations between measures of immune functions and cytokine profiles with behavioral measures in ASD (**Table 2**). Significant correlations were shown between certain behavioral indices and the chemokine's, macrophage chemoattractant MCP-1, macrophage inflammatory protein (MIP)-1β, eotaxin, and "regulated upon activation normal T-cell expressed and secreted" factor (RANTES) (31). RANTES was associated with lethargy, stereotypy, and hyperactivity. Eotaxin was associated with hyperactivity, visual perception, fine motor control, expressive language, communication and daily living skills, and socialization. MCP-1 was associated with visual perception. These associations, if proven to be functional, raise many questions pertaining to the immune system's connectivity to the nervous system and involvement in neurobehavioral illnesses (for summary of immunological findings relating to behavior in ASD, see **Table 2**). Of importance here is the probability of immune involvement in the core features of ASD. These findings also raise the possibility of assessing behavioral changes in ASD through a quantitative measure.

NEUROLOGICAL ABNORMALITIES IN ASD

With the exception of neuroinflammatory changes, most reported neurobiological abnormalities in ASD are inconsistent.

Structurally, abnormalities have been described in the cerebellum, hippocampus, amygdala, and insular cortex (32). Abnormal brain volume has also been identified [for review see Ref. (33)]. A

Table 2 | Behavior and immune functions in ASD [adapted from Ref. (84)].

Studies	*n*	Age	Assessment method	Immune measure	Behavior measure
Ashwood et al. (28)	143	2–5	ADI-R, ADOS, SCQ, VABS, MSEL, and ABC	Plasma levels of active TGFβ1	Lower TGFβ1 levels were associated with lower adaptive behaviors and worse behavioral symptoms
Iwata et al. (89)	37	20–25	ADI-R	Plasma levels of P-selectin	Lower levels of P-selectin associated with poor social development
Heuer et al. (90)	271	2–5	ADI-R, ADOS, and ABC	IgG levels in plasma	Decreased IgG associated with increased aberrant behaviors
Grigorenko et al. (91)	1059	n/s	ADI-R and ADOS	Genotyping of the MIF gene and plasma levels of MIF ($n = 20$)	Plasma MIF levels were positively correlated with worse scores on ADOS for social impairment and imaginative skills
Onore et al. (92)	60	2–5	ADOS, ADI-R, MSEL, VABS, and ABC	Induced cytokine response to PHA	Negative correlation between PHA induced IL-23 production and sociability scores of the ADOS
Enstrom et al. (93)	30	2–5	ADI-R, ADOS, SCQ, VABS, MSEL, and ABC	Monocyte TLR ligand stimulation	More impaired social behaviors and non-verbal communication are associated with increased production of IL-1β and IL-6 after TLR4 stimulation
Ashwood et al. (94)	139	2–5	ADI-R, ADOS, SCQ, VABS, MSEL, and ABC	Induced cytokine response to PHA and LPS	Pro-inflammatory or TH1 cytokines were associated with greater impairments in core features of ASD as well as aberrant behaviors; GM-CSF and TH2 cytokines were associated with better cognitive and adaptive function
Goines et al. (95)	466	2–5	ADI-R, ADOS, SCQ, VABS, MSEL, and ABC	Antibodies directed against a 45 or 62 kDa cerebellum protein	Children with antibodies directed against a 45-kDa cerebellum protein had increased lethargy and stereotypy; children with antibodies against a 62-kDa cerebellum protein showed increased aberrant behaviors on the VABS composite standard score
Kajizuka et al. (96)	62	6–19	ADI-R	Serum levels of PDGF	Increased serum levels of PDGF-BB homodimers positively associated with increased restricted, repetitive, and stereotyped patterns of behavior and interests
Ashwood et al. (31)	175	2–5	ADI-R, ADOS, SCQ, VABS, MSEL, and ABC	Plasma chemokines CCL2, CCL5, and eotaxin	Plasma chemokine levels associated with higher aberrant behavior scores and more impaired developmental and adaptive function
Ashwood et al. (97)	223	2–5	ADI-R, ADOS, SCQ, VABS, MSEL, and ABC	Plasma levels of cytokines IL-1β, IL-6, IL-8, and IL-12p40	Elevated cytokine levels in plasma were associated with more impaired communication and aberrant behaviors
Ross et al. (98)	16	3-31	ADI-R	GM-CSF, INFγ, IL-12p70, IL-1β, IL-6, IL-8, TNFα, and IL-10	Elevation of cytokines correlated with autistic symptoms in patients with 22q11.2 deletion syndrome

meta-analysis reported on an average of 13% smaller brain volume at birth, an average of 10% larger brain volume at 1 year of age than controls, and 2% larger in adolescence (33). An increase in gray matter with a reduced unit density has been quite reliably identified in this cohort (33). CSF volume has also been reported to be increased with enlarged ventricles (34) and mini-columnar size is decreased (35). It has been proposed that such structural variation may affect adaptation and hence learning, and may account for the heterogeneity and wide-ranging functional deficits seen in ASD (36). Disordered neural connectivity has been discussed for some time (37). The evidence supports under-connectivity between sensory cortices and association cortices in moderate to severe ASD, essentially leading to a failure to assimilate sensory information into a working environmental context, and a lack of connectivity of associative cortices to the frontal cortex in higher functioning autism (38). This helps explain associated learning difficulties in low functioning autism, and the poor fine motor control and impaired imitation identified in higher functioning autism (39–41).

AUTONOMIC DYSFUNCTION

Autonomic involvement in ASD has been widely reported for over 30 years (42–52). A recent controlled trial explored in detail the nature and type of autonomic involvement (49). Real-time variability together with continuous monitoring of blood pressure and breathing rhythms were assessed in an ASD cohort versus controls. Over 80% of the ASD cohorts were found to have a reduced vagal tone, highly suggestive of low central parasympathetic activity and, significantly, in a separate study, vagal tone in the neonate was found to predict neurodevelopmental outcome more accurately than birth weight, socio-economic status, or co-morbid medical conditions (50). Given that the autonomic nervous system (ANS) is responsible for the majority of sensory information received by the central nervous system, any disruption to the ANS is likely to have wide-ranging effects on higher cortical development. In a longitudinal follow-up study, Goytag et al. examined the order of cortical development using repeat MRI and concluded: higher-order association cortices mature only after lower-order somatosensory and visual cortices, the functions of which they integrate, are developed (53). The development of a normal parasympathetic tone is thus likely to be crucial for adequate neurodevelopment [for review see Ref. (50)]. More research is required.

ENVIRONMENTAL ASPECTS OF ASD

Hertz-Picciotto et al. provide a detailed review of developmental immunotoxicity (DIT) in relation to neurodevelopment disorders (54). Xenobiotic exposure in early life may lead to altered immune function throughout life, a persistent neuroinflammatory response and systemic immune dysregulation, and the possibility of a neurobehavioral manifestation of the disease (54).

The type of immune dysfunction relates to the type of xenobiotic involved and the timing of xenobiotic exposure with dose-dependent effects not as applicable in the developing immune system but specific neurological development depends on signaling from the immune system (55). Such conveyance of environmental state to the nervous system from the immune system is advantageous and essential, but is incompatible with adequate neurodevelopment in poor environmental conditions. Whether there is a single type of xenobiotic involved in the etiology of ASD or whether the pathophysiology involves exposure to general environmental pollution remains a keenly researched area. Pesticides, flame retardants, heavy metals, traffic fumes, and endotoxins have all been implicated (56–61). The apparent lack of consistency is further compounded by difficulties in measuring chronic toxicity and toxin-induced disruption particularly if the xenobiotic exposure is no longer present.

Dietert et al. describes several similarities between early-life immune insults (ELII), including DIT and ASD with gender differences, time-windows for immune development, and the corresponding variable presentation in both ELII and ASD making a compelling argument (62). Studying DIT and indeed developmental neurotoxicity requires functional measures and a history of significant exposure. Complicating matters further is the modest, but significant genomic variation in xenobiotic metabolism and hence resistance or vulnerability to environmental exposures.

ABNORMALITIES IN GUT MICROFLORA IN ASD

Abnormal clostridia species have been found repeatedly in ASD (63–67). The theory of clostridia involvement was postulated by Bolte in 1998 who suggested that clostridia toxin adversely affected neurotransmitter function that could result in neurobehavioral changes presenting as autism (68). Supporting this hypothesis, Parracho et al. outlined robust measures of microflora abnormalities in ASD cases suffering from bowel problems using PCR analysis and found a clear and consistent abnormality in the clostridia species present in ASD sufferers versus controls. *Clostridium histolytica* were found in higher levels in the ASD group versus healthy unrelated controls ($p < 0.01$) and healthy related controls ($p < 0.05$) (65).

A clinical trial was carried out to assess the bowel and behavioral impact of anti-microbial therapy directed against these abnormal clostridia species (69). Oral vancomycin was used for 6 weeks. Behavioral measurements were carried out before and after, as well as clinical assessment of bowel symptoms. The numbers were low but the response to intervention was reported as statistically significant. 8 of the 10 patients studied improved in terms of behavior and bowel symptoms with some scoring within the neurotypical range. Discontinuation of vancomycin after the 6-week trial period led to a gradual regression in bowel and behavioral symptoms in all participants (69) suggesting that gut environment gives preference to these abnormal species. As yet, there has been no investigation of the combined approach of anti-microbial therapy and other interventions targeted at altering microbiota composition.

Williams et al. recently reported consistently abnormal Firmicutes to Bacteriodetes ratios from biopsy specimens in children with ASD versus inflammatory bowel disease (IBD) controls. This was linked to reduced disaccharidases (starch digesting enzymes), which in the same study were also found to be low in the ASD group. Williams et al. postulated a link between high carbohydrate transit to the large intestine in ASD leading to alteration in the proportion of Firmicutes to Bacteriodetes. The appearance of this "compositional dysbiosis" was highly correlated in the ASD group with Firmicutes to Bacteriodetes ratio of 31:69 (versus controls

27:73) in the ileal biopsies ($p < 0.0006$) and 32:68 (versus controls 25:75) in the cecal biopsies ($p < 0.022$) (66).

Although microflora are known to alter host immune function, including cytokine production [for review see Ref. (70–73)], to our knowledge there has, to date, been no investigation of the relationship between abnormal microflora and cytokine production in ASD, although a few studies have examined cytokines in ASD patients with bowel symptoms and found positive correlations (72–74).

DISCUSSION

It is the wide heterogeneity of ASD that poses the greatest challenge. Identifying a common pathophysiology is hampered by such diversity as is the identification of management strategies, both behavioral and medical. Equally those faced with patient care often struggle to discern the range of presentations and the impact this has on management. ASD shares simply, a marked impairment with any of the faculties required for social integration; this can present with a lethargic, disinterested child or an agitated, distracted child or any number of features leading ultimately to impaired social integration. It may be that in order to determine treatment response, we must first delineate/categorize treatable groups. Indeed if some form of environmental insult occurs early on in development (be it infection, toxicant, or other environmental stressor), then it may not only cause variable manifestations based on timing, nature, and genomic individuality, it may also leave no discernible or at least easily discernible trace. It may, as Hertz-Piciotta et al. (54) and Dietert et al. (62) suggest, merely be an event that primes or disrupts a critical window in development. Given the wide-ranging heterogeneity of the disorder and the many faculties required for social integration, it may be neither the insulting agent, the timing, the genomic vulnerability nor the system(s) affected that remain static or, when ASD is taken as a single consequential expression, statistically identifiable.

Within the developing neurological, immunological, and neuroimmunological systems, there is vulnerability to environmental insult. Depending on the nature, timing, and duration of insult, neurological, immunological, or neuroimmunological abnormalities may predominate, and the relative proportion each system is affected will vary accordingly (see **Figure 1**).

Socialization and speech are complex neurological functions. ASD may represent impairment in any system/faculty required to facilitate such complex neurological functions. There is likely ample opportunity for an environmental insult to disrupt one or more of the mechanisms leading to the impairment of the higher-order processes of social integration and along the way disrupt a number of other physiological mechanisms that may contribute or indeed cause the additional and variable behavioral manifestations within the spectrum of disease. As troublesome as the notion may be, and granted there will be reasonable pathophysiological correlations identified particularly within sub-groups, the greatest commonality in ASD may be etiological, and even then it may merely be a trend in human–environment relationship versus an exact noxious substance.

Similar hypotheses have been presented by others: e.g., Dietert et al. (47), Hertz-Picotta et al. (46), Goines and Ashwood (75), and Unwin et al. (76). The central theme is the presence of a variable insult leading to the variable presentation of ASD. In recognition of these previous studies, the hypothesis presented here is referred to as the variable insult model of ASD. Such hypotheses are critical to providing a framework to identify sub-types within the ASD group, building in some predictability both for researchers and for those faced with clinical management. Such sub-typing can be based on the dominant system pathophysiology involved or one can attempt clinical classification. **Table 3** is an example of such an attempt at clinical sub-typing based on the variable insult model of ASD.

The sub-categories presented in **Table 3** are broad and overlap considerably. More specific sub-typing seems probable, perhaps relating to the intensity of the insult and perhaps more specifically to the offending agent, as suggested recently by Unwin et al. (76). Already abnormal RNA transcription has been identified in ASD children correlating with environmental toxicants versus controls with similar levels of toxicants (77, 78). The transcription abnormalities are specific to the toxicant, raising the possibility of different etiological agents triggering different initial pathophysiological mechanisms sharing only the secondary consequences. The factors involved in the different gene expression in ASD, whether they be linked to genomic individuality, previous exposure, some kind of immunological priming, or abnormal GI flora, raises interesting questions, but in these current considerations the mere difference in RNA transcription between different xenobiotics and also between ASD patients versus control groups raises important questions about accurate delineation of sub-types and the different pathophysiological mechanisms involved in the eventual ASD outcome.

Variable pathophysiological pathways leading to ASD seem likely, and recent advancements in scientific techniques carry the capacity to differentiate each pathway with relevance to the prevention and clinical management of the condition. For example, PCR analysis of GI microflora continues to reveal deeper insights into the common GI abnormalities prevalent in ASD (65, 66, 81). Evidence demonstrates the importance of such microflora on immune and neurological function, and the evolution of GI microflora composition over the first few years of life (82, 83). The compositional dysbiosis discovered by Williams et al. (66) in ASD patients may reflect another common manifestation of ASD due perhaps to similar complexities as is involved in social integration with genomic, neurological, immunological, and neuroimmunological systems required to select and regulate the GI microflora. This may explain the frequently reported presence of abnormal species in ASD and the diversity of such abnormal microflora/pathogens [for review see Ref. (65, 81)]; the selection and regulation processes are also part of the developmental process and are vulnerable to a variety of insults at a variety of levels. ASD diagnosis may be more scientifically sound should it move toward a formulation including environmental exposure, genomic vulnerability, and the identification of the system(s) pathophysiology with treatment interventions based on such measurable criteria. Animal models can serve such ever increasing sub-categorization, modeled to reflect each category and utilized to identify novel therapeutic interventions at specific groups. Without such an appreciation of the variability associated with ASD, it may be difficult to achieve

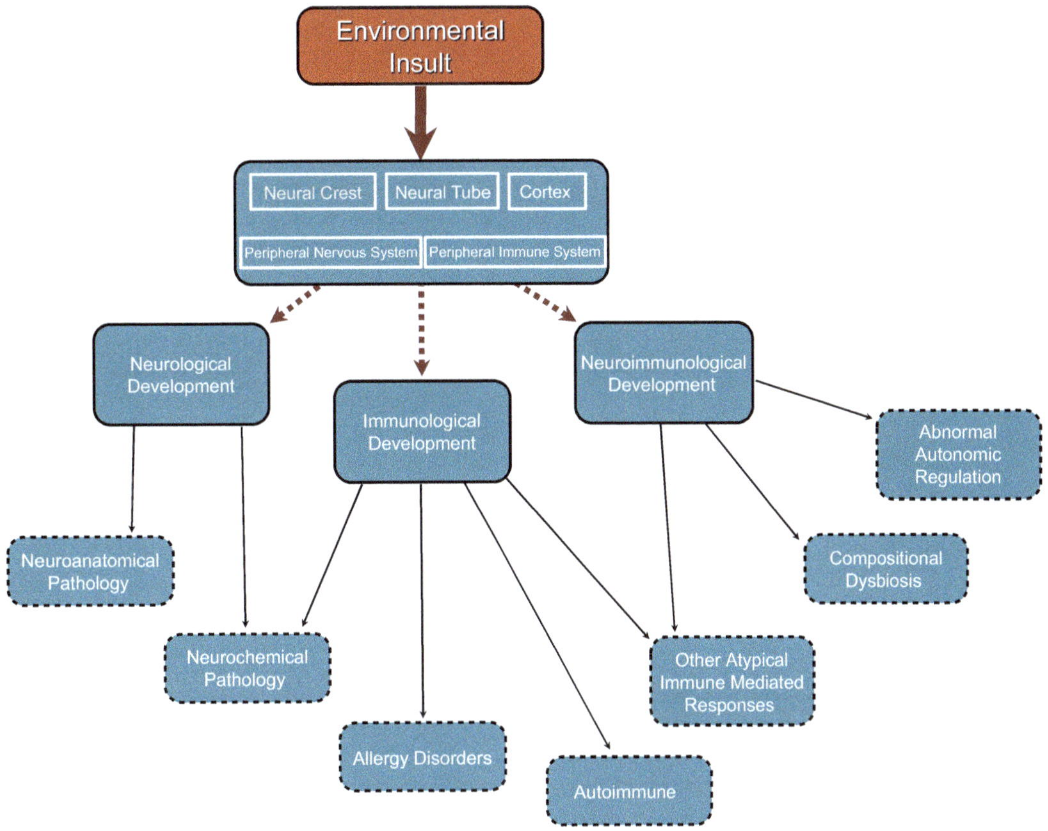

FIGURE 1 | Cascade of effects originating in neurodevelopmental insults occurring at different points in development. Insults can occur at any point in neurodevelopment from embryonic through to juvenile and perhaps even adulthood. Insults to neural crest and neural tube development in the embryo would have structural and functional outcomes in all peripheral neural elements including autonomic (sympathetic, parasympathetic), peripheral sensory system, and enteric (gut) nervous system. Neural tube effects might also produce changes in central autonomic functions and/or set points for physiological control systems resident in the hypothalamus and brain stem autonomic nuclei. Factors affecting cortical development would have an impact on higher cortical functions including psychosocial, sensory processing, and motor functioning. Any of these neurodevelopmental effects would have cascading effects through the sensory and neuro-immune pathways to neurological, neuro-immune, and immune functions.

statistical significance in treatment trials targeted at specific deficits.

The variable insult hypothesis predicts diverse immune-related abnormalities, probability of poor GI microflora regulation, variable autonomic function with impaired/disordered autonomic reactivity, and variable neuroanatomical findings. Further, the variable insult model predicts that ASD animal models could be established through a variety of mechanisms. Valproate with an acute single dose administered gestationally at E12.5 leads to ASD symptomatology in rats (79), as does valproate administered in a sub-chronic dosing given between post-natal days P6–12, albeit the sub-chronic dosing may have more sensory issues (80). Unwin et al. (76) proposed that homogeneity may be found by identifying the etiological agent, and presents the differences in associative symptomatology in children with ASD who had either perinatal exposure to selective serotonin re-uptake inhibitor (SSRI) or who had low birth weight (LBW). The SSRI group seemed to have more gastrointestinal disturbance, although it was not clear whether this was a depression effect or drug effect, and the LBW group had more sleep and breathing disturbance. Within the variable insult model of ASD, SSRI exposure may represent greater disruption to the peripheral ANS, perhaps during neural crest formation and development, whereas the LBW group may have suffered more pronounced central autonomic disruption. Difficulties with sensory processing may then affect both groups through different mechanisms with similar social outcomes.

If we start to look at the etiological agents contributing to the development of ASD, then perhaps we can start to find sub-groups. Such an approach brings more complexity to the clinical assessment of patients suffering from ASD but perhaps such a complex condition requires greater effort and more complex formulations prior to predicting prognosis and response to medical or behavioral management. If we go further still and delineate the various pathophysiologies that can lead to ASD symptomatology through animal and human experiments, then early identification of the system(s) requiring attention may be possible and may then better guide harm reduction strategies. Prevention remains the priority, but harm reduction through focused scientific investigation could reduce the burden of disease going forward. For example,

Table 3 | Broad clinical sub-categories of ASD.

	Prenatal – birth		Infant – early child (birth to 3 years)	
	Early acute insult	Early chronic insult	Late acute insult	Late chronic insult
Congenital abnormalities	++++	+++	+	+
Severe dysmotility	++++	+++	++	++
Sudden regression	+	++	++++	+++
Insidious regression	++	+++	+	++++
Early immune-related issues	+++	++++	++	++
Motor delays	++++	+++	+	+
Family history of autoimmunity	++	++	++++	+++
Gestational exposure	++++	+++	+	+
Early infancy exposure	+	++	++++	++++

The number of crosses indicates the severity/frequency of each measure relative to age of exposure and its duration. Early acute insult refers to a sudden or relatively sudden, usually marked exposure to xenobiotic, infection, or other environmental stressor during prenatal or gestational periods. Early chronic insult refers to a sustained usually moderate level of exposure over a period of months during prenatal and/or gestational period. Late acute insult refers to a sudden or relatively sudden, usually marked exposure to xenobiotic, infection, or other environmental stressor in infancy to early childhood (birth to 3 years). Late chronic insult refers to a sustained moderate level of exposure over a period of months during infancy to early childhood.

in Unwin et al.'s SSRI group, early intervention relating to GI pathology could allow correction of the dysfunctional peripheral autonomic input and thus permit greater sensory integration, and thus improved developmental outcome. Equally addressing the breathing dysrhythmias in the LBW group may improve autonomic reactivity improving both sensory integration and neuroimmune responsiveness. Elsewhere, we present clinical data to support such a possibility through improved autonomic function following management of co-morbid health conditions and the subsequent improvement in ASD symptoms.

CLINICAL APPLICATION

The pathophysiology of ASD remains largely unknown. Evidence so far suggests prognosis is not pre-determined and there is a dynamic component of the disease. The greater frequency of extra-CNS disease(s) (85–88), increased respiratory and GI-related childhood mortality, and substantially greater risk of progressive seizure disorders (20–22) together with the frequently reported neuroinflammatory changes (2–5) in ASD suggests ongoing disease activity, and whilst targeted treatment trials are awaited these tangible aspects of disease must be the focus of clinical intervention. Actively seeking extra-CNS disease in ASD and pro-actively managing such conditions, with the appreciation that presentation of such disease and response to intervention may not be typical or, whilst the pathophysiology remains ill-defined, predictable, is a pillar of harm reduction. Delineating sub-groups further will hopefully help predict the areas requiring further attention in each patient group.

SUMMARY

Autism spectrum disorder is a severe neurological condition with variable presentation, disease evolution, and variable, albeit generally poor, functional outcomes. Patients with ASD have greater risk of physical and mental health complications, and also a greater mortality. Neuroinflammation, peripheral immune abnormalities, and environmental factors have consistently been identified, further supporting the need for research that prioritizes disease prevention and harm reduction. The results from large epidemiological studies are awaited to identify potential key areas for this research.

Heterogeneity has been a significant barrier to successful intervention in ASD. It may be that the commonality of impaired social integration represents dysfunction of a wide variety of systems and faculties during a crucial developmental period required for the complexities of social integration and as such the commonality is merely etiological. Similar levels of intricacy may explain the propensity to abnormal acquisition of GI flora during an equally important microbiota developmental period. Here, we reviewed the most promising research findings to explain the diverse neurological, immunological, and neuroimmunological abnormalities in ASD within consideration of variable environmental insults. In our opinion, this provides a useful framework to understand and further explore this devastating neurodevelopmental condition.

REFERENCES

Hallmayer J, Cleveland S, Torres A, Phillips J, Cohen B, Torigoe T, et al. Genetic heritability and shared environmental factors among twin pairs with autism. *Arch Gen Psychiatry* (2011) 76:v1. doi:10.1001/archgenpsychiatry.2011.76

Vargas DL, Nascimbene C, Krishnan C, Zimmerman AW, Pardo CA. Neuroglial activation and neuroinflammation in the brain of patients with autism. *Ann Neurol* (2005) 57(1):67–81. doi:10.1002/ana.20315

Suzuki K, Sugihara G, Ouchi Y, Nakamura K, Futatsubashi M, Takebayashi K, et al. Microglial activation in young adults with autism spectrum disorder. *JAMA Psychiatry* (2013) 70(1):49–58. doi:10.1001/jamapsychiatry.2013.272

Tetreault NA, Hakeem AY, Jiang S, Williams BA, Allman E, Wold BJ, et al. Microglia in the cerebral cortex in autism. *J Autism Dev Disord* (2012) 42(12):2569–84. doi:10.1007/s10803-012-1513-0

Morgan JT, Chana G, Pardo CA, Achim C, Semendeferi K, Buckwalter J, et al. Microglial activation and increased microglial density observed in the dorsolateral prefrontal cortex in autism. *Biol Psychiatry* (2010) 68(4):368–76. doi:10.1016/j.biopsych.2010.05.024

Coleman M. Clinical review: medical differential diagnosis and treatment of the autistic syndrome. *Eur Child Adolesc Psychiatry* (1993) 2(3):161–8. doi:10.1007/BF02125571

Steffenburg S. Neuropsychiatric assessment of children with autism: a population based study. *Dev Med Child Neurol* (1991) 33(6):495–511. doi:10.1111/j.1469-8749.1991.tb14915.x

Lawler CP. The environmental for autism research: signs of improvement? *Environ Health Perspect* (2008) 116(10):A416. doi:10.1289/ehp.12107

Interagency Autism Coordinating Committee. *2011 IACC Strategic Plan for Autism Spectrum Disorder Research*. Washington, DC: US Department of Health and Human Services (2011).

Combating Autism Act, US Public Law 109-416 (2006).

Coleman M, Gillberg C. *The Autisms*. New York: Oxford University Press (2012).

Kanner L. Autistic disturbances of affective contact. *Nervous child* (1943) 2(3):217–50.

Kanner L. Problems of nosology and psychodynamics of early infantile autism. *Am J Orthopsychiatry* (1949) 19(3):416–26. doi:10.1111/j.1939-0025. 1949. tb05441.x

Kanner L. Follow-up study of eleven autistic children originally reported in 1943. *J Autism Dev Disord* (1971) 1(2):119–45. doi:10.1007/BF01537953

Seltzer MM, Shattuck P, Abbeduto L, Greenberg JS. Trajectory of development in adolescents and adults with autism. *Ment Retard Dev Disabil Res Rev* (2004) 10:234–47. doi:10.1002/mrdd.20038

Lotter V. Epidemiology of autistic conditions in young children: 1. Prevalence. *Soc Psychiatry* (1966) 1:124–37. doi:10.1007/BF00584048

Kuehn BM. CDC: autism spectrum disorders common. *JAMA* (2007) 297(9):940–940. doi:10.1001/jama.297.9.940

Autism and Developmental Disabilities Monitoring Network Surveillance Year 2008 Principal Investigators, Centers for Disease Control and Prevention. Preva- lence of autism spectrum disorders – autism and developmental disabilities monitoring network, 14 sites, United States, 2008. *MMWR Surveill Summ* (2012) 61(3):1–19.

Baron-Cohen S, Scott FJ, Allison C, Williams J, Bolton P, Matthews FE, et al. Prevalence of autism-spectrum conditions: UK school-based population study. *Br J Psychiatry* (2009) 194(6):500–9. doi:10.1192/bjp.bp.108.059345

Shavelle RM, Strauss DJ, Pickett J. Causes of death in autism. *J Autism Dev Disord* (2001) 31(6):569–76. doi:10.1023/A:1013247011483

Gillberg C, Billstedt E, Sundh V, Gillberg IC. Mortality in autism: a prospective longitudinal community-based study. *J Autism Dev Disord* (2010) 40(3):352–7. doi:10.1007/s10803-009-0883-4

Mouridsen SE, Brønnum-Hansen H, Rich B, Isager T. Mortality and causes of death in autism spectrum disorders. *Autism* (2008) 12(4):403–14. doi:10.1177/ 1362361308091653

Turner LM, Stone WL. Variability in outcome for children with an ASD diagnosis at age 2. *J Child Psychol Psychiatry* (2007) 48(8):793–802. doi:10.1111/j.1469-7610.2007.01744.x

Levy A, Perry A. Outcomes in adolescents and adults with autism: a review of the literature. *Res Autism Spectr Disord* (2011) 5(4):1271–82. doi:10.1016/j.rasd. 2011.01.023

Newschaffer CJ, Croen LA, Daniels J, Giarelli E, Grether JK, Levy SE, et al. The epidemiology of autism spectrum disorders. *Annu Rev Public Health* (2007) 28:235–58.

Schendel DE, Diguiseppi C, Croen LA, Fallin MD, Reed PL, Schieve LA, et al. The study to explore early development (SEED): a multisite epidemiologic study of autism by the Centres for Autism and Developmental Disabilities Research and Epidemiology (CADDRE) Network. *J Autism Dev Disord* (2012) 42:1–20. doi:10.1007/s10803-012-1461-8

Pardo CA, Vargas DL, Zimmerman AW. Immunity, neuroglia and neuroinflammation in autism. *Int Rev Psychiatry* (2005) 17(6):485–95. doi:10.1080/02646830500381930

Ashwood P, Enstrom A, Krakowiak P, Hertz-Picciotto I, Hansen RL, Croen LA, et al. Decreased transforming growth factor beta1 in autism: a potential link between immune dysregulation and impairment in clinical behavioral out- comes. *J Neuroimmunol* (2008) 204(12):149–53. doi:10.1016/j.jneuroim.2008. 07.006

Enstrom AM, Lit L, Onore CE, Gregg JP, Hansen RL, Pessah IN, et al. Altered gene expression and function of peripheral blood natural killer cells in children with autism. *Brain Behav Immun* (2009) 23(1):124–33. doi:10.1016/j.bbi.2008.08.001

Dalziel SR, Thompson JM, Macias CG, Fernandes RM, Johnson DW, Waisman Y, et al. Predictors of severe H1N1 infection in children presenting within Pedi- atric Emergency Research Networks (PERN): retrospective case-control study. *BMJ* (2013) 347:f4836. doi:10.1136/bmj.f4836

Ashwood P, Krakowiak P, Hertz-Picciotto I, Hansen R, Pessah IN, Van deWater J. Associations of impaired behaviors with elevated plasma chemokines in autism spectrum disorders. *J Neuroimmunol* (2011) 232(1):196–9. doi:10.1016/ j.jneuroim.2010.10.025

Pardo CA, Eberhart CG. The neurobiology of autism. *Brain Pathol* (2007) 17:434–47. doi:10.1111/j.1750-3639.2007.00102.x

Herbert MR. Large brains in autism: the challenge of pervasive abnormality. *Neuroscientist* (2005) 11:417–40. doi:10.1177/0091270005278866

Hallahan B, Daly EM, McAlonan G, Loth E, Toal F, O'Brien F, et al. Brain morphometry volume in autistic spectrum disorder: a magnetic resonance imaging study of adults. *Psychol Med* (2009) 39(02):337–46. doi:10.1017/S0033291708003383

Casanova M, Buxhoeveden D, Switala A, Roy E. Minicolumnar pathology in autism. *Neurology* (2002) 58(3):428–32. doi:10.1212/WNL.58.3.428

Casanova MF. The significance of minicolumnar size variability in autism: a perspective from comparative anatomy. In: Zimmerman AW, editor. *Autism*. Totowa, NJ: Humana Press (2008) p. 349–60. doi:10.1007/978-1-60327- 489-0_16

Minshew NJ, Payton JB. New perspectives in autism, Part II: the differential diagnosis and neurobiology of autism. *Curr Probl Pediatr* (1988) 18:613–94. doi:10.1016/0045-9380(88)90017-5

Minshew NJ, Williams DL. The new neurobiology of autism. *Arch Neurol* (2007) 64:945–50. doi:10.1001/archneur.64.7.945

Baird AD, Scheffer IE, Wilson SJ. Mirror neuron system involvement in empathy: a critical look at the evidence. *Soc Neurosci* (2011) 6(4):327–35. doi:10.1080/17470919.2010.547085

Gowen E, Hamilton A. Motor abilities in autism: a review using a computa- tional context. *J Autism Dev Disord* (2013) 43(2):323–44. doi:10.1007/s10803- 012-1574-0

Gowen E. Imitation in autism: why action kinematics matter. *Front Integr Neurosci* (2012) 6:117. doi:10.3389/fnint.2012.00117

Hutt C, Forrest SJ, Richer J. Cardiac arrhythmia and behaviour in autistic chil- dren. *Acta Psychiatr Scand* (1975) 51(5):361–72. doi:10.1111/j.1600-0447.1975. tb00014.x

Kootz JP, Cohen DJ. Modulation of sensory intake in autistic children: cardiovas- cular and behavioral indices. *J Am Acad Child Psychiatry* (1981) 20(4):692–701. doi:10.1097/00004583-198102000-00002

Kootz JP, Marinelli B, Cohen DJ. Modulation of response to environmental stimulation in autistic children. *J Autism Dev Disord* (1982) 12(2):185–93. doi:10.1007/BF01531308

Zahn TP, Rumsey JM, Van Kammen DP. Autonomic nervous system activity in autistic, schizophrenic, and normal men: effects of stimulus significance. *J Abnorm Psychol* (1987) 96(2):135. doi:10.1037/0021-843X.96.2.135

James AL, Barry RJ. Respiratory and vascular responses to simple visual stimuli in autistics, retardates and normals. *Psychophysiology* (1980) 17(6):541–7. doi:10.1111/j.1469-8986.1980.tb02294.x

Cohen DJ, Johnson WT. Cardiovascular correlates of attention in normal and psychiatrically disturbed children: blood pressure, peripheral blood flow, and peripheral vascular resistance. *Arch Gen Psychiatry* (1977) 34(5):561. doi:10.1001/archpsyc.1977.01770170071006

Palkovitz RJ, Wiesenfeld AR. Differential autonomic responses of autistic and normal children. *J Autism Dev Disord* (1980) 10(3):347–60. doi:10.1007/BF02408294

Ming X, Julu PO, Brimacombe M, Connor S, Daniels ML. Reduced cardiac parasympathetic activity in children with autism. *Brain Dev* (2005) 27(7):509–16. doi:10.1016/j.braindev.2005.01.003

Field T, Diego M. Vagal activity, early growth and emotional development. *Infant Behav Dev* (2008) 31(3):361–73. doi:10.1016/j.infbeh.2007.12.008

Kushki A, Drumm E, Pla Mobarak M, Tanel N, Dupuis A, Chau T, et al. Investigating the autonomic nervous system response to anxiety in children with autism spectrum disorders. *PLoS One* (2013) 8(4):e59730. doi:10.1371/journal. pone.0059730

James AL, Barry RJ. Cardiovascular and electrodermal responses to simple stimuli in autistic, retarded and normal children. *Int J Psychophysiol* (1984) 1(2):179–93. doi:10.1016/0167-8760(84)90037-0

Gogtay N, Giedd JN, Lusk L, Hayashi KM, Greenstein D, Vaituzis AC, et al. Dynamic mapping of human cortical development during childhood through early adulthood. *Proc Natl Acad Sci U S A* (2004) 101(21):8174. doi:10.1073/pnas.0402680101

Hertz-Picciotto I, Park HY, Dostal M, Kocan A, Trnovec T, Sram R. Pre- natal exposures to persistent and non-persistent organic compounds and effects on immune system development. *Basic Clin Pharmacol Toxicol* (2008) 102(2):146–54. doi:10.1111/j.1742-7843.2007.00190.x

West LJ. Defining critical windows in the development of the human immune system. *Hum Exp Toxicol* (2002) 21:499–505. doi:10.1191/0960327102ht288oa

Volk HE, Hertz-Picciotto I, Delwiche L, Lurmann F, McConnell R. Residential proximity to freeways and autism in the CHARGE study. *Environ Health Perspect* (2011) 119(6):873. doi:10.1289/ehp.1002835

Hertz-Picciotto I, Bergman A, Fängström B, Rose M, Krakowiak P, Pessah I, et al. Polybrominated diphenyl ethers in relation to autism and developmental delay: a case-control study. *Environ Health* (2011) 10:1. doi:10.1186/1476-069X- 10-1

Toms LM, Sjödin A, Harden F, Hobson P, Jones R, Edenfield E, et al. Serum polybrominated diphenyl ether (PBDE) levels are higher in children (25 years of age) than in infants and adults. *Environ Health Perspect* (2009) 117(9):1461. doi:10.1289/ehp.0900596

Roberts EM, English PB, Grether JK, Windham GC, Somberg L, Wolff C. Mater- nal residence near agricultural pesticide applications and autism spectrum dis- orders among children in the California Central Valley. *Environ Health Perspect* (2007) 115(10):1482. doi:10.1289/ehp.10168

Eskenazi B, Rosas LG, Marks AR, Bradman A, Harley K, Holland N, et al. Pesticide toxicity and the developing brain. *Basic Clin Pharmacol Toxicol* (2008) 102(2):228–36. doi:10.1111/j.1742-7843.2007.00171.x

Rosas LG, Eskenazi B. Pesticides and child neurodevelopment. *Curr Opin Pediatr* (2008) 20(2):191. doi:10.1097/MOP.0b013e3282f60a7d

Dietert RR, Dietert JM. Potential for early-life immune insult including developmental immunotoxicity in autism and autism spectrum disorders: focus on critical windows of immune vulnerability. *J Toxicol Environ Health B Crit Rev* (2008) 11(8):660–80. doi:10.1080/10937400802370923

Finegold SM, Molitoris D, Song Y, Liu C, Vaisanen ML, Bolte E, et al. Gastrointestinal microflora studies in late-onset autism. *Clin Infect Dis* (2002) 35(Suppl 1):S6–16. doi:10.1086/341914

Song Y, Liu C, Finegold SM. Real-time PCR quantitation of clostridia in feces of autistic children. *Appl Environ Microbiol* (2004) 70(11):6459–65. doi:10.1128/AEM.70.11.6459-6465.2004

Parracho HM, Bingham MO, Gibson GR, McCartney AL. Differences between the gut microflora of children with autistic spectrum disorders and that of healthy children. *J Med Microbiol* (2005) 54(10):987–91. doi:10.1099/jmm.0. 46101-0

Williams BL, Hornig M, Buie T, Bauman ML, Cho Paik M, Wick I, et al. Impaired carbohydrate digestion and transport and mucosal dysbiosis in the intestines of children with autism and gastrointestinal disturbances. *PLoS One* (2011) 6(9):e24585. doi:10.1371/journal.pone.0024585

Martirosian G, Ekiel A, Aptekorz M, Wiechuła B, Kazek B, Jankowska-Steifer E, et al. Fecal lactoferrin and *Clostridium* spp. in stools of autistic children. *Anaer- obe* (2011) 17(1):43–5. doi:10.1016/j.anaerobe.2010.12.003

Bolte ER. Autism and *Clostridium tetani*. *Med Hypotheses* (1998) 51(2):133–44. doi:10.1016/S0306-9877(98)90107-4

Sandler RH, Finegold SM, Bolte ER, Buchanan CP, Maxwell AP, Väisänen ML, et al. Short-term benefit from oral vancomycin treatment of regressive-onset autism. *J Child Neurol* (2000) 15(7):429–35. doi:10.1177/088307380001500701

Noverr MC, Huffnagle GB. Review: the 'microflora hypothesis' of allergic diseases. *Clin Exp Allergy* (2005) 35(12):1511–20. doi:10.1111/j.1365-2222.2005.02379.x

Round JL, Mazmanian SK. The gut microbiota shapes intestinal immune responses during health and disease. *Nat Rev Immunol* (2009) 9:313–23. doi:10.1038/nri2515

Jyonouchi H, Geng L, Streck DL, Toruner GA. Children with autism spec- trum disorders (ASD) who exhibit chronic gastrointestinal (GI) symptoms and marked fluctuation of behavioral symptoms exhibit distinct innate immune abnormalities and transcriptional profiles of peripheral blood (PB) monocytes. *J Neuroimmunol* (2011) 238(1–2):73–80. doi:10.1016/j.jneuroim.2011.07.001

Jyonouchi H, Geng L, Ruby A, Reddy C, Zimmerman-Bier B. Evaluation of an association between gastrointestinal symptoms and cytokine production against common dietary proteins in children with autism spectrum disorders. *J Pediatr* (2005) 146(5):605–10. doi:10.1016/j.jpeds.2005.01.027

Jyonouchi H, Geng L, Ruby A, Zimmerman-Bier B. Dysregulated innate immune responses in young children with autism spectrum disorders: their relation- ship to gastrointestinal symptoms and dietary intervention. *Neuropsychobiology* (2005) 51(2):77–85. doi:10.1159/000084164

Goines PE, Ashwood P. Cytokine dysregulation in autism spectrum disorders (ASD): possible role of the environment. *Neurotoxicol Teratol* (2013) 36:67–81. doi:10.1016/j.ntt.2012.07.006

Unwin LM, Maybery MT, Wray JA, Whitehouse AJO. A"bottom-up" approach to aetiological research in autism spectrum disorders. *Front Hum Neurosci* (2013) 7:606. doi:10.3389/fnhum.2013.00606

Tian Y, Green PG, Stamova B, Hertz-Picciotto I, Pessah IN, Hansen R, et al. Correlations of gene expression with blood lead levels in children with autism compared to typically developing controls. *Neurotox Res* (2011) 19(1):1–13. doi:10.1007/s12640-009-9126-x

Stamova B, Green PG, Tian Y, Hertz-Picciotto I, Pessah IN, Hansen R, et al. Correlations between gene expression and mercury levels in blood of boys with and without autism. *Neurotox Res* (2011) 19(1):31–48. doi:10.1007/s12640-009- 9137-7

Kamila M, Markram H. The intense world theory – a unifying theory of the neurobiology of autism. *Front Hum Neurosci* (2010) 4:224. doi:10.3389/fn-hum. 2010.00224

Reynolds S, Millette A, Devine DP. Sensory and motor characterization in the postnatal valproate rat model of autism. *Dev Neurosci* (2012) 34:258–67. doi:10.1159/000336646

Finegold Sydney M, Downes J, Summanen PH. Microbiology of regressive autism. *Anaerobe* (2012) 18(2):260–2. doi:10.1016/j.anaerobe.2011.12.018

Ley RE, Peterson DA, Gordon JI. Ecological and evolutionary forces shaping microbial diversity in the human intestine. *Cell* (2006) 124(4):837–48. doi:10.1016/j.cell.2006.02.017

Palmer C, Bik EM, DiGiulio DB, Relman DA, Brown PO. Development of the human infant intestinal microbiota. *PLoS Biol* (2007) 5:e177. doi:10.1371/journal.pbio.0050177

Onore C, Careaga M, Ashwood P. The role of immune dysfunction in the patho- physiology of autism. *Brain Behav Immun* (2012) 26(3):383–92. doi:10.1016/j. bbi.2011.08.007

Schieve LA, Gonzalez V, Boulet SL, Visser SN, Rice CE, Van Naarden Braun K, et al. Concurrent medical conditions and health care use and needs among children with learning and behavioral developmental disabilities, National Health Interview Survey, 2006-2010. *Res Dev Disabil* (2012) 33(2):467–76. doi:10.1016/j.ridd.2011.10.008

Kohane IS, McMurry A, Weber G, MacFadden D, Rappaport L, Kunkel L, et al. The comorbidity burden of children and young adults with autism spectrum disorders. *PLoS One* (2012) 7(4):e33224. doi:10.1371/journal.pone.0033224

Buie T, Fuchs GJ III, Furuta GT, Kooros K, Levy J, Lewis JD, et al. Recommendations for evaluation and treatment of common gastrointestinal problems in children with ASDs. *Pediatrics* (2010) 125(Suppl 1):S19–29. doi:10.1542/peds. 2009-1878D

Buie T, Campbell DB, Fuchs GJ III, Furuta GT, Levy J, Van de Water J, et al. Evaluation, diagnosis, and treatment of gastrointestinal disorders in individ- uals with ASDs: a consensus report. *Pediatrics* (2010) 125(Suppl 1):S1–18. doi:10.1542/peds.2009-1878C

Iwata Y, Tsuchiya KJ, Mikawa S, Nakamura K, Takai Y, Suda S, et al. Serum levels of P-selectin in men with high-functioning autism. *Br J Psychiatry* (2008) 193:338–9. doi:10.1192/bjp.bp.107.043497

Heuer L, Ashwood P, Schauer J, Goines P, Krakowiak P, Hertz-Picciotto I, et al. Reduced levels of immunoglobulin in children with autism correlates with behavioral symptoms. *Autism Res* (2008) 1:275–83. doi:10.1002/aur.42

Grigorenko EL, Han SS, Yrigollen CM, Leng L, Mizue Y, Anderson GM, et al. Macrophage migration inhibitory factor and autism spectrum disorders. *Pedi- atrics* (2008) 122:e438–45. doi:10.1542/peds.2007-3604

Onore C, Enstrom A, Krakowiak P, Hertz-Picciotto I, Hansen R, Van de Water J, et al. Decreased cellular IL-23 but not IL-17 production in chil- dren with autism spectrum disorders. *J Neuroimmunol* (2009) 216:126–34. doi:10.1016/j.jneuroim.2009.09.005

Enstrom AM, Onore CE, Van de Water JA, Ashwood P. Differential monocyte responses to TLR ligands in children with autism spectrum disorders. *Brain Behav Immun* (2010) 24:64–71. doi:10.1016/j.bbi.2009.08.001

Ashwood P, Krakowiak P, Hertz-Picciotto I, Hansen R, Pessah IN, Van de Water Altered T cell responses in children with autism. *Brain Behav Immun* (2010) 25(5):840–9. doi:10.1016/j.bbi.2010.09.002

Goines P, Haapanen L, Boyce R, Duncanson P, Braunschweig D, Delwiche L, et al. Autoantibodies to cerebellum in children with autism associate with behavior. *Brain Behav Immun* (2011) 25:514–23. doi:10.1016/j.bbi.2010.11.017

Kajizuka M, Miyachi T, Matsuzaki H, Iwata K, Shinmura C, Suzuki K, et al. Serum levels of platelet-derived growth factor BB homodimers are increased in male children with autism. *Prog Neuropsychopharmacol Biol Psychiatry* (2010) 34:154–8. doi:10.1016/j.pnpbp.2009.10.017

Ashwood P, Krakowiak P, Hertz-Picciotto I, Hansen R, Pessah I, Van de Water Elevated plasma cytokines in autism spectrum disorders provide evidence of immune dysfunction and are associated with impaired behavioral outcome. *Brain Behav Immun* (2011) 25:40–45. doi:10.1016/j.bbi.2010.08.003

6

Stress modulates intestinal secretory immunoglobulin A

Rafael Campos-Rodríguez[1], Marycarmen Godínez-Victoria[1], Edgar Abarca-Rojano[1], Judith Pacheco-Yépez[1], Humberto Reyna-Garfias[1], Reyna Elizabeth Barbosa-Cabrera[1], Maria Elisa Drago-Serrano[2]*

[1] *Sección de Posgrado e Investigación, Escuela Superior de Medicina, Instituto Politécnico Nacional, Distrito Federal, México*
[2] *Departamento de Sistemas Biológicos, Unidad Xochimilco, Universidad Autónoma Metropolitana, Distrito Federal, México*

Edited by:
Emilio Domínguez-Salazar, Universidad Autónoma Metropolitana, Unidad Iztapalapa, México

Reviewed by:
Antonio Pereira, Federal University of Rio Grande do Norte, Brazil
Emilio Domínguez-Salazar, Universidad Autónoma Metropolitana, Unidad Iztapalapa, México

***Correspondence:**
Maria Elisa Drago-Serrano, Departamento de Sistemas Biológicos, Unidad Xochimilco, Universidad Autónoma Metropolitana, Calzada del Hueso No. 1100, Colonia Villa Quietud, CP 04960, México City, Distrito Federal, México
e-mail: dragome@yahoo.com

Stress is a response of the central nervous system to environmental stimuli perceived as a threat to homeostasis. The stress response triggers the generation of neurotransmitters and hormones from the hypothalamus pituitary adrenal axis, sympathetic axis and brain gut axis, and in this way modulates the intestinal immune system. The effects of psychological stress on intestinal immunity have been investigated mostly with the restraint/immobilization rodent model, resulting in an up or down modulation of SIgA levels depending on the intensity and time of exposure to stress. SIgA is a protein complex formed by dimeric (dIgA) or polymeric IgA (pIgA) and the secretory component (SC), a peptide derived from the polymeric immunoglobulin receptor (pIgR). The latter receptor is a transmembrane protein expressed on the basolateral side of gut epithelial cells, where it uptakes dIgA or pIgA released by plasma cells in the lamina propria. As a result, the IgA-pIgR complex is formed and transported by vesicles to the apical side of epithelial cells. pIgR is then cleaved to release SIgA into the luminal secretions of gut. Down modulation of SIgA associated with stress can have negative repercussions on intestinal function and integrity. This can take the form of increased adhesion of pathogenic agents to the intestinal epithelium and/or an altered balance of inflammation leading to greater intestinal permeability. Most studies on the molecular and biochemical mechanisms involved in the stress response have focused on systemic immunity. The present review analyzes the impact of stress (mostly by restraint/immobilization, but also with mention of other models) on the generation of SIgA, pIgR and other humoral and cellular components involved in the intestinal immune response. Insights into these mechanisms could lead to better therapies for protecting against pathogenic agents and avoiding epithelial tissue damage by modulating intestinal inflammation.

Keywords: SIgA, pIgR, intestinal mucosa, restraint-stress, glucocorticoids, brain-gut axis

INTRODUCTION

Stress is a response of the central nervous system (CNS) to environmental stimuli perceived as a threat to homeostasis. The stress response involves a complex network of mechanisms essential for survival, mediated by neurotransmitters, peptidic hormones and endocrine hormones from the enteric nervous system (ENS), a branch of the autonomic nervous system that among other functions affects the production of interleukins (ILs). These molecules in turn modulate the humoral and cellular components of the intestinal immune system. The ENS contains both vagal and spinal sensory neurons, which play an essential role in the transference of information from the CNS to ENS and vice versa (de Jonge, 2013).

Experimental assays have evidenced that the stress modulates the generation of secretory immunoglobulin A (SIgA; Jarillo-Luna et al., 2007; Martínez-Carrillo et al., 2011) and the expression of pIgR (Reyna-Garfias et al., 2010). Through transcytosis this receptor transports immunoglobin-pIgR complexes (dIgA-pIgR and pIgA-pIgR) across gut epithelial cells. Upon reaching the apical side of these cells, pIgR is cleaved to release SIgA or SC, a pIgR derived peptide into the intestinal lumen (Brandtzaeg, 2009). Along with the gut microflora, both SIgA and pIgR have an essential role in two important intestinal processes. They protect against pathogenic agents that colonize and/or invade the intestinal epithelium, and modulate the gut inflammatory response to maintain homeostasis (Michetti et al., 1992; Uren et al., 2003; Sait et al., 2007; Bruno et al., 2010; Drago-Serrano et al., 2010).

Few studies have explored the effect of stress on SIgA and pIgR, or the capacity of these molecules to maintain homeostasis in the intestine. Most studies involving molecular and biochemical mechanisms of the stress response have focused on systemic rather than intestinal immunity.

The aim of the present review is to explore the impact of stress on the humoral and cellular components of the intestinal immune response, especially IgA, SIgA and pIgR. Although most of the evidence is from studies involving rodent models of restraint/immobilization, other stress-producing protocols affecting SIgA are mentioned, including loud noise, alternating home and metabolic cages, exposure to heat, repeated electric foot shock, and the mixing of newborns from distinct litters (**Table 1**).

Table 1 | Impact of stress on intestinal immunity.

Animal model	Effect	Reference
Alternating home/metabolic cages (male rats)	↓SIgA; fecal/urine corticosterone excretion unchanged	Eriksson et al. (2004)
Heat stress (rats)	↓SIgA; ↓ IL-2,-4, and -10 in small gut; ↑CD8+ T cells in MLN	Liu et al. (2012)
Repeated electric foot shock (mice)	↓IFN-γ released by gut IEL and α/β TCR+ cells; ↑glucocorticoids	Zhang et al. (2005)
Electric foot shock (EFS) and psychological stress (PS) (rats)	↓SIgA (PS); ↑IgA (EFS) in MLN; ↑corticosterone (EFS)	Yamamoto et al. (2009)
Repeated restraint stress (mice)	↓SIgA; lamina propria IgA+ plasm a cell levels unchanged; ↓gut intraepithelial lymphocytes via adrenal hormones	Jarillo-Luna et al. (2007, 2008)
Restraint stress (mice)	↓T cell and B cells; ↑apoptosis in PP; ↑glucocorticoids	Sudo et al. (2001)
Chronic restraint stress (mice)	↓SIgA+ plasma cells, CD8+T and B cells in PP	Martínez-Carrillo et al. (2011)
Immobilization and acoustic stress (CB1R ko mice)	↓SIgA; ↑ bacterial translocation	Zoppi et al. (2012)
Repeated immobilization (rats with MCAO)	↓SIgA; ↑ bacterial translocation, colon inflammation	Caso et al. (2009)
Acute immobilization stress (rats)	↓SIgA; ↑colon inflammation	Ponferrada et al. (2007)
Repeated restraint stress (rats)	↑SIgA and α- chain mRNA in proximal and distal gut	Reyna-Garfias et al. (2010)
Weaning, cold stress, mix of piglets infected with ETEC	↑SIgA and ETEC fecal shedding	Jones et al. (2001)

↓ down modulation; ↑ up modulation; EFS, electric foot shock; IgA, immunoglobulin A; IFN-γ, interferon-γ; IL, interleukin; IEL, intraepithelial lymphocytes; MCAO, middle cerebral artery occlusion; mRNA messenger ribonucleic acid; MLN, mesenteric lymph node; PP, Peyer's patches; SIgA, secretory IgA; TCR, T cell receptor; TNF, tumor necrosis factor; CB1R ko, cannabinoid 1 receptor knock out; Mix, mixing newborns from distinct litters; ETEC, enterotoxigenic E. coli.

THE NERVOUS SYSTEM AND THE INTESTINAL IMMUNE RESPONSE

The mutual influence of the nervous system and the intestinal immune response has been widely studied using experimental models of stress. ILs and microbiota from the gut can modulate the nervous system. On the other hand, the nervous system can modulate intestinal immunity by several pathways (de Jonge, 2013).

For instance, the nervous system regulates immune function through the hypothalamic pituitary adrenal axis (HPA). In response to stress, the hypothalamus releases the corticotrophin releasing factor (CRF) into the anterior pituitary, causing the release of adrenocorticotropic hormone (ACTH) into the blood flow. ACTH stimulates the generation of glucocorticoids (cortisol in humans and corticosterone in mice) in the cortex of the adrenal medulla (McClennen et al., 1998; Jezova et al., 1999), which are then released into the blood. Additionally, the nervous system modulates intestinal immunity through the sympathetic autonomic nervous system by triggering the release of catecholamines (adrenaline and noradrenaline) from the adrenal gland medulla (Kvetnanský et al., 1995; Jezova et al., 1999; **Figure 1**).

Stress also triggers the response of a plethora of peptide hormones and neurotransmitters by intrinsic innervation of the ENS. The ENS is connected bidirectionally to the CNS through sympathetic and parasympathetic nerve pathways forming the brain-gut axis (BGA; de Jonge, 2013). The autonomic ENS comprises sympathetic (noradrenergic) and parasympathetic (cholinergic) fibers that interact directly with the CNS through parasympathetic (vagal) and sympathetic splanchnic fibers. Within the ENS the intrinsic nerve fibers are organized in myenteric (Auerbach's plexus), submucosal (Meissner's plexus) and mucosal plexus. The latter contain nerve endings that can make contact with antigen presenting cells (APCs) to control gut immune responses (de Jonge, 2013). Regulation of the BGA is accomplished by the integration of four control levels. Control level one is accomplished by the ENS endowed with local innervations that functionally are independent of the extrinsic nervous connections. Level two entails the prevertebral sympathetic ganglia where peripheral reflex pathways are influenced by preganglionic sympathetic fibers from the spinal cord. Levels three and four are within the CNS. In the level three sympathetic and parasympathetic fibers outflow to the gut is determined in part by reflex with sensory fibers that travel with autonomic nerves. The level four includes higher nerve centers that supply descending signals that are integrated with incoming sensory signals at the level three (**Figure 2**).

At the intestinal level the bilateral communication between the nervous system and intestinal immune response occurs through sympathetic innervations, which influence (i) the differential distribution of immunocytes in different regions of the small intestine (Ke et al., 2011), (ii) the migration of lymphocytes towards Peyer's patches and mesenteric lymphoid nodules (MLN; Gonzalez-Ariki and Husband, 1998), and (iii) the ontogeny of IgA+ B cells populating the intestinal lamina propria (Gonzalez-Ariki and Husband, 2000).

Mouse gut is innervated by fibers expressing adrenergic receptors (Hirafuji et al., 2001; Nasser et al., 2006). Upon interacting with an agonist, these receptors enable enterochromaffin cells to release neuropeptides that affect IgA levels. The secretion of IgA is also influenced by the interaction of peptidic innervations inside Peyer's patches with immunocytes, and of nerve fibers from the

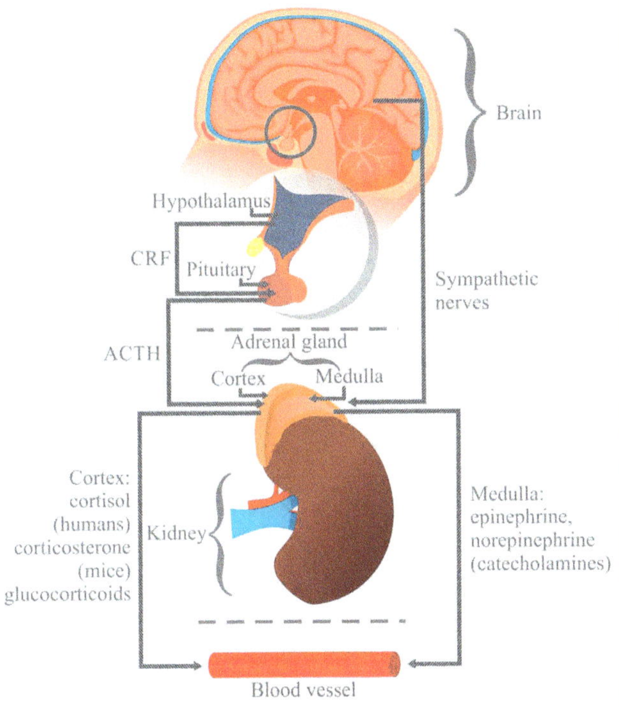

FIGURE 1 | In response to stress, the hypothalamus (H) releases the corticotrophin releasing factor (CRF) into the anterior pituitary (P), causing the release of adrenocorticotropic hormone (ACTH) into the blood flow. ACTH stimulates the generation of glucocorticoids (cortisol in humans and corticosterone in mice) in the cortex of the adrenal gland (A), which are then released into the blood. Stress also activates the autonomic sympathetic nerves in the medulla of the adrenal gland to elicit the production of catecholamines, norepinephrine and epinephrine, which are then released into the blood. Glucocorticoids and catecholamines influence the generation of interleukins, which are involved in the viability and proliferation of immunocompetent gut cells via receptors.

gut basement membrane with IgA+ cells (Hisajima et al., 2005; Vulchanova et al., 2007). Moreover, the release of norepinephrine (Schmidt et al., 2007), acetylcholine (Wilson et al., 1982; Schmidt et al., 2007) and neuropeptides (Schmidt et al., 1999) by gut nerve fibers modulates the secretion of intestinal IgA and the expression of pIgR (Cox et al., 2007). Additionally, gut nerve fibers release the vasoactive intestinal peptide, neuropeptide Y (Mongardi Fantaguzzi et al., 2009) and somatostatin (Schmidt et al., 1999), which all help modulate the intestinal production of SIgA (Shibata et al., 2008).

THE GENERATION OF INTESTINAL IgA

From an immunological point of view, intestinal SIgA is produced by a multistage process modulated by ILs. This process involves the activation and class switch recombination of IgM+ to IgA+ B cells, the latter of which are committed to IgA synthesis either by a T-cell dependent or T-cell independent pathway (Cerutti, 2008).

The T-dependent pathway is induced in follicular areas of Peyer's patches after the interaction between the APCs and helper Th2 lymphocytes (**Figure 3**). On their surface, APCs (like dendritic cells) express the CD40 antigen and a peptide-derived antigen associated with the major histocompatibility class II molecule (MHC-II). The CD40 antigen interacts with CD40L on Th2 cells, and the peptide-MHC-II complex with the Th2 cell receptor (TCR). In either case, immunological synapses lead to the release of the transforming growth factor (TGF)-β1 by Th2 cells, which is an essential step for the activation and class switch recombination of IgM+ B cells to IgA+ B lymphocytes.

Other Th2-derived ILs, including IL-4,-5,-6, and -10, promote the proliferation of IgA+ B cells and their differentiation into IgA secreting plasma cells. In the presence of retinoic acid, IgA+ B cells express gut-homing receptors, such as α4β7 integrin, CCR9 and CCR10, and cause these cells to migrate from Peyer's patches to the MLN via the circulation of efferent lymphatic vessels. From the MLN these cells go to the thoracic duct, enter the bloodstream, and finally home to the lamina propria, the effector site of the gut immune system.

Epithelial cells that line the lamina propria express mucosal address in cell adhesion molecule 1 (MadCAM1) and the chemokines CCL25 and CCL28, which are the ligands for α4β7 integrin, CCR9 and CCR10, respectively, on B cells. In the lamina propria IgA+ B cells mature to plasma cells capable of releasing dimers or polymers of IgA joined to J-chain (Brandtzaeg, 2009; **Figure 3**).

The T-independent pathway for the production of intestinal IgA occurs in extra-follicular structures, including isolated lymphoid follicles and lamina propria. The class switch recombination of IgM+ B cells to IgA+ B lymphocytes takes place through two pathways, and both involve a T-independent antigen. IgM+ B lymphocytes express B cell receptors (BCRs) and Toll-like receptors (TLRs). Polysaccharides interact with BCRs and bacterial lipopolysaccharide (LPS) and/or nucleic acids with TLRs (Cerutti, 2008). In the lamina propria IgA+ B cells further differentiate into IgA+ plasma cells.

THE TRANSPORT OF INTESTINAL IgA

The expression of pIgR is necessary for the transport (transcytosis) of dIgA or pIgA across the epithelial layer. pIgR is a 120 kDa transmembrane protein consisting of five extracellular immunoglobulin (Ig) homology domains, a transmembrane region and a cytoplasmic domain. The amino (NH_2) terminal of this protein chain is oriented to the extracellular space, while the carboxyl (COOH) terminal has an intracellular orientation and contains signals for intracellular sorting and endocytosis (Asano and Komiyama, 2011; Johansen and Kaetzel, 2011).

pIgR is expressed on the basolateral surface of epithelial cells. Its expression can be constitutive or regulated at a transcriptional level by IL-4 and pro-inflammatory cytokines, the latter including tumor necrosis factor α (TNF-α) and interferon γ (IFN-γ; Johansen and Kaetzel, 2011). IgA transcytosis begins when pIgR uptakes dIgA or pIgA released in the lamina propria by plasma cells (Cerutti, 2008). The dIgA-pIgR or pIgA-pIgR complex is transported by vesicles across the epithelial cell, and upon reaching the apical side pIgR is cleaved to render SC bound to dIgA/pIgA. The resulting SIgA is released into the intestinal lumen (Asano and Komiyama, 2011).

The cleavage of pIgR to yield SC occurs at the linker that connects domain 5 to the transmembrane region (**Figure 4**).

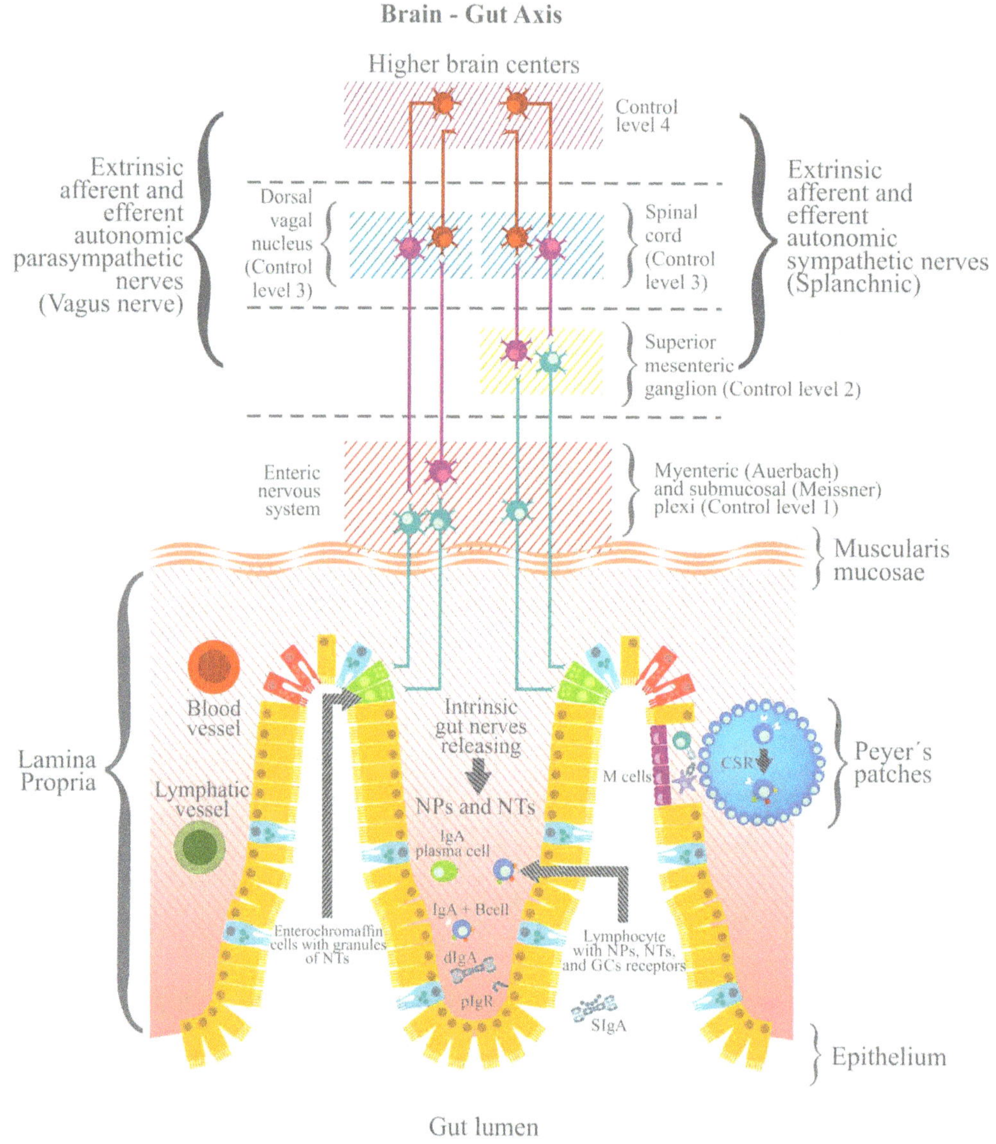

FIGURE 2 | Stress also triggers the activation of the enteric nervous system, including afferent and efferent intrinsic intestinal nerves (afferent nerves send signals from periphery to the brain; efferent nerves from the brain to the periphery) and extrinsic innervations, whether sympathetic (splanchnic) or parasympathetic (Vagus nerve). The enteric nervous system is connected to the CNS via sympathetic and parasympathetic pathways, forming the brain-gut axis (BGA). Four levels for the control of BGA are shown (Wood et al., 1999). The stress response of the BGA influences the generation of dIgA and/or the pIgR mediated trancytosis. NTs, neurotransmitters; NPs, neuropeptides; GCs, glucocorticoids.

Biochemically and morphologically, trancytosis involves: (i) the endocytosis of dIgA from clathrin coated pits and its delivery to basolateral endosomes, (ii) microtubule dependent translocation to apical recycling endosomes, and (iii) delivery of the plasma membrane to apical endosomes (Johansen and Kaetzel, 2011).

THE ROLE OF SIgA AND pIgR

Both SIgA and pIgR have an essential role in immune exclusion, which protects against infections caused by enteropathogens. This role has been explored in the murine model of *Salmonella typhimurium* infection (Michetti et al., 1992; Drago-Serrano et al., 2010).

SIgA helps to limit the adhesion of luminal antigens to the epithelium. These antigens, if not excluded in gut secretions, are able to elicit the release of cell derived inflammatory cytokines, which can enhance permeability and disrupt the functional integrity of the gut. As a result of increased gut permeability, penetration of luminal antigens into the systemic compartment may cause a strong and even life-threatening systemic inflammatory response (Brandtzaeg, 2009; Corthésy, 2007).

pIgA and the different forms of IgA also have anti-inflammatory role. For instance, pIgA and dIgA protect host tissue by neutralizing pro-inflammatory antigens inside and below the

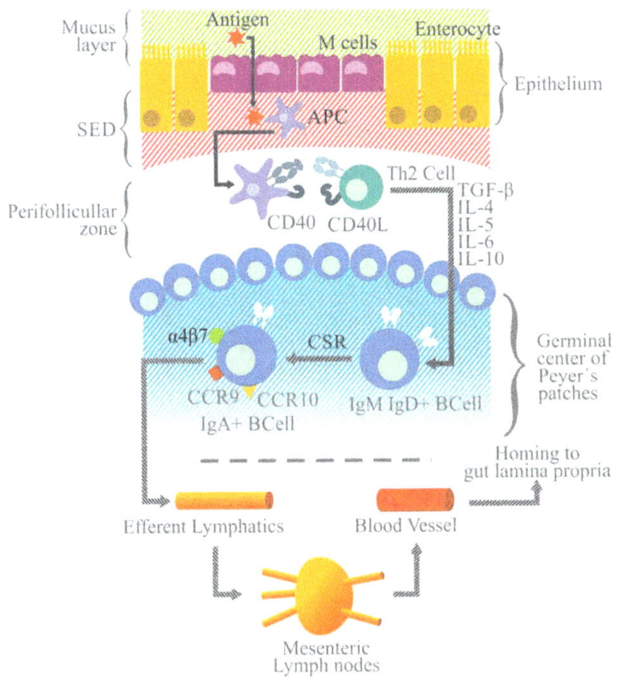

FIGURE 3 | Simplified model of IgA generation. Antigen presenting cells and dendritic cells are located in the subepithelial dome (SED) beneath M cells. After sampling, luminal antigen is processed and expressed on the surface as an antigen-derived peptide associated with the MHC-II molecule. Dendritic cells with the MCH II peptide and the CD40 antigen on the surface migrate to the perifollicular zone of Peyer's patches to interact with Th2 lymphocytes endowed with TCRs and CD40 ligand (CD40L) on their surface. Immunological synapsis between APC and Th2 cells via the binding of the MHC-II peptide to TCR and of CD40 to CD40L leads to the activation of Th2 and the release of TGF-β. Along with signals elicited by the CD40/CD40L binding, TGF-β is a Th2-derived IL essential for the class switch recombination of IgM+ B cells to generate IgA+ B cells, occurring in the germinal center of Peyer's patches (highlighted in blue). Other Th2 ILs (e.g., IL-4, -5, -6, and -10) favor the differentiation and maturation of IgA+ B cells into IgA+ plasma cells. IgA+ B lymphocytes acquire the expression of gut-homing receptors, such as α4β7, CCR9 and CCR10, and migrate toward efferent lymphatic vessels and mesenteric lymphoid nodules. From there they can reach the blood stream and migrate to the lamina propria (the gut effector site). Gut epithelial cells express the MadCAM1 ligand for α4β7, and release CCL25 and CCL28, chemokines that are ligands for the CCR9 and CCR10 receptors, respectively.

gut epithelium layer. On the other hand, dIgA and pIgA are unable to elicit the production of pro-inflammatory cytokines on cells by binding with receptors specific for the Fc α-domain (Corthésy, 2007). Furthermore, SIgA and pIgR, along with the intestinal microflora, contribute to gut homeostasis by maintaining the intestinal inflammatory response within the normal physiological limit (Uren et al., 2003; Sait et al., 2007; Bruno et al., 2010). Since the gut microbiota and SIgA are bilaterally modulated, an alteration in one may affect intestinal homeostasis and lead to intestinal inflammation (Suzuki et al., 2004; Bruno et al., 2010).

Hence, the generation of IgA+ B cells in Peyer's patches, the homing of IgA+ B cells to the gut lamina propria, and the transcytosis of dIgA/pIgA via pIgR are all potential targets of stress-related effects that can alter SIgA levels.

THE RESTRAINT MODEL AND THE INFLUENCE OF STRESS IN THE INTESTINE

Assays based on the restraint model have provided important insights into the influence of stress on the humoral and cellular components involved in the intestinal immune response via neuroendocrine pathways. In the restraint procedure, a rodent is placed (without forced squeezing) inside a cylindrical plastic tube. This represents mainly psychological stress, as the perception of confinement mimics a collapsed tunnel for these burrow-dwelling animals (Dhabhar and Viswanathan, 2005). Another restraint procedure, known as immobilization, involves adhering outstretched rodent limbs on a board with tape. Compared to restraint in a plastic tube, this model has elicited a much more robust stress response through the generation of neuroendocrine mediators (e.g., glucocorticoids and catecholamines; Glavin et al., 1994).

The restraint stress model has provided evidence of intricate neurological pathways underlying the regulation of SIgA. Such pathways involve neurotransmitters and endocrine hormones released from the blood flow or produced locally (e.g., glucocorticoids released by intestinal epithelial cells), and their interaction with the receptors of target cells (Cima et al., 2004).

It is now known that modulation of SIgA production is influenced by the duration (acute or chronic) and intensity of stress. Generally at a systemic level, acute stress (represented by a single session lasting a few minutes to a few hours) tends to upregulate the number of immune cells. Contrarily, the multiple sessions over a period of several days, weeks or months that represent chronic stress (Dhabhar, 2009) tend to downregulate the systemic immune response. Experimental assays with skin delay type hypersensitivity response in rats corroborate this same general pattern of acute and chronic stress (Dhabhar and McEwen, 1997).

Intensity of stress is another factor that can influence the result on the immune response. It is measured by the increase in levels of adrenal hormones, neurotransmitters and physiological parameters (e.g., heart rate and blood pressure), as well as the period of time that these changes persist (during and after the stress-inducing event; Dhabhar, 2009). This assays on mice have shown that (i) the acute stress response elicited by intense running promotes the accumulation of T lymphocytes in Peyer's patches via adrenergic mechanisms, evidenced by the fact that this exercise-dependent increase was blocked by α- (phentolamine) or β- (nadolol) adrenoceptor antagonists (Krüger et al., 2008), and (ii) repeated sessions of chronic restraint stress have a negative influence on intestinal levels of SIgA, which may be due to the capability of corticosteroids to decrease the trancytosis of SIgA via pIgR (Jarillo-Luna et al., 2007). Another study on mice reported that corticosteroids decrease pIgA levels in mucosal secretions and increase such levels in serum. This effect is due in part to the greater production in serum of SC, which is derived from hepatic pIgR. The binding of SC to pIgA retards the clearance of the latter from the blood by the liver (Wira et al., 1990).

In addition to reducing intestinal SIgA levels, repeated stress has a negative influence on the number of lymphoid cells in Peyer's patches and the intestinal intraepithelial compartment. These suppressive effects of restraint stress were mimicked by the administration of pharmacological dose of catecholamines and glucocorticoids, results suggested the activation of two

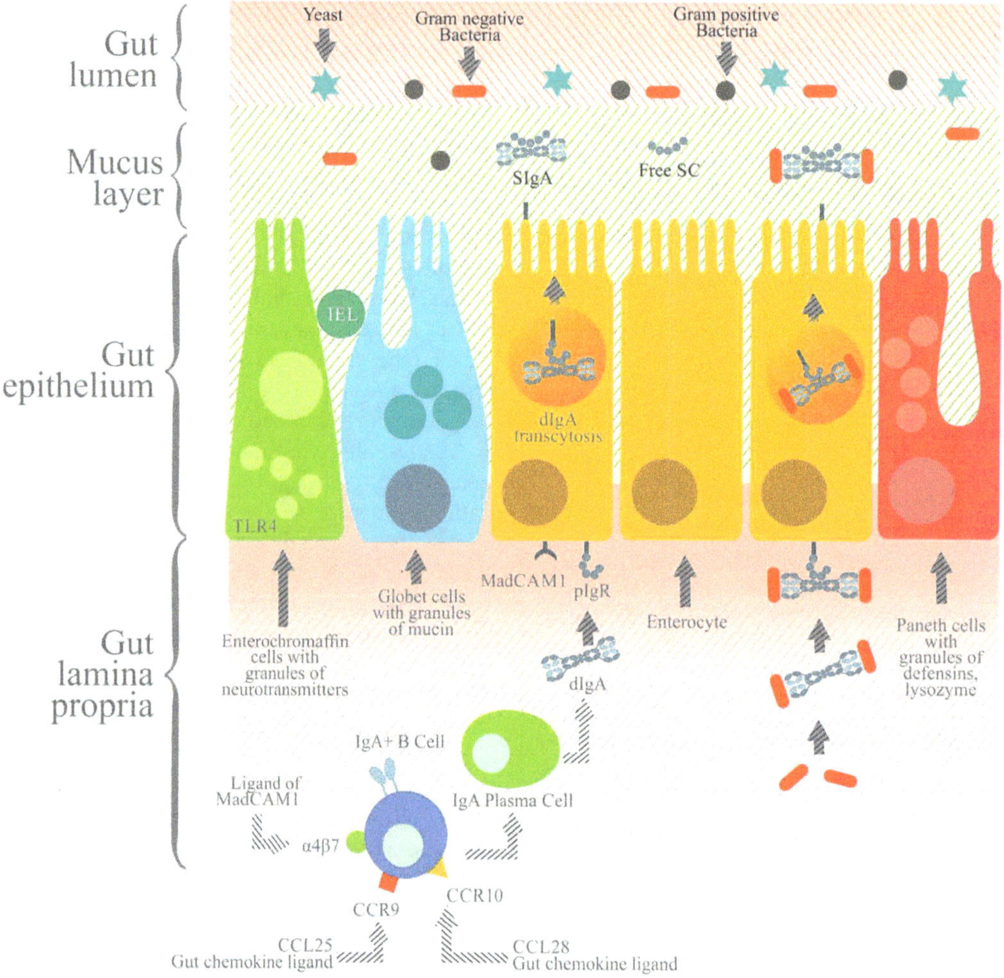

FIGURE 4 | In the gut lamina propria, IgA+ B cells further differentiate into IgA+ plasma cells that secrete dIgA or pIgA antibodies joined by the J chain. dIgA or pIgA are captured by the polymeric immunoglobulin receptor (pIgR), a transmembrane receptor with five extracellular domains and an intracellular tail expressed at the basolateral side of the enterocytes. The dIgA-pIgR complex is internalized and transported by transcytosis to the apical side, and the extracellular portion of pIgR with five domains is proteolytically cleaved from the transmembrane region. The former is then released to the gut lumen as secretory component (SC) bound to dIgA to yield secretory IgA (SIgA). SIgA and SC secreted into the mucus layer prevent the direct adhesion to the epithelium of pathogenic agents, which are eventually cleared from the lumen. Apart from enterocytes, other cell components of the gut epithelium include enterochromaffin cells with granules of neurotransmitters, Paneth cells with granules containing defensins and lysozyme, and goblet cells with mucin granules and IEL.

pathways— the sympathetic autonomic nervous system and the HPA axis (Jarillo-Luna et al., 2007, 2008; Martínez-Carrillo et al., 2011). In another study, the endogenous production of glucocorticoids, triggered by a continuous 12-h period of restraint stress, decreased the number of T and B cells in Peyer's patches, which is in line with a reduction in the levels of intestinal SIgA and lymphocytes (Sudo et al., 2001).

Other experimental stress protocols have been reported to have a negative influence on the gut immune response (**Table 1**). The stress produced in rats by exposure to heat negatively affected some intestinal parameters, including the levels of CD3+ and CD4+ T lymphocytes, the expression of TLR-2 and TLR-4, as well as the transcriptional mRNA expression of IFN-γ and IL-2, -4, and -10 (Liu et al., 2012). Assays on rats with an electric shock protocol showed that stress suppressed the production of IFN-γ through T cells with TCRαβ in the intraepithelial compartment, while at the same time elevating the level of endogenous glucocorticoids (Zhang et al., 2005). Studies on rodents under psychological stress have also reported a decrease in levels of intestinal SIgA, caused by: (i) an expectation of electric foot shock (Yamamoto et al., 2009), (ii) a continuous back and forth transference from housing cages to metabolic cages (Eriksson et al., 2004), and (iii) immobilization, in some cases combined with exposure to loud noise (Ponferrada et al., 2007; Caso et al., 2009; Zoppi et al., 2012).

THE IMMUNOMODULATORY MECHANISMS OF STRESS (TABLE 2)

CELL MIGRATION

The aforementioned stress-related changes in the levels of IgA, IgA secreting cells and IgA producing ILs may be related to cell

Table 2 | Mechanisms of immune modulation by stress.

Effect	Mechanism	Reference
↓SIgA levels by acute immobilization stress	↓ SIgA attenuated by peroxisome proliferator-activated receptor- γ (PPAR)-γ activation	Ponferrada et al. (2007)
↓SIgA levels by immobili-zation and acoustic stress	↓ SIgA attenuated by cannabinoid 1 receptor (CB1R) activation	Zoppi et al. (2012)
↓ activation/migration of T cells induced by restraint stress	Alterations of cytoskeletal actin and plasma membrane factors by stress hormones	Flint et al. (2011)
↓ number of lymphocytes in spleen by restraint stress	Apoptosis through p53 and PI3K/NF-κB pathways	Zhang et al. (2008a)
↓ number of T lymphocytes in Peyer's patches by exercise associated stress	Fas/FasL apoptosis pathway	Krüger et al. (2009)
↓ number of lymphocytes in spleen by chronic restraint stress	μ-receptor mediated apoptosis, dependent on endogenous opioids and independent of glucocorticoids from activation of HPA axis	Wang et al. (2002)
↓ number of splenocytes by chronic restraint stress	CD95 (Fas/APO-1) mediated apoptosis, dependent on endogenous opioids but independent of the activation of HPA axis	Yin et al. (2000)
↑Immunosuppression by chronic restraint stress	Apoptosis via TLR4/PI3K signaling	Zhang et al. (2008b)
↑Immunosupression by restraint stress	↓ MHC-II expression in peritoneal macrophages along with ↑corticosterone levels	Zwilling et al. (1990)
↑Immunosupression by restraint stress	↓ MHC-II expression influenced by corticosterone and some hormones not associated with the activation of HPA axis	Zwilling et al. (1993)
↑ T cell proliferation or apoptosis by restraint stress	Activation of *GADD45g* and *pura* genes, responsible for apoptosis and proliferation, respectively	Flint et al. (2005)
↑ SIgA levels and ETEC proliferation following stress by weaning and short term exposure to cold	Catecholamines enable iron acquisition that promotes bacterial proliferation	Jones et al. (2001), Lyte et al. (2011)

↓ down modulation; ↑up modulation; MHC-II, major histocompatibility complex class II; PI3K/NF-κB, phosphoinositide 3 kinase/nuclear factor κB; TLR4, Toll-like receptor 4; HPA, hypothalamus-pituitary-adrenal axis; GADD45g, growth arrest and DNA-damage inducible gamma; pura, purine rich element binding protein A; ETEC, Enterotoxigenic Escherichia coli; SIgA, secretory immunoglobuline A.

migration, a phenomenon that has been studied mostly in the systemic response (Bauer et al., 2001). Acute restraint stress decreases the number of peripheral helper T lymphocytes, upregulates the expression of adhesion molecules (CD11a and CD11b) on T cells, and increases the levels of circulating NK cells and glucocorticoids. These changes were not found in mice previously exposed to chronic intermittent restraint stress, suggesting an adaptation response to prolonged stress.

One presumable mechanism entails greater restraint-induced levels of glucocorticoids and/or catecholamines, which influence lymphocyte trafficking through the expression of adhesion molecules on endothelial cells (Dietrich, 2004; Krüger and Mooren, 2007; Krüger et al., 2008). This effect was found in mice under stress caused by exercise (Krüger et al., 2008). It seems that stress hormones influence lymphocyte migration and function through specific alterations in the actin cytoskeleton, an effect also found in mice under restraint stress (Flint et al., 2011).

CELL VIABILITY AND T CELL ACTIVATION

Another downmodulatory mechanism related to restraint stress is a decrease in cell viability and/or T cell activation. For instance, at a systemic level the restraint stress protocol elicits a reduction in splenic lymphocytes by apoptosis through the activation of p53 and PI3K/NFκB pathways (Zhang et al., 2008a). p53 is a pro-apoptotic factor which upmodulates the expression of Fas. Phosphoinositide 3 kinases (PI3K) are signal transduction enzymes involved in regulating cell proliferation, and the nuclear factor κB (NFκB) modulates the expression of genes involved in the innate and adaptive immune responses, as well as in cell survival and death (Zhang et al., 2008a).

At the intestinal level, the decreased number of viable lymphocytes in Peyer's patches induced by restraint stress may also lead to apoptosis (Sudo et al., 2001), which seems to be dependent on the Fas/Fas ligand activation signal, as evidenced by T cells in Peyer's patches of mice under stress by intense exercise (Krüger et al., 2009). One report suggested that glucocorticoids are the main apoptotic inducers involved in the decreased number of intestinal intraepithelial lymphocytes (Brunner et al., 2001), which is in agreement with other studies. The molecular mechanisms of glucocorticoid-induced apoptosis are highly dependent on the binding of this ligand with its receptor (Schmidt et al., 2004), which is a cytosolic ligand-dependent transcription factor. After binding to the ligand, the glucocorticoid receptor dissociates from the protein complex, dimerizes and translocates into the nucleus, where it then binds to regulate the transcription of apoptotic genes (Schmidt et al., 2004).

Another presumable mechanism of lymphocyte apoptosis induced by restraint stress relies on signals triggered by the interaction of endogenous opioids with μ-opioid (Wang et al., 2002) and CD95 receptors (Yin et al., 2000). Cell death caused by the binding of endogenous opioids with CD95 (also known as Fas or apo1) or μ-opioid seems to be independent of the HPA axis (Yin et al., 2000). The binding of CD95 with specific agonists induces the activation of a cascade of caspases, and ultimately nucleases, that results in apoptotic cell death (Yin et al., 2000). Endogenous opioid peptides (endorphins, enkephalins and endomorphins) play a critical modulatory role in emotional stress-induced changes in the immune system (Bodnar, 2012).

An additional mechanism by which restraint stress downmodulates lymphocytes is through the activation of TLR-4, which in turn inhibits the activation of the PI3K (Zhang et al., 2008b). While inhibition of the PI3K signaling pathway induces lymphocyte apoptosis (Yin et al., 2006), its activation inhibits the same (Wu et al., 2000). TLR-4 can also mediate signaling that leads to cell death through the interaction of the death domain of myeloid differentiation factor 88 (MyD88) with the Fas associated death domain (FADD; Haase et al., 2003).

THE INHIBITION OF MHC-II

Expression of the MHC-II glycoprotein by APC is essential for the initiation of the immune response by CD4+ T cells (Blum et al., 2013). A stress-induced decrease in MHC-II expression is carried out by elevated levels of corticosterone (Zwilling et al., 1990) and other hormones not associated with the HPA axis (Zwilling et al., 1993). It seems that a higher level of corticosterone triggered by restraint stress diminishes the number of IFN-γ receptors on macrophages. Since the binding of IFN-γ to its receptor triggers the signaling necessary for MHC-II expression (Zwilling et al., 1992), a reduction in the expression of this receptor decreases the expression of MHC-II.

ENDOGENOUS RECEPTORS CAN ATTENUATE THE STRESS-INDUCED DOWN REGULATION OF SIgA

Assays conducted on mice under a protocol of immobilization, in some cases with exposure to loud noise, evidenced that the immunosuppressive influence of stress on SIgA can be attenuated by the activation of the cannabinoid 1 receptor (CB1R; Zoppi et al., 2012) and the peroxisome proliferator-activated receptor (PPAR)-γ (Ponferrada et al., 2007). Both the CB1R (Hill and McEwen, 2010) and PPAR-γ nuclear receptors (Dubuquoy et al., 2006) have an essential role in the modulation of colon inflammation by stress.

Cannabinoid 1 receptor is one of the most prominent receptors for cannabinoids distributed in the CNS and peripherally in immune cells. It is a G-protein coupled receptor whose endogenous ligands are arachidonate derived lipophilic molecules, N-arachidonylethanolamine anandamide and 2- arachidonylglycerol, which affect emotional behavior (Hill and McEwen, 2010).

Peroxisome proliferator-activated receptor-γ is a nuclear receptor expressed in the colon that forms a heterodimer with the retinoid X receptor (RXR). It is activated by natural endogenous ligands, polyunsaturated fatty acids (PUFAs) and eicosanoids, allowing for its heterodimerization with RXR and its binding to the nuclear peroxisome proliferator response element (PPRE). PPAR-γ and RXR play a central role in the regulation of inflammatory signaling pathways by acting on kinases and transcription factors, such as NFkB, and by inhibiting mucosal production of inflammatory cytokines (Dubuquoy et al., 2006). When PPAR-γ expression in intestinal epithelial cells is induced by LPS-activated TLR-4, it leads to the regulation of NFkB and MAPK pathways and modulation of the inflammatory response. Up regulation of TLR-4 expression together with impaired expression of PPAR-γ in epithelial cells may lead to superficial colonic inflammation in patients with ulcerative colitis.

THE UPMODULATORY EFFECTS OF STRESS

Although stress has been regarded as immunosuppressive, it can enhance the levels of IgA (Yamamoto et al., 2009) and CD3+/CD8+ T lymphocytes in the MLN of rats under stress by electric foot shock or exposure to heat (Liu et al., 2012). The capacity of restraint stress to activate the gene expression of purine rich element binding protein A (*pura*) has been reported to be responsible for priming T cells to undergo proliferation (Flint et al., 2005). Thus, the upmodulatory effects of restraint stress hormones on SIgA levels and on mRNA expression of pIgR should not be surprising (Reyna-Garfias et al., 2010). Indeed, at the molecular level it has been reported that glucocorticoids upmodulate the transcriptional mRNA expression of pIgR via a glucocorticoid DNA response element located in the 5'upstream region of the pIgR gene in rat duodenum (Li et al., 1999).

Experimental studies have evidenced that stress can trigger SIgA secretion in response to an enhanced bacterial proliferation, as reported in feces from piglets infected with ETEC under protocols involving weaning and short-term exposure to cold (Jones et al., 2001). In this case, the presumable influence of stress in promoting bacterial proliferation may be related to catecholamines, which can make iron available to bacteria by removing it from host proteins like transferrin and lactoferrin (Lyte et al., 2011).

Although the context of the development of the immune response in the intestine and systemic compartments is different, the modulatory influence of the stress response may share some mechanisms in both cases.

CONCLUSION AND PERSPECTIVES

Gut homeostasis results from neuroimmune modulation by anti- and pro-inflammatory ILs, neurotransmitters and endocrine hormones, all of which influence the generation of intestinal SIgA. This immunoglobin in turn affects intestinal inflammation and permeability, which are essential factors in the functional integrity of the gut under stress conditions. Experimental studies with the restraint/immobilization rodent model have resulted in an up or down modulation of SIgA levels depending on the intensity and time of exposure to stress. In the case of down regulation, there is an increased susceptibility to infection and intestinal inflammation. Pharmacological modulation of the cannabinoid system and the PPAR-γ may be therapeutically useful for intestinal dysfunctions resulting from a stress-induced decrease in SIgA levels. Future studies should explore the adaptation of experimental models for the evaluation of therapeutic and preventive strategies to control intestinal inflammation and/or infection in patients with high vulnerability to stress.

REFERENCES

Asano, M., and Komiyama, K. (2011). Polymeric immunoglobulin receptor. *J. Oral Sci.* 53, 147–156. doi: 10.2334/josnusd.53.147

Bauer, M. E., Perks, P., Lightman, S. L., and Shanks, N. (2001). Are adhesion molecules involved in stress-induced changes in lymphocyte distribution? *Life Sci.* 69, 1167–1179. doi: 10.1016/S0024-3205(01)01200-0

Blum, J. S., Wearsch, P. A., and Cresswell, P. (2013). Pathways of antigen processing. *Annu. Rev. Immunol.* 31, 443–473. doi: 10.1146/annurev-immunol-032712-095910

Bodnar, R. J. (2012). Endogenous opiates and behavior: 2011. *Peptides* 38, 463–522. doi: 10.1016/j.peptides.2012.09.027

Brandtzaeg, P. (2009). Mucosal immunity: induction, dissemination, and effector functions. *Scand. J. Immunol.* 70, 505–515. doi: 10.1111/j.1365-3083.2009.02319.x

Brunner, T., Arnold, D., Wasem, C., Herren, S., and Frutschi, C. (2001). Regulation of cell death and survival in intestinal intraepithelial lymphocytes. *Cell Death Differ.* 8, 706–714. doi: 10.1038/sj.cdd.4400854

Bruno, M. E., Rogier, E. W., Frantz, A. L., Stefka, A. T., Thompson, S. N., and Kaetzel, C. S. (2010). Regulation of the polymeric immunoglobulin receptor in intestinal epithelial cells by Enterobacteriaceae: implications for mucosal homeostasis. *Immunol. Invest.* 39, 356–382. doi: 10.3109/08820131003622809

Caso, J. R., Hurtado, O., Pereira, M. P., García-Bueno, B., Menchén, L., Alou, L., et al. (2009). Colonic bacterial translocation as a possible factor in stress-worsening experimental stroke outcome. *Am. J. Physiol. Regul. Integr. Comp. Physiol.* 296, R979–R985. doi: 10.1152/ajpregu.90825.2008

Cerutti, A. (2008). The regulation of IgA class switching. *Nat. Rev. Immunol.* 8, 421–434. doi: 10.1038/nri2322

Cima, I., Corazza, N., Dick, B., Fuhrer, A., Herren, S., Jakob, S., et al. (2004). Intestinal epithelial cells synthesize glucocorticoids and regulate T cell activation. *J. Exp. Med.* 200, 1635–1646. doi: 10.1084/jem.20031958

Corthésy, B. (2007). Roundtrip ticket for secretory IgA: role in mucosal homeostasis? *J. Immunol.* 178, 27–32.

Cox, S. W., Ebersole, L. E., Carpenter, G. H., and Proctor, G. B. (2007). Effects of autonomic agonists and immunomodulatory cytokines on polymeric immunoglobulin receptor expression by cultured rat and human salivary and colonic cell lines. *Arch. Oral Biol.* 52, 411–416. doi: 10.1016/j.archoralbio.2006.10.006

de Jonge, W. J. (2013). The gut's little brain in control of intestinal immunity. *ISRN Gastroenterol.* 2013, Article ID 630159. doi: 10.1155/2013/630159

Dhabhar, F. S. (2009). Enhancing versus suppressive effects of stress on immune function: implications for immunoprotection and immunopathology. *Neuroimmunomodulation* 16, 300–317. doi: 10.1159/000216188

Dhabhar, F. S., and McEwen, B. S. (1997). Acute stress enhances while chronic stress suppresses cell-mediated immunity in vivo: a potential role for leukocyte trafficking. *Brain Behav. Immun.* 11, 286–306. doi: 10.1006/brbi.1997.0508

Dhabhar, F. S., and Viswanathan, K. (2005). Short-term stress experienced at time of immunization induces a long-lasting increase in immunologic memory. *Am. J. Physiol. Regul. Integr. Comp. Physiol.* 289, R738–R744. doi: 10.1152/ajpregu.00145.2005

Dietrich, J. B. (2004). Endothelial cells of the blood-brain barrier: a target for glucocorticoids and estrogens? *Front. Biosci.* 9:684–693. doi: 10.2741/1272

Drago-Serrano, M. E., Rivera-Aguilar, V., Reséndiz-Albor, A. A., and Campos-Rodríguez, R. (2010). Lactoferrin increases both resistance to *Salmonella typhimurium* infection and the production of antibodies in mice. *Immunol. Lett.* 134, 35–46. doi: 10.1016/j.imlet.2010.08.007

Dubuquoy, L., Rousseaux, C., Thuru, X., Peyrin-Biroulet, L., Romano, O., Chavatte, P., et al. (2006). PPARgamma as a new therapeutic target in inflammatory bowel diseases. *Gut* 55, 1341–1349. doi: 10.1136/gut.2006.093484

Eriksson, E., Royo, F., Lyberg, K., Carlsson, H. E., and Hau, J. (2004). Effect of metabolic cage housing on immunoglobulin A and corticosterone excretion in faeces and urine of young male rats. *Exp. Physiol.* 89, 427–433. doi: 10.1113/expphysiol.2004.027656

Flint, M. S., Budiu, R. A., Teng, P. N., Sun, M., Stolz, D. B., Lang, M., et al. (2011). Restraint stress and stress hormones significantly impact T lymphocyte migration and function through specific alterations of the actin cytoskeleton. *Brain Behav. Immun.* 25, 1187–1196. doi: 10.1016/j.bbi.2011.03.009

Flint, M. S., Carroll, J. E., Jenkins, F. J., Chambers, W. H., and Han, M. L., Baum, A. (2005). Genomic profiling of restraint stress-induced alterations in mouse T lymphocytes. *J. Neuroimmunol.* 167, 34–44. doi: 10.1016/j.jneuroim.2005.06.012

Glavin, G. B., Paré, W. P., Sandbak, T., Bakke, H. K., and Murison, R. (1994). Restraint stress in biomedical research: an update. *Neurosci. Biobehav. Rev.* 18, 223–249. doi: 10.1016/0149-7634(94)90027-2

Gonzalez-Ariki, S., and Husband, A. J. (1998). The role of sympathetic innervation of the gut in regulating mucosal immune responses. *Brain Behav. Immun.* 12, 53–63. doi: 10.1006/brbi.1997.0509

Gonzalez-Ariki, S., and Husband, A. J. (2000). Ontogeny of IgA(+) cells in lamina propria: effects of sympathectomy. *Dev. Comp. Immunol.* 24, 61–69. doi: 10.1016/S0145-305X(99)00056-7

Haase, R., Kirschning, C. J., Sing, A., Schröttner, P., Fukase, K., Kusumoto, S., et al. (2003). A dominant role of Toll-like receptor 4 in the signaling of apoptosis in bacteria-faced macrophages. *J. Immunol.* 171, 4294–4303.

Hill, M. N., and McEwen, B. S. (2010). Involvement of the endocannabinoid system in the neurobehavioural effects of stress and glucocorticoids. *Prog. Neuropsychopharmacol. Biol. Psychiatry* 34, 791–797. doi: 10.1016/j.pnpbp.2009.11.001

Hirafuji, M., Ogawa, T., Kato, K., Hamaue, N., Endo, T., Parvez, H., et al. (2001). Noradrenaline stimulates 5-hydroxytryptamine release from mouse ileal tissues via alpha(2)-adrenoceptors. *Eur. J. Pharmacol.* 432, 149–152. doi: 10.1016/S0014-2999(01)01474-1

Hisajima, T., Kojima, Y., Yamaguchi, A., Goris, R. C., and Funakoshi, K. (2005). Morphological analysis of the relation between immunoglobulin A production in the small intestine and the enteric nervous system. *Neurosci. Lett.* 381, 242–246. doi: 10.1016/j.neulet.2005.02.047

Jarillo-Luna, A., Rivera-Aguilar, V., Garfias, H. R., Lara-Padilla, E., Kormanovsky, A., and Campos-Rodríguez, R. (2007). Effect of repeated restraint stress on the levels of intestinal IgA in mice. *Psychoneuroendocrinology* 32, 681–692. doi: 10.1016/j.psyneuen.2007.04.009

Jarillo-Luna, A., Rivera-Aguilar, V., Martìnez-Carrillo, B. E., Barbosa-Cabrera, E., Garfias, H. R., and Campos-Rodríguez, R. (2008). Effect of restraint stress on the population of intestinal intraepithelial lymphocytes in mice. *Brain Behav. Immun.* 22, 265–275. doi: 10.1016/j.bbi.2007.08.004

Jezova, D., Ochedalski, T., Glickman, M., Kiss, A., and Aguilera, G. (1999). Central corticotropin-releasing hormone receptors modulate hypothalamic-pituitary-adrenocortical and sympathoadrenal activity during stress. *Neuroscience* 94, 797–802. doi: 10.1016/S0306-4522(99)00333-4

Johansen, F. E., and Kaetzel, C. S. (2011). Regulation of the polymeric immunoglobulin receptor and IgA transport: new advances in environmental factors that stimulate pIgR expression and its role in mucosal immunity. *Mucosal Immunol.* 4, 598–602. doi: 10.1038/mi.2011.37

Jones, P. H., Roe, J. M., and Miller, B. G. (2001). Effects of stressors on immune parameters and on the faecal shedding of enterotoxigenic *Escherichia coli* in piglets following experimental inoculation. *Res. Vet. Sci.* 70, 9–17. doi: 10.1053/rvsc.2000.0436

Ke, Y., Liu, W., Wang, Z., Dong, Y., and Chen, Y. (2011). The role of sympathectomy on the distribution of intraepithelial lymphocyte, mast cell, IgA^{+}, $CD4^{+}$ and $CD8^{+}$ cell in intestine of mice. *Asian J. Anim. Vet. Adv.* 6, 935–943. doi: 10.3923/ajava.2011.935.943

Krüger, K., Frost, S., Most, E., Völker, K., Pallauf, J., and Mooren, F. C. (2009). Exercise affects tissue lymphocyte apoptosis via redox-sensitive and Fas-dependent signaling pathways. *Am. J. Physiol. Regul. Integr. Comp. Physiol.* 296, R1518–R1527. doi: 10.1152/ajpregu.90994.2008

Krüger, K., Lechtermann, A., Fobker, M., Völker, K., and Mooren, F. C. (2008). Exercise-induced redistribution of T lymphocytes is regulated by adrenergic mechanisms. *Brain Behav. Immun.* 22, 324–338. doi: 10.1016/j.bbi.2007.08.008

Krüger, K., and Mooren, F. C. (2007). T cell homing and exercise. *Exerc. Immunol. Rev.* 13, 37–54.

Kvetnanský, R., Pacák, K., Fukuhara, K., Viskupic, E., Hiremagalur, B., Nankova, B., et al. (1995). Sympathoadrenal system in stress. Interaction with the hypothalamic-pituitary-adrenocortical system. *Ann. N. Y. Acad. Sci.* 771, 131–158. doi: 10.1111/j.1749-6632.1995.tb44676.x

Li, T. W., Wang, J., Lam, J. T., Gutierrez, E. M., Solorzano-Vargus, R. S., Tsai, H. V., et al. (1999). Transcriptional control of the murine polymeric IgA receptor promoter by glucocorticoids. *Am. J. Physiol.* 276, G1425–G1434.

Liu, X., Li, H., Lu, A., Zhong, Y., Hou, X., Wang, N., et al. (2012). Reduction of intestinal mucosal immune function in heat-stressed rats and bacterial translocation. *Int. J. Hyperthermia* 28, 756–765. doi: 10.3109/02656736.2012.729173

Lyte, M., Vulchanova, L., and Brown, D. R. (2011). Stress at the intestinal surface: catecholamines and mucosa-bacteria interactions. *Cell Tissue Res.* 343, 23–32. doi: 10.1007/s00441-010-1050-0

Martínez-Carrillo, B. E., Godinez-Victoria, M., Jarillo-Luna, A., Oros-Pantoja, R., Abarca-Rojano, E., Rivera-Aguilar, V., et al. (2011). Repeated restraint stress reduces the number of IgA-producing cells in Peyer's patches. *Neuroimmunomodulation* 18, 131–141. doi: 10.1159/000322625

McClennen, S. J., Cortright, D. N., and Seasholtz, A. F. (1998). Regulation of pituitary corticotropin-releasing hormone-binding protein messenger ribonucleic acid levels by restraint stress and adrenalectomy. *Endocrinology* 139, 4435–4441. doi: 10.1210/en.139.11.4435

Michetti, P., Mahan, M. J., Slauch, J. M., Mekalanos, J. J., and Neutra, M. R. (1992). Monoclonal secretory immunoglobulin IgA protects mice against oral challenge with the invasive pathogen *Salmonella typhimurium*. *Infect. Immun.* 60, 1786–1792.

Mongardi Fantaguzzi, C., Thacker, M., Chiocchetti, R., and Furness, J. B. (2009). Identification of neuron types in the submucosal ganglia of the mouse ileum. *Cell Tissue Res.* 336, 179–189. doi: 10.1007/s00441-009-0773-2

Nasser, Y., Ho, W., and Sharkey, K. A. (2006). Distribution of adrenergic receptors in the enteric nervous system of the guinea pig, mouse, and rat. *J. Comp. Neurol.* 495, 529–553. doi: 10.1002/cne.20898

Ponferrada, A., Caso, J. R., Alou, L., Colón, A., Sevillano, D., Moro, M. A., et al. (2007). The role of PPARgamma on restoration of colonic homeostasis after experimental stress-induced inflammation and dysfunction. *Gastroenterology* 132, 1791–1803. doi: 10.1053/j.gastro.2007.02.032

Reyna-Garfias, H., Miliar, A., Jarillo-Luna, A., Rivera-Aguilar, V., Pacheco-Yepez, J., Baeza, I., et al. (2010). Repeated restraint stress increases IgA concentration in rat small intestine. *Brain Behav. Immun.* 24, 110–118. doi: 10.1016/j.bbi.2009.09.005

Sait, L. C., Galic, M., Price, J. D., Simpfendorfer, K. R., Diavatopoulos, D. A., Uren, T. K., et al. (2007). Secretory antibodies reduce systemic antibody responses against the gastrointestinal commensal flora. *Int. Immunol.* 19, 257–265. doi: 10.1093/intimm/dxl142

Schmidt, L. D., Xie, Y., Lyte, M., Vulchanova, L., and Brown, D. R. (2007). Autonomic neurotransmitters modulate immunoglobulin A secretion in porcine colonic mucosa. *J. Neuroimmunol.* 185, 20–28. doi: 10.1016/j.jneuroim.2006.10.028

Schmidt, P. T., Eriksen, L., Loftager, M., Rasmussen, T. N., and Holst, J. J. (1999). Fast acting nervous regulation of immunoglobulin A secretion from isolated perfused porcine ileum. *Gut* 45, 679–685. doi: 10.1136/gut.45.5.679

Schmidt, S., Rainer, J., Ploner, C., Presul, E., Riml, S., and Kofler, R. (2004). Glucocorticoid-induced apoptosis and glucocorticoid resistance: molecular mechanisms and clinical relevance. *Cell Death Differ.* 11(Suppl. 1), S45–S55. doi: 10.1038/sj.cdd.4401456

Shibata, M., Hisajima, T., Nakano, M., Goris, R. C., and Funakoshi, K. (2008). Morphological relationships between peptidergic nerve fibers and immunoglobulin A-producing lymphocytes in the mouse intestine. *Brain Behav. Immun.* 22, 158–166. doi: 10.1016/j.bbi.2007.08.013

Sudo, N., Oyama, N., Yu, X. N., and Kubo, C. (2001). Restraint stress-induced elevation of endogenous glucocorticoids decreases Peyer's patch cell numbers via mechanisms that are either dependent or independent on apoptotic cell death. *Neuroimmunomodulation* 9, 333–339. doi: 10.1159/000059391

Suzuki, K., Meek, B., Doi, Y., Muramatsu, M., Chiba, T., Honjo, T., et al. (2004). Aberrant expansion of segmented filamentous bacteria in IgA-deficient gut. *Proc. Natl. Acad. Sci. U.S.A.* 101, 1981–1986. doi: 10.1073/pnas.0307317101

Uren, T. K., Johansen, F. E., Wijburg, O. L., Koentgen, F., Brandtzaeg, P., and Strugnell, R. A. (2003). Role of the polymeric Ig receptor in mucosal B cell homeostasis. *J. Immunol.* 170, 2531–2539.

Vulchanova, L., Casey, M. A., Crabb, G. W., Kennedy, W. R., and Brown, D. R. (2007). Anatomical evidence for enteric neuroimmune interactions in Peyer's patches. *J. Neuroimmunol.* 185, 64–74. doi: 10.1016/j.jneuroim.2007.01.014

Wang, J., Charboneau, R., Barke, R. A., Loh, H. H., and Roy, S. (2002). Mu-opioid receptor mediates chronic restraint stress-induced lymphocyte apoptosis. *J. Immunol.* 169, 3630–3636.

Wilson, I. D., Soltis, R. D., Olson, R. E., and Erlandsen, S. L. (1982). Cholinergic stimulation of immunoglobulin A secretion in rat intestine. *Gastroenterology* 83, 881–888.

Wira, C. R., Sandoe, C. P., and Steele, M. G. (1990). Glucocorticoid regulation of the humoral immune system. I. In vivo effects of dexamethasone on IgA and IgG in serum and at mucosal surfaces. *J. Immunol.* 144, 142–146.

Wood, J. D., Alpers, D. H., and Andrews, P. L. (1999). Fundamentals of neurogastroenterology. *Gut* 45(Suppl. 2), II6–II16. doi: 10.1136/gut.45.2008.ii6

Wu, W., Lee, W. L., Wu, Y. Y., Chen, D., Liu, T. J., Jang, A., et al. (2000). Expression of constitutively active phosphatidylinositol 3-kinase inhibits activation of caspase 3 and apoptosis of cardiac muscle cells. *J. Biol. Chem.* 275, 40113–40119. doi: 10.1074/jbc.M004108200

Yamamoto, S., Motomura, A., Akahoshi, A., Takahashi, K., and Minami, H. (2009). Immunoglobulin secretions in the mesenteric lymph node in stressed rats. *J. Nutr. Sci. Vitaminol. (Tokyo)* 55, 191–194. doi: 10.3177/jnsv.55.191

Yin, D., Tuthill, D., Mufson, R. A., and Shi, Y. (2000). Chronic restraint stress promotes lymphocyte apoptosis by modulating CD95 expression. *J. Exp. Med.* 191, 1423–1428. doi: 10.1084/jem.191.8.1423

Yin, D., Woodruff, M., Zhang, Y., Whaley, S., Miao, J., Ferslew, K., et al. (2006). Morphine promotes Jurkat cell apoptosis through pro-apoptotic FADD/P53 and anti-apoptotic PI3K/Akt/NF-kappaB pathways. *J. Neuroimmunol.* 174, 101–107. doi: 10.1016/j.jneuroim.2006.02.001

Zhang, X., Okutsu, M., Kanemi, O., and Nagatomi, R. (2005). Effect of foot shock stress on the interferon-gamma production of murine intestinal intraepithelial lymphocytes. *Immunol. Lett.* 100, 170–176. doi: 10.1016/j.imlet.2005.03.011

Zhang, Y., Foster, R., Sun, X., Yin, Q., Li, Y., Hanley, G., et al. (2008a). Restraint stress induces lymphocyte reduction through p53 and PI3K/NF-kappaB pathways. *J. Neuroimmunol.* 200, 71–76. doi: 10.1016/j.jneuroim.2008.06.014

Zhang, Y., Zhang, Y., Miao, J., Hanley, G., Stuart, C., Sun, X., et al. (2008b). Chronic restraint stress promotes immune suppression through toll-like receptor 4-mediated phosphoinositide 3-kinase signaling. *J. Neuroimmunol.* 204, 13–19. doi: 10.1016/j.jneuroim.2008.08.011

Zoppi, S., Madrigal, J. L., Pérez-Nievas, B. G., Marín-Jiménez, I., Caso, J. R., Alou, L., et al. (2012). Endogenous cannabinoid system regulates intestinal barrier function in vivo through cannabinoid type 1 receptor activation. *Am. J. Physiol. Gastrointest. Liver Physiol.* 302, G565–G571. doi: 10.1152/ajpgi.00158.2011

Zwilling, B. S., Brown, D., Feng, N., Sheridan, J., and Pearl, D. (1993). The effect of adrenalectomy on the restraint stressed induced suppression of MHC class II expression by murine peritoneal macrophages. *Brain Behav. Immun.* 7, 29–35. doi: 10.1006/brbi.1993.1003

Zwilling, B. S., Brown, D., and Pearl, D. (1992). Induction of major histocompatibility complex class II glycoproteins by interferon-gamma: attenuation of the effects of restraint stress. *J. Neuroimmunol.* 37, 115–122. doi: 10.1016/0165-5728(92)90162-E

Zwilling, B. S., Dinkins, M., Christner, R., Faris, M., Griffin, A., Hilburger, M., et al. (1990). Restraint stress-induced suppression of major histocompatibility complex class II expression by murine peritoneal macrophages. *J. Neuroimmunol.* 29, 125–130. doi: 10.1016/0165-5728(90)90154-F

Conflict of Interest Statement: The authors declare that the research was conducted in the absence of any commercial or financial relationships that could be construed as a potential conflict of interest.

7

Immune mechanisms in cerebral ischemic tolerance

Lidia Garcia-Bonilla, Corinne Benakis, Jamie Moore, Costantino Iadecola and Josef Anrather*

Brain and Mind Research Institute, Weill Cornell Medical College, New York, NY, USA

Edited by:
Adam Denes, University of Manchester, UK

Reviewed by:
Sophie Layé, Université Bordeaux, France
Craig J. Smith, Salford Royal NHS Foundation Trust, UK

***Correspondence:**
Josef Anrather, Brain and Mind Research Institute, Weill Cornell Medical College, 407 East 61st Street, RR-409, New York, NY 10065, USA
e-mail: joa2006@med.cornell.edu

Stressor-induced tolerance is a central mechanism in the response of bacteria, plants, and animals to potentially harmful environmental challenges. This response is characterized by immediate changes in cellular metabolism and by the delayed transcriptional activation or inhibition of genetic programs that are not generally stressor specific (cross-tolerance). These programs are aimed at countering the deleterious effects of the stressor. While induction of this response (preconditioning) can be established at the cellular level, activation of systemic networks is essential for the protection to occur throughout the organs of the body. This is best signified by the phenomenon of remote ischemic preconditioning, whereby application of ischemic stress to one tissue or organ induces ischemic tolerance (IT) in remote organs through humoral, cellular and neural signaling. The immune system is an essential component in cerebral IT acting simultaneously both as mediator and target. This dichotomy is based on the fact that activation of inflammatory pathways is necessary to establish IT and that IT can be, in part, attributed to a subdued immune activation after index ischemia. Here we describe the components of the immune system required for induction of IT and review the mechanisms by which a reprogrammed immune response contributes to the neuroprotection observed after preconditioning. Learning how local and systemic immune factors participate in endogenous neuroprotection could lead to the development of new stroke therapies.

Keywords: preconditioning, ischemic tolerance, stroke, TLR, epigenetics, microRNAs, TNF, inflammation

INTRODUCTION

Inflammation is a central component in the pathophysiology of cerebral ischemia. Brain ischemia triggers both a local and systemic inflammatory response. These responses play contradictory roles: contributing to progression of the ischemic lesion on one hand, and to processes of tissue repair in the injured brain on the other (Iadecola and Anrather, 2011a; Macrez et al., 2011). Since post-ischemic inflammation shows detrimental and beneficial aspects, anti-inflammatory therapies that indiscriminately target both arms of this immune response have not been successful (Iadecola and Anrather, 2011a; Macrez et al., 2011). Therefore, a deeper understanding of post-ischemic inflammation is needed in order to harness its beneficial effects for therapeutic purposes.

In addition to its beneficial role in the repair and regeneration of ischemic tissue, inflammatory pathways are also involved in evoking neuroprotective mechanisms that lead to ischemic tolerance (IT). The brain is equipped with a remarkable capacity to mount self-protective programs that are tuned to limit the deleterious effects of ischemia, commonly referred to as endogenous neuroprotection (Iadecola and Anrather, 2011b). These protective programs can be evoked by preconditioning (PC) stimuli (**Table 1**), such as sublethal stressors, resulting in IT (Kirino, 2002; Narayanan et al., 2013). Thus, understanding the endogenous inflammatory pathways involved in brain IT may lead to novel therapeutic strategies for the prevention and repair of neuronal damage in stroke patients (Shpargel et al., 2008; Macrez et al., 2011).

Cerebral IT can be acquired by several stimuli including short episodes of transient focal and global cerebral ischemia, remote organ ischemia, hypoxia, hypothermia, hyperthermia, exposure to inhalation anesthetics, cortical spreading depression (CSD), brief episodes of seizures or by exposure to low-dose bacterial lipopolysaccharide (LPS) prior to cerebral ischemia (Gidday, 2006; Kunz et al., 2007; Shpargel et al., 2008). IT is characterized by the activation of evolutionary conserved programs that serve to increase the resistance of the brain to ischemia. In the case of early preconditioning, these programs can be activated through preexisting signaling modules that converge in the mitochondria to improved mitochondrial function and energy metabolism during the ischemic event (Dirnagl and Meisel, 2008). In contrast, delayed PC involves gene transcription and protein synthesis (Kitagawa et al., 1990). Because activation of transcription is the main mechanism by which many pro-inflammatory signaling cascades induce a specific cellular response, inflammation is thought to be a significant component of delayed PC. **Table 2** summarizes the inflammatory pathways involved in IT achieved by different PC stimuli (**Table 1**). Inflammation is activated by innate immune receptors such as Toll-like receptors (TLRs) or cytokines receptors such as tumor necrosis factor receptor 1 (TNFR1) and interleukin-1 receptor (IL-1R). Activation of these pathways results in the induction of inflammatory genes that are mediators or effectors of the PC stimulus. In addition to conferring cytoprotection directly, the acquired IT protects the brain by suppressing post-ischemic proinflammatory gene expression,

Table 1 | List of preconditioning stimuli inducing ischemic tolerance.

Abbreviation	Preconditioning stimulus	Achieved by
IPC	Ischemic preconditioning	Transient focal and global cerebral ischemia
RIPC	Remote ischemic preconditioning	Transient occlusion of femoral arteries, mesenteric artery or renal artery
HPC	Hypoxic preconditioning	Exposure to a hypoxic gas mixture
HBO-PC	Hyperoxia or hyperbaric oxygen preconditioning	Exposure to hyperoxia (high oxygen tension) or hyperbaricity (high atmospheric pressure)
Hypo- or hyper-thermic PC	Hypothermic or hyperthermic preconditioning	Decrease or increase of body temperature, respectively
Anesthetic PC	Anesthetic preconditioning	Inhalation of low dose isoflurane or halothane
CSD-PC	Cortical spreading depression preconditioning	Propagation of depolarization wave across the cortical surface
Seizure PC	Seizure preconditioning	Kainic acid injections that induce mild epileptic activity
Exercise PC	Exercise preconditioning	Motor training (treadmill)
TLR-PC	Toll-like receptor preconditioning	Administration of low dose of TLR ligands
LPS-PC	Lipopolysaccharide preconditioning	Administration of low dose of bacterial lipopolysaccharide endotoxin

microglial and endothelial activation and leukocyte infiltration (Huang et al., 2006; Iadecola and Anrather, 2011b).

In this review we will focus on inflammatory pathways leading to cerebral IT. We will review the signaling cascades involved in immune activation in different PC modalities and highlight the molecular components involved. Lastly, this review will highlight the importance of epigenetic modifications and microRNAs in PC-induced reprogramming of the immune system.

EVIDENCE FOR A ROLE OF INFLAMMATORY PATHWAYS IN DIFFERENT PC PARADIGMS

A wide variety of preconditioning stimuli trigger the activation of inflammatory pathways that lead to brain IT (**Table 2**). The receptors, transducers and effector elements of these pathways are shared among different preconditioning paradigms. For example, TLRs are potent mediators of both ischemic (Pradillo et al., 2009; Wang et al., 2010) and endotoxic PC (acquired by systemic administration of LPS) (Tasaki et al., 1997; Ahmed et al., 2000; Vartanian et al., 2011). Likewise, the TNF pathway is involved in ischemic, hypoxic, hyperthermic and exercise-induced PC. Although inflammatory pathways are not independently sufficient for the induction of IT, there is evidence that several PC modalities are dependent upon the induction of such pathways.

ISCHEMIC, HYPOXIC, AND HYPEROXIC PC

Short non-damaging episodes of ischemia prior to a lethal ischemic episode leads to IT (Kirino, 2002). Cerebral IT can be acquired by local PC, mediated either by global (Kitagawa et al., 1990) or focal cerebral ischemia (Barone et al., 1998), or by remote ischemic PC (RIPC), typically achieved by limb ischemia (Tapuria et al., 2008). Although both TLR2 and TLR4 have been implicated in the post-ischemic inflammatory response (Cao et al., 2007; Abe et al., 2010; Brea et al., 2011; Shichita et al., 2012), only TLR4 has been shown to participate in ischemic preconditioning (IPC) (Konstantinov et al., 2004; Pradillo et al., 2009). TLR4 signaling activates transcription nuclear factor-κB (NF-κB) leading to the expression of TNF, inducible nitric oxide (iNOS) and cyclooxygenase-2 (COX-2), which are required to evoke a PC effect (see **Table 2**). Similarly, TNFR1, another central receptor of the innate immune system and activator of NF-κB, is essential for the induction of IPC (Konstantinov et al., 2004; Pradillo et al., 2005; **Figure 1**).

IT is not limited to the organ to which a stressor is applied. A PC stimulus applied to one organ also leads to IT in other organs, referred to remote PC (for reviews see Tapuria et al., 2008; Anrather and Hallenbeck, 2013; Hess et al., 2013). Remote ischemia can be achieved in rodents by transient occlusion of one or both femoral arteries, the mesenteric artery or the renal artery prior to cerebral ischemia. RIPC results in a decrease of the infarct volume following cerebral ischemia [for a comprehensive list in animal model see (Hess et al., 2013) and (Anrather and Hallenbeck, 2013)]. The effect of RIPC on circulating immune cells has been investigated in humans following forearm transient ischemia (**Table 2**). These studies showed that the expression of pro-inflammatory genes is down-regulated in circulating leukocytes (Konstantinov et al., 2004) and neutrophil function is altered (Shimizu et al., 2010).

Hypoxic-ischemic brain damage is mediated by TLRs (Stridh et al., 2011). Therefore, TLRs might also trigger inflammatory signaling in hypoxic PC (HPC), although no report to date has confirmed their involvement. To induce HPC in rodents, animals are placed in chambers and exposed to a hypoxic gas mixture, usually 8% oxygen and 92% nitrogen, for 3–4 h (Yin et al., 2007; Wacker et al., 2012). Hypoxia-inducible factor 1 (HIF-1) and NF-κB are activated in the brain after HPC (Yin et al., 2007;

Table 2 | Molecular inflammatory mechanisms of brain preconditioning.

PC stimulus	PC type	Receptors	Transducers and effectors induced by PC	References
Ischemia	BCCAo	TLR4	NF-κB, TNF-α, iNOS, COX-2 (48 h)	Pradillo et al., 2009
	MCAo	TNFR1	TACE/TNF-α, NF-κB (48 h)	Pradillo et al., 2005
			TNF-α/TACE (48 h)	Cárdenas et al., 2002
			HO-1, COX-2/PGE_2/ PI3K/Akt (24 h)	Park et al., 2008
			IL-1β gene (6 h), IL-1ra (6 and 24 h)	Shin et al., 2009
			IL-1β (6 h)	Wang et al., 2000
	Remote forearm ischemia	TLR4, TNFR6	HSP70, Calpastatin, TIMP1, ↓caspase-8; PI3KCA, SNAP-23 (24 h)	Konstantinov et al., 2004
			↓neutrophil adhesion and phagocytosis, IL-1β, IL-10 (24 h and 10 days)	Shimizu et al., 2010
			↓platelet activation (PMAs) (5 and 45 min)	Pedersen et al., 2011
	Remote femoral artery ischemia		↑reperfusion (possible protection of endothelium) (48 h)	Vlasov et al., 2005
Hypoxia	8% oxygen, 20 min to 4 h		TNF-α, ceramide (24 h)	Liu et al., 2000
			SphK/S1P (2–4 h), HIF, SphK2, CCL2 (12–24 h)	Wacker et al., 2012
			neuronal CCL2 (12 h), endothelial CCL2 (2 days)	Stowe et al., 2012
			PI3K/Akt/GSK-3β, NF-κB (1–24 h) (post-hypoxic ischemia)	Yin et al., 2007
HBO-PC	Hyperbaric		COX-2 (1–3 days) (post-global ischemia)	Cheng et al., 2011
			HIF-1α, EPO (12 h) (post-MCAo)	Peng et al., 2008
	Normobaric hyperoxia		TNF-α, TACE (24 h)	Bigdeli and Khoshbaten, 2008
Hypothermia	33.0°C, 4 h of reperfusion		↓PMN leucocytes, intercellular adhesion molecule-1 mRNA (4–22 h) (post-MCAo)	Kawai et al., 2000
Hyperthermia	41.5–42°C, 15 min		↑Cortisol (possible prevention of BBB disruption) (24 h)	Ikeda et al., 1999
	38 or 40°C, 6 h		↑HIF-1 alpha expression, HIF-1 binding activity (astrocytes) (0 h)	Du et al., 2010
	42–43°C, 2 h		↑HSP70 (glial, endothelial cells) (24 h)	Ota et al., 2000
Anesthetics	Isoflurane or halothane		↑iNOS (6–24 h)	Kapinya et al., 2002; Zhao and Zuo, 2004
			↑HO-1, NO and TNF-α (macrophages) (24 h)	Li et al., 2009
CSD	0.5 M KCl		↑ERK and COX-2 expression (0–8 h and 2–3 days)	Horiguchi et al., 2005, 2006
	3 M KCl	NMDA receptor	↑TNF-α, IL-1β (4 h)	Jander et al., 2001
Seizure	Kainic acid, bicuculline methiodide, or electrical stimulation		Unknown	Vezzani et al., 2002

(Continued)

Table 2 | Continued

PC stimulus	PC type	Receptors	Transducers and effectors induced by PC	References
Exercise	Treadmill		↑TNF-α (0 h)	Ding et al., 2005
TLR ligands	LPS	TLR4	NF-κB suppression; IRF3, Ship1, Tollip, p105 (post-MCAo) (72 h)	Sly et al., 2004; Vartanian et al., 2011
			Genes related to TLR pathway and cytokine–cytokine receptor interaction pathway (3 h)	Marsh et al., 2009b; Stevens et al., 2011
			IRF3, IFNβ (3 and 24 h)	Marsh et al., 2009b
			↑Ceramide (6–12 and 48 h)	Zimmermann et al., 2001
			↑PMN infiltration (post-MCAo) (6 and 24 h)	Ahmed et al., 2000
	CpG ODN	TLR9	IRF3, IRF7, type I IFN gene expression (post-MCAo) (3 and 24 h); TNF-α (serum) (1 h)	Stevens et al., 2008, 2011
	GDQ	TLR7, IFNAR	IRF7, IFNα (1–2 h)	Leung et al., 2012
	Poly-ICLC	TLR3	↑plasma levels of IL-1β, IL-6, IL-12, TNF-α, and IFNγ compared to LPS-PC (3 h)	Packard et al., 2012
			↑IFN-β (protein 6–8 h and mRNA 6–24 h), preservation of BBB endothelial cell	Gesuete et al., 2012
	Pam3CSK4	TLR2	↑zonula occludens-1 (ZO-1), no loss of occludin protein inducing preservation of BBB (6 and 24 h)	Hua et al., 2008

A PC stimulus (column 1) may be divided in several PC types (column 2) that through the stimulation of several receptors (column 3), activate different transducers and effectors of inflammatory pathways (column 4), accounting for the protective mechanism of the brain. Time points in brackets indicate the time point of analysis relative to the PC induction; post-MCAo indicates that the analysis was performed after induction of index ischemia.

ATA, atmosphere abolute pressure; BBB, Blood Brain Barrier; BCCAo, Bilateral Common Carotid Artery Occlusion; CCL2, chemokine (C-C motif) ligand; CCR1, 5, Chemokine Receptor 1, 5; COX-2, Cyclooxygenase 2; CpG ODN, cytosine-guanine oligodeoxynucleotides; CSD, Cortical Spreading Depression, EPO, Erythropoietin; GDQ, Gardiquimod; GSK-3β, Glycogen Synthase Kinase 3; HBO-PC, Hyperbaric Oxygen Preconditioning; HIF, Hypoxia-Inducible Factor; HO-1, Heme Oxygenase-1; HSP70, Heat Shock Protein 70; IFN, Interferon; IFNAR, type I interferon receptor; IL-1β, Interleukin 1β; IL-1ra, IL-1 receptor antagonist; iNOS, Inducible Nitric Oxidase Synthase; IPC, Ischemic Preconditioning; IRF, Interferon Regulatory Factor; KCl, Chloride potassium; LPS, lipopolysaccharide; MCAo, Middle Cerebral Artery occlusion; MCPIP1, Monocyte Chemotactic Protein–Induced Protein 1; MyD88, Myeloid differentiation primary response 88; NF-κB, Nuclear Factor-κB; NMDA, N-methyl-D-aspartate; NO, Nitric Oxide; ODN, oligodeoxynucleotide; Pam3CSL4, Pam3CysSerLys4; PGE_2, Prostaglandin E2; PI3K, Phosphatidylinositol 3-Kinase; PI3KCA-γ, PI3K catalytic subunit gamma isoform; PMA, platelet–monocyte aggregates; PMN, polymorphonuclear; Poly-ICLC, polyinosinic polycytidylic acid; RANTES, Regulated on Activation, Normal T Cell Expressed and Secreted; S1P, Sphingosine-1-phosphate; Ship1, Src homology-2 domain-containing inositol 5-phosphatase 1; SNAP-23, Synaptosome-associated protein-23; SphK2, Sphingosine Kinase 2; TACE, Tumor Necrosis factor-alpha-Converting Enzyme; TIMP1, Tissue inhibitor of metalloproteinase 1; TLR, Toll-Like Receptor; TNFR, Tumor necrosis factor receptor; TNF-α, Tumor necrosis factor alpha; Tollip, toll interacting protein; TRIF, TIR-domain-containing adapter-inducing interferon-β.

Wacker et al., 2012) leading to the expression of iNOS (Jung et al., 2000), TNF-α (Liu et al., 2000) and chemokine (C-C motif) ligand 2 (CCL2) (Stowe et al., 2012), which have been implicated in establishing IT after HPC (see below section Molecular Components of the Immune System Involved in PC).

The immune system is also involved in hyperoxic PC, which can be achieved by either normobaric hyperoxia or hyperbaric oxygen PC (HBO-PC). Delivering a gas mixture containing 90–95% oxygen induces normobaric hyperoxia. HBO-PC consists of the inspiration of an oxygen-containing gas mixture at higher than one atmospheric absolute pressure (ATA), usually 2–2.5 ATA. Bigdeli et al. showed that rats subjected to 16 h of normobaric hyperoxia had reduced infarct volume after Middle Cerebral Artery occlusion (MCAo) and that the TNF-α converting enzyme (TACE)/TNF-α/NF-κB pathway is associated with the protective effect (Bigdeli and Khoshbaten, 2008). Moreover, COX-2 has also been reported to be a mediator of HBO-PC (Cheng et al., 2011). Administration of the specific COX-2 inhibitor, NS-398, before HBO exposure reversed the protective effect of HBO-PC. Cheng et al. further identified COX-2-dependent upregulation of HIF-1α as a possible down-stream mediator of HBO-PC.

HYPOTHERMIC AND HYPERTHERMIC PC

Hypothermia induced during and/or after ischemia has a well-established protective effect in acute ischemic stroke (Wu and Grotta, 2013) and may be partly due the inhibition of the inflammatory response occurring during stroke (Ceulemans et al.,

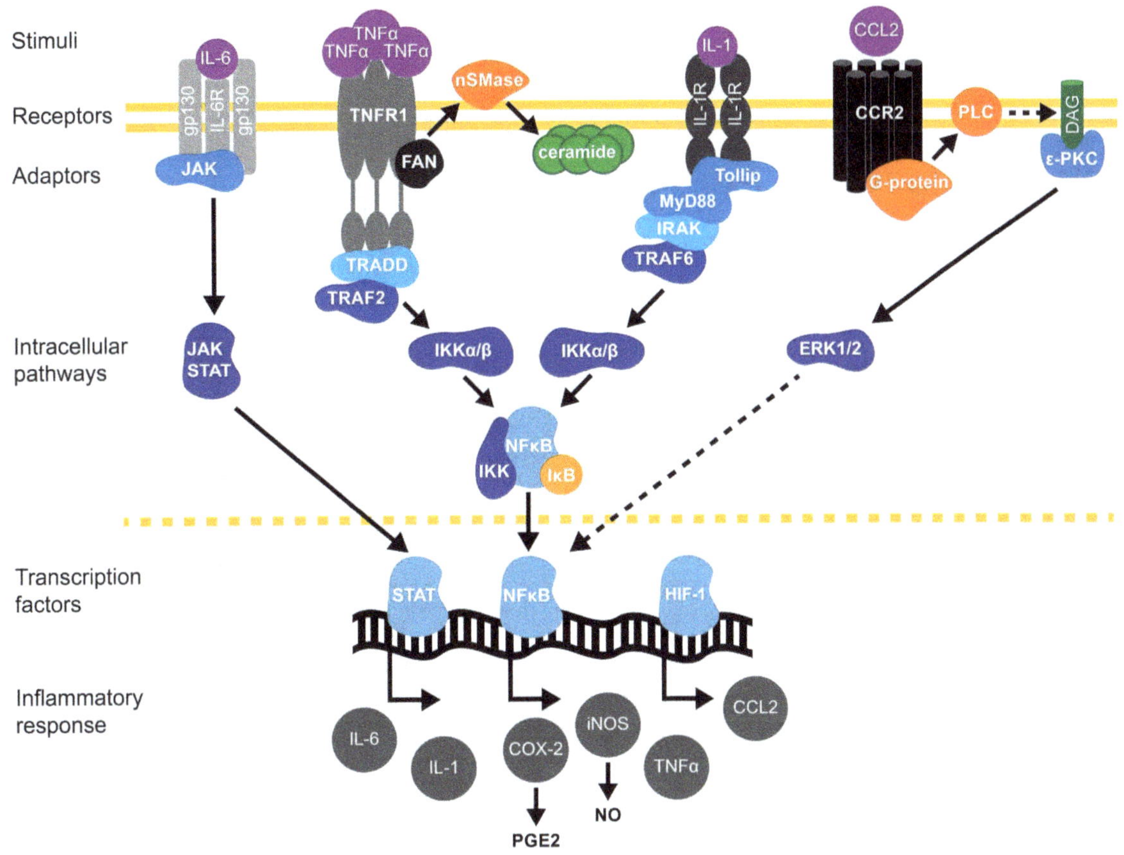

FIGURE 1 | Cytokine signaling pathways in brain preconditioning. Following preconditioning (PC), the increase in tumor necrosis factor (TNF)-α, interleukin (IL)-1β and IL-6 and chemokine (C-C motif) ligand 2 (CCL2) leads to the activation of inflammatory cascades and induction of gene expression such as inducible nitric oxide synthase (iNOS) and cyclooxygenase (COX)-2, mediators of delayed PC. IL-6/IL-6R activates Janus kinase (JAK)-signal transducer and activator of transcription (STAT) pathway. Phosphorylation and nuclear translocation of STAT induces iNOS and COX-2 up-regulation (Dawn et al., 2004). TNF-α activates TNF receptor 1(TNFR1)/Tumor necrosis factor receptor type 1-associated DEATH domain protein (TRADD)/TNF-α receptor–associated factor 2 (TRAF2) pathway (Hallenbeck, 2002; Pradillo et al., 2005). Furthermore, TNF-α activation promotes ceramide synthesis that also mediates TNFα-preconditioning (Liu et al., 2000; Ginis et al., 2002). The neutral sphingomyelinase domain (NSD) of TNFR1 recruits factor associated with neutral sphingomyelinase activation (FAN). FAN activates neutral sphingomyelinase (nSMase) in the outer leaflet of the plasma membrane to produce ceramide (Hallenbeck, 2002). IL-1R activates toll interacting protein (tollip)/myeloid differentiation primary response 88 (MyD88)-IL-1R-associated kinase (IRAK)/TRAF6 signaling. TRAF mediates the activation of inhibitor of κB kinase (IKK), which triggers the phosphorylation-induced proteasomal degradation of the IκB, NF-κB activation and subsequent iNOS and COX-2 expression. CCL2/CCR2 activation promotes phospholipase-C (PLC)-diacylglycerol (DAG)-protein kinase C (PKC) pathway that leads to extracellular signal-regulated kinases (ERK1/2) activation and ultimately causes NF-κB activation (Rehni and Singh, 2012). In addition, HIF-1-induced expression of CCL-2 confers cerebral ischemic tolerance (Stowe et al., 2012). COX-2-derived prostaglandin E2 (PGE_2) (Horiguchi et al., 2006) and iNOS-derived nitric oxide (NO) (Cho et al., 2005) are molecular mediators of PC.

2010). Brief exposure to hyperthermia represents an additional method of PC (**Table 2**). In animal model of stroke, transient hypothermia prior an ischemic insult (Nishio et al., 2000; Yunoki et al., 2003) or during reperfusion (Kawai et al., 2000) reduces infarct volume. The latter study has reported a decrease number of polymorphonuclear leucocytes during reperfusion—shown by a reduced myeloperoxidase activity in rats subjected to hypothermia (Kawai et al., 2000). Hyperthermic PC reduces brain damage in newborn rats as well (Ota et al., 2000). The protective mechanism of hyperthermic PC has been linked to the induction of the heat shock protein 70 (HSP70) within glial and endothelial cells (Ota et al., 2000). In addition to its role as an intracellular chaperon, HSP70 acts as an endogenous ligand of TLR4. Extracellular HSP70 is released from damaged cells and serves as a damage-associated molecular pattern (DAMPs) molecule (Bianchi, 2007). It has been shown that HSP70 mediates endotoxin tolerance by signaling through the TLR4/CD14 pathway (Vabulas et al., 2002; Aneja et al., 2006), similar to the canonical TLR4 ligand LPS. Thus, induction of HSP70 following hyperthermia could be a factor in the establishment of IT.

ANESTHETIC PC

Inhalation anesthetics are strong inducers of IT and can directly modulate immune functions in neutrophils, monocytes and lymphocytes (Clarkson, 2007; Wang et al., 2008). Rats pretreated with low dose isoflurane or halothane were protected after permanent MCAo (Kapinya et al., 2002). The protective effect was attributed to increased iNOS expression after anesthetic PC, and was reversed by treating the animals with the iNOS inhibitor aminoguanidine. Volatile anesthetics might directly alter the response of immune cells to inflammatory stimuli. Isoflurane PC of mouse macrophages induced the expression of heme oxygenase-1 (HO-1) and decreased NO and TNF-α release after subsequent LPS exposure (Li et al., 2009).

CORTICAL SPREADING DEPRESSION, BRAIN STIMULATION, AND SEIZURES

CSD is an electrophysiological phenomenon characterized by a slowly propagating depolarization wave across the cortical surface that confers delayed IT (Yanamoto et al., 1998; Horiguchi et al., 2006; Shpargel et al., 2008). In animal models, CSD PC is elicited by either topical application or superfusion of the cortical surface with a 0.5–5 M KCl solution that induces IT lasting 1–15 days (Kawahara et al., 1995; Yanamoto et al., 1998; Horiguchi et al., 2006). The delayed tolerance induced by CSD is protein synthesis dependent and has been linked to the up-regulation of trophic factors and glial cell activation (Kawahara et al., 1999). On the other hand, spreading depression in organotypic hippocampal slice cultures increases the expression of several pro-inflammatory cytokines including TNF-α, IL-1β, IL-1α, and IL-6 (Kunkler et al., 2004). Indeed, *in vivo* experiments found an early induction of both TNF-α and IL-1β after CSD (Jander et al., 2001). Pre-treatment with the non-competitive N-methyl-D-aspartate (NMDA) receptor antagonist MK-801 completely abolished the upregulation of these cytokines, implicating NMDA receptors as a critical element driving their production. Additionally, Horiguchi et al. reported that CSD-induced neuroprotection against ischemic injury resulting from MCAo is dependent upon increased COX-2 expression (Horiguchi et al., 2005, 2006), supporting the involvement of the inflammatory response in CSD PC.

Electrical stimulation of the cerebellar fastigial nucleus, but not other cerebellar nuclei, can induce potent and long-lasting protection from focal or global cerebral ischemic injury (Reis et al., 1991, 1998; Golanov et al., 1998). At the same time, fastigial nucleus stimulation evokes a strong anti-inflammatory response and suppresses post-ischemic iNOS expression and brain inflammation after cortical IL-1β injection (Galea et al., 1998a,b). The effect is mediated, at least in part, by increasing the tolerance of mitochondria to calcium overload, and suppressing the release of mitochondrial pro-apoptototic factors induced by cerebral ischemia (Zhou et al., 2005). The molecular mechanisms of the protective effects on mitochondria involve upregulation of prohibitin, an integral protein of the inner mitochondrial membrane, which protects mitochondrial structure and function during cell stress (Zhou et al., 2012). Consistent with its role in PC, overexpression of prohibitin renders neurons more resistant to injury in a wide variety of models (Zhou et al., 2012).

Neuroprotection against cerebral damage induced by lethal ischemic/hypoxia or global ischemia can also be acquired through induction of mild epileptic activity elicited by kainic acid injections (Plamondon et al., 1999; Towfighi et al., 1999). Although the mechanisms are unknown, synthesis and release of TNF-α, IL-1β, IL-1α, and IL-6 by glia might contribute to this tolerance modality (Vezzani et al., 2002).

EXERCISE PC

Physical exercise prevents stroke and forced exercise training affords neuroprotection against ischemic injury (Endres et al., 2003). Experimentally, exercise PC can be achieved by training rodents on a motor driven treadmill for 1–3 weeks (Wang et al., 2001; Ding et al., 2005; Curry et al., 2010). Among other mechanisms, such as protection against the blood-brain barrier (BBB) disruption, promotion of angiogenesis and inhibition of apoptosis, exercise PC involves activation of the immune system (Zhang et al., 2011). The skeletal muscle is an important source of several cytokines, often referred to as myokines, including IL-6, IL-8, IL-15, BDNF, LIF, and FGF21 (Pedersen, 2011). The release of these myokines into circulation might be responsible for the systemic effects of exercise, including its neuroprotective potential (Iadecola and Anrather, 2011b). Downstream mediators of exercise PC may include TNF-α (Ding et al., 2005) and extracellular signal-regulated kinases 1 and 2 (ERK1/2) (Guo et al., 2008; Curry et al., 2010). In one study, exercised rats submitted to MCAo showed reduced infarct volume when compared to non-exercised rats and this protection was associated with a gradual increase in the level of TNF-α in the brain over the 3 week course of treadmill exercise (Ding et al., 2005). Pre-ischemic blockage of TNF-α signaling with an anti-TNF-α antibody or inhibition of ERK1/2 activation abolished the protective effect (Guo et al., 2008). Exercise PC can also change the expression of innate immunity receptors. Treadmill exercise decreased cerebral TLR4 receptor expression in rats, although the importance of this finding as a mechanism for cerebral IT has not been investigated to date (Zwagerman et al., 2010).

MOLECULAR COMPONENTS OF THE IMMUNE SYSTEM INVOLVED IN PC

Inflammatory signaling is governed by a complex array of molecules that not only modulate the response of the target cell, but also change the local microenvironment and cellular tissue composition by recruiting cell types that are not normally present in that tissue. This inflammatory cascade is driven by cytokines, chemokines and their receptors and is regulated by immunomodulatory molecules. Several of these components have been implicated in PC. Evidence for direct involvement of some of these immune factors in cerebral IT is summarized in **Table 3**.

TLRs

The Toll receptor was first described in the context of Drosophila embryogenesis (Anderson et al., 1985). Subsequently, it was discovered that the Toll pathway is activated upon Drosophila fungal infection revealing a role of Toll receptors in the immune response (Lemaitre et al., 1996). Exposure of immune cells to certain pathogens activates these receptors resulting, in the activation of intracellular signaling pathways that lead to the expression of genes involved in the inflammatory response. In vertebrates, TLRs, named for their homology to the *toll* gene in Drosophila, are transmembrane proteins containing domains that are able to recognize viral or microbial components known as pathogen-associated molecular patterns (PAMPs) (Wang et al., 2011). Peptidoglycans (PGN), lipoproteins, lipoteichoic acids (LTA),

Table 3 | Evidence for the involvement of inflammatory mediators in PC.

Inflammatory mediators	Deletion/ Inhibitor	PC type (dose)/time of application prior to brain ischemia	Index ischemia	Species	Outcome	References
Chemokine receptors	CCL2 KO	HPC 2 days prior	tMCAo	Mouse	Reversed	Stowe et al., 2012
	CCL2 antibody	HPC 2 days prior	tMCAo	Mouse	Reversed	Stowe et al., 2012
Cytokines recpetors	TNF-α KO	LPS (0.2 mg/Kg) 3 days prior	tMCAo	Mouse	Reversed	Rosenzweig et al., 2007
	TNF-α KO	CpG ODN (1.6 mg/Kg) 3 days prior	tMCAo	Mouse	Reversed	Stevens et al., 2008
	TNFbp	LPS (0.2 mg/Kg) 2–4 days prior	pMCAo	SHR	Reversed	Tasaki et al., 1997
	IL-1ra	BCCo 3 days prior	BCCAo	Gerbil	Reversed	Ohtsuki et al., 1996
TLR receptors	TLR2 KO	Pam3CSK4 1 h prior	tMCAo	Mouse	Reversed	Lu et al., 2011
	TLR4 KO	BCCAo 2 days prior	pMCAo	Mouse	Partially reversed	Pradillo et al., 2009
	TLR7 KO	GDQ (40 μg/mouse) 3 days prior	tMCAo	Mouse	Reversed	Leung et al., 2009
TLRs adaptors	TRIF KO	LPS (0.4 mg/Kg) 3 days prior	tMCAo	Mouse	Reversed	Vartanian et al., 2011
	IRF3 KO	LPS (0.5 mg/Kg) 3 days prior	tMCAo	Mouse	Reversed	Marsh et al., 2009b
	IRF3 KO	CpG ODN (1.6 mg/Kg) 3 days prior	tMCAo	Mouse	Reversed	Stevens et al., 2011
	IRF3 KO	tMCAo 3 days prior	tMCAo	Mouse	Partially reversed	Stevens et al., 2011
	IRF7 KO	LPS (1 mg/Kg) 3 days prior	tMCAo	Mouse	Reversed	Stevens et al., 2011
	IRF7 KO	CpG ODN (1.6 mg/Kg) 3 days prior	tMCAo	Mouse	Reversed	Stevens et al., 2011
	IRF7 KO	tMCAo 3 days prior	tMCAo	Mouse	Partially reversed	Stevens et al., 2011
iNOS	iNOS KO	tMCAo 1 day prior	tMCAo	Mouse	Reversed	Cho et al., 2005
	Amino- guanidine (iNOS)	tMCAO 1 day prior	tMCAo	Mouse	Reversed	Cho et al., 2005
	Amino- guanidine (iNOS)	LPS (0.5 mg/Kg) 1 day prior	tMCAo	Mouse	Reversed	Cho et al., 2005
	Amino- guanidine (iNOS)	Isoflurane 1 day prior	pMCAo	Rat	Reversed	Kapinya et al., 2002
COX-2	NS-398 (COX-2)	HBO 5 days prior	4VO	Rat	Reversed	Cheng et al., 2011
	Rofecoxib (COX-2)	tMCAO 8 h prior	pMCAo	Rat	Reversed	Park et al., 2008
NF-κB pathway	DTTC (NF-κB)	4VO 3 days prior	4VO	Rat	Reversed	Blondeau et al., 2001
	κB decoy DNA (NF-κB)	4VO 3 days prior	4VO	Rat	Reversed	Blondeau et al., 2001
	DTTC (NF-κB)	linolenic acid (500 nmol/Kg) 3 days prior	4VO	Rat	Reversed	Blondeau et al., 2001
	κB decoy DNA (NF-κB)	linolenic acid (500 nmol/Kg) 3 days prior	4VO	Rat	Reversed	Blondeau et al., 2001

The deletion or inhibition of chemokines, cytokines, or TLR receptors, iNOS and COX-2 molecules and TLR or NF-κB signaling components described in the table, are able to abolish the preconditioning effect, unveiling the role of inflammatory pathways involved in IT.

4VO, 4 Vessel Occlusion; BCCAo, Bilateral Common Carotid Artery occlusion; COX-2, cyclooxygenase-2; CpG ODN, cytosine-guanine oligodeoxynucleotides; DTTC, diethyldithiocarbamate; GDQ, Gardiquimod; HBO-PC, Hyperbaric Oxygen Preconditioning; HPC, hypoxic preconditioning; IL-1ra, Interleukin 1 Receptor Antagonist; iNOS, inducible Nitric Oxide Synthase; IRF, Interferon (IFN)-regulatory factor; LPS, Lipopolysaccharide; pMCAo, permanent Middle Cerebral Artery occlusion; TLR, Toll-Like Receptor; SHR, Spontaneously Hypertensive Rats; tMCAo, transient Middle Cerebral Artery occlusion; TNFbp, Tumor Necrosis Factor binding protein; TNF-α, Tumor Necrosis Factor α; TRIF, TIR-domain-containing adapter-inducing interferon-β.

lipopolysaccharides (LPS), as well as viral and bacterial nucleic acids, serve as PAMPs recognized by individual TLRs (Akira, 2009). To date 13 members of the TLR family have been identified in mammals. Among the most extensively studied TLRs are TLR2 which binds to LTA component of Gram-positive bacteria and TLR4, which recognizes LPS on the cell wall of Gram-negative bacteria (Verstak et al., 2007). Upon ligand binding, TLRs further signal by recruiting intracellular Toll/IL-1R (TIR)-homology domain containing adaptor proteins, which selectively activate signaling cascades that lead to immune responses. Several TLR adapter molecules that are associated with functionally different signaling cascades, such as myeloid differentiation factor-88 (MyD88) and TIR domain containing adaptor protein inducing interferon β (TRIF), are known to date. With the exception of TLR3, TLRs signal through MyD88-dependent pathways, while TLR4 can activate both MyD88-dependent and—independent pathways (Wang et al., 2011; Mallard, 2012).

MyD88 mobilizes members of the IL-1R-associated kinase family (IRAK) leading to nuclear translocation of the transcription factor NF-κB. NF-κB is a major regulator of the inflammatory response (Li and Verma, 2002) and is responsible for the induction of various inflammatory genes including cytokines, chemokines, adhesion molecules, proinflammatory enzymes, and growth factors (Pahl, 1999). NF-κB is commonly found as a heterodimer consisting of p50 (NFKB1) and p65 (RelA) subunits. In resting cells, the inactive form of NF-κB is located in the cytoplasm by association with inhibitor proteins, IκBα and IκBβ (Baeuerle and Henkel, 1994). Upon stimulation, IκB proteins are phosphorylated and proteolytically degraded, and NF-κB dimers are able to translocate to the nucleus and bind to the promoter region of target genes initiating their transcription (Baldwin, 1996). NF-κB is activated in many cell types including cells of the central nervous system (Kaltschmidt et al., 1994). In the rodent brain, NF-κB can be activated by numerous factors known to be induced after ischemia-reperfusion, such as glutamate, increased intracellular Ca^{2+}, reactive oxygen species (ROS) and inflammatory cytokines (Harari and Liao, 2010). Furthermore, target genes of NF-κB have been implicated in the pathogenesis of cerebral ischemia, such as IL-1, IL-6, TNF-α, ICAM-1, MMP9, COX-2, and iNOS (Baeuerle and Henkel, 1994; Allan et al., 2005; Kaltschmidt et al., 2005; Harari and Liao, 2010). Thus, it has been postulated that stimulation of signaling pathways that lead to NF-κB activation are associated with detrimental outcome in cerebral ischemia (Stephenson et al., 2000). Supporting this notion, inhibition of NF-κB using pharmacologic agents results in reduced infarct size after stroke in rodents (Clemens et al., 1998; Nurmi et al., 2004). It has also been shown that mice lacking the p50 NF-κB subunit have reduced ischemic damage (Schwaninger et al., 1999; Nurmi, 2004). However, subsequent studies have also revealed a deleterious effect of NF-κB inhibition in neonatal hypoxia (Nijboer et al., 2008) and an increase of neuronal death after transient ischemia in p50 deficient mice (Duckworth et al., 2006) raising the possibility for a dual role of NF-κB in stroke.

TLR4 stimulation also leads to the activation of MyD88-independent pathways. In this case, binding of the adaptor molecule TRIF activates the transcription factors interferon regulatory factor 3 (IRF3) and 7 (IRF7), resulting in expression of IFNα and IFNβ type I IFN genes (Marsh et al., 2009a; Wang et al., 2011; Mallard, 2012) (**Figure 2**). Type I IFNs are released in the extracellular space and signal in an auto- or paracrine manner through a single heterodimeric receptor, IFNAR, to activate the JAK/STAT pathway, leading to the expression of several chemokines such as CCL2, CCL7, and CXCL10, while inhibiting CXCL1 and CXCL2 expression. Depending on the concentration of IFN and type of target cell, the resulting immune response can be pro- or anti-inflammatory (Trinchieri, 2010).

Aside from binding to PAMPs, TLRs also recognize endogenous molecules known as DAMPs, which are released during ischemic cellular injury (Chen and Nuñez, 2010). Prototypical DAMPs released from injured cells include high-mobility group box 1 (HMGb1) protein that activates TLR2, 4, and 9; heat shock proteins (HSPs; TLR2, 4); RNA (TLR3); mitochondrial DNA (TLR9); hyaluronic acid (TLR2, TLR4) and peroxiredoxins (TLR2, TLR4) (Chen and Nuñez, 2010; Patel et al., 2012; Shichita et al., 2012). HMGb1 and peroxiredoxins have been reported to increase cerebral ischemic injury by augmenting the post-ischemic inflammatory response (Kim, 2006; Yang et al., 2011; Shichita et al., 2012). While the role of DAMPs in cerebral IT has not been addressed, it has been shown that systemic administration of HMGb1 protects against myocardial ischemia–reperfusion injury and liver ischemia-reperfusion injury, a process that involves TLR4 (Izuishi et al., 2006; Hu et al., 2010). Additionally, HSP70 mediates endotoxin tolerance by signaling through TLR4 receptors (Aneja et al., 2006). Therefore, these findings support DAMPs to participate in the PC effect through TLRs activation. In contrast to the detrimental effect of TLR activation in response to ischemia (Wang et al., 2011), stimulation of some TLRs prior to ischemia provides robust neuroprotection (Marsh et al., 2009a; Wang et al., 2011). The ability of TLR ligands to induce cerebral IT was first demonstrated after systemic administration of low-dose LPS, the major TLR4 ligand, causing spontaneously hypertensive rats to become tolerant to subsequent ischemic brain damage induced by MCAo (Tasaki et al., 1997). Subsequently, LPS-induced tolerance to brain ischemia has been demonstrated in several experimental stroke models in mice, gerbils and pigs (Rosenzweig et al., 2004; Hickey et al., 2007; Yu et al., 2010). A dose below 1 mg/Kg of LPS administered 1–3 days prior to cerebral ischemia is generally used in rodents to induce IT. Furthermore, TLR4-mutant mice were refractory to IPC, indicating that TLR4 plays an universal role in establishing IT (Pradillo et al., 2009). Comparable to TLR4, pre-treatment with the TLR2 lipopetide ligand Pam3CysSerLys4 (Pam3CSK4) resulted in significantly decreased cerebral infarct volume after focal cerebral ischemia/reperfusion in mice (Hua et al., 2008). Preservation of the BBB has been suggested to play a role in this PC mechanism. Similarly, stimulation of TLR7 by administration of its agonist gardiquimod, an imidazoquinoline compound, provides neuroprotection against ischemic injury and was associated with the up-regulation of the IFN pathway and IFNα production (Leung et al., 2012). Interestingly and in contrast to TLR4 and TLR9 induced PC, TLR7-mediated PC was abolished in IFNAR mutant mice. Finally, activation of TLR9 by unmethylated CpG oligodeoxynucleotides induced IT after transient MCAo in mice (Stevens et al., 2008). Similar to LPS-PC, the protective effect after TLR9 stimulation lasted for up to a week and was dependent on the expression of TNF-α (**Figure 2A**) (Stevens et al., 2008; Marsh et al., 2009a). Accordingly, CpG oligodeoxynucleotides administration to TNF-α null mice failed to induce IT.

IT induced by TLR activation involves the reprogramming of inflammatory pathways. This is achieved by at least two different mechanisms. Concomitantly with induction of pro-inflammatory

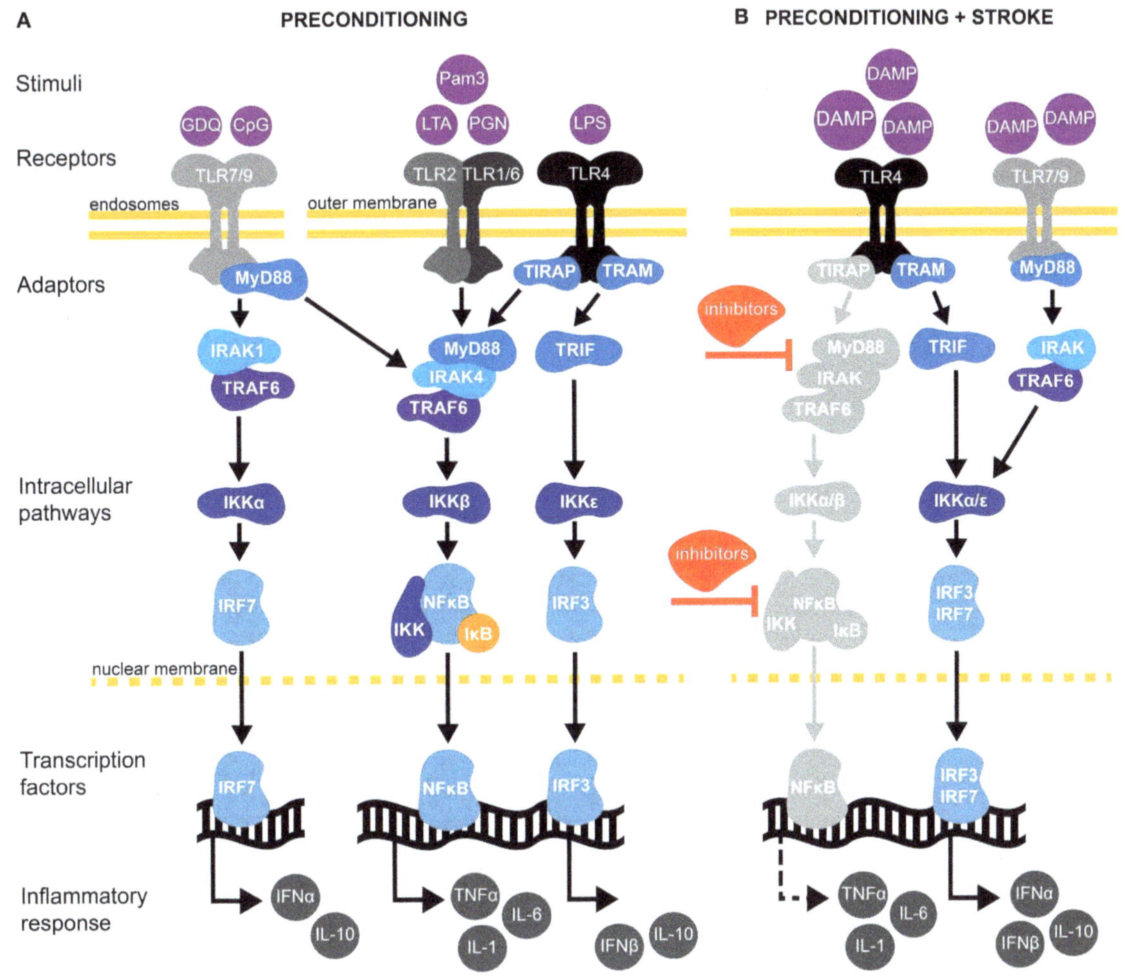

FIGURE 2 | TLR signaling pathways in cerebral IT. (A) Preconditioning through TLRs may be afford by exposure with low dose of pathogen-associated molecular pattern (PAMPs) molecules (Mallard, 2012). TLRs are localized either at the outer cell surface (TLR1, TLR2, TLR4, and TLR6) or within endosomes (TLR7 and TLR9) (Marsh et al., 2009a). TLR2 dimerizes with TLR1 or TLR6 and is activated upon binding of PAMPs such as the synthetic lipopeptide Pam3CysSerLys4 (Pam3CSK4), the non-peptide ligand lipoteichoic acid (LTA) or peptidoglycans (PGN). TLR4 predominantly recognizes lipopolysaccharides (LPS) from Gram-negative bacteria. TLR7 and TRL9 can be activated by the synthetic imidazoquinoline Gardiquimod (GDQ) or small DNA such as non-methylated cytosine-guanosine (CpG), respectively (Wang et al., 2011). Preconditioning of TLRs will favor the activation of the myeloid differentiation factor-88 (MyD88)-dependent pathway. Upon binding of ligands, MyD88 is activated either directly (TLR7/9) or via the toll-interleukin 1 receptor (TIR) domain containing adaptor protein TIRAP (TLR2/4). The latter further mobilizes members of the IL-1R-associated kinase family (IRAK) leading to the subsequent binding/activation of TNF receptor associated factor-6 (TRAF6), the inhibitor of κB kinase (IKK) complex (composed of IKKα and IKKβ) and IκB. Once IκB is phosphorylated and degraded by the proteasome, nuclear factor-κB (NF-κB) translocates to the nucleus leading to low level of pro-inflammatory cytokine synthesis, such as TNF-α. TLR PC also induces the production of several negative inhibitors of TLR signaling, targeting mainly MyD88 and NF-κB pathways. Induction of proinflammatory cytokines and activation of such inhibitors are required to induce a state of ischemic tolerance (Marsh et al., 2009a; Vartanian and Stenzel-Poore, 2010; Wang et al., 2011). In addition to activating the MyD88-dependent pathway, TLR4 signals through the MyD88-independent pathway to activate IRF3 by sequential recruiting of the adaptor molecule TIR inducing interferon β (TRIF) and IKKε resulting in expression of anti-inflammatory type I interferon (IFN) genes, including IFNβ (Marsh et al., 2009b). Type I IFNγ genes are also induced by TLR7/9 activation through the TRAF6/IKKα pathway (Hoshino et al., 2006). **(B)** Damage-associated molecular pattern (DAMPs) molecules are endogenous ligands of TLRs produced in response to ischemic injury (Vabulas et al., 2002). Following preconditioning, activation of TLR4/7/9 by DAMPs will fail to activate MyD88 and the subsequent signaling molecules, such as IRAK and NF-κB. Indeed, several inhibitors produced during the first exposition of TLRs to exogenous stimuli will block the signaling of TLRs to NF-κB. Whether pro-inflammatory cytokines are suppressed or up-regulated is controversial and might be model specific (Marsh et al., 2009a; Vartanian and Stenzel-Poore, 2010). On one hand, TLR preconditioning induces a down-regulation of NF-κB. On the other hand, it has been shown that neuroprotection following cerebral ischemia is achieved by an up-regulation of the TLR-IRF axis generating an increase of TGF-β, IL-10, IFNα, and IFNβ anti-inflammatory cytokines (Stevens et al., 2011; Leung et al., 2012). Thus, TLR preconditioning induces a reorganization of the TLR signaling pathways after cerebral ischemia toward TRIF/IRF signaling that may confer protection of the brain against ischemic damage.

mediators, activation of the MyD88-dependent pathway will result in the upregulation of negative regulators, which prevent the interaction of several adaptors along the TLR4-MyD88 pathway (**Figure 2A**) (Sly et al., 2004). At the same time, activating the MyD88-independent pathway evokes a type I IFN response. Indeed, recent studies have found a neuroprotective role of the MyD88-independent pathway in TLR-induced IT after stroke (Marsh et al., 2009a). It has been postulated that pretreatment with LPS induces a switch in the transcriptional response to subsequent TLR4 stimulation by increasing the expression of the IRF3-induced cytokine IFNβ (Veldhuis et al., 2003) (**Figure 2B**). Consistent with this hypothesis, gene expression analysis following LPS-PC revealed upregulation of inhibitors of the Myd88-dependent and NF-κB pathways (Vartanian et al., 2011). Interestingly, the expression of pro-inflammatory genes related to the NF-κB signaling pathway was similar in both mice undergoing LPS-PC and in control mice following cerebral ischemia (**Figure 2B**). However, the study showed that LPS-PC increased IRF3 activity following ischemia and evoked the upregulation of anti-inflammatory genes including TGF-β and IL-10 (Vartanian et al., 2011). The importance of the MyD88-independent pathway in establishing IT is further supported by the fact that LPS-PC was unable to induce IT in TRIF- but not in Myd88-deficient mice (Vartanian et al., 2011).

CYTOKINES

Cytokines are secreted proteins with growth, differentiation, and activation functions that shape the nature of the immune response. Among the more than 70 candidate cytokines, TNF-α, IL-1, IL-6, and IL-17 play major roles in initiating and amplifying the post-ischemic inflammatory response, while IL-10 and TGF-β are the main anti-inflammatory factors (Iadecola and Anrather, 2011a). Since immune cells, including monocytes/macrophages, in the periphery and microglia in the brain express TLR receptors (Downes and Crack, 2010), they are capable of responding to systemic TLR agonists used as a preconditioning stimulus and modify cytokine expression or secretion (Rosenzweig et al., 2004; Ransohoff and Brown, 2012). Accordingly, several cytokines secreted by cells of the innate immune system have been implicated in PC. For example, TNF-α has been identified as an essential mediator of LPS-PC. It has been shown that LPS-preconditioned TNF-α null mice were not protected from ischemic brain injury (Rosenzweig et al., 2007). This study confirmed previous findings demonstrating that administration of a specific TNF antagonist reversed the protective effect of LPS PC in a model of permanent focal ischemia in mice (Tasaki et al., 1997). Similarly, upregulation of IL-1α and IL-1β after bilateral common carotid artery occlusion (BCCAo) triggered tolerance to global ischemia (Ohtsuki et al., 1996; Shin et al., 2009). Ohtsuki et al. also showed that systemic delivery of either IL-1α or IL-1β was sufficient to induce IT to a subsequent episode of lethal global ischemia and that intraperitoneal injection of recombinant human IL-1 receptor antagonist prior to IPC abolished the neuroprotective effect.

In addition to systemic administration of cytokines, neuroprotection has also been reported with direct delivery of cytokines to the brain before ischemia. Previous intracerebrovascular injection of IL-6 in rats subjected to permanent ischemia protects from cell death (Loddick et al., 1998). Likewise, intracisternal administration of TNF-α in mice before distal MCAo is neuroprotective (Nawashiro et al., 1997). However, in the same study, both intravenous and intraperitoneal routes of TNF-α administration failed to exert neuroprotection against cerebral ischemia. While differences in modality of administration and stroke models may account for the observed disparities in outcome, it remains unclear how systemic cytokines exert their effect within the brain. TNF-α, IL-1β, and IL-6 are transported unidirectionally across the BBB (Banks, 2005). Thus, systemic induction of cytokines can lead to an increase of them in the brain. For instance, IL-1 expression in the brain has been documented after an increase of circulating IL-1 induced by LPS PC (Gabellec et al., 1995). On the other hand, inducers of PC, such as LPS and cytokines, can act through interaction with receptors in circumventricular organs that lack a BBB, triggering upregulation of cytokine levels in the brain. Accordingly, it has been shown that perivascular cells and neurons in the circumventricular organs produce TNF-α in response to systemically administered LPS (Breder et al., 1994).

CHEMOKINES

Chemokines are small molecules involved in the recruitment of immune cells to sites of inflammation or injury (Charo and Ransohoff, 2006). In the central nervous system, chemokines are highly upregulated in neuropathologic conditions. Neurons, astrocytes, microglia, endothelial cells as well as circulating leukocytes are potential sources of chemokines. Several chemokines have been linked to the pathogenesis of ischemic brain injury (Jaerve and Müller, 2012). Upon release, they exacerbate tissue injury by increasing leukocyte and monocytes/macrophages infiltration, potentiating neuronal injury. However, chemokines also possess neuroprotective and neurotrophic functions (Semple et al., 2009). The prevalence of beneficial or detrimental effects may depend on various factors, including the type of the chemokine, its concentration, the time course of production relative to the time of injury and the target cell type (Semple et al., 2009). The contribution of chemokines to PC has been investigated in several models of IT. For instance, HPC or BCCAo prior to transient or global MCAo resulted in reduced infarct size attributed to CCL2 (MCP-1), a leukocyte-derived pro-inflammatory chemokine (Rehni and Singh, 2012; Stowe et al., 2012). Following HPC, expression of CCL2 increased in both neurons and cerebral endothelial cells prior to the induction of the ischemic injury. Moreover, the induction of IT was blocked by CCL2 neutralizing antibodies and was not observed in CCL2-knockout mice (Stowe et al., 2012). Although the protection conferred by HPC is associated with the number of $CCR2^+$ monocytes in blood and leaving the circulation, their direct protective role in brain IT needs to be further characterized. Rehni et al. have shown that IT induced by BCCAo PC was lost after treatment with a selective antagonist of CCR2 (Rehni and Singh, 2012), corroborating the role of CCL2 chemokines and its receptor in IT.

CANNABINOIDS

The endocannabinoid system consists of the cannabinoid type 1 (CB1) and type 2 (CB2) receptors and their ligands (Howlett et al., 2002). The expression of these two receptor subtypes varies among tissues. CB1 receptors are abundant in the CNS and are also present in several peripheral tissues, albeit to a lesser extent (Matsuda et al., 1990; Galiègue et al., 1995). Although also present in the brain (Gong et al., 2006), CB2 is mostly expressed in immune cells (Galiègue et al., 1995). Cannabinoid receptors may be activated upon binding of their endogenous ligands arachidonoyl ethanolamide or anandamide (AEA), 2-arachidonoylglycerol (2-AG), and 2-arachidonyl glyceryl ether (noladin ether), or synthetic analogs which are derivatives of herbal cannabinoids, such as the terpenoid Δ^9-tetrahydrocannabinol (THC), the active compound of the cannabis plant (Di Marzo et al., 1998). Both CB1 and CB2 receptors are members of the seven-transmembrane G-protein coupled receptor superfamily. They may initiate downstream signaling pathways that activate potassium channels, phosphatidylinositol-3-kinase and mitogen-activated protein kinases (Di Marzo et al., 1998). The CNS endocannabinoid system has a variety of physiological roles, which are mainly mediated by CB1 receptors. These include, but are not limited to: psychotropic effect, pain inhibition, memory function and increased appetite (Ameri, 1999; Pacher and Haskó, 2008). Modulation of immune responses and the release of inflammatory mediators have been primarily attributed to CB2 receptors (Pacher et al., 2006; Ullrich et al., 2007; Elliott et al., 2011).

The endocannabinoid system has been implicated in ischemic injury (Pacher and Haskó, 2008). Several studies have shown a neuroprotective effect of CB activation in brain ischemia (Nagayama et al., 1999; Panikashvili et al., 2001) by decreasing intracellular Ca^{2+} (Zhuang et al., 2005), modulating brain temperature (Leker et al., 2003), inhibiting pro-inflammatory signaling cascades (Panikashvili et al., 2005) and by preventing endothelial cell activation and leukocyte adhesion (Zhang et al., 2007, 2009). There is emerging evidence that cannabinoids also play a role in PC. Induction of IT by electroacupuncture PC improves neuronal survival in a rat model of focal ischemia (Wang et al., 2005, 2009; Ma et al., 2011). While early PC in this model was dependent on the activation of CB1 receptors as demonstrated by the reversal of the protective effect after administration of the CB1 receptor antagonist AM251 or CB1 siRNA (Wang et al., 2009), delayed PC was dependent upon the activation of CB2 receptors (Ma et al., 2011). It was shown that IT was partially reversed when animals were treated with the specific CB2 antagonist AM630. Inhibition of the CB1 receptor, however, did not block the induction of delayed IT. Although the cellular components of this response have not been investigated, the nearly exclusively expression of CB2 receptors on immune cells makes it possible that modulation of the immune response accounts for the observed neuroprotection.

iNOS

Nitric oxide (NO) is produced by nitric oxidase synthase (NOS) through oxidation of the guanidino nitrogen of L-arginine. Endothelial (eNOS), neuronal (nNOS) and inducible or inflammatory (iNOS) isoforms are found in the brain, and play important roles in IT (for recent review see (Iadecola et al., 2011). iNOS is specifically expressed under pathological conditions, typically those associated with inflammation (Nathan, 1997). Data from our laboratory have shown that iNOS mediates IT following either IPC or LPS-PC in a mouse model of transient MCAo (Cho et al., 2005). PC-mediated neuroprotection was abolished when the selective inhibitor, aminoguanidine, was delivered prior to PC, or when iNOS null mice were used. iNOS expression and accumulation of peroxynitrite in cerebral blood vessels was observed 24 h after IPC (Cho et al., 2005), whereas LPS-PC was associated with accumulation of peroxynitrite in neurons and vessels (Kunz et al., 2007). The role of iNOS in PC has also been reported with anesthetic preconditioning (Kapinya et al., 2002). Prior treatment with isoflurane or halothane, which reduces infarct volume after permanent MCAo, induced iNOS expression in the cortex 18–24 h after PC. Analogous to the studies mentioned above, anesthetic PC was blocked when animals were treated with the iNOS inhibitor aminoguanidine.

COX-2

Similar to iNOS, brain cycloxygenase-2 (COX-2) is markedly upregulated during post-ischemic inflammation and its reaction products contribute to the evolution of ischemic damage (Iadecola et al., 2001). Likewise, the role of COX-2 has been investigated in several PC paradigms. Increased brain levels of COX-2 following PC by CSD, was associated with the development of cerebral IT in a rat model of MCAo (Horiguchi et al., 2006). IPC by transient MCAo induced COX-2 and HO-1 expression, and significantly reduced infarct volume after index MCAo. Administration of the COX-2-selective inhibitor rofecoxib abolished the neuroprotective effect of IPC, indicating a key role of COX-2 in establishing IT (Park et al., 2008). More recently, the role of COX-2 in PC induced by HBO has also been reported (Cheng et al., 2011). COX-2 induction is associated with protection against subsequent global cerebral occlusion in rats and IT was abolished by treatment with COX-2 selective inhibitor NS-398. Contrary to IPC, no role of COX-2 in LPS PC was found in a excitotoxic model of brain injury induced by NMDA (Kawano et al., 2007).

ROS

ROS play a key role in the pathogenesis of the ischemic cascade. ROS are mainly generated after cerebral ischemia by the injured tissue during the acute phase (minutes-hours) and by infiltrating leukocytes during the sub-acute ischemic phase (Chan, 2001; Kahles et al., 2007). For example, neutrophils that infiltrate the ischemic brain produce excessive superoxide via NADPH oxidase, contributing to the exacerbation of ischemic injury (Kunz et al., 2006; Chen et al., 2009; Pun et al., 2009). In preconditioning, the role of ROS via inflammatory mechanisms has also been reported. Kunz et al. showed improvement of cerebrovascular function after transient MCAo in LPS preconditioned mice, an effect associated with peroxynitrite formation (Kunz et al., 2007). Interestingly, peroxynitrite was specifically formed after PC from the reaction of iNOS-derived NO and Nox2 (NADPH oxidase)-derived superoxide, and was not observed in iNOS or Nox2-null mice. Moreover, peroxynitrite was also found to be beneficial in the tolerance induced by LPS-PC to brain injury resulting from cortical injection with NMDA (Kawano et al., 2007).

EPIGENETIC MECHANISMS

In delayed PC, the time window during which IT is observed can last for days or even weeks. This contrasts with the limited duration of inflammatory signaling where responses are often short lived, and several negative feedback loops are in place to restrict the duration of the inflammatory response. This is achieved by the expression of a series of cellular inhibitors that are concomitantly produced along with pro-inflammatory molecules, leading to a timely termination of gene expression after the stimulus subsides. These inhibitors can directly target transcription factors, as is the case with NF-κB, which is sequestered in the cytoplasm by newly synthetized IκB proteins—or, by inactivating key proteins within the pro-inflammatory signaling cascade. For example, A20, an ubiquitin editing enzyme that is highly inducible by pro-inflammatory stimuli, targets several proteins in the TNFR signaling cascades by removing K63-linked ubiquitin chains from TRAF2, TRAF6 and NEMO. It results in suppression of NF-κB signaling, and by replacing K63- with K48-linked ubiquitin chains in RIP1, thus targeting it for proteasomal degradation (Verstrepen et al., 2010). Similarly, suppressor of cytokine signaling (SOCS), a family of 40 related proteins, and PIAS (protein inhibitor of activated STAT) target primarily the JAK (Janus kinase)/STAT (signal transducer and activator of transcription) pathway, which is the main cellular transducer of cytokine signals (Yoshimura et al., 2007). Accordingly, short-acting inflammatory signals, as applied during PC protocols, are transient, and not suitable to alter the cellular state for an extended period of time. This view is supported by experimental data in ischemic and LPS preconditioned animals, that show transient global alterations of gene expression profiles after PC, which have largely dissipated by the time of index ischemia (Stenzel-Poore et al., 2003; Marsh et al., 2009b). This raises the question of how the "memory" of the PC event is preserved if the attendant mRNA response has already subsided. An essential feature of such a mechanism, is its persistence beyond the initial stimulation and its decay over time, thus, equipping the cell or organ with a relatively short lived memory of a previous exposure to a potentially lethal stressor. One possibility is that the protein products of the subsided transcriptional activity are still present at the time of induction of ischemia, which could steer the response from injury toward protection. Another possibility is that the transcriptional response to PC induces longer lasting epigenetic changes that shape the genetic response when injurious ischemia occurs. Epigenetic mechanisms include all processes that regulate gene expression without alteration of the underlying DNA sequence, and include, for example, histone modifications, DNA methylation, and non-coding RNAs.

HISTONE AND DNA MODIFICATIONS IN PRECONDITIONING OF THE IMMUNE SYSTEM AND THE BRAIN

Histone modifications by methylation, acetylation, phosphorylation, ubiquitination, and sumoylation are key events in regulating chromatin structure and gene expression. The mechanism by which these modifications alter gene expression is not entirely understood, but may involve tethering of chromatin remodeling machinery, transcriptional repressors and activators. While acetylation of N-terminal histone tails are a hallmark of actively transcribed genes, it is less likely that histone acetylation plays a major role in imprinting a lasting memory from a previous exposure. Supporting this view is the fact that histone deacetylase (HDAC) is recruited early to the promoter of induced genes, in most cases during the gene activation process itself, resulting in a high turnover rate of acetylation marks in the order of minutes and fast disposal of this modification once transcription of the particular gene subsides (Hazzalin and Mahadevan, 2005). On the other hand, DNA methylation is a very thermostable epigenetic mark and, with the possible exception of 5-hydroxymethylcytosine, refractory to environmental stimuli. Therefore, DNA methylation is unsuited to act as an on-off switch for epigenetic memory (Qureshi and Mehler, 2010). Histone H3 tri-methylation at lysine 4 (H3K4me3), in contrast, has been shown to mark active or poised enhancers for an extended period of time. In a model of Candida albicans infected macrophages, persistent H3K4me3 modifications in the enhancer regions of inflammatory genes was associated with a more robust inflammatory response and reduced re-infection rate upon re-exposure (Quintin et al., 2012). Notably, the K4 trimethylation was observed for up to a week after deposition. The importance of H3K4me3 in changing transcriptional responses has been shown in LPS-preconditioned macrophages (Foster et al., 2007). Macrophages pre-exposed to LPS responded to a second LPS exposure with a transcriptional program distinct from that of naïve macrophages exposed to LPS. Genes could be divided into "tolerizeable" genes (T), which were suppressed in tolerant macrophages, and "non-tolerizeable" genes (NT), expressed at higher levels in tolerant than non-tolerant macrophages. It was found that promoter regions of T-class genes were refractory to histone H4 acetylation and H3K4 trimethylation, two modifications positively correlated with transcriptional activity, upon the second LPS challenge (Foster et al., 2007). Depending on the chromatin status in the resting state, genes can be divided in primary and secondary response genes (Ramirez-Carrozzi et al., 2006). Primary genes show a chromatin structure that is suited for immediate transcription and their activation is independent of new protein synthesis. Secondary genes show histone modifications characteristic of inactivated genes and the removal of this block and gene induction is protein synthesis dependent. Interestingly, this study found that LPS-PC changed many genes from secondary to primary response genes upon LPS re-stimulation, further implicating that epigenetic memory has been established in this model.

Several histone modifiers have been implicated in the PC response of the brain, including sirtuin family HDACs (Morris et al., 2011) and polycomb group proteins (PcG), a multimeric protein complex that mediates gene silencing and PC (Stapels et al., 2010). In addition to their role in neuronal physiology, both protein families have been implicated in the regulation of immune function (Swigut and Wysocka, 2007; Gallí et al., 2011). Whether they also regulate the immune signaling during PC, however, has not been directly addressed thus far.

MICRORNAS AND LONG NON-CODING RNAS

microRNAs (miRNAs) are small non-coding RNAs (18- to 24- nucleotides) that repress translation of mRNAs. Mature miRNAs are excised from a precursor RNA by the activity of Dicer and are guided to the 3′-untranslated region (3′-UTR) of mRNAs targets by the RNA-induced silencing complex (RISC). This leads to the down-regulation of gene expression via degradation or translational inhibition (Bartel, 2009). miRNAs have an essential quality that makes them compatible with the maintenance of preconditioning memory, namely their stability (Rüegger and Großhans, 2012). In addition, they are inducible by environmental stimuli, and are regulated at the levels of transcription, biogenesis, stability and decay. Supportive for a role of some miRNAs in establishing epigenetic memory, is the fact that they are extremely long lived, more than 12 days in the case of miR-208 in the heart (van Rooij et al., 2007). Furthermore, ablation of many miRNAs is well tolerated in the mouse, with these mutant animals only developing substantially altered phenotypes after being subjected to some kind of stress. These observations suggest that the persistence of inducible miRNAs due to their long half-lives after initial stimulation, may enable the maintenance of gene-expression programs that enhance the resistance of cells to repeated stress-exposure. When such "memory" miRNAs are absent (such as in animals depleted of the genes encoding the miRNAs), aberrant phenotypes become apparent (Leung and Sharp, 2010). The findings that miRNA can be actively secreted and transferred from cell-to-cell via microvesicles makes it possible that miRNA can work at a distance by transferring epigenetic signatures from a stimulus-exposed cell to a cell that has not encountered the particular environmental stressor (Valadi et al., 2007).

It is estimated that 500–1000 different miRNAs are expressed in mammalian cells and several miRNAs have been implicated in the regulation of the immune response and inflammation (O'Connell et al., 2012). Certain miRNAs, for instance, miR-9, -21, -146a, -147, -203, are induced in response to TLR activation, and serve as negative feedback regulators of the MyD88-dependent TLR signaling pathway and NF-κB activity (O'Neill et al., 2011). Conversely, miR-155 enhances the inflammatory response by down-regulating negative regulators Src Homology-2 domain-containing inositol-5′-phosphatase 1 (SHIP1) and SOCS1 leading to prolonged activation of AKT and IFN signaling pathways (O'Connell et al., 2009).

Cerebral ischemia-reperfusion injury alters the expression of several miRNAs (Dharap et al., 2009; Wang et al., 2013). Interestingly, IPC and HPC have been shown to rapidly alter miRNA levels in the brain (Dharap and Vemuganti, 2010; Lee et al., 2010; Liu et al., 2012). Although it is unknown if these alterations directly affect immune pathways participating in PC, the finding that expression of miRNAs involved in inflammatory signaling is altered by IPC in mice, is suggestive for such a role. For example, miR-17-5p, an inhibitor of monocyte maturation, and the TLR4-targeting miRNA let-7e were down-regulated in the cerebral cortex of mice after IPC (Lusardi et al., 2010). Furthermore, the peroxisome proliferator-activated receptor gamma (PPARγ)-targeting miR-27b and miR-146a, which regulates Traf6, IRAK1, and IRAK2 expression, were up-regulated after PC by transient MCAo in rats (Dharap and Vemuganti, 2010). The same study showed down-regulation of miR-145, which targets the essential TLR4-associated signaling molecule MyD88-adapter-like (MAL). Tellingly, monocyte chemotactic protein-induced protein 1 (MCPIP1), a multifunctional protein with RNAse activity that antagonizes Dicer, and thereby inhibits miRNA biogenesis (Suzuki et al., 2011), has been shown to abrogate the effects of LPS-PC in a mouse model of transient cerebral ischemia (Liang et al., 2011). Taken together, although PC-induced regulation of immune components by miRNA has not been conclusively shown to contribute to cerebral IT, the correlative data gathered so far are supportive for a role of miRNAs in regulation of immune pathways during PC.

Long non-coding RNAs range from 200 bp to several kb, and are expressed in a cell type specific manner (Mercer et al., 2009). Although most of these molecules have not been functionally characterized, they may have diverse roles ranging from regulation of chromosome inactivation to control of gene expression (Mercer et al., 2009). Because several long non-coding RNAs have been shown to be inducible and are involved in regulating immune cell activity and inflammatory signaling, they constitute another potential player by which epigenetic processes can establish a cellular memory. Their role in PC has yet to be investigated.

CONCLUSIONS

Although post-ischemic inflammation is considered a major pathogenic factor in stroke, emerging evidence supports a beneficial role of selected inflammatory pathways. One such mechanism is the induction of endogenous neuroprotection through ischemic PC (**Figure 3**). The evidence summarized in this review indicates that the immune system plays a central role in the mechanisms eliciting neuroprotective responses after PC. While activation of IT-inducing immune pathways shows robust neuroprotection in animal models, the clinical translation of such approaches is complicated by side effects including systemic inflammation and immunodepression (Meisel et al., 2005; McColl et al., 2009). The identification of specific pathways and effector molecules involved in establishing inflammatory PC will help to design targeted PC protocols that can be potentially translated into clinical practice (Keep et al., 2010; Anrather and Hallenbeck, 2013; Narayanan et al., 2013). Notably, immune pathways are not only involved in PC induced by inflammatory mediators, but have also been implicated in several PC paradigms that are not triggered by inflammatory signals, such as ischemic and anesthetic PC, attesting a pivotal role for the immune system in mediating and/or establishing IT. Because of the involvement of inflammatory pathways in a wide variety of diseases, many of the immune components involved in PC are prime therapeutic targets and subjects of extensive drug development. Several proteins involved in PC, such as type I IFNs, are currently in clinical use, and re-purposing them for stroke therapy or prevention could provide a fast track for clinical translation. However, much remains to be learned. For example, few studies have investigated the role of specific immune cells in IT, an area of research that could result in cell-specific therapies and would therefore mitigate the likelihood of adverse effects associated with administration

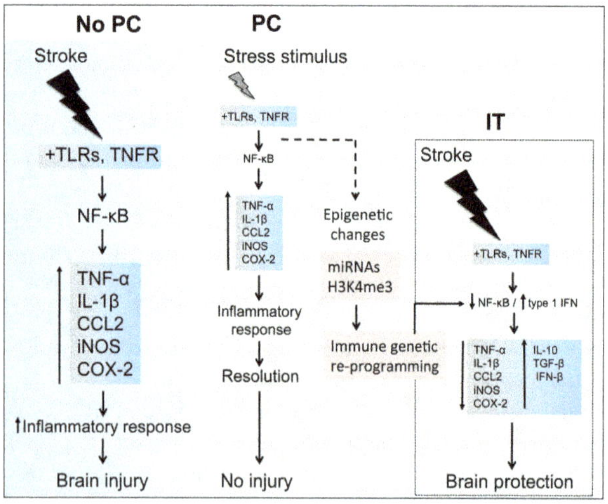

FIGURE 3 | Inflammatory components in stroke and preconditioning. Stroke induces a major inflammatory response through toll-like receptors (TLRs) and tumor necrosis factor receptor (TNFR) signaling, which activate nuclear factor-κB (NF-κB) resulting in upregulation of inflammatory molecules, such as TNF-α, interleukin (IL)-1β, CCL2, inducible nitric oxidase synthase (iNOS) and cyclooxygenase (COX)-2, contributing to the ischemic brain injury. In preconditioning (PC), the exposure to a wide range of stressors activates inflammatory pathways and leads to upregulation of inflammatory molecules similarly to those induced by stroke. After the effects of the stressor have subsided, the inflammatory response is resolved during the early phase of PC and gene expression returns to basal levels. However, longer lasting epigenetic changes induced in the immune system components by micro-RNAs (miRNAs) and histone methylation (i.e., histone H3 trimethylation at lysine 4, H3K4me3) may reprogram inflammatory pathways to respond differently after an episode of severe ischemia, for instance favoring the expression of anti-inflammatory cytokines (IL-10, tumor growth factor-(TGF)-β and interferon-(IFN)-β that induces ischemic tolerance (IT).

of inflammatory cytokines. In addition, a better understanding of the epigenetic mechanisms involved in IT could lead to therapies that preserve PC-induced epigenetic changes, thereby substantially extending the time frame in which IT is observed.

ACKNOWLEDGMENTS

This work was supported by National Institutes of Health (NIH) Grants NS34179 (Costantino Iadecola) and NS081179 (Josef Anrather). Corinne Benakis was supported by grant P3SMP3 148367 from the Swiss National Science Foundation and the Swiss Foundation for Grants in Biology and Medicine (SFGBM).

REFERENCES

Abe, T., Shimamura, M., Jackman, K., Kurinami, H., Anrather, J., Zhou, P., et al. (2010). Key role of CD36 in Toll-like receptor 2 signaling in cerebral ischemia. *Stroke* 41, 898–904. doi: 10.1161/STROKEAHA.109.572552

Ahmed, S. H., He, Y. Y., Nassief, A., Xu, J., Xu, X. M., Hsu, C. Y., et al. (2000). Effects of lipopolysaccharide priming on acute ischemic brain injury. *Stroke* 31, 193–199. doi: 10.1161/01.STR.31.1.193

Akira, S. (2009). Pathogen recognition by innate immunity and its signaling. *Proc. Jpn. Acad. Ser. B Phys. Biol. Sci.* 85, 143–156. doi: 10.2183/pjab.85.143

Allan, S. M., Tyrrell, P. J., and Rothwell, N. J. (2005). Interleukin-1 and neuronal injury. *Nat. Rev. Immunol.* 5, 629–640. doi: 10.1038/nri1664

Ameri, A. (1999). The effects of cannabinoids on the brain. *Prog. Neurobiol.* 58, 315–348. doi: 10.1016/S0301-0082(98)00087-2

Anderson, K. V., Bokla, L., and Nüsslein-Volhard, C. (1985). Establishment of dorsal-ventral polarity in the Drosophila embryo: the induction of polarity by the Toll gene product. *Cell* 42, 791–798. doi: 10.1016/0092-8674(85)90275-2

Aneja, R., Odoms, K., Dunsmore, K., Shanley, T. P., and Wong, H. R. (2006). Extracellular heat shock protein-70 induces endotoxin tolerance in THP-1 cells. *J. Immunol.* 177, 7184–7192.

Anrather, J., and Hallenbeck, J. M. (2013). Biological networks in ischemic tolerance—rethinking the approach to clinical conditioning. *Transl. Stroke Res.* 4, 114–129. doi: 10.1007/s12975-012-0244-z

Baeuerle, P. A., and Henkel, T. (1994). Function and activation of NF-kappaB in the immune system. *Annu. Rev. Immunol.* 12, 141–179. doi: 10.1146/annurev.iy.12.040194.001041

Baldwin, A. S. (1996). The NF-kappa B and I kappa B proteins: new discoveries and insights. *Annu. Rev. Immunol.* 14, 649–683. doi: 10.1146/annurev.immunol.14.1.649

Banks, W. A. (2005). Blood-brain barrier transport of cytokines: a mechanism for neuropathology. *Curr. Pharm. Des.* 11, 973–984. doi: 10.2174/1381612053381684

Barone, F. C., White, R. F., Spera, P. A., Ellison, J., Currie, R. W., Wang, X., et al. (1998). Ischemic preconditioning and brain tolerance: temporal histological and functional outcomes, protein synthesis requirement, and interleukin-1 receptor antagonist and early gene expression. *Stroke* 29, 1937–1950. discussion: 1950–1951.

Bartel, D. P. (2009). MicroRNAs: target recognition and regulatory functions. *Cell* 136, 215–233. doi: 10.1016/j.cell.2009.01.002

Bianchi, M. E. (2007). DAMPs, PAMPs and alarmins: all we need to know about danger. *J. Leukocyte Biol.* 81, 1–5. doi: 10.1189/jlb.0306164

Bigdeli, M. R., and Khoshbaten, A. (2008). *In vivo* preconditioning with normobaric hyperoxia induces ischemic tolerance partly by triggering tumor necrosis factor-alpha converting enzyme/tumor necrosis factor-alpha/nuclear factor-kappaB. *Neuroscience* 153, 671–678. doi: 10.1016/j.neuroscience.2008.02.064

Blondeau, N., Widmann, C., Lazdunski, M., and Heurteaux, C. (2001). Activation of the nuclear factor-kappaB is a key event in brain tolerance. *J. Neurosci.* 21, 4668–4677.

Brea, D., Blanco, M., Ramos-Cabrer, P., Moldes, O., Arias, S., Pérez-Mato, M., et al. (2011). Toll-like receptors 2 and 4 in ischemic stroke: outcome and therapeutic values. *J. Cereb. Blood Flow Metab.* 31, 1424–1431. doi: 10.1038/jcbfm.2010.231

Breder, C. D., Hazuka, C., Ghayur, T., Klug, C., Huginin, M., Yasuda, K., et al. (1994). Regional induction of tumor necrosis factor alpha expression in the mouse brain after systemic lipopolysaccharide administration. *Proc. Natl. Acad. Sci. U.S.A.* 91, 11393–11397. doi: 10.1073/pnas.91.24.11393

Cao, C.-X., Yang, Q.-W., Lv, F.-L., Cui, J., Fu, H.-B., and Wang, J.-Z. (2007). Reduced cerebral ischemia-reperfusion injury in Toll-like receptor 4 deficient mice. *Biochem. Biophys. Res. Commun.* 353, 509–514. doi: 10.1016/j.bbrc.2006.12.057

Cárdenas, A., Moro, M. A., Leza, J. C., O'Shea, E., Dávalos, A., Castillo, J., et al. (2002). Upregulation of TACE/ADAM17 after ischemic preconditioning is involved in brain tolerance. *J. Cereb. Blood Flow Metab.* 22, 1297–1302. doi: 10.1097/00004647-200211000-00002

Ceulemans, A.-G. A., Zgavc, T. T., Kooijman, R. R., Hachimi-Idrissi, S. S., Sarre, S. S., and Michotte, Y. Y. (2010). The dual role of the neuroinflammatory response after ischemic stroke: modulatory effects of hypothermia. *J. Neuroinflammation* 7, 74–74. doi: 10.1186/1742-2094-7-74

Chan, P. H. (2001). Reactive oxygen radicals in signaling and damage in the ischemic brain. *J. Cereb. Blood Flow Metab.* 21, 2–14. doi: 10.1097/00004647-200101000-00002

Charo, I. F., and Ransohoff, R. M. (2006). The many roles of chemokines and chemokine receptors in inflammation. *N. Engl. J. Med.* 354, 610–621. doi: 10.1056/NEJMra052723

Chen, G. Y., and Nuñez, G. (2010). Sterile inflammation: sensing and reacting to damage. *Nat. Rev. Immunol.* 10, 826–837. doi: 10.1038/nri2873

Chen, H., Song, Y. S., and Chan, P. H. (2009). Inhibition of NADPH oxidase is neuroprotective after ischemia-reperfusion. *J. Cereb. Blood Flow Metab.* 29, 1262–1272. doi: 10.1038/jcbfm.2009.47

Cheng, O., Ostrowski, R. P., Wu, B., Liu, W., Chen, C., and Zhang, J. H. (2011). Cyclooxygenase-2 mediates hyperbaric oxygen preconditioning in the rat model of transient global cerebral ischemia. *Stroke* 42, 484–490. doi: 10.1161/STROKEAHA.110.604421

Cho, S., Park, E.-M., Zhou, P., Frys, K., Ross, M. E., and Iadecola, C. (2005). Obligatory role of inducible nitric oxide synthase in ischemic preconditioning. *J. Cereb. Blood Flow Metab.* 25, 493–501. doi: 10.1038/sj.jcbfm.9600058

Clarkson, A. N. (2007). Anesthetic-mediated protection/preconditioning during cerebral ischemia. *Life Sci.* 80, 1157–1175. doi: 10.1016/j.lfs.2006.12.022

Clemens, J. A., Stephenson, D. T., Yin, T., Smalstig, E. B., Panetta, J. A., Little, S. P., et al. (1998). Drug-induced neuroprotection from global ischemia is associated with prevention of persistent but not transient activation of nuclear factor-B in rats editorial comment. *Stroke* 29, 677–682. doi: 10.1161/01.STR.29.3.677

Curry, A., Guo, M., Patel, R., Liebelt, B., Sprague, S., Lai, Q., et al. (2010). Exercise pre-conditioning reduces brain inflammation in stroke via tumor necrosis factor-α, extracellular signal-regulated kinase 1/2 and matrix metalloproteinase-9 activity. *Neurol. Res.* 32, 756–762. doi: 10.1179/174313209X459101

Dawn, B., Xuan, Y.-T., Guo, Y., Rezazadeh, A., Stein, A. B., Hunt, G., et al. (2004). IL-6 plays an obligatory role in late preconditioning via JAK-STAT signaling and upregulation of iNOS and COX-2. *Cardiovasc. Res.* 64, 61–71. doi: 10.1016/j.cardiores.2004.05.011

Dharap, A., Bowen, K., Place, R., Li, L.-C., and Vemuganti, R. (2009). Transient focal ischemia induces extensive temporal changes in rat cerebral MicroRNAome. *J. Cereb. Blood Flow Metab.* 29, 675–687. doi: 10.1038/jcbfm.2008.157

Dharap, A., and Vemuganti, R. (2010). Ischemic pre-conditioning alters cerebral microRNAs that are upstream to neuroprotective signaling pathways. *J. Neurochem.* 113, 1685–1691. doi: 10.1111/j.1471-4159.2010.06735.x

Di Marzo, V., Melck, D., Bisogno, T., and De Petrocellis, L. (1998). Endocannabinoids: endogenous cannabinoid receptor ligands with neuromodulatory action. *Trends Neurosci.* 21, 521–528. doi: 10.1016/S0166-2236(98)01283-1

Ding, Y.-H., Young, C. N., Luan, X., Li, J., Rafols, J. A., Clark, J. C., et al. (2005). Exercise preconditioning ameliorates inflammatory injury in ischemic rats during reperfusion. *Acta Neuropathol.* 109, 237–246. doi: 10.1007/s00401-004-0943-y

Dirnagl, U., and Meisel, A. (2008). Endogenous neuroprotection: mitochondria as gateways to cerebral preconditioning? *Neuropharmacology* 55, 334–344. doi: 10.1016/j.neuropharm.2008.02.017

Downes, C. E., and Crack, P. J. (2010). Neural injury following stroke: are Toll-like receptors the link between the immune system and the CNS? *Br. J. Pharmacol.* 160, 1872–1888. doi: 10.1111/j.1476-5381.2010.00864.x

Du, F., Zhu, L., Qian, Z.-M., Wu, X.-M., Yung, W.-H., and Ke, Y. (2010). Hyperthermic preconditioning protects astrocytes from ischemia/reperfusion injury by up-regulation of HIF-1 alpha expression and binding activity. *Biochim. Biophys. Acta* 1802, 1048–1053. doi: 10.1016/j.bbadis.2010.06.013

Duckworth, E. A. M., Butler, T., Collier, L., Collier, S., and Pennypacker, K. R. (2006). NF-κB protects neurons from ischemic injury after middle cerebral artery occlusion in mice. *Brain Res.* 1088, 167–175. doi: 10.1016/j.brainres.2006.02.103

Elliott, M. B., Tuma, R. F., Amenta, P. S., Barbe, M. F., and Jallo, J. I. (2011). Acute effects of a selective cannabinoid-2 receptor agonist on neuroinflammation in a model of traumatic brain injury. *J. Neurotrauma* 28, 973–981. doi: 10.1089/neu.2010.1672

Endres, M., Gertz, K., Lindauer, U., Katchanov, J., Schultze, J., Schröck, H., et al. (2003). Mechanisms of stroke protection by physical activity. *Ann. Neurol.* 54, 582–590. doi: 10.1002/ana.10722

Foster, S. L., Hargreaves, D. C., and Medzhitov, R. (2007). Gene-specific control of inflammation by TLR-induced chromatin modifications. *Nature* 447, 972–978. doi: 10.1038/nature05836

Gabellec, M. M., Griffais, R., Fillion, G., and Haour, F. (1995). Expression of interleukin 1 alpha, interleukin 1 beta and interleukin 1 receptor antagonist mRNA in mouse brain: regulation by bacterial lipopolysaccharide (LPS) treatment. *Brain Res. Mol. Brain Res.* 31, 122–130. doi: 10.1016/0169-328X(95)00042-Q

Galea, E., Glickstein, S. B., Feinstein, D. L., Golanov, E. V., and Reis, D. J. (1998a). Stimulation of cerebellar fastigial nucleus inhibits interleukin-1beta-induced cerebrovascular inflammation. *Am. J. Physiol.* 275, H2053–H2063.

Galea, E., Golanov, E. V., Feinstein, D. L., Kobylarz, K. A., Glickstein, S. B., and Reis, D. J. (1998b). Cerebellar stimulation reduces inducible nitric oxide synthase expression and protects brain from ischemia. *Am. J. Physiol.* 274, H2035–H2045.

Galiègue, S., Mary, S., Marchand, J., Dussossoy, D., Carrière, D., Carayon, P., et al. (1995). Expression of central and peripheral cannabinoid receptors in human immune tissues and leukocyte subpopulations. *Eur. J. Biochem.* 232, 54–61. doi: 10.1111/j.1432-1033.1995.tb20780.x

Gallí, M., Van Gool, F., and Leo, O. (2011). Sirtuins and inflammation: friends or foes? *Biochem. Pharmacol.* 81, 569–576. doi: 10.1016/j.bcp.2010.12.010

Gesuete, R., Packard, A. E. B., Vartanian, K. B., Conrad, V. K., Stevens, S. L., Bahjat, F. R., et al. (2012). Poly-ICLC preconditioning protects the blood-brain barrier against ischemic injury *in vitro* through type I interferon signaling. *J. Neurochem.* 123(Suppl. 2), 75–85. doi: 10.1111/j.1471-4159.2012.07946.x

Gidday, J. M. (2006). Cerebral preconditioning and ischaemic tolerance. *Nat. Rev. Neurosci.* 7, 437–448. doi: 10.1038/nrn1927

Ginis, I., Jaiswal, R., Klimanis, D., Liu, J., Greenspon, J., and Hallenbeck, J. M. (2002). TNF-alpha-induced tolerance to ischemic injury involves differential control of NF-kappaB transactivation: the role of NF-kappaB association with p300 adaptor. *J. Cereb. Blood Flow Metab.* 22, 142–152. doi: 10.1097/00004647-200202000-00002

Golanov, E. V., Liu, F., and Reis, D. J. (1998). Stimulation of cerebellum protects hippocampal neurons from global ischemia. *Neuroreport* 9, 819–824. doi: 10.1097/00001756-199803300-00010

Gong, J.-P., Onaivi, E. S., Ishiguro, H., Liu, Q.-R., Tagliaferro, P. A., Brusco, A., et al. (2006). Cannabinoid CB2 receptors: immunohistochemical localization in rat brain. *Brain Res.* 1071, 10–23. doi: 10.1016/j.brainres.2005.11.035

Guo, M., Lin, V., Davis, W., Huang, T., Carranza, A., Sprague, S., et al. (2008). Preischemic induction of TNF-alpha by physical exercise reduces blood-brain barrier dysfunction in stroke. *J. Cereb. Blood Flow Metab.* 28, 1422–1430. doi: 10.1038/jcbfm.2008.29

Hallenbeck, J. M. (2002). The many faces of tumor necrosis factor in stroke. *Nat. Med.* 8, 1363–1368. doi: 10.1038/nm1202-1363

Harari, O. A., and Liao, J. K. (2010). NF-κB and innate immunity in ischemic stroke. *Ann. N.Y. Acad. Sci.* 1207, 32–40. doi: 10.1111/j.1749-6632.2010.05735.x

Hazzalin, C. A., and Mahadevan, L. C. (2005). Dynamic acetylation of all lysine 4-methylated histone H3 in the mouse nucleus: analysis at c-fos and c-jun. *PLoS Biol.* 3:e393. doi: 10.1371/journal.pbio.0030393

Hess, D. C., Hoda, M. N., and Bhatia, K. (2013). Remote limb perconditioning and postconditioning: will it translate into a promising treatment for acute stroke? *Stroke* 44, 1191–1196. doi: 10.1161/STROKEAHA.112.678482

Hickey, E. J., You, X., Kaimaktchiev, V., Stenzel-Poore, M., and Ungerleider, R. M. (2007). Lipopolysaccharide preconditioning induces robust protection against brain injury resulting from deep hypothermic circulatory arrest. *J. Thorac. Cardiovasc. Surg.* 133, 1588–1596. doi: 10.1016/j.jtcvs.2006.12.056

Horiguchi, T., Snipes, J. A., Kis, B., Shimizu, K., and Busija, D. W. (2005). The role of nitric oxide in the development of cortical spreading depression-induced tolerance to transient focal cerebral ischemia in rats. *Brain Res.* 1039, 84–89. doi: 10.1016/j.brainres.2005.01.047

Horiguchi, T., Snipes, J. A., Kis, B., Shimizu, K., and Busija, D. W. (2006). Cyclooxygenase-2 mediates the development of cortical spreading depression-induced tolerance to transient focal cerebral ischemia in rats. *Neuroscience* 140, 723–730. doi: 10.1016/j.neuroscience.2006.02.025

Hoshino, K., Sugiyama, T., Matsumoto, M., Tanaka, T., Saito, M., Hemmi, H., et al. (2006). IkappaB kinase-alpha is critical for interferon-alpha production induced by Toll-like receptors 7 and 9. *Nature* 440, 949–953. doi: 10.1038/nature04641

Howlett, A. C. A., Barth, F. F., Bonner, T. I. T., Cabral, G. G., Casellas, P. P., Devane, W. A. W., et al. (2002). International union of pharmacology. XXVII. Classification of cannabinoid receptors. *Pharmacol. Rev.* 54, 161–202. doi: 10.1124/pr.54.2.161

Hu, X., Jiang, H., Cui, B., Xu, C., Lu, Z., and He, B. (2010). Preconditioning with high mobility group box 1 protein protects against myocardial ischemia-reperfusion injury. *Int. J. Cardiol.* 145, 111–112. doi: 10.1016/j.ijcard.2009.05.057

Hua, F., Ma, J., Ha, T., Kelley, J., Williams, D. L., Kao, R. L., et al. (2008). Preconditioning with a TLR2 specific ligand increases resistance to cerebral ischemia/reperfusion injury. *J. Neuroimmunol.* 199, 75–82. doi: 10.1016/j.jneuroim.2008.05.009

Huang, J., Upadhyay, U. M., and Tamargo, R. J. (2006). Inflammation in stroke and focal cerebral ischemia. *Surg. Neurol.* 66, 232–245. doi: 10.1016/j.surneu.2005.12.028

Iadecola, C., and Anrather, J. (2011a). The immunology of stroke: from mechanisms to translation. *Nat. Med.* 17, 796–808. doi: 10.1038/nm.2399

Iadecola, C., and Anrather, J. (2011b). Stroke research at a crossroad: asking the brain for directions. *Nat. Neurosci.* 14, 1363–1368. doi: 10.1038/nn.2953

Iadecola, C., Kahles, T., Gallo, E. F., and Anrather, J. (2011). Neurovascular protection by ischaemic tolerance: role of nitric oxide. *J. Physiol. (Lond.)* 589, 4137–4145. doi: 10.1113/jphysiol.2011.210831

Iadecola, C., Niwa, K., Nogawa, S., Zhao, X., Nagayama, M., Araki, E., et al. (2001). Reduced susceptibility to ischemic brain injury and N-methyl-D-aspartate-mediated neurotoxicity in cyclooxygenase-2-deficient mice. *Proc. Natl. Acad. Sci. U.S.A.* 98, 1294–1299. doi: 10.1073/pnas.98.3.1294

Ikeda, T., Xia, X. Y., Xia, Y. X., and Ikenoue, T. (1999). Hyperthermic preconditioning prevents blood-brain barrier disruption produced by hypoxia-ischemia in newborn rat. *Brain Res. Dev. Brain Res.* 117, 53–58. doi: 10.1016/S0165-3806(99)00097-8

Izuishi, K., Tsung, A., Jeyabalan, G., Critchlow, N. D., Li, J., Tracey, K. J., et al. (2006). Cutting edge: high-mobility group box 1 preconditioning protects against liver ischemia-reperfusion injury. *J. Immunol.* 176, 7154–7158.

Jaerve, A., and Müller, H. W. (2012). Chemokines in CNS injury and repair. *Cell Tissue Res.* 349, 229–248. doi: 10.1007/s00441-012-1427-3

Jander, S., Schroeter, M., Peters, O., Witte, O. W., and Stoll, G. (2001). Cortical spreading depression induces proinflammatory cytokine gene expression in the rat brain. *J. Cereb. Blood Flow Metab.* 21, 218–225. doi: 10.1097/00004647-200103000-00005

Jung, F., Palmer, L. A., Zhou, N., and Johns, R. A. (2000). Hypoxic regulation of inducible nitric oxide synthase via hypoxia inducible factor-1 in cardiac myocytes. *Circ. Res.* 86, 319–325. doi: 10.1161/01.RES.86.3.319

Kahles, T., Luedike, P., Endres, M., Galla, H.-J., Steinmetz, H., Busse, R., et al. (2007). NADPH oxidase plays a central role in blood-brain barrier damage in experimental stroke. *Stroke* 38, 3000–3006. doi: 10.1161/STROKEAHA.107.489765

Kaltschmidt, B., Widera, D., and Kaltschmidt, C. (2005). Signaling via NF-kappaB in the nervous system. *Biochim. Biophys. Acta* 1745, 287–299. doi: 10.1016/j.bbamcr.2005.05.009

Kaltschmidt, C., Kaltschmidt, B., Neumann, H., Wekerle, H., and Baeuerle, P. A. (1994). Constitutive NF-kappa B activity in neurons. *Mol. Cell Biol.* 14, 3981–3992.

Kapinya, K. J., Löwl, D., Fütterer, C., Maurer, M., Waschke, K. F., Isaev, N. K., et al. (2002). Tolerance against ischemic neuronal injury can be induced by volatile anesthetics and is inducible NO synthase dependent. *Stroke* 33, 1889–1898. doi: 10.1161/01.STR.0000020092.41820.58

Kawahara, N., Ruetzler, C. A., and Klatzo, I. (1995). Protective effect of spreading depression against neuronal damage following cardiac arrest cerebral ischaemia. *Neurol. Res.* 17, 9–16.

Kawahara, N., Ruetzler, C. A., Mies, G., and Klatzo, I. (1999). Cortical spreading depression increases protein synthesis and upregulates basic fibroblast growth factor. *Exp. Neurol.* 158, 27–36. doi: 10.1006/exnr.1999.7091

Kawai, N. N., Okauchi, M. M., Morisaki, K. K., and Nagao, S. S. (2000). Effects of delayed intraischemic and postischemic hypothermia on a focal model of transient cerebral ischemia in rats. *Stroke* 31, 1982–1989. doi: 10.1161/01.STR.31.8.1982

Kawano, T., Kunz, A., Abe, T., Girouard, H., Anrather, J., Zhou, P., et al. (2007). iNOS-derived NO and nox2-derived superoxide confer tolerance to excitotoxic brain injury through peroxynitrite. *J. Cereb. Blood Flow Metab.* 27, 1453–1462. doi: 10.1038/sj.jcbfm.9600449

Keep, R. F., Wang, M. M., Xiang, J., Hua, Y., and Xi, G. (2010). Is there a place for cerebral preconditioning in the clinic? *Transl. Stroke Res.* 1, 4–18. doi: 10.1007/s12975-009-0007-7

Kim, J. B. (2006). HMGB1, a novel cytokine-like mediator linking acute neuronal death and delayed neuroinflammation in the postischemic brain. *J. Neurosci.* 26, 6413–6421. doi: 10.1523/JNEUROSCI.3815-05.2006

Kirino, T. (2002). Ischemic tolerance. *J. Cereb. Blood Flow Metab.* 22, 1283–1296. doi: 10.1097/00004647-200211000-00001

Kitagawa, K., Matsumoto, M., Tagaya, M., Hata, R., Ueda, H., Niinobe, M., et al. (1990). "Ischemic tolerance" phenomenon found in the brain. *Brain Res.* 528, 21–24. doi: 10.1016/0006-8993(90)90189-I

Konstantinov, I. E., Arab, S., Kharbanda, R. K., Li, J., Cheung, M. M. H., Cherepanov, V., et al. (2004). The remote ischemic preconditioning stimulus modifies inflammatory gene expression in humans. *Physiol. Genomics* 19, 143–150. doi: 10.1152/physiolgenomics.00046.2004

Kunkler, P. E., Hulse, R. E., and Kraig, R. P. (2004). Multiplexed cytokine protein expression profiles from spreading depression in hippocampal organotypic cultures. *J. Cereb. Blood Flow Metab.* 24, 829–839. doi: 10.1097/01.WCB.0000126566.34753.30

Kunz, A., Anrather, J., Zhou, P., Orio, M., and Iadecola, C. (2006). Cyclooxygenase-2 does not contribute to postischemic production of reactive oxygen species. *J. Cereb. Blood Flow Metab.* 27, 545–551. doi: 10.1038/sj.jcbfm.9600369

Kunz, A., Park, L., Abe, T., Gallo, E. F., Anrather, J., Zhou, P., et al. (2007). Neurovascular protection by ischemic tolerance: role of nitric oxide and reactive oxygen species. *J. Neurosci.* 27, 7083–7093. doi: 10.1523/JNEUROSCI.1645-07.2007

Lee, S.-T., Chu, K., Jung, K.-H., Yoon, H.-J., Jeon, D., Kang, K.-M., et al. (2010). MicroRNAs induced during ischemic preconditioning. *Stroke* 41, 1646–1651. doi: 10.1161/STROKEAHA.110.579649

Leker, R. R., Gai, N., Mechoulam, R., and Ovadia, H. (2003). Drug-induced hypothermia reduces ischemic damage: effects of the cannabinoid HU-210. *Stroke* 34, 2000–2006. doi: 10.1161/01.STR.0000079817.68944.1E

Lemaitre, B., Nicolas, E., Michaut, L., Reichhart, J. M., and Hoffmann, J. A. (1996). The dorsoventral regulatory gene cassette spätzle/Toll/cactus controls the potent antifungal response in Drosophila adults. *Cell* 86, 973–983. doi: 10.1016/S0092-8674(00)80172-5

Leung, A. K. L., and Sharp, P. A. (2010). MicroRNA functions in stress responses. *Mol. Cell* 40, 205–215. doi: 10.1016/j.molcel.2010.09.027

Leung, P. Y., Packard, A. E., and Stenzel-Poore, M. P. (2009). It's all in the family: multiple Toll-like receptors offer promise as novel therapeutic targets for stroke neuroprotection. *Future Neurol.* 4, 201–208. doi: 10.2217/14796708.4.2.201

Leung, P. Y., Stevens, S. L., Packard, A. E. B., Lessov, N. S., Yang, T., Conrad, V. K., et al. (2012). Toll-like receptor 7 preconditioning induces robust neuroprotection against stroke by a novel type I interferon-mediated mechanism. *Stroke* 43, 1383–1389. doi: 10.1161/STROKEAHA.111.641522

Li, Q., and Verma, I. M. (2002). NF-kappaB regulation in the immune system. *Nat. Rev. Immunol.* 2, 725–734. doi: 10.1038/nri910

Li, Q.-F., Zhu, Y.-S., Jiang, H., Xu, H., and Sun, Y. (2009). Heme oxygenase-1 mediates the anti-inflammatory effect of isoflurane preconditioning in LPS-stimulated macrophages. *Acta Pharmacol. Sin.* 30, 228–234. doi: 10.1038/aps.2008.19

Liang, J., Wang, J., Saad, Y., Warble, L., Becerra, E., and Kolattukudy, P. E. (2011). Participation of MCP-induced protein 1 in lipopolysaccharide preconditioning-induced ischemic stroke tolerance by regulating the expression of proinflammatory cytokines. *J. Neuroinflammation* 8:182. doi: 10.1186/1742-2094-8-182

Liu, C., Peng, Z., Zhang, N., Yu, L., Han, S., Li, D., et al. (2012). Identification of differentially expressed microRNAs and their PKC-isoform specific gene network prediction during hypoxic pre-conditioning and focal cerebral ischemia of mice. *J. Neurochem.* 120, 830–841. doi: 10.1111/j.1471-4159.2011.07624.x

Liu, J., Ginis, I., Spatz, M., and Hallenbeck, J. M. (2000). Hypoxic preconditioning protects cultured neurons against hypoxic stress via TNF-alpha and ceramide. *Am. J. Physiol. Cell Physiol.* 278, C144–C153.

Loddick, S. A., Turnbull, A. V., and Rothwell, N. J. (1998). Cerebral interleukin-6 is neuroprotective during permanent focal cerebral ischemia in the rat. *J. Cereb. Blood Flow Metab.* 18, 176–179. doi: 10.1097/00004647-199802000-00008

Lu, C., Liu, L., Chen, Y., Ha, T., Kelley, J., Schweitzer, J., et al. (2011). TLR2 ligand induces protection against cerebral ischemia/reperfusion injury via activation of phosphoinositide 3-kinase/Akt signaling. *J. Immunol.* 187, 1458–1466. doi: 10.4049/jimmunol.1003428

Lusardi, T. A., Farr, C. D., Faulkner, C. L., Pignataro, G., Yang, T., Lan, J., et al. (2010). Ischemic preconditioning regulates expression of microRNAs and a predicted target, MeCP2, in mouse cortex. *J. Cereb. Blood Flow Metab.* 30, 744–756. doi: 10.1038/jcbfm.2009.253

Ma, L., Zhu, Z., Zhao, Y., Hou, L., Wang, Q., Xiong, L., et al. (2011). Cannabinoid receptor type 2 activation yields delayed tolerance to focal cerebral ischemia. *Curr. Neurovasc. Res.* 8, 145–152. doi: 10.2174/156720211795495394

Macrez, R., Ali, C., Toutirais, O., Le Mauff, B., Defer, G., Dirnagl, U., et al. (2011). Stroke and the immune system: from pathophysiology to new therapeutic strategies. *Lancet Neurol.* 10, 471–480. doi: 10.1016/S1474-4422(11)70066-7

Mallard, C. (2012). Innate immune regulation by toll-like receptors in the brain. *ISRN Neurol.* 2012:701950. doi: 10.5402/2012/701950

Marsh, B., Stevens, S. L., Packard, A. E. B., Gopalan, B., Hunter, B., Leung, P. Y., et al. (2009b). Systemic lipopolysaccharide protects the brain from ischemic injury by reprogramming the response of the brain to stroke: a critical role for IRF3. *J. Neurosci.* 29, 9839–9849. doi: 10.1523/JNEUROSCI.2496-09.2009

Marsh, B. J., Williams-Karnesky, R. L., and Stenzel-Poore, M. P. (2009a). Toll-like receptor signaling in endogenous neuroprotection and stroke. *Neuroscience* 158, 1007–1020. doi: 10.1016/j.neuroscience.2008.07.067

Matsuda, L. A., Lolait, S. J., Brownstein, M. J., Young, A. C., and Bonner, T. I. (1990). Structure of a cannabinoid receptor and functional expression of the cloned cDNA. *Nature* 346, 561–564. doi: 10.1038/346561a0

McColl, B. W., Allan, S. M., and Rothwell, N. J. (2009). Systemic infection, inflammation and acute ischemic stroke. *Neuroscience* 158, 1049–1061. doi: 10.1016/j.neuroscience.2008.08.019

Meisel, C., Schwab, J. M., Prass, K., Meisel, A., and Dirnagl, U. (2005). Central nervous system injury-induced immune deficiency syndrome. *Nat. Rev. Neurosci.* 6, 775–786. doi: 10.1038/nrn1765

Mercer, T. R., Dinger, M. E., and Mattick, J. S. (2009). Long non-coding RNAs: insights into functions. *Nat. Rev. Genet.* 10, 155–159. doi: 10.1038/nrg2521

Morris, K. C., Lin, H. W., Thompson, J. W., and Perez-Pinzon, M. A. (2011). Pathways for ischemic cytoprotection: role of sirtuins in caloric restriction, resveratrol, and ischemic preconditioning. *J. Cereb. Blood Flow Metab.* 31, 1003–1019. doi: 10.1038/jcbfm.2010.229

Nagayama, T. T., Sinor, A. D. A., Simon, R. P. R., Chen, J. J., Graham, S. H. S., Jin, K. K., et al. (1999). Cannabinoids and neuroprotection in global and focal cerebral ischemia and in neuronal cultures. *J. Neurosci.* 19, 2987–2995.

Narayanan, S. V., Dave, K. R., and Perez-Pinzon, M. A. (2013). Ischemic preconditioning and clinical scenarios. *Curr. Opin. Neurol.* 26, 1–7. doi: 10.1097/WCO.0b013e32835bf200

Nathan, C. (1997). Inducible nitric oxide synthase: what difference does it make? *J. Clin. Invest.* 100, 2417–2423. doi: 10.1172/JCI119782

Nawashiro, H., Tasaki, K., Ruetzler, C. A., and Hallenbeck, J. M. (1997). TNF-alpha pretreatment induces protective effects against focal cerebral ischemia in mice. *J. Cereb. Blood Flow Metab.* 17, 483–490. doi: 10.1097/00004647-199705000-00001

Nijboer, C. H., Heijnen, C. J., Groenendaal, F., May, M. J., van Bel, F., and Kavelaars, A. (2008). A dual role of the NF-kappaB pathway in neonatal hypoxic-ischemic brain damage. *Stroke* 39, 2578–2586. doi: 10.1161/STROKEAHA.108.516401

Nishio, S., Yunoki, M., Chen, Z. F., Anzivino, M. J., and Lee, K. S. (2000). Ischemic tolerance in the rat neocortex following hypothermic preconditioning. *J. Neurosurg.* 93, 845–851. doi: 10.3171/jns.2000.93.5.0845

Nurmi, A. (2004). Nuclear factor-B contributes to infarction after permanent focal ischemia. *Stroke* 35, 987–991. doi: 10.1161/01.STR.0000120732.45951.26

Nurmi, A., Vartiainen, N., Pihlaja, R., Goldsteins, G., Yrjanheikki, J., and Koistinaho, J. (2004). Pyrrolidine dithiocarbamate inhibits translocation of nuclear factor kappa-B in neurons and protects against brain ischaemia with a wide therapeutic time window. *J. Neurochem.* 91, 755–765. doi: 10.1111/j.1471-4159.2004.02756.x

O'Connell, R. M., Chaudhuri, A. A., Rao, D. S., and Baltimore, D. (2009). Inositol phosphatase SHIP1 is a primary target of miR-155. *Proc. Natl. Acad. Sci. U.S.A.* 106, 7113–7118. doi: 10.1073/pnas.0902636106

O'Connell, R. M., Rao, D. S., and Baltimore, D. (2012). microRNA regulation of inflammatory responses. *Annu. Rev. Immunol.* 30, 295–312. doi: 10.1146/annurev-immunol-020711-075013

Ohtsuki, T., Ruetzler, C. A., Tasaki, K., and Hallenbeck, J. M. (1996). Interleukin-1 mediates induction of tolerance to global ischemia in gerbil hippocampal CA1 neurons. *J. Cereb. Blood Flow Metab.* 16, 1137–1142. doi: 10.1097/00004647-199611000-00007

O'Neill, L. A., Sheedy, F. J., and McCoy, C. E. (2011). MicroRNAs: the fine-tuners of Toll-like receptor signalling. *Nat. Rev. Immunol.* 11, 163–175. doi: 10.1038/nri2957

Ota, A., Ikeda, T., Xia, X. Y., Xia, Y. X., and Ikenoue, T. (2000). Hypoxic-ischemic tolerance induced by hyperthermic pretreatment in newborn rats. *J. Soc. Gynecol. Investig.* 7, 102–105. doi: 10.1016/S1071-5576(00)00038-1

Pacher, P., Bátkai, S., and Kunos, G. (2006). The endocannabinoid system as an emerging target of pharmacotherapy. *Pharmacol. Rev.* 58, 389–462. doi: 10.1124/pr.58.3.2

Pacher, P., and Haskó, G. (2008). Endocannabinoids and cannabinoid receptors in ischaemia-reperfusion injury and preconditioning. *Br. J. Pharmacol.* 153, 252–262. doi: 10.1038/sj.bjp.0707582

Packard, A. E. B., Hedges, J. C., Bahjat, F. R., Stevens, S. L., Conlin, M. J., Salazar, A. M., et al. (2012). Poly-IC preconditioning protects against cerebral and renal ischemia-reperfusion injury. *J. Cereb. Blood Flow Metab.* 32, 242–247. doi: 10.1038/jcbfm.2011.160

Pahl, H. L. (1999). Activators and target genes of Rel/NF-kappaB transcription factors. *Oncogene* 18, 6853–6866. doi: 10.1038/sj.onc.1203239

Panikashvili, D., Mechoulam, R., Beni, S. M., Alexandrovich, A., and Shohami, E. (2005). CB1 cannabinoid receptors are involved in neuroprotection via NF-κB inhibition. *J. Cereb. Blood Flow Metab.* 25, 477–484. doi: 10.1038/sj.jcbfm.9600047

Panikashvili, D., Simeonidou, C., Ben-Shabat, S., Hanus, L., Breuer, A., Mechoulam, R., et al. (2001). An endogenous cannabinoid (2-AG) is neuroprotective after brain injury. *Nature* 413, 527–531. doi: 10.1038/35097089

Park, M. K., Kang, Y. J., Lee, H. S., Kim, H. J., Seo, H. G., Lee, J. H., et al. (2008). The obligatory role of COX-2 expression for induction of HO-1 in ischemic preconditioned rat brain. *Biochem. Biophys. Res. Commun.* 377, 1191–1194. doi: 10.1016/j.bbrc.2008.10.149

Patel, H., Shaw, S. G., Shi-Wen, X., Abraham, D., Baker, D. M., and Tsui, J. C. S. (2012). Toll-like receptors in ischaemia and its potential role in the pathophysiology of muscle damage in critical limb ischaemia. *Cardiol. Res. Pract.* 2012:121237. doi: 10.1155/2012/121237

Pedersen, B. K. (2011). Exercise-induced myokines and their role in chronic diseases. *Brain Behav. Immun.* 25, 811–816. doi: 10.1016/j.bbi.2011.02.010

Pedersen, C. M., Cruden, N. L., Schmidt, M. R., Lau, C., Bøtker, H. E., Kharbanda, R. K., et al. (2011). Remote ischemic preconditioning prevents systemic platelet activation associated with ischemia-reperfusion injury in humans. *J. Thromb. Haemost.* 9, 404–407. doi: 10.1111/j.1538-7836.2010.04142.x

Peng, Z., Ren, P., Kang, Z., Du, J., Lian, Q., Liu, Y., et al. (2008). Up-regulated HIF-1α is involved in the hypoxic tolerance induced by hyperbaric oxygen preconditioning. *Brain Res.* 1212, 71–78. doi: 10.1016/j.brainres.2008.03.027

Plamondon, H., Blondeau, N., Heurteaux, C., and Lazdunski, M. (1999). Mutually protective actions of kainic acid epileptic preconditioning and sublethal global ischemia on hippocampal neuronal death: involvement of adenosine A1 receptors and K(ATP) channels. *J. Cereb. Blood Flow Metab.* 19, 1296–1308. doi: 10.1097/00004647-199912000-00002

Pradillo, J. M., Fernández-López, D., García-Yébenes, I., Sobrado, M., Hurtado, O., Moro, M. A., et al. (2009). Toll-like receptor 4 is involved in neuroprotection afforded by ischemic preconditioning. *J. Neurochem.* 109, 287–294. doi: 10.1111/j.1471-4159.2009.05972.x

Pradillo, J. M., Romera, C., Hurtado, O., Cárdenas, A., Moro, M. A., Leza, J. C., et al. (2005). TNFR1 upregulation mediates tolerance after brain ischemic preconditioning. *J. Cereb. Blood Flow Metab.* 25, 193–203. doi: 10.1038/sj.jcbfm.9600019

Pun, P. B. L., Lu, J., and Moochhala, S. (2009). Involvement of ROS in BBB dysfunction. *Free Radic. Res.* 43, 348–364. doi: 10.1080/10715760902751902

Quintin, J., Saeed, S., Martens, J. H. A., Giamarellos-Bourboulis, E. J., Ifrim, D. C., Logie, C., et al. (2012). Candida albicans infection affords protection against reinfection via functional reprogramming of monocytes. *Cell Host Microbe* 12, 223–232. doi: 10.1016/j.chom.2012.06.006

Qureshi, I. A., and Mehler, M. F. (2010). Emerging role of epigenetics in stroke: part 1: DNA methylation and chromatin modifications. *Arch. Neurol.* 67, 1316–1322. doi: 10.1001/archneurol.2010.275

Ramirez-Carrozzi, V. R., Nazarian, A. A., Li, C. C., Gore, S. L., Sridharan, R., Imbalzano, A. N., et al. (2006). Selective and antagonistic functions of SWI/SNF and Mi-2beta nucleosome remodeling complexes during an inflammatory response. *Genes Dev.* 20, 282–296. doi: 10.1101/gad.1383206

Ransohoff, R. M., and Brown, M. A. (2012). Innate immunity in the central nervous system. *J. Clin.l Invest.* 122, 1164–1171. doi: 10.1172/JCI58644

Rehni, A. K., and Singh, T. G. (2012). Involvement of CCR-2 chemokine receptor activation in ischemic preconditioning and postconditioning of brain in mice. *Cytokine* 60, 83–89. doi: 10.1016/j.cyto.2012.05.009

Reis, D. J., Berger, S. B., Underwood, M. D., and Khayata, M. (1991). Electrical stimulation of cerebellar fastigial nucleus reduces ischemic infarction elicited by middle cerebral artery occlusion in rat. *J. Cereb. Blood Flow Metab.* 11, 810–818. doi: 10.1038/jcbfm.1991.139

Reis, D. J., Kobylarz, K., Yamamoto, S., and Golanov, E. V. (1998). Brief electrical stimulation of cerebellar fastigial nucleus conditions long-lasting salvage from focal cerebral ischemia: conditioned central neurogenic neuroprotection. *Brain Res.* 780, 161–165. doi: 10.1016/S0006-8993(97)01017-2

Rosenzweig, H. L., Lessov, N. S., Henshall, D. C., Minami, M., Simon, R. P., and Stenzel-Poore, M. P. (2004). Endotoxin preconditioning prevents cellular inflammatory response during ischemic neuroprotection in mice. *Stroke* 35, 2576–2581. doi: 10.1161/01.STR.0000143450.04438.ae

Rosenzweig, H. L., Minami, M., Lessov, N. S., Coste, S. C., Stevens, S. L., Henshall, D. C., et al. (2007). Endotoxin preconditioning protects against the cytotoxic effects of TNFalpha after stroke: a novel role for TNFalpha in LPS-ischemic tolerance. *J. Cereb. Blood Flow Metab.* 27, 1663–1674. doi: 10.1038/sj.jcbfm.9600464

Rüegger, S., and Großhans, H. (2012). MicroRNA turnover: when, how, and why. *Trends Biochem. Sci.* 37, 436–446. doi: 10.1016/j.tibs.2012.07.002

Schwaninger, M., Schneider, A., Martin-Villalba, A., Weih, F., Vogel, J., and Wirth, T. (1999). NF-kappaB is activated and promotes cell death in focal cerebral ischemia. *Nat. Med.* 5, 554–559. doi: 10.1038/8432

Semple, B. D., Kossmann, T., and Morganti-Kossmann, M. C. (2009). Role of chemokines in CNS health and pathology: a focus on the CCL2/CCR2 and CXCL8/CXCR2 networks. *J. Cereb. Blood Flow Metab.* 30, 459–473. doi: 10.1038/jcbfm.2009.240

Shichita, T., Hasegawa, E., Kimura, A., Morita, R., Sakaguchi, R., Takada, I., et al. (2012). Peroxiredoxin family proteins are key initiators of post-ischemic inflammation in the brain. *Nat. Med.* 18, 911–917. doi: 10.1038/nm.2749

Shimizu, M., Saxena, P., Konstantinov, I. E., Cherepanov, V., Cheung, M. M. H., Wearden, P., et al. (2010). Remote ischemic preconditioning decreases adhesion and selectively modifies functional responses of human neutrophils. *J. Surg. Res.* 158, 155–161. doi: 10.1016/j.jss.2008.08.010

Shin, J. A., Park, E.-M., Choi, J.-S., Seo, S.-M., Kang, J. L., Lee, K.-E., et al. (2009). Ischemic preconditioning-induced neuroprotection is associated with differential expression of IL-1beta and IL-1 receptor antagonist in the ischemic cortex. *J. Neuroimmunol.* 217, 14–19. doi: 10.1016/j.jneuroim.2009.06.001

Shpargel, K. B., Jalabi, W., Jin, Y., Dadabayev, A., Penn, M. S., and Trapp, B. D. (2008). Preconditioning paradigms and pathways in the brain. *Cleve. Clin. J. Med.* 75(Suppl. 2), S77–S82. doi: 10.3949/ccjm.75.Suppl_2.S77

Sly, L. M., Rauh, M. J., Kalesnikoff, J., Song, C. H., and Krystal, G. (2004). LPS-Induced Upregulation of SHIP is essential for endotoxin tolerance. *Immunity* 21, 227–239. doi: 10.1016/j.immuni.2004.07.010

Stapels, M., Piper, C., Yang, T., Li, M., Stowell, C., Xiong, Z. G., et al. (2010). Polycomb group proteins as epigenetic mediators of neuroprotection in ischemic tolerance. *Sci. Signal.* 3, ra15–ra15. doi: 10.1126/scisignal.2000502

Stenzel-Poore, M. P., Stevens, S. L., Xiong, Z., Lessov, N. S., Harrington, C. A., Mori, M., et al. (2003). Effect of ischaemic preconditioning on genomic response to cerebral ischaemia: similarity to neuroprotective strategies in hibernation and hypoxia-tolerant states. *Lancet* 362, 1028–1037. doi: 10.1016/S0140-6736(03)14412-1

Stephenson, D., Yin, T., Smalstig, E. B., Hsu, M. A., Panetta, J., Little, S., et al. (2000). Transcription factor nuclear factor-kappa B is activated in neurons after focal cerebral ischemia. *J. Cereb. Blood Flow Metab.* 20, 592–603. doi: 10.1097/00004647-200003000-00017

Stevens, S. L., Ciesielski, T. M. P., Marsh, B. J., Yang, T., Homen, D. S., Boule, J.-L., et al. (2008). Toll-like receptor 9: a new target of ischemic preconditioning in the brain. *J. Cereb. Blood Flow Metab.* 28, 1040–1047. doi: 10.1038/sj.jcbfm.9600606

Stevens, S. L., Leung, P. Y., Vartanian, K. B., Gopalan, B., Yang, T., Simon, R. P., et al. (2011). Multiple preconditioning paradigms converge on interferon regulatory factor-dependent signaling to promote tolerance to ischemic brain injury. *J. Neurosci.* 31, 8456–8463. doi: 10.1523/JNEUROSCI.0821-11.2011

Stowe, A. M., Wacker, B. K., Cravens, P. D., Perfater, J. L., Li, M. K., Hu, R., et al. (2012). CCL2 upregulation triggers hypoxic preconditioning-induced protection from stroke. *J. Neuroinflammation* 9:33. doi: 10.1186/1742-2094-9-33

Stridh, L., Smith, P. L. P., Naylor, A. S., Wang, X., and Mallard, C. (2011). Regulation of toll-like receptor 1 and -2 in neonatal mice brains after hypoxia-ischemia. *J. Neuroinflammation* 8:45. doi: 10.1186/1742-2094-8-45

Suzuki, H. I., Arase, M., Matsuyama, H., Choi, Y. L., Ueno, T., Mano, H., et al. (2011). MCPIP1 ribonuclease antagonizes dicer and terminates microRNA biogenesis through precursor microRNA degradation. *Mol. Cell* 44, 424–436. doi: 10.1016/j.molcel.2011.09.012

Swigut, T., and Wysocka, J. (2007). H3K27 demethylases, at long last. *Cell* 131, 29–32. doi: 10.1016/j.cell.2007.09.026

Tapuria, N., Kumar, Y., Habib, M. M., Abu-Amara, M., Seifalian, A. M., and Davidson, B. R. (2008). Remote ischemic preconditioning: a novel protective method from ischemia reperfusion injury—a review. *J. Surg. Res.* 150, 304–330. doi: 10.1016/j.jss.2007.12.747

Tasaki, K., Ruetzler, C. A., Ohtsuki, T., Martin, D., Nawashiro, H., and Hallenbeck, J. M. (1997). Lipopolysaccharide pre-treatment induces resistance against subsequent focal cerebral ischemic damage in spontaneously hypertensive rats. *Brain Res.* 748, 267–270. doi: 10.1016/S0006-8993(96)01383-2

Towfighi, J., Housman, C., Mauger, D., and Vannucci, R. C. (1999). Effect of seizures on cerebral hypoxic-ischemic lesions in immature rats. *Brain Res. Dev. Brain Res.* 113, 83–95. doi: 10.1016/S0165-3806(99)00004-8

Trinchieri, G. (2010). Type I interferon: friend or foe? *J. Exp. Med.* 207, 2053–2063. doi: 10.1084/jem.20101664

Ullrich, O., Merker, K., Timm, J., and Tauber, S. (2007). Immune control by endocannabinoids—new mechanisms of neuroprotection? *J. Neuroimmunol.* 184, 127–135. doi: 10.1016/j.jneuroim.2006.11.018

Vabulas, R. M., Ahmad-Nejad, P., Ghose, S., Kirschning, C. J., Issels, R. D., and Wagner, H. (2002). HSP70 as endogenous stimulus of the Toll/interleukin-1 receptor signal pathway. *J. Biol. Chem.* 277, 15107–15112. doi: 10.1074/jbc.M111204200

Valadi, H., Ekström, K., Bossios, A., Sjöstrand, M., Lee, J. J., and Lötvall, J. O. (2007). Exosome-mediated transfer of mRNAs and microRNAs is a novel mechanism of genetic exchange between cells. *Nat. Cell Biol.* 9, 654–659. doi: 10.1038/ncb1596

van Rooij, E., Sutherland, L. B., Qi, X., Richardson, J. A., Hill, J., and Olson, E. N. (2007). Control of stress-dependent cardiac growth and gene expression by a microRNA. *Science* 316, 575–579. doi: 10.1126/science.1139089

Vartanian, K., and Stenzel-Poore, M. (2010). Toll-like receptor tolerance as a mechanism for neuroprotection. *Transl. Stroke Res.* 1, 252–260. doi: 10.1007/s12975-010-0033-5

Vartanian, K. B., Stevens, S. L., Marsh, B. J., Williams-Karnesky, R., Lessov, N. S., and Stenzel-Poore, M. P. (2011). LPS preconditioning redirects TLR signaling following stroke: TRIF-IRF3 plays a seminal role in mediating tolerance to ischemic injury. *J. Neuroinflammation* 8:140. doi: 10.1186/1742-2094-8-140

Veldhuis, W. B., Derksen, J. W., Floris, S., van der Meide, P. H., de Vries, H. E., Schepers, J., et al. (2003). Interferon-beta blocks infiltration of inflammatory cells and reduces infarct volume after ischemic stroke in the rat. *J. Cereb. Blood Flow Metab.* 1029–1039. doi: 10.1097/01.WCB.0000080703.47016.B6

Verstak, B., Hertzog, P., and Mansell, A. (2007). Toll-like receptor signalling and the clinical benefits that lie within. *Inflamm. Res.* 56, 1–10. doi: 10.1007/s00011-007-6093-7

Verstrepen, L., Verhelst, K., van Loo, G., Carpentier, I., Ley, S. C., and Beyaert, R. (2010). Expression, biological activities and mechanisms of action of A20 (TNFAIP3). *Biochem. Pharmacol.* 80, 2009–2020. doi: 10.1016/j.bcp.2010.06.044

Vezzani, A., Moneta, D., Richichi, C., Aliprandi, M., Burrows, S. J., Ravizza, T., et al. (2002). Functional role of inflammatory cytokines and antiinflammatory molecules in seizures and epileptogenesis. *Epilepsia* 43(Suppl. 5), 30–35. doi: 10.1046/j.1528-1157.43.s.5.14.x

Vlasov, T. D., Korzhevskii, D. E., and Polyakova, E. A. (2005). Ischemic preconditioning of the rat brain as a method of endothelial protection from ischemic/repercussion injury. *Neurosci. Behav. Physiol.* 35, 567–572. doi: 10.1007/s11055-005-0095-0

Wacker, B. K., Perfater, J. L., and Gidday, J. M. (2012). Hypoxic preconditioning induces stroke tolerance in mice via a cascading HIF, sphingosine kinase, and CCL2 signaling pathway. *J. Neurochem.* 123, 954–962. doi: 10.1111/jnc.12047

Wang, F., Birch, S. E., He, R., Tawadros, P., Szaszi, K., Kapus, A., et al. (2010). Remote ischemic preconditioning by hindlimb occlusion prevents liver ischemic/reperfusion injury. *Ann. Surg.* 251, 292–299. doi: 10.1097/SLA.0b013e3181bfda8c

Wang, L., Traystman, R. J., and Murphy, S. J. (2008). Inhalational anesthetics as preconditioning agents in ischemic brain. *Curr. Opin. Pharmacol.* 8, 104–110. doi: 10.1016/j.coph.2007.09.005

Wang, Q., Peng, Y., Chen, S., Gou, X., Hu, B., Du, J., et al. (2009). Pretreatment with electroacupuncture induces rapid tolerance to focal cerebral ischemia through regulation of endocannabinoid system. *Stroke* 40, 2157–2164. doi: 10.1161/STROKEAHA.108.541490

Wang, Q., Xiong, L., Chen, S., Liu, Y., and Zhu, X. (2005). Rapid tolerance to focal cerebral ischemia in rats is induced by preconditioning with electroacupuncture: window of protection and the role of adenosine. *Neurosci. Lett.* 381, 158–162. doi: 10.1016/j.neulet.2005.02.019

Wang, R. Y., Yang, Y. R., and Yu, S. M. (2001). Protective effects of treadmill training on infarction in rats. *Brain Res.* 922, 140–143. doi: 10.1016/S0006-8993(01)03154-7

Wang, X., Li, X., Currie, R. W., Willette, R. N., Barone, F. C., and Feuerstein, G. Z. (2000). Application of real-time polymerase chain reaction to quantitate induced expression of interleukin-1beta mRNA in ischemic brain tolerance. *J. Neurosci. Res.* 59, 238–246. doi: 10.1016/S1385-299X(00)00015-5

Wang, Y., Wang, Y., and Yang, G.-Y. (2013). MicroRNAs in cerebral ischemia. *Stroke Res. Treat.* 2013:276540. doi: 10.1155/2013/276540

Wang, Y.-C., Lin, S., and Yang, Q.-W. (2011). Toll-like receptors in cerebral ischemic inflammatory injury. *J. Neuroinflammation* 8:134. doi: 10.1186/1742-2094-8-134

Wu, T.-C., and Grotta, J. C. (2013). Hypothermia for acute ischaemic stroke. *Lancet Neurol.* 12, 275–284. doi: 10.1016/S1474-4422(13)70013-9

Yanamoto, H., Hashimoto, N., Nagata, I., and Kikuchi, H. (1998). Infarct tolerance against temporary focal ischemia following spreading depression in rat brain. *Brain Res.* 784, 239–249. doi: 10.1016/S0006-8993(97)01344-9

Yang, Q.-W., Lu, F.-L., Zhou, Y., Wang, L., Zhong, Q., Lin, S., et al. (2011). HMBG1 mediates ischemia-reperfusion injury by TRIF-adaptor independent Toll-like receptor 4 signaling. *J. Cereb. Blood Flow Metab.* 31, 593–605. doi: 10.1038/jcbfm.2010.129

Yin, W., Signore, A. P., Iwai, M., Cao, G., Gao, Y., Johnnides, M. J., et al. (2007). Preconditioning suppresses inflammation in neonatal hypoxic ischemia via Akt activation. *Stroke* 38, 1017–1024. doi: 10.1161/01.STR.0000258102.18836.ca

Yoshimura, A., Naka, T., and Kubo, M. (2007). SOCS proteins, cytokine signalling and immune regulation. *Nat. Rev. Immunol.* 7, 454–465. doi: 10.1038/nri2093

Yu, J. T., Lee, C. H., Yoo, K.-Y., Choi, J. H., Li, H., Park, O. K., et al. (2010). Maintenance of anti-inflammatory cytokines and reduction of glial activation in the ischemic hippocampal CA1 region preconditioned with lipopolysaccharide. *J. Neurol. Sci.* 296, 69–78. doi: 10.1016/j.jns.2010.06.004

Yunoki, M., Nishio, S., Ukita, N., Anzivino, M. J., and Lee, K. S. (2003). Hypothermic preconditioning induces rapid tolerance to focal ischemic injury in the rat. *Exp. Neurol.* 181, 291–300. doi: 10.1016/S0014-4886(03)00056-6

Zhang, F., Wu, Y., and Jia, J. (2011). Exercise preconditioning and brain ischemic tolerance. *Neuroscience* 177, 170–176. doi: 10.1016/j.neuroscience.2011.01.018

Zhang, M., Adler, M. W., Abood, M. E., Ganea, D., Jallo, J., and Tuma, R. F. (2009). CB2 receptor activation attenuates microcirculatory dysfunction during cerebral ischemic/reperfusion injury. *Microvasc. Res.* 78, 86–94. doi: 10.1016/j.mvr.2009.03.005

Zhang, M., Martin, B. R., Adler, M. W., Razdan, R. K., Jallo, J. I., and Tuma, R. F. (2007). Cannabinoid CB2 receptor activation decreases cerebral infarction in a mouse focal ischemia/reperfusion model. *J. Cereb. Blood Flow Metab.* 27, 1387–1396. doi: 10.1038/sj.jcbfm.9600447

Zhao, P., and Zuo, Z. (2004). Isoflurane preconditioning induces neuroprotection that is inducible nitric oxide synthase-dependent in neonatal rats. *Anesthesiology* 101, 695–703. doi: 10.1097/00000542-200409000-00018

Zhou, P., Qian, L., D'Aurelio, M., Cho, S., Wang, G., Manfredi, G., et al. (2012). Prohibitin reduces mitochondrial free radical production and protects brain cells from different injury modalities. *J. Neurosci.* 32, 583–592. doi: 10.1523/JNEUROSCI.2849-11.2012

Zhou, P., Qian, L., Zhou, T., and Iadecola, C. (2005). Mitochondria are involved in the neurogenic neuroprotection conferred by stimulation of cerebellar fastigial nucleus. *J. Neurochem.* 95, 221–229. doi: 10.1111/j.1471-4159.2005.03358.x

Zhuang, S.-Y., Bridges, D., Grigorenko, E., McCloud, S., Boon, A., Hampson, R. E., et al. (2005). Cannabinoids produce neuroprotection by reducing intracellular calcium release from ryanodine-sensitive stores. *Neuropharmacology* 48, 1086–1096. doi: 10.1016/j.neuropharm.2005.01.005

Zimmermann, C., Ginis, I., Furuya, K., Klimanis, D., Ruetzler, C., Spatz, M., et al. (2001). Lipopolysaccharide-induced ischemic tolerance is associated with increased levels of ceramide in brain and in plasma. *Brain Res.* 895, 59–65. doi: 10.1016/S0006-8993(01)02028-5

Zwagerman, N., Plumlee, C., Guthikonda, M., and Ding, Y. (2010). Toll-like receptor-4 and cytokine cascade in stroke after exercise. *Neurol. Res.* 32, 123–126. doi: 10.1179/016164109X12464612122812

8

Immune responses at brain barriers and implications for brain development and neurological function in later life

Helen B. Stolp[1,2]*, Shane A. Liddelow[3,4], Inês Sá-Pereira[5], Katarzyna M. Dziegielewska[4] and Norman R. Saunders[4]

[1] Department of Perinatal Imaging and Health, King's College London, London, UK
[2] Department of Physiology, Anatomy and Genetics, University of Oxford, Oxford, UK
[3] Department of Neurobiology, Stanford University, Stanford, CA, USA
[4] Department of Pharmacology and Therapeutics, University of Melbourne, Parkville, VIC, Australia
[5] Department of Pharmacology, University of Oxford, Oxford, UK

Edited by:
Beatriz Gomez-Gonzalez, Universidad Autonoma Metropolitana, Unidad Iztapalapa, Mexico

Reviewed by:
Rick Meeker, University of North Carolina, USA
Tobias Tenenbaum, University Children's Hospital Mannheim, Germany

****Correspondence:***
Helen B. Stolp, Department of Perinatal Imaging and Health, St. Thomas' Hospital, King's College London, London SE1 7EH, UK
e-mail: helen.stolp@dpag.ox.ac.uk

For a long time the brain has been considered an immune-privileged site due to a muted inflammatory response and the presence of protective brain barriers. It is now recognized that neuroinflammation may play an important role in almost all neurological disorders and that the brain barriers may be contributing through either normal immune signaling or disruption of their basic physiological mechanisms. The distinction between normal function and dysfunction at the barriers is difficult to dissect, partly due to a lack of understanding of normal barrier function and partly because of physiological changes that occur as part of normal development and ageing. Brain barriers consist of a number of interacting structural and physiological elements including tight junctions between adjacent barrier cells and an array of influx and efflux transporters. Despite these protective mechanisms, the capacity for immune-surveillance of the brain is maintained, and there is evidence of inflammatory signaling at the brain barriers that may be an important part of the body's response to damage or infection. This signaling system appears to change both with normal ageing, and during disease. Changes may affect diapedesis of immune cells and active molecular transfer, or cause rearrangement of the tight junctions and an increase in passive permeability across barrier interfaces. Here we review the many elements that contribute to brain barrier functions and how they respond to inflammation, particularly during development and aging. The implications of inflammation–induced barrier dysfunction for brain development and subsequent neurological function are also discussed.

Keywords: blood-brain barrier, choroid plexus, cerebrospinal fluid, inflammation, development

INTRODUCTION

It is a long-held belief that the central nervous system (CNS) is an immune-privileged site, due in part to the muted inflammatory response and presence of several protective brain barriers at the CNS-peripheral interface. In contrast to this earlier dogma, it is now evident that the CNS does contain immune capabilities, and that neuroinflammation is likely to play an important role in most, if not all, neurological disorders. In addition, the protective barriers of the brain contribute to these altered functions through either normal immune signaling, or disruption of the basic physiological barrier mechanisms. Recent work has shown that the peripheral immune response contributes to neuroinflammatory conditions (Anthony et al., 2011). This has been particularly well-established in conditions such as multiple sclerosis (and the corresponding animal model—experimental autoimmune encephalomyelitis, EAE) and similar findings have been reported in models of amyotrophic lateral sclerosis, stroke, and epilepsy among others (Campbell et al., 2007b, 2010; Serres et al., 2009; Auvin et al., 2010).

In all these conditions, changes in blood-brain barrier structure and function have been reported. The brain barriers play an important role in maintaining the homeostatic environment of the CNS, and damage to the various structural and functional components of the barrier systems may contribute significantly to disease etiology or progression. What is currently unclear is how (a) the brain barriers themselves contribute to inflammatory signaling in neurological disease? and (b) which specific barrier mechanisms are altered in response to inflammation? Of particular interest to us is the importance of these pathological mechanisms in the developing brain.

In a typical adult inflammatory state, cells mediating the inflammatory response arrive at the site of inflammation or infection and release a large number of mediators that act to control the accumulation and activation of other cell types (both locally and migrating). The key features of CNS inflammation include a range of responses: glial activation, edema, major histocompatibility complex expression, systemic acute phase response (general

Abbreviations: CSF, cerebrospinal fluid; CNS, central nervous system; EAE, experimental autoimmune encephalitis; E, embryonic; Itga6, integrin a6; JAM, junctional adhesion molecule; IL, interleukin; PGP, P-glycoprotein; PKC, protein kinase C; SVZ, subventricular zone; TNF, tumor necrosis factor; VCAM, vascular cell adhesion molecule; VZ, ventricular zone, ZO, zonular occludin.

inflammation and acute phase protein synthesis), complement activation, synthesis of inflammatory mediators (e.g., cytokines, free radicals, prostaglandins) expression of adhesion molecules and the invasion of circulating immune cells (Perry et al., 1995). Due to the protective nature of both the blood-brain and blood-CSF barriers, there are two questions for consideration. Firstly, are mediators of the inflammatory response captured within the CNS space unable to be removed rapidly by the bloodstream? And secondly, does the functional tightness of the barrier impede the entry of immune cells, thereby slowing the immune response? Though the brain can mount its own defense by the activation of resident cells such as astrocytes and microglia (both cell types that are able to produce and secrete and number of cytokines), there is still a major reliance on peripheral immune cells. There is a continued argument about the balance between protection and damage in the CNS that results from a neuroinflammatory response, given its limited regenerative capacity (Aguzzi et al., 2013).

Differentiating the role of inflammatory mediators in pathogenesis is particularly difficult early in development, as a number of immune mediators play an important role in normal brain development. Neuropoietic cytokines contribute to proliferation of neural precursors, fate determination and differentiation, migration of neurons and glia, as well as cell survival and activity-dependent alteration of synaptic function (Stolp, 2013). Inflammation during development therefore, may cause widespread injury to the brain—not only due to the damaging effects of the inflammatory response itself, but also by interfering with the normal balance of cytokine signaling and therefore CNS development.

It is now well-documented that the barrier systems in the brain are well-established during early development and are essential for the normal functioning of the brain (see Saunders et al., 2012 for review). However, other research suggests that the brain barriers may be more susceptible to inflammation-induced changes in the developing brain (Anthony et al., 1997; Stolp et al., 2005a) in turn contributing to the pathology of serious neurodevelopmental disorders such as autism, cerebral palsy and epilepsy (Stolp and Dziegielewska, 2009). Alterations in signaling through barrier systems following inflammatory injury may lead to changes in many elements of brain development—contributing to these serious developmental disorders [reviewed by Stolp (2013)] or they may change the susceptibility of the brain to later onset conditions such as schizophrenia or neurodegenerative disease [reviewed by Stolp and Dziegielewska (2009); Bilbo and Schwarz (2012)].

The aim of this review is to introduce the brain barrier mechanisms and the response and contribution of these barriers to inflammation in the CNS. We shall initially discuss these issues in the context of adult disease, before exploring the developmental barrier systems and their contribution to neurodevelopmental disorders.

BARRIER MECHANISMS IN THE ADULT AND DEVELOPING BRAIN

The brain develops and functions within a well-defined internal environment, which is determined by regulation of interchange between the main compartments of the CNS, brain, cerebrospinal fluid (CSF) and the blood, by a combination of physical and functional mechanisms. These mechanisms, often referred to by the generic term of "blood-brain barrier," are present at three main interfaces in the brain, both in the adult and in the embryo, although there are some important age-related differences between them. These interfaces, illustrated in **Figure 1**, are: (i) the blood-brain barrier proper at the level of the cerebral endothelial cells, (ii) the blood-CSF barrier at the epithelial cells of the choroid plexuses within the four cerebral ventricles and (iii) the pia arachnoid. There is also an additional barrier interface (iv), present only in the early brain development, between the CSF and the brain interstitial fluid. In both the adult and developing brain the essential morphological feature of the blood-brain barrier proper (i) lies in the presence of tight junctions between the cerebral endothelial cells of the vasculature of the brain both within the parenchyma and over the surface in the pia-arachnoid. Compared with other blood vessels there is also a lack of pinocytotic vesicles in the cerebral endothelial cells, although there is some evidence that they may be more frequent in endothelial cells in the developing brain (Dziegielewska et al., 1979). In the choroid plexuses (ii), tight junctions are found between intimately apposed epithelial cells. The tight junctions prevent the intercellular (paracellular) passage of small molecules even in the very early stages of the developing brain (Ek et al., 2003, 2006). An important functional consequence of this is that the presence of tight intercellular junctions enables the cerebral endothelial cells and choroid plexus epithelial cells to have effective one-way transport mechanisms (Liddelow et al., 2009; Ek et al., 2010), which are essential for establishing and maintaining the internal environment of the brain separate from that of the rest of the organism. The morphology of the barrier interface over the surface of the brain (iii) is more complex during early development. Thus, in addition to the adult barrier of tight junctions linking the endothelial cells of blood vessels in the pia arachnoid, there is a wide array of specialized intercellular junctions over the pial surface of the brain, which has been described in the rat embryo (Balslev et al., 1997). From embryonic day 14 (E14), the progressive appearance of distinct junctional structures between the glial end feet was observed. Analysis of albumin distribution at the electron microscopic level suggested that these junctions may contribute to restriction of diffusion between the subarachnoid space and the brain interstitial space. However, at E12 and E14, the intercellular basis for this barrier appeared incomplete, so it was suggested that basement membrane may be an important component of this functionally effective barrier interface (Balslev et al., 1997). At the CSF-brain interface (iv) lining the cerebral ventricles, early in embryonic development, the cells of the neuroependyma (neuroepithelium) are linked by strap junctions (Møllgård et al., 1987), which are an effective limitation to intercellular diffusion at least for large molecules (Fossan et al., 1985). During brain development these strap junctions disappear, and in the adult the cells lining the ventricles (ependymal cells) are linked by gap junctions (Møllgård et al., 1987) that do not provide a significant restraint to diffusion of even large molecules from CSF to brain interstitial fluid (Fossan et al., 1985). Consequently, in the embryonic brain only, there appear to be barrier mechanisms that restrict entry of proteins from CSF into the brain interstitial fluid. These proteins may be contributing to some aspects of early brain development such as neurogenesis and cellular differentiation in the ventricular zone (VZ), either by uptake of individual proteins or ligands bound to them (see below).

In terms of functional exchanges at the brain barrier interfaces, these have only been studied in any detail at the blood-brain and blood-CSF barriers, although much less so during early development than in the adult brain. Some recent studies have used molecular screening techniques to elucidate the range of genes coding for various proteins involved in transport mechanisms that are expressed at these interfaces during fetal or neonatal stages of brain development. Daneman et al. (2010) used Affymetrix genechip arrays to compare expression patterns in neonatal and adult mouse cerebral endothelial cells, while Liddelow et al. (2012, 2013) used both Affymetrix arrays and high-throughput RNA sequencing to compare gene expression in mice and rats from E15 embryos and adult choroid plexuses. These studies are complimented by those of Kratzer et al. (2012) who used Affymetrix arrays to study gene expression in rat choroid plexus at several ages between E18 and adult, and by Marques et al. (2009) of adult mouse choroid plexus using Illumina whole genome beadchips. Collectively, these studies have revealed expression of an astonishing array of transcripts for proteins known to be associated with tight junctions, transporters (both influx and efflux) and ion channels, as well as numerous enzymes in various metabolic and signal transduction pathways. Many of these genes are expressed at a higher level (in some cases two orders of magnitude higher) in the developing cerebral endothelial and choroid plexus epithelial cells than in the adult. A major problem, however, is determining whether these high levels of expression also reflect a higher level of transport. By comparing published data from *in vivo* transport from blood to brain or CSF, for example for glucose and amino acids in neonatal animals (such experiments in fetuses have so far proved to be a technically intractable problem), it is clear that these high levels of expression are likely to reflect higher levels of transport in the developing brain (Saunders et al., 2013). However, because of the overlap in substrates for different transporters it is not yet possible to be sure that higher expression always equates to greater transport. Some examples comparing expression of individual transporter genes with data on *in vivo* transport of various amino acids are shown in **Table 1**.

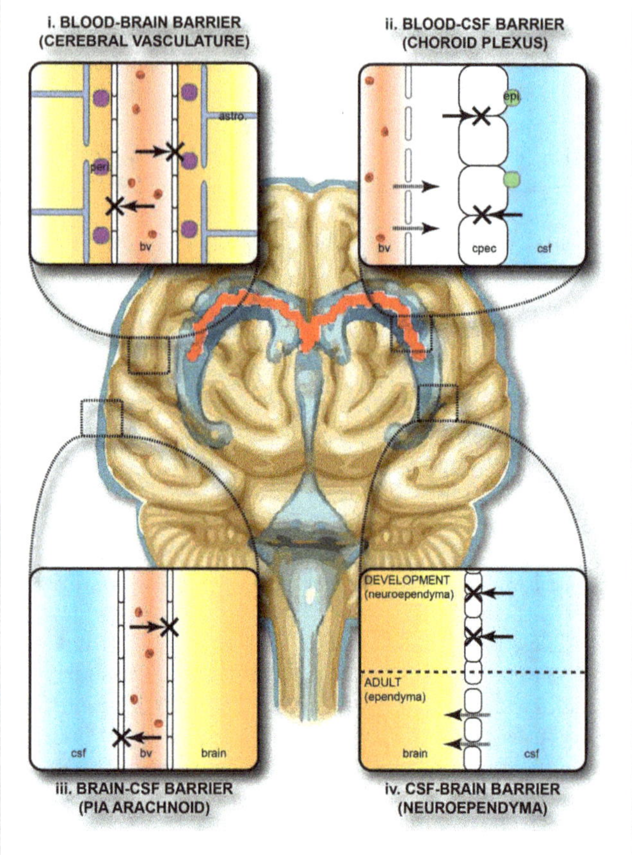

FIGURE 1 | Protective barriers of the brain. The collective term "blood-brain barrier" is used to describe four main interfaces between the central nervous system and the periphery. (i) The blood-brain barrier proper formed by tight junctions between the endothelial cells of the cerebral vasculature. It is thought that pericytes (peri.) are sufficient to induce some barrier characteristics in endothelial cells, while astrocytes (astro.) are able to maintain the integrity of the blood-brain barrier postnatally. (ii) The blood-CSF barrier formed by tight junctions between epithelial cells of the choroid plexus epithelial cells (note the plexus vasculature is fenestrated). Resident epiplexus (epi.) immune cells are present on the CSF-surface of the plexus epithelium. (iii) The outer CSF-brain barrier and the level of the pia arachnoid, formed by tight junctions between endothelial cells of the arachnoid vessels. (iv) The inner CSF-brain barrier, present only in early development, formed by strap junctions between the neuroependymal cells lining the ventricular surfaces. In the adult this barrier is no longer present. Both the blood-brain and CSF-brain barriers extend down the spinal cord. The CSF-filled ventricular system is depicted in blue, while CNS brain tissue is in brown. The lateral ventricular choroid plexuses are shown in red. Abbreviations: astro, astrocyte; bv, blood vessel; cpec, choroid plexus epithelial cell; csf, cerebrospinal fluid; peri, pericytes.

Early in brain development, the choroid plexuses are much more substantial structures compared to the limited level of vascularization of the brain (Saunders et al., 2013). It seems reasonable to propose that the plexuses may be more important than the sparse blood vessels for the supply of nutrients and other essential molecules to the early developing brain [as originally proposed by Klosovskii and Zhukova (1963)]. If this is the case, it is not clear whether the access for these materials or immune cells to the CNS is via diffusion across the CSF-brain interfaces (internal and external) or if there are also transport mechanisms in the cells of these interfaces. Such a mechanism for plasma proteins has recently been proposed for choroid plexus epithelial cells (Liddelow et al., 2012).

So very little is known about the cellular and molecular properties of the CSF-brain interface in the developing brain that is not even clear if the transport mechanisms at this interface function similarly to other barriers. It is known that at some early stages of brain development, at a time when strap junctions are present at the CSF-brain interface (see above), plasma-derived proteins found in the CSF (which are present in a much higher concentration than in adult CSF, Dziegielewska et al., 1988) are taken up by some of the neuroependymal cells lining the ventricular system (**Figure 2**). This phenomenon has been described for both endogenous proteins (e.g., alpha 2-HS glycoprotein in human fetuses—Møllgård et al., 1988) and exogenously administered non-native proteins (e.g., human albumin injected into the wallaby—Dziegielewska et al., 1988; or rat—Balslev et al., 1997). Examples of plasma protein staining in different animal species are shown in **Figure 2**. It is not known, however, if this is selective with respect to individual proteins (as is seen in the choroid plexus, Liddelow et al., 2009), regions of the ventricular system or stage of brain development. It is also unclear whether the functional significance of this protein uptake lies in the ligands known to be bound to many of these proteins (e.g., growth factors, vitamins) or in some specific properties of the individual proteins themselves. It is also unknown if this internal barrier is able to impede any CNS immune response.

As a result of the complex array of barrier mechanisms (both physical and biochemical) that surround the brain both in the adult and during development, there is great control of both the passive barrier to diffusion, and of the dynamic transport system controlling the internal environment of the CNS. As more evidence is provided for the movement of ions, plasma proteins, drugs and other molecules both into and out of the CNS, there is increasing support for the notion that an interaction with the immune system is additionally one of the many functions of these barrier systems.

Table 1 | Comparison of expression of influx transporters and published reports on transport function in the developing brain.

Transporter	Fold change	Transport function
Slc16a10	66.8	Iodothyronines T3, T4[a]
Slc6a15	11.4	Neutral amino acids[b]
**Slc40a1*	9.6	Iron[c]
Slc7a11	7.1	Cysteine, glutamate[b]
Slc4a1	5.5	Anion transporter[d], (Cl^--HCO_3 exchange)[e]
Slc6a13	4.6	GABA transporter[f]
Slc1a4	4.4	Glutamate, neutral amino acids[g]
Slc38a4	4.2	Acidic and neutral amino acids[b,g]
Slc6a6	4.1	Taurine[b]
Slc4a4	4.1	Na^+-HCO_3^- cotransporter[d]
Slc7a1	4.1	Acidic amino acids[b]
Slc39a8	3.3	Zinc transporter[h]

*Expression levels for the E15 and adult mouse choroid plexus. Fold change in expression compares E15 with adult choroid plexus (positive values are enriched in the embryo). Superscript numbers indicate published studies showing transport into developing brain or CSF. *Gene product ferroportin-1 identified in choroid plexus. References: [a](Porterfield and Hendrich, 1992); [b](Lefauconnier and Trouve, 1983); [c](Morgan and Moos, 2002); [d](Damkier et al., 2010); [e](Amtorp and Sorensen, 1974); [f](Al-Sarraf et al., 1997); [g](Al-Sarraf, 2002); [h](Chowanadisai et al., 2005). Data from Liddelow et al. (2012), adapted from Saunders et al. (2013).*

ADULT RESPONSE TO INFLAMMATION

CELLULAR INFILTRATION INTO THE BRAIN

The CNS is continuously monitored by resident microglia and blood-borne immune cells such as macrophages, dendritic cells and T cells that are able to detect damaging agents that would disrupt homeostasis and optimal functioning of neurons and glia. Normal immune mechanisms in the CNS are often thought of in a manner different from that seen in the periphery—for instance the immune response in the brain can be substantial (e.g., in response to meningitis) but by contrast, a loss of immunity is also reported (e.g., cerebral infections) (for review see Ousman and Kubes, 2012) and the muted inflammatory response in the brain following injury (Andersson et al., 1992) was the original rational behind the concept of the CNS being an immune-privileged site. The developing, and ageing, brain appears to have an exacerbated immune response compared to that normally seen in the adult (Perry et al., 1995; Campbell et al., 2007a). An important example of the interaction of peripheral immune cells with the CNS is the myeloid origin of the innate CNS immune cells—microglia (Aguzzi et al., 2013). Additionally, resident bone marrow-derived perivascular cells inhabit the perivascular space, which directly communicates with the CSF-filled subarachnoid space. These cells are able to respond rapidly to inflammatory injury and

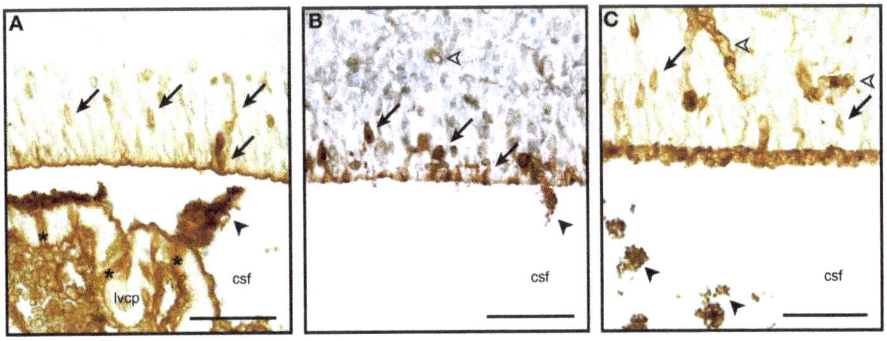

FIGURE 2 | Neuroependymal cell uptake of plasma proteins from the CSF. Coronal, paraffin-embedded section of lateral ventricular wall from sheep fetuses at embryonic day 40 (E40, **A**), E60 **(B)**, and E15 mouse **(C)** stained to detect endogenous plasma protein. The migrating neurons in the ventricular zone are strongly stained (arrows), blood vessels also show a positive staining reaction (unfilled arrowhead). Protein is also seen precipitated in the CSF (filled arrowheads). Extensive precipitation of CSF plasma protein can be seen in the embryonic mouse example displayed in panel **(C)** (arrowheads, also in **A,B**). Choroid plexus epithelial cells individually positive for protein can also be seen in panel **(A)** (asterisks). Abbreviations: csf, cerebrospinal fluid; lvcp, lateral ventricular choroid plexus. Scale bars 50 μm in each.

are continuously replaced by peripheral monocytes (Hickey and Kimura, 1988). It is therefore essential that the brain-barriers are able to facilitate entry of these cells into the CNS as part of normal function. This mechanism for facilitating peripheral immune cell entry to the CNS, however, appears to be up-regulated in cases of neuroinflammation (e.g., during stroke and multiple sclerosis), and is associated with deleterious effects on pathology (Vexler et al., 2006; De Vries et al., 2012). There is, therefore, a fine line between a "helpful" inflammatory response to injury in the CNS and pathological neuroinflammatory state.

There is still controversy in the field whether or not resident perivascular cells are able to remove themselves from the CNS to instigate a peripheral immune reaction following failure of the CNS to mount an adequate immune response (Matyszak and Perry, 1998). It has been demonstrated that CNS-derived antigens can leave the CNS via drainage through lymph nodes—potentially making CNS antigens available to the periphery without the need for the movement of cells across the blood-brain barrier (Harling-Berg et al., 1989). An acute phase response can be initiated in the liver to induced cerebral inflammation, as a direct result of this type of signaling (Anthony et al., 2011). From recent evidence it seems more likely that perivascular cells contribute to multiple sclerosis disease progression (or EAE in animal models) by reactivation of encephalitogenic T-cells (Mcmahon et al., 2005). Multiple sclerosis is characterized by substantial diapedesis of T-cells across the blood-brain barrier, contributing to demyelinating plaques associated with the disease (Engelhardt and Coisne, 2011; Zaguia et al., 2013). It is currently unclear whether this is a normal immune/blood-brain barrier response to myelin antigen presentation (even if the presence of these antigens themselves is abnormal), or whether during diseases like multiple sclerosis they are exacerbated as a result of an abnormal and exaggerated response from the cerebral vasculature. Activated T-cells leave lymph nodes and are likely able to gain additional entry to the CNS across the choroid plexuses into CSF where they are re-stimulated by meningeal and choroid plexus antigen presenting cells (Kolmer's epiplexus macrophage cells) and produce cytokines. The mechanism for the entry of these cells across the choroid plexus is unclear, evidence supporting it has been recently reviewed by Engelhardt and Sorokin (2009). Choroid plexus epithelial cells constitutively express ICAM-1 and VCAM-2, and MADCAM1 (mucosal vascular addressin cell adhesion molecule 1) during inflammation on their apical surfaces. This localization means therefore, that they are not available for the basolateral to apical migration of the immune cells (blood-to-CSF direction; Wolburg et al., 1999). This is counterintuitive, considering the high number of leukocytes frequently observed in the CSF under neuroinflammatory conditions. A recent study has suggested CCR6$^+$ T-cells may use chemokine CC ligand 20 (CCL20) expressed by the choroid plexus epithelial cells to migrate across the CNS (Reboldi et al., 2009) rather than more traditional adhesion molecules, though P-selectin has also been identified at the choroid plexus epithelial barrier (Wolburg et al., 1999). Following entry of activated T-cells into the CNS, subpial vessels are activated and expression of adhesion molecules and chemokines increases, facilitating the process of T cell entry into the CNS. Typically in a disease such as multiple sclerosis, these cells will remain in the abluminal perivascular space unless further activated by interactions with perivascular macrophages and microglia, allowing them to invade the parenchyma (Ransohoff and Engelhardt, 2012). An additional new finding proposes that the choroid plexus epithelial tight junctions lack *Claudin3* (Liddelow et al., 2013), which when knocked out in mice blood-brain barrier endothelial cells causes increased peripheral immune cell diapedesis (Wolburg et al., 2003) suggesting that the choroid plexus has the junctional make-up to allow infiltration of peripherally derived immune cells and monitoring, without a destruction of other barrier mechanisms—important for the maintenance of the CNS internal milieu.

Immune surveillance, in the absence of specific inflammatory signals is therefore likely to occur primarily through the blood-CSF barrier, facilitated by the specific composition of the junctions between epithelial cells. Importantly, junctional rearrangement appears to be an essential element of inflammation-induced cellular recruitment to the brain.

The passage of immune cells through the blood-brain barrier is not a simple process and requires a sequential interaction between different type of molecules on the surfaces of immune cells and endothelial cells. This process has been well described and extensively reviewed (see Banks and Erickson, 2010; Engelhardt and Coisne, 2011; Greenwood et al., 2011). Briefly, adhesion molecules including VCAM-1 on endothelial cells bind to leukocyte integrins, initiating a number of signaling processes that ultimately combine with a number of adhesion molecules allowing a firm attachment between the cell types, and reorganization of the endothelial cytoskeleton to allow diapedisis to occur. This may include changing the interactions between the paracellular tight junctions (Greenwood et al., 2003; Carman and Springer, 2004) facilitating diapedisis via a paracellular route, as well as transcellular route, and potentially causing increased permeability to the solutes in plasma as well as the white blood cells. To facilitate this process, inflammatory stimuli can induce redistribution of junctional adhesion molecule A (JAM-A/*F11r*) away from the cell-to-cell junctions between endothelial cells. Inhibition of this redistribution can reduce the migration of monocytes and neutrophils (Stamatovic et al., 2012), supporting the concept that rearrangement of tight junction proteins facilitates infiltration of leukocytes into the brain via a paracellular route during inflammation. The earlier onset of EAE in *Pecam1* knock-out mice also suggests that weak junctional attachments between cells may sensitize the barrier to injury (Graesser et al., 2002). However, in this instance only increased white blood cell infiltration has been reported rather than increased permeability to solutes (discussed below). Peripheral cytokines stimulate this whole process by causing endothelial cells to increase expression of cell adhesion molecules on their surface, including selectins, ICAM-1, and VCAM-1 (Meager, 1999), in turn causing alterations in the effectiveness of immune cell penetration to the CNS. It has been shown that during the induction of EAE, endothelial cells forming the blood-brain barrier display an increase in the level of CCL2 proteins (also known as monocyte chemoattractant protein 1, MCP-1). CCL2 is the ligand of the activated mononuclear immune cell receptor, CCR2, effectively increasing the number/rate entry of these peripheral immune cells across the blood-brain barrier (Sagar et al., 2012).

Upon entry to the CNS, immune cells can either set up residence in the glia limitans and monitor the health of CNS cells (as is the case with perivascular cells—see above) or they can immediately move further into the nervous tissue to stage further immune responses. If no inflammatory mediator/antigen is present upon entry to the glia limitans, these cells return to the periphery (Hickey et al., 1991). An equivalent phenomenon has been recognized in systemic vascular beds (Proebstl et al., 2012; Alon and Nourshargh, 2013).

CHANGES IN BARRIER PERMEABILITY

Besides the active role of the brain barriers in immune cell infiltration into the brain, it is thought that inflammation causes pathological changes, which result in increased passive permeability of brain barrier to solutes, contributing to exacerbation of the neuro-inflammatory response. Even in multiple sclerosis, where a focus is normally placed on cellular infiltration, the disruption of the blood-brain barrier tight junctions precedes the formation of sclerotic lesions (Minagar and Alexander, 2003; De Vries et al., 2012). Altered zonular occludin 1 (ZO-1) presence in cerebral microvessels in multiple sclerosis affected brains has been observed in both normal-appearing white matter and inactive lesions, in addition to areas with active lesions (Plumb et al., 2002; Kirk et al., 2003). Altered ZO-1 presence was associated with fibrinogen entry into the brain parenchyma even in the absence of leukocyte recruitment in active lesions (Kirk et al., 2003). Altered vessel distribution of tight junction proteins has also been observed in cases of cerebral amyloid angiopathy (Carrano et al., 2012). No white blood cell infiltration has been reported associated with vessels lacking tight junction proteins, though clumps of microglia in the nearby tissue support the inflammatory nature of these changes. Increased fibrinogen in the brain parenchyma suggests, as described above for multiple sclerosis that the loss or altered distribution of tight junction proteins can be associated with increased permeability to solutes from the blood, without associated cellular infiltration (Carrano et al., 2012). The blood-CSF barrier may also be affected by inflammation in this manner, though this barrier has been less extensively studied (in terms of both solute permeability studies and assessment of tight junction integrity) compared to the blood-brain barrier. In *in vitro* experiments, choroid plexus epithelial cell monolayers showed altered tight junction protein distribution for CLAUDIN-2 and OCCLUDIN when the cells were exposed to retrovirally-activated T-cells (Khuth et al., 2005). This cellular interaction or direct administration of pro-inflammatory cytokines also caused deficits in both active influx transport and efflux systems in the choroid plexus epithelial cells. *In vivo* peripheral inflammation caused by administration of lipopolysaccharide reduced expression of *Claudin3, 5* and *11* in the adult mouse choroid plexus epithelium (Marques et al., 2009). These *in vivo* results are very useful, though it should be noted that other authors (e.g., Liddelow et al., 2013) when using next generation RNA sequencing reported no expression of *Claudin3* or *5* in the choroid plexus epithelial cells.

The mechanism by which inflammation causes this change in tight junction integrity, particularly in the absence of leukocyte infiltration, is not completely understood. A study from Rigor et al. (2012) demonstrated protein kinase C-θ (PKC-θ) mediated barrier dysfunction via IL-1β treatment. The authors report increased PKC-θ activation in an *in vitro* model of the blood-brain barrier, followed by decreased transendothelial electrical resistance. It was proposed that ZO-1 protein phosphorylation and consequent tight junction disorganization might explain the low transendothelial electrical resistance after IL-1β exposure (Rigor et al., 2012). Although suggestive, these *in vitro* results require *in vivo* substantiation of this mechanism. PKC isozymes are capable of phosphorylating a variety of proteins that regulate diverse cellular signaling pathways: some proteins related with cytoskeleton rearrangement, which can affect tight junctions organization, may be activated as shown via TNFα modulated of p115RhoGEF phosphorylation (via PKC-α) and consequently RhoA activation. This activation promotes F-actin rearrangement and increased endothelial cell permeability *in vitro* (Peng et al., 2011), but has not been demonstrated *in vivo*.

In addition to increased permeability to solutes through the paracellular pathway following tight junction disruption, new evidence suggests that up-regulation of pinocytotic activity may contribute to increased solutes of permeability via a trancellular route, with no alteration in tight junction morphology (Armulik et al., 2010). This phenomenon is a well-recognized transport mechanism in the other biological systems and appears to be regulated by inflammation [as described, for example by Chidlow and Sessa (2010)], and needs to be investigated further at the brain barriers.

INFLAMMATION INDUCED CHANGES IN TRANSPORTERS AT THE BLOOD-BRAIN BARRIERS

The endothelial cells of the blood-brain barrier and epithelial cells of the choroid plexus blood-CSF barrier are studded with many influx and efflux transporters (for review see Saunders et al., 2013) Transport across the blood–brain barrier and blood–CSF barrier is directional, with different classes of transporters involved in movement into (e.g., most SLC transporters) and out of (e.g., ABC efflux pumps) the brain. Together, these combined transporters have different effects, ranging from removing solutes from the brain, preventing their entry into the brain (efflux mechanisms), setting up ion gradients or delivering specific nutrients, ions and other required molecules to the brain cells (influx mechanisms). These transporters function normally to maintain the internal homeostatic milieu of the CNS, however, many transporters at the barrier are altered during inflammation and can contribute to the overall inflammatory response (Khuth et al., 2005; Von Wedel-Parlow et al., 2009; Erickson et al., 2012).

Alteration in the expression of barrier transporters is not consistent across diseases or disease models. In multiple sclerosis, endothelial cells display reduced expression of the efflux transporter P-glycoprotein (PGP; Kooij et al., 2010), while in the SOD1 mouse model of amyotrophic lateral sclerosis, PGP is enriched on vessels within neurodegenerative regions (Jablonski et al., 2012). In isolated rat brain capillaries, increases of both PGP activity and protein levels were observed 6 h after TNFα and endothelin-1 exposure (Bauer et al., 2007), while *in vivo* experiments in adult rats evidence suggests that inflammation after endothelin-1 intrathecal injection increases PGP and BCRP activity only, without changing the protein levels (Harati et al., 2012). In contrast, Parkinson's disease patients present with alterations in one of the active transport processes at the blood-brain barrier that associate with disease etiology. Polymorphisms in the *Abcb1* gene have been recognized in Parkinson's disease patients (Westerlund et al., 2009), and PET studies have shown decreased function of PGP in Parkinson's disease (Kortekaas et al., 2005; Bartels et al., 2008). It is hypothesized that this may contribute to pathology by increasing the cerebral burden of iron, as well as sensitizing the brain to damage following pesticide exposure (Bartels, 2011). Developmentally, there are changes in both gene expression and protein presence of many of these transporters at both the blood-CSF and blood-brain barriers. Ek and colleagues (2010) showed in the rat that PGP (*Abcb1*) expression in both the forebrain and brainstem increased between E13 embryos and adults. MRP1 (*Abcc1*) expression peaked at birth and MRP4 (*Abcc4*) at 1 week postnatally, while BCRP (*Abcg2*) levels remained constant through development. This was in contrast to the choroid plexus epithelium, which displayed a large decrease (20-fold) in *Abcg2* (BCRP) expression, and increases in *Abcc1* (MRP1) and *Abcc4* (MRP4) levels. The authors were able to also show these changes using immunohistochemistry of protein levels, suggesting the transcript was active. More recent studies show that the absolute levels of these transcripts are much higher at the choroid plexus when compared with the blood vessel endothelium (Daneman et al., 2010; Liddelow et al., 2012, 2013).

No study to date has investigated the alterations in transcript or protein following inflammation in developing brain barriers. Increased efflux activity following inflammation, for example by up-regulation of ABC transporters may be an important protective mechanism. However, increased expression does not necessarily equate to increased function. Thus, these data highlight the importance of not only looking at gene expression and protein levels, but also transporter activity to try to unveil the contribution of efflux pumps to inflammation pathophysiology. Therefore, it is important to keep in mind the different steps in the inflammatory response and the different inflammation scenarios that can modulate how brain barriers may contribute in protective or harmful ways. Thus, due to the effects of inflammation on various transporters, brain barriers can contribute to changes in the CNS environment independently, beyond the changes produced as an associated effect of the activation of immune cells within the brain.

INFLAMMATORY SIGNALING IN CEREBRAL ENDOTHELIAL AND EPITHELIAL CELLS

In ischemic stroke, compromised endothelial cells produce inflammatory cytokines and chemokines including the interleukins IL-1β, IL-8, and CCL2. These cytokines induce expression of cell adhesion molecules by endothelial cells, facilitating the movement of peripheral immune cells into the CNS (Stanimirovic and Satoh, 2000) and potentially contributing to the initiation of cellular responses to inflammation by microglia and astrocytes within the brain parenchyma.

Daneman et al. (2010) investigated the transcriptome of purified blood-brain barrier endothelial cells in postnatal mice and reported up-regulation of the LPS/IL-1 mediated inhibition of retinoic x receptor (RXR) pathway in brain endothelial cells when compared to lung and liver endothelium. Downstream genes of RXRα were also enriched in cerebral endothelium, while inhibitory molecules of the receptor were reported only in peripheral blood vessels. RXRα nuclear receptor can activate the transcription of numerous molecules and can be inhibited by a kinase cascade initiated by LPS, IL-1, or TNFα signals. These data suggest that the RXR pathway may play an important role in the maintenance of blood-brain barrier immunogenic properties. As outlined above, however, this pathway has not been investigated in CNS inflammation to confirm its role in blood-brain barrier function and dysfunction.

The choroid plexus blood-CSF barrier may also respond to inflammation by producing different inflammatory mediators, activating different pathways. Microarray analysis was able to identify a high number of genes that were up-regulated after peripheral injection of LPS in adult mice (Marques et al., 2009). Chemokines, including *Ccl4, Ccl5, Ccl7*, and *Cxcl1* as well as interleukins, *Il1β*, *Il6*, and *Il15*, cell adhesion molecules and many transporter molecules were enriched. Moreover, genes of the MAPK, NFκB, interferon signaling, and IL-10 pathways were also identified.

There is increasing evidence that the brain barriers are able to mount, at least an initial response to peripheral inflammation—either in reaction to infiltration of inflammatory mediators to the CNS, or due to the effects of infiltration of activated peripheral immune cells, and that this vascular inflammatory response may in itself contribute significantly to neuroinflammatory disease.

DEVELOPMENTAL INFLAMMATORY MEDIATORS AT THE BRAIN BARRIERS

Recent reports on the transcriptome of the blood-brain (Daneman et al., 2010) and blood-CSF (Liddelow et al., 2012, 2013; Kratzer et al., 2013) barriers during early development highlight the alterations in expression levels of a range of transcripts that are involved in the inflammatory response. Combined with studies looking at brain barrier cells following inflammatory insults (Marques et al., 2009) it is apparent that the brain barriers are able to take a more active role in responding to both peripheral and central immune responses than previously believed. Perinatal brain injury frequently complicates preterm birth and can lead to significant long-term morbidity. Cytokines and inflammatory cells are mediators in the common pathways associated with perinatal brain injury induced by a variety of insults, such as hypoxic-ischemic injury, reperfusion injury, toxin-mediated injury, and infection—all of which cause a rapid and sometimes sustained immune response. In addition to movement of peripherally produced inflammatory mediators across the brain barriers, the infiltration of peripheral immune cells can also alter throughout development. The differential expression of *Icam1* (intercellular adhesion molecule 1) is higher at the blood-brain barrier than at the blood-CSF barrier (Daneman et al., 2010; Liddelow et al., 2012; Saunders et al., 2013). The developmental changes in expression of *Icam1* are also different between the two main brain barriers—with no developmental change in expression in the cerebral vasculature, but a slight increase in expression in the adult choroid plexus epithelium. Another transcript with product likely to be involved in the extravasations of peripheral cells, integrin α6 (*Itga6*) was also expressed at a higher level at the blood-brain barrier and was enriched in the adult when compared to postnatal mice (Daneman et al., 2010). In the choroid plexus *Itga6* transcript, though with lower expression than the cerebral vasculature, was enriched in the embryonic mouse over 7-fold (Liddelow et al., 2013) highlighting the potential developmental difference in the role of the choroid plexus and blood vessels in the contribution to immune surveillance of the brain and the response to inflammation.

The level of peripherally-derived, blood-borne cytokines entering the brain is low, however, it is comparable to other water-soluble molecules that are known to cross the brain barriers to a degree sufficient to affect brain function (e.g., morphine, Banks et al., 1995). There are a large number of transport systems for common inflammatory mediators that are present on both the blood-brain and blood-CSF barriers. IL-1, a pro-inflammatory cytokine, is able to exert a range of effects on the brain, including mediating key host defenses in response to many chronic CNS diseases. The functional family of IL-1 contains the agonists (IL-1α and IL-1β), the receptors (IL-1RT1 and IL-1RT2) and a naturally occurring antagonist molecule (IL-1RN). At the blood-brain barrier, endothelial cells contain measurable levels of IL-1β and IL-1RT2 (the receptor with a higher affinity for IL-1β) while levels of transcript for IL-1α and the type 1 receptor (IL-1RT1) fall below levels of detection (Daneman et al., 2010). Levels of transcript do not appear to change through development, at least in the mouse. In contrast choroid plexus epithelial cell expression of IL-1 members shows the predominant receptor transcript that is detected is IL-1RT1, with over a 10-fold increase in expression between the embryo and the adult (Liddelow et al., 2012).

Similar to IL-1, IL-6 signals through a cell-surface type I cytokine receptor complex. It is made up of the ligand-binding IL-6RA segment (*Il6r*) and the signal-transduction IL-6RB component (*Il6st*). It should be noted that IL-6RB is also a common signal-transducer for other cytokines (e.g., LIF, CNTF, IL-11, among others). *Il6* ligand transcript is low in endothelial cells, however, *Il6r* and *Il6st* are high from very early in development and do not change into adulthood. A similar lack of developmental expression changes was seen in the choroid plexus with low *Il6* and *Il6st* expression in both embryonic and adult mice (Liddelow et al., 2012), however, no expression for *Il6r* was detected in this study. A more recent RNA sequencing study by these authors, however, reports expression of *Il6r* in choroid plexus epithelium (Liddelow et al., 2013), highlighting the importance of validation of microarray genechip experiments to ensure no false positive or negative results.

The levels of transcript for TNFα by barrier cells (both cerebral endothelium and plexus epithelium) are extremely low, suggesting the majority of TNFα in the CNS is provided by local production from other cells types (e.g., microglia—though it is likely they only produce measurable levels of TNFα following injury), or by transport from the periphery. Having said this, following induction of a peripheral inflammatory response, levels of TNFα (as well as IL-1β) transcript in choroid plexus epithelial cells and meningeal endothelium increased (Quan et al., 1999). Knock-out animal models for TNFα receptors *Tnfrsf1a* (TNFR1/p55 receptor) and *Tnfrsf1b* (TNFR2/p75 receptor) have shown a reduction of the ligand penetrating the blood-brain barrier into the spinal cord, but not into the brain of single knock-out animals (Pan and Kastin, 2002). Double knock-out animals of both *Tnfrsf1a* and *Tnfrsf1b* showed a complete abolition of TNFα penetration—suggesting that both receptors are necessary for transporting the ligand into the CNS (Pan and Kastin, 2002). Genechip data from the blood-brain barrier (Daneman et al., 2010) show a high expression of both *Tnfrsf1a* and *Tnfrsf1b*, as well as several other TNFα receptor family members (*Tnfrs11a, 12a, 19,* and 21) with no change in expression between early postnatal and adult mice. At the blood-CSF barrier, plexus epithelial expression of TNFα receptor family transcripts is low, however, there is embryonic enrichment of *Tnfsf1b* and *Tnfrsf21.*

It therefore appears that while the barrier systems may not produce a vast array of cytokines under resting conditions, both in development and adulthood, they express many receptors for inflammatory mediators and signal amplifiers, indicating the importance of an early vascular response to inflammatory signaling. Barrier cells also appear able to rapidly up-regulate the expression, and likely release, of some cytokines following an inflammatory insult in as little as a few short hours. The capacity of the barrier cells to respond to inflammatory signaling may be an important confounding factor in the developmental response of the brain to inflammation. While it is beyond the scope of this review, it is important to note that the systemic immune response is also changing over this time, and may contribute to the differences observed in the CNS response to inflammation/injury during development.

DEVELOPMENTAL INFLAMMATORY RESPONSE

It is now clear that the vasculature in the developing brain is primed to respond to inflammatory stimuli. Despite this, little work has been done to investigate the blood-brain barrier response to inflammation throughout CNS development. This is presumably partly due to the historical misconception that the blood-brain barrier is functionally immature in the developing brain. However, it has been well-established (as described above) that the structural and functional mechanism that contribute to the blood-brain barrier are present from very early in embryogenesis. Work from the last 10 years also suggests that the response of the blood-brain barrier to inflammation is selective and specific depending on the age at the time of insult and the location of the inflammatory signals (discussed below).

Work from our laboratories has shown that systemic inflammation causes a specific increase in the permeability of the blood-brain barrier in vessels in the periventricular white matter tract in neonatal rats (Stolp et al., 2005a). The reasons for the increased permeability in these blood vessels is not yet clear, though numerous explanations have been presented, including a developmental delay in the maturity of these vessels or a specific susceptibility to increased vascular flow. Regarding potential immaturity of cerebral vessels, work from Virgintino et al. (2004) and Anstrom et al. (2007) have clearly shown variation in the complexity of tight junction proteins in the microvasculature of the human brain with different developmental ages and brain regions. While the complexity of the tight junctions has been much discussed in the context of brain development, it is not yet clear how well this correlates with barrier permeability (Møllgård et al., 1979). It is suggested that a delayed maturation of the vessel structure in the germinal matrix and periventricular white matter may lead to increased susceptibility of these brain regions to damage during premature birth, hypoxia, or inflammatory insults (Anstrom et al., 2007). This is an appealing hypothesis, which recognizes a maturation process that may be sufficient, for example in the controlled intrauterine environment, for normal function but which could be easily damaged by changes in blood pressure or some other environmental challenge. It has been established, however, that changes in cerebral blood flow are in themselves insufficient to account for damage in these brain regions following hypoxia-ischemia (Mcclure et al., 2008). Additionally, the age specific increase in blood-brain barrier permeability reported by Stolp et al. (2005a) is not easily explained if the complexity of the tight junction structure is the only contributing factor in the vascular response to insult. When a marsupial species was used to repeat experiments studying the age-specific response to inflammation, so that a longer developmental period could be assessed in a postnatal systemic inflammation paradigm, it was determined that the increased permeability of the periventricular white matter vessels was limited to a specific stage of development, rather than a general response of the developing brain (Stolp et al., 2005a). There are two potential explanations for this: the first that the inflammatory response at the earliest times is not sufficiently developed to stimulate the signaling pathway responsible for the increased permeability; or secondly, that there is a specific combination of factors that occur at the equivalent of the first post-natal week in the rat which combine to produce the susceptibility of the barrier in these specific vessels. There is certainly a substantial increase in the number of activated and migrating microglia and astrocytes in the white matter at this stage of development (Stolp et al., 2009; Verney et al., 2010, 2012), which may contribute to the central inflammatory response and increase the sensitivity of the nearby vessels to the inflammatory signals. The transcriptome of astrocytes activated following peripheral LPS inflammation in adults show a marked increase in the expression of many receptors to cytokines such as TNFα and TGFβ, however, there is not the same increase in the expression of the ligands themselves (Zamanian et al., 2012). There is, however, a relatively high expression of the lipocalin 2 receptor, *Slc22a17*, which is not present on choroid plexus epithelium (Liddelow et al., 2013), but is on cerebral endothelium (Daneman et al., 2010) in close association with astrocytic endfeet. Lipocalin 2 is involved in the innate immune response by sequestrating iron, in turn limiting bacterial growth (Yang et al., 2002), and has recently been shown to be the highest enriched transcript in reactive astrocytes (Zamanian et al., 2012), suggesting an astrocytic role in the innate immune system and the acute phase response to infection in the CNS, and therefore a potential for an atypical cerebral inflammatory response when astrocytes are apparently activated by migration during development.

Interestingly, different developmental barrier susceptibility has been identified in response to directly induced intracerebral inflammation. Injection of IL-1β into the striatum of postnatal day 2 (P2), P21, and adult rats produced a substantial difference in the inflammatory response (Anthony et al., 1997). A small increase in neutrophil accumulation was observed at P2 and in adult animals and a small increase in permeability of vessels to horseradish peroxidase within the injection site, as well as in the meningeal vessels. However, in P21 animals there was a significant increase in permeability of all the vessels in the injected hemisphere associated with a substantial increase in neutrophil extravasation into the brain. Subsequent experiments showed that the changes in permeability were neutrophil dependent, as neutrophil depletion by x-irradiation of the bone marrow prevented this response (Anthony et al., 1997). A neutrophil specific alteration in blood-brain barrier permeability has also been described in a model of stroke (Fernandez-Lopez et al., 2012). However, in this case the early postnatal brain appeared to be protected against altered blood-brain barrier permeability and neutrophil infiltration, compared to the adult. While various small changes in vascular structure (e.g., high basal levels of basement membrane proteins) and activation processes (variable adhesion molecule expression following stroke) were recognized, Fernandez-Lopez and colleagues (2012) determined that the reduced response in neonates was not due to a lack of capacity for neutrophil migration in early development, but instead may be due to altered ratios of chemoattractant molecules between the systemic and central systems. This highlights important differences between models of developmental brain injuries and the etiological mechanisms involved. There is a clear need for further research in this area to tease apart specific signaling systems. Particularly given the completely different response to that seen in the neonatal rat following systemic inflammation, where no neutrophil infiltration has been reported in relation to an age and location specific change in barrier permeability (Stolp et al., 2005a).

The observed developmental differences in the CNS response to inflammation are likely to reflect a combination of many aspects of brain development as well as maturation of the systemic inflammatory response. Specific studies are still lacking on the interactions between these two systems in development, as has been done in adult neuroinflammatory disease (see Anthony et al., 2011).

CONSEQUENCES FOR DISEASE AND AGEING

The consequence of the inflammatory signaling process and the potential association of changes in blood-brain barrier permeability may be widespread in the developing brain. The specific changes within the developing brain appear to vary depending on the timing of insult and reflect a mixture of the developmental stage of the CNS, as well as the specialities of the immune signaling response of the barrier systems at the time of insult.

In the second half of gestation in the rodent, equivalent to the 1st—2nd trimester in humans (Clancy et al., 2001), there is no evidence of blood-brain barrier disruption associated with experimentally induced inflammation. However, there is substantial evidence for changes to the developing brain, which reflect changes in immune signaling. There is a reported decrease in (VZ) proliferation, but not the subventricular zone (SVZ), in response to low dose LPS-induced inflammation in mice at E13.5 of gestation (Stolp et al., 2011). The change in proliferation in the VZ but not the SVZ implies a variable contribution of the vasculature and the CSF for central immune signaling following induction of the systemic maternal inflammatory response (discussed further below), and indicate that the progenitor cells in the VZ and SVZ are in different environmental niches (**Figure 3**). Additional studies confirm the sensitivity of the VZ cell population to immune signaling, indicating presence of receptors to specific cytokines (e.g., IL-1β) or pathogen associated molecules (including TLR2 and 3) and stimulation of these receptors decrease neurogenesis and may alter cellular differentiation (Lathia et al., 2008; Okun et al., 2010; Crampton et al., 2012).

The change in permeability of the ventricular surface in concert with the decreased proliferation in the VZ (Stolp et al., 2011) but an absence of altered permeability at the blood-brain barrier supports the idea of a CSF-brain specific signaling mechanism regulating the proliferation of cells in the VZ in early development. Recent work by Lehtinen et al. (2011) shows that insulin-like growth factor 1 produced by the choroid plexus in late gestation in the mouse modulates proliferation of the VZ progenitors. Additionally, a selective fourth ventricle OTX-induced choroid plexus deletion, which significantly changes the composition of the CSF, also modifies proliferation in the cortical VZ throughout gestation (Johansson et al., 2013). Cunningham et al. (2013) hypothesize that microglia in the developing brain may be integral to the modulation of proliferation in the progenitor zones of the developing brain, however, their observations are true for both the VZ and the SVZ and may reflect an additional level of control, separate to CSF-specific inflammatory signaling pathways. Substantial changes in the number of F4/80 positive monocytes/microglia within the developing brain were not observed in a study of low-dose maternal immune regulation (Stolp HB, unpublished data). The presence of strap junctions between the neuroependymal cells in early fetal development but not in the adult (Møllgård et al., 1987), suggest a developmentally important role of junctions between the progenitor cells in the VZ. It has been suggested that junctions between these cells are important for regulation of polarity and therefore proliferation in the VZ (Huttner and Brand, 1997). It is possible that these junctions are modified in response to inflammation in a similar manner to that described for adult barrier junctions. Although the presence of strap junctions forming the inner CSF-brain barrier is only present early in development, there is still specific uptake of proteins by these neuroependymal VZ cells (**Figure 2**)—reiterating the importance of protein-cargo trafficking into the CSF and thence the brain during development (Knott et al., 1997; Liddelow et al., 2012).

A different response is seen slightly later in the process of brain development. In early postnatal rodents [approximately P1–7, equivalent to the 2nd—3rd trimester of human pregnancy, (Clancy et al., 2001)] increased permeability of the blood-brain barrier is observed specifically in the periventricular white matter and associated with damage (Stolp et al., 2005a,b, 2009). It is currently unclear how much the damage in this area of the brain is directly related to increased barrier permeability or other associated phenomenon. Large quantities of plasma proteins in the brain, as occurs with blood-brain barrier breakdown, have been associated with increased cell death (Nordborg et al., 1991; Wagner et al., 2002) and altered neuronal function, potentially leading to epileptic-type activity (Friedman, 2011; Tomkins et al., 2011). It is suggested, however, that changes in blood-brain barrier permeability associated with systemic inflammation in postnatal animals is not enough to account for the white matter damage alone, as it requires increased microglial activation (Stolp et al., 2009). Increased numbers of microglia, particularly with the morphological appearance of activation, have been

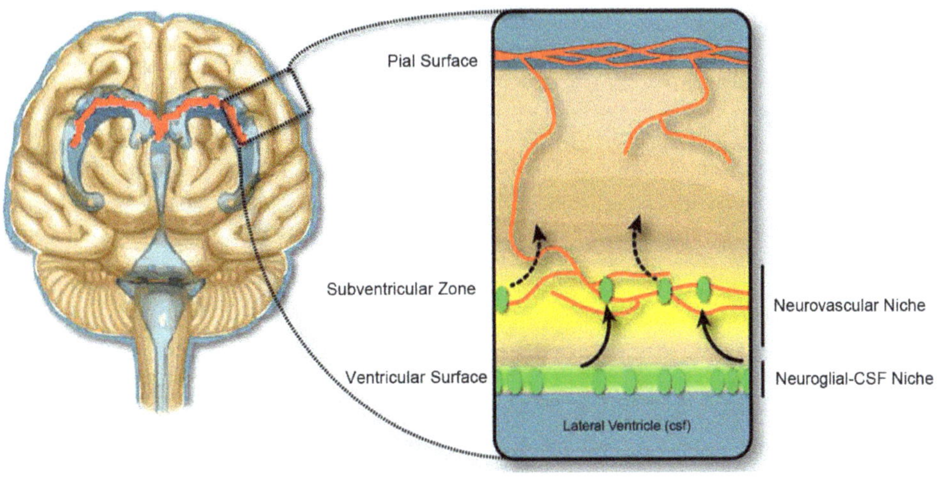

FIGURE 3 | Neurogenic niches in the developing brain. Dividing cells in the subventricular zone are closely associated with blood vessels, and the concept of a neurovascular niche (yellow), which reflects a zone of influence of vascular factors on neural progenitor cells, suggested in the adult and developmental subventricular zone. In early development, the dividing cells in the ventricular zone are not closely associated with the blood vasculature, but may be affected by trophic factors produced in the CSF, and therefore exist in a neuroglial-CSF niche. Cells from the ventricular zone migrate toward the neurovascular niche, before differentiating and migrating to outer cortical layers of the brain.

associated with the peak periods of white matter damage (Verney et al., 2010, 2012; Supramaniam et al., 2013). It is possible that the large number of migrating, activated microglia within the white matter tracts are primed to respond to inflammatory signaling transferred through blood vessels, or to the presence of systemic proteins following blood-brain barrier breakdown, and it is these immune cells that interact with oligodendrocytes in the developing white matter to cause injury.

These two scenarios indicate changes to the brain that are an immediate cause in systemic inflammation and inflammatory signaling into the developing brain. There are likely to be many more examples like this, as numerous immune mediators are important for the regulation of maturation processes in the brain (e.g., CXCR4 and CXCL7 as key migration cues). It is, however, necessary to also consider subtle changes that may alter the response of the maturing/ageing brain to insults later in life. One example of this is a long-term alteration in blood-brain barrier function that occurs following systemic inflammation early in life. In this case, the magnitude/prolonged nature of the inflammatory response is key—and long-term changes in barrier function only occur after prolonged exposure to systemic inflammatory (Stolp et al., 2005b).

Given the contribution of the blood-brain barrier to adult neuroinflammatory diseases (as discussed above), any structural deficits within the barrier junctions that exist as a result of injury in early life may increase the risk of early or delayed onset of neurodegenerative conditions [reviewed by Stolp and Dziegielewska (2009)].

SUMMARY REMARKS

(1) The brain, both in the adult and in development, is surrounded by a complex array of barrier mechanisms comprised of morphological (tight junctions), biochemical, and physiological (influx and efflux transporters) components that control and determine its internal environment. There is increasing evidence that one important function is an interaction with the immune system. Any structural deficits within the barrier junctions that exist as a result of injury in early life may increase the risk of early onset of neurodegenerative conditions.

(2) Evidence suggests that normal immune surveillance, which is likely to occur primarily through the blood-CSF barrier, is facilitated by the specific composition of the junctions between epithelial cells. Junctional rearrangement appears to be an essential element of inflammation-induced cellular recruitment to the brain.

(3) Transporters constitutively present at brain barriers can be affected by inflammation, therefore contributing to changes in the CNS environment alone or in association with the changes produced by the activation of immune cells.

(4) There is increasing evidence that the brain barriers are able to mount a response to peripheral inflammation and that this vascular inflammatory response may in itself contribute significantly to neuroinflammatory disease.

(5) The developmentally controlled CNS response to inflammation is a combination of many aspects of maturation processes of both the brain and the systemic inflammatory response itself. Specific study of the interactions between these two systems in development, as has been done in adult disease, is very important for proper understanding of normal and pathological mechanisms involved.

CONCLUSION

The brain barrier systems provide an essential interface between the periphery and the brain, which is intrinsically involved in the communication of inflammatory signals between these two compartments. Though very little is known about the responses of individual cells forming these barriers during inflammation, especially during development and ageing, it is apparent that they respond differentially to disease. We can say with confidence therefore that immunity is an active and fluid component of normal brain-barrier function. What we cannot say with a similar level of confidence, however, is how this function is altered under stress, or how one should approach these alterations from a clinical setting. There is still a substantial amount of work required before specific aspects of changes in the plethora of barrier mechanisms contributing to neuropathological conditions arising during development and in old age can be defined. More attention needs to be paid to changes in cellular-based barrier mechanisms, rather than focus on the integrity of tight junctions, which has been the emphasis of much of the research effort in this field so far.

ACKNOWLEDGMENTS

The authors would like to acknowledge the support on this project from the European Union Seventh Framework Programme [FP7/2007–2013] under grant agreement n° HEALTH-F2-2009-241778.

REFERENCES

Aguzzi, A., Barres, B. A., and Bennett, M. L. (2013). Microglia: scape goat, saboteur, or something else? *Science* 339, 156–161. doi: 10.1126/science.1227901

Alon, R., and Nourshargh, S. (2013). Learning in motion: pericytes instruct migrating innate leuko- cytes. *Nat. Immunol.* 14, 14–15. doi: 10.1038/ni.2489

Al-Sarraf, H. (2002). Transport of 14C-gamma-aminobutyric acid into brain, cerebrospinal fluid and choroid plexus in neonatal and adult rats. *Brain Res. Dev. Brain Res.* 139, 121–129. doi: 10.1016/S0165-3806(02)00537-0

Al-Sarraf, H., Preston, J. E., and Segal, M. B. (1997). Acidic amino acid accumulation by rat choroid plexus during development. *Brain Res. Dev. Brain Res.* 102, 47–52. doi: 10.1016/S0165-3806(97)00075-8

Amtorp, O., and Sorensen, S. C. (1974). The ontogenetic development of concentration differences for pro- tein and ions between plasma and cerebrospinal fluid in rabbits and rats. *J. Physiol.* 243,387–400.

Andersson, P. B., Perry, V. H., and Gordon, S. (1992). The acute inflammatory response to lipopolysaccharide in CNS parenchyma differs from that in other body tissues. *Neuroscience* 48, 169–186. doi: 10.1016/0306-4522(92)90347-5

Anstrom, J. A., Thore, C. R., Moody, D. M., and Brown, W. R. (2007). Immunolocalization of tight junc- tion proteins in blood vessels in human germinal matrix and cortex. *Histochem. Cell Biol.* 127, 205–213. doi: 10.1007/s00418-006- 0232-z

Anthony, D. C., Bolton, S. J., Fearn, S., and Perry, V. H. (1997). Age- related effects of interleukin-1 beta on polymorphonuclear neutrophil-dependent increases in blood-brain barrier permeability in rats. *Brain* 120(Pt 3), 435–444. doi: 10.1093/brain/120.3.435

Anthony, D. C., Couch, Y., Losey, P., and Evans, M. C. (2011). The systemic response to brain injury and disease. *Brain Behav. Immun.* 26, 534–540. doi: 10.1016/j.bbi. 2011.10.011

Armulik, A., Genove, G., Mae, M., Nisancioglu, M. H., Wallgard, E., Niaudet, C., et al. (2010). Pericytes regulate the blood-brain barrier. *Nature* 468, 557–561. doi: 10.1038/nature09522

Auvin, S., Mazarati, A., Shin, D., and Sankar, R. (2010). Inflammation enhances epileptogenesis in the developing rat brain. *Neurobiol. Dis.* 40, 303–310. doi: 10.1016/j.nbd. 2010.06.004

Balslev, Y., Saunders, N. R., and Møllgård, K. (1997). Ontogenetic development of diffusional restriction to protein at the pial surface of the rat brain: an electron microscopical study. *J. Neurocytol.* 26, 133–148. doi: 10.1023/A:1018527928760

Banks, W. A., and Erickson, M. A. (2010). The blood-brain barrier and immune function and dysfunc- tion. *Neurobiol. Dis.* 37, 26–32. doi: 10.1016/j. nbd.2009.07.031

Banks, W. A., Kastin, A. J., and Broadwell, R. D. (1995). Passage of cytokines across the blood-brain barrier. *Neuroimmunomodulation* 2, 241–248. doi: 10.1159/000097202

Bartels, A. L. (2011). Blood-brain barrier P-glycoprotein function in neurodegenerative disease. *Curr. Pharm. Des.* 17, 2771–2777. doi: 10.2174/138161211797440122

Bartels, A. L., Willemsen, A. T., Kortekaas, R., De Jong, B. M., De Vries, R., De Klerk, O., et al. (2008). Decreased blood-brain barrier P-glycoprotein function in the progression of Parkinson's disease, PSP and MSA. *J. Neural. Transm.* 115, 1001–1009. doi: 10.1007/s00702-008-0030-y

Bauer, B., Hartz, A. M., and Miller, D. S. (2007). Tumor necrosis factor alpha and endothelin-1 increase P-glycoprotein expression and transport activity at the blood- brain barrier. *Mol. Pharmacol.* 71, 667–675. doi: 10.1124/ mol.106. 029512

Bilbo, S. D., and Schwarz, J. M. (2012). The immune system and developmental programming of brain and behavior. *Front. Neuroendocrinol.* 33, 267–286. doi: 10.1016/j.yfrne.2012.08.006

Campbell, S. J., Carare-Nnadi, R. O., Losey, P. H., and Anthony, D. C. (2007a). Loss of the atypical inflammatory response in juve- nile and aged rats. *Neuropathol. Appl. Neurobiol.* 33, 108–120. doi: 10.1111/j.1365-2990.2006.00773.x

Campbell, S. J., Jiang, Y., Davis, A. E., Farrands, R., Holbrook, J., Leppert, D., et al. (2007b). Immunomodulatory effects of etan- ercept in a model of brain injury act through attenuation of the acute-phase response. *J. Neurochem.* 103, 2245–2255. doi: 10.1111/j. 1471-4159.2007.04928.x

Campbell, S. J., Meier, U., Mardiguian, S., Jiang, Y., Littleton, E. T., Bristow, A., et al. (2010). Sickness behaviour is induced by a peripheral CXC- chemokine also expressed in multiple sclerosis and EAE. *Brain Behav. Immun.* 24, 738–746. doi: 10.1016/j.bbi.2010.01.011

Carman, C. V., and Springer, T. A. (2004). A transmigratory cup in leukocyte diapedesis both through individual vascular endothe- lial cells and between them. *J. Cell Biol.* 167, 377–388. doi: 10.1083/jcb.200404129

Carrano, A., Hoozemans, J. J., Van Der Vies, S. M., Van Horssen, J., De Vries, H. E., and Rozemuller, A. J. (2012). Neuroinflammation and blood-brain barrier changes in capillary amyloid angiopathy. *Neurodegener. Dis.* 10, 329–331. doi: 10.1159/000334916

Chidlow, J. H. Jr., and Sessa, W. C. (2010). Caveolae, caveolins, and cavins: complex control of cellu- lar signalling and inflammation. *Cardiovasc. Res.* 86, 219–225. doi: 10.1093/cvr/cvq075

Chowanadisai, W., Kelleher, S. L., and Lonnerdal, B. (2005). Zinc defi- ciency is associated with increased brain zinc import and LIV-1 expres- sion and decreased ZnT-1 expres- sion in neonatal rats. *J. Nutr.* 135, 1002–1007.

Clancy, B., Darlington, R. B., and Finlay, B. L. (2001). Translating developmental time across mammalian species. *Neuroscience* 105, 7–17. doi: 10.1016/S0306-4522(01)00171-3

Crampton, S. J., Collins, L. M., Toulouse, A., Nolan, Y. M., and O'keeffe, G. W. (2012). Exposure of foetal neural progenitor cells to IL-1beta impairs their proliferation and alters their differentiation—a role for maternal inflammation? *J. Neurochem.* 120, 964–973.

Cunningham, C. L., Martinez Cerdeno, V., and Noctor, S. C. (2013). Microglia regulate the number of neural precursor cells in the developing cerebral cortex. *J. Neurosci.* 33, 4216–4233. doi: 10.1523/JNEUROSCI.3441-12.2013

Damkier, H. H., Brown, P. D., and Praetorius, J. (2010). Epithelial pathways in choroid plexus electrolyte transport. *Physiology (Bethesda)* 25, 239–249. doi: 10.1152/physiol.00011.2010

Daneman, R., Zhou, L., Agalliu, D., Cahoy, J. D., Kaushal, A., and Barres, B. A. (2010). The mouse blood-brain barrier transcriptome: a new resource for understand- ing the development and func- tion of brain endothelial cells. *PLoS ONE* 5:e13741. doi: 10.1371/jour- nal.pone.0013741

De Vries, H. E., Kooij, G., Frenkel, D., Georgopoulos, S., Monsonego, A., and Janigro, D. (2012). Inflammatory events at blood- brain barrier in neuroinflammatory and neurodegenerative disorders: implications for clinical disease. *Epilepsia* 53(Suppl. 6), 45–52. doi: 10.1111/j.1528-1167.2012.03702.x

Dziegielewska, K. M., Evans, C. A., Malinowska, D. H., Møllgård, K., Reynolds, J. M., Reynolds, L., et al. (1979). Studies of the development of brain barrier systems to lipid insoluble molecules in fetal sheep. *J. Physiol.* 292, 207–231.

Dziegielewska, K. M., Hinds, L. A., Møllgård, K., Reynolds, M. L., and Saunders, N. R. (1988). Blood- brain, blood-cerebrospinal fluid and cerebrospinal fluid-brain barriers in a marsupial (*Macropus eugenii*) dur- ing development. *J. Physiol.* 403, 367–388.

Ek, C. J., Dziegielewska, K. M., Stolp, H., and Saunders, N. R. (2006). Functional effectiveness of the blood-brain barrier to small water- soluble molecules in developing and adult opossum (*Monodelphis domestica*). *J. Comp. Neurol.* 496, 13–26. doi: 10.1002/cne.20885

Ek, C. J., Habgood, M. D., Dziegielewska, K. M., and Saunders, R. (2003). Structural charac- teristics and barrier properties of the choroid plexuses in developing brain of the opossum (Monodelphis domestica). *J. Comp. Neurol.* 460, 451–464. doi: 10.1002/cne.10661

Ek, C. J., Wong, A., Liddelow, S. A., Johansson, P. A., Dziegielewska, K. M., and Saunders, N. R. (2010). Efflux mechanisms at the developing brain barriers: ABC-transporters in the fetal and postnatal rat. *Toxicol. Lett.* 197, 51–59. doi: 10.1016/j.toxlet.2010. 04.025

Engelhardt, B., and Coisne, C. (2011). Fluids and barriers of the CNS establish immune privilege by con- fining immune surveillance to a two-walled castle moat surrounding the CNS castle. *Fluids Barriers CNS* 8:4. doi: 10.1186/2045-8118-8-4

Engelhardt, B., and Sorokin, L. (2009). The blood-brain and the blood-cerebrospinal fluid barriers: function and dysfunction. *Semin. Immunopathol.* 31, 497–511. doi: 10.1007/s00281-009-0177-0

Erickson, M. A., Hartvigson, P. E., Morofuji, Y., Owen, J. B., Butterfield, D. A., and Banks, W. A. (2012). Lipopolysaccharide impairs amyloid beta efflux from brain: altered vascular sequestration, cerebrospinal fluid reabsorption, peripheral clearance and trans- porter function at the blood-brain barrier. *J. Neuroinflammation* 9, 150. doi: 10.1186/1742-2094-9-150

Fernandez-Lopez, D., Faustino, J., Daneman, R., Zhou, L., Lee, S. Y., Derugin, N., et al. (2012). Blood-brain barrier permeability is increased after acute adult stroke but not neonatal stroke in the rat. *J. Neurosci.* 32, 9588–9600. doi: 10.1523/JNEUROSCI.5977-11.2012

Fossan, G., Cavanagh, M. E., Evans, C. A., Malinowska, D. H., Møllgård, K., Reynolds, M. L., et al. (1985). CSF- brain permeability in the immature sheep fetus: a CSF-brain barrier. *Brain Res.* 350, 113–124.

Friedman, A. (2011). Blood-brain barrier dysfunction, status epilep- ticus, seizures, and epilepsy: a puzzle of a chicken and egg? *Epilepsia* 52(Suppl. 8), 19–20. doi: 10.1111/j.1528-1167.2011.03227.x

Graesser, D., Solowiej, A., Bruckner, M., Osterweil, E., Juedes, A., Davis, S., et al. (2002). Altered vascular permeability and early onset of experimental autoimmune encephalomyelitis in PECAM-1- deficient mice. *J. Clin. Invest.* 109, 383–392.

Greenwood, J., Amos, C. L., Walters, C. E., Couraud, P. O., Lyck, R., Engelhardt, B., et al. (2003). Intracellular domain of brain endothelial intercellular adhe- sion molecule-1 is essential for T lymphocyte-mediated signaling and migration. *J. Immunol.* 171, 2099–2108.

Greenwood, J., Heasman, S. J., Alvarez, J. I., Prat, A., Lyck, R., and Engelhardt, B. (2011). sReview: leucocyte-endothelial cell crosstalk at the blood-brain barrier: a pre- requisite for successful immune cell entry to the brain. *Neuropathol. Appl. Neurobiol.* 37, 24–39. doi: 10.1111/j.1365-2990.2010.01140.x

Harati, R., Villegier, A. S., Banks, W. A., and Mabondzo, A. (2012). Susceptibility of juvenile and adult blood-brain barrier to endothelin- 1: regulation of P-glycoprotein and breast cancer resistance protein expression and transport activity. *J. Neuroinflammation* 9, 273. doi: 10.1186/1742-2094-9-273

Harling-Berg, C., Knopf, P. M., Merriam, J., and Cserr, H. F. (1989). Role of cervical lymph nodes in the systemic humoral immune response to human serum albumin microin- fused into rat cerebrospinal fluid. *J. Neuroimmunol.* 25, 185–193. doi: 10.1016/0165-5728(89)90136-7

Hickey, W. F., Hsu, B. L., and Kimura, H. (1991). T-lymphocyte entry into the central nervous system. *J. Neurosci. Res.* 28, 254–260. doi: 10.1002/jnr.490280213

Hickey, W. F., and Kimura, H. (1988). Perivascular microglial cells of the CNS are bone marrow- derived and present antigen *in vivo*. *Science* 239, 290–292. doi: 10.1126/science.3276004

Huttner, W. B., and Brand, M. (1997). Asymmetric division and polar- ity of neuroepithelial cells. *Curr. Opin. Neurobiol.* 7, 29–39. doi: 10.1016/S0959-4388(97)80117-1

Johansson, P. A., Irmler, M., Acampora, D., Beckers, J., Simeone, A., and Gotz, M. (2013). The transcrip- tion factor Otx2 regulates choroid plexus development and function. *Development* 140, 1055–1066. doi: 10.1242/dev.090860

Khuth, S. T., Strazielle, N., Giraudon, P., Belin, M. F., and Ghersi-Egea, J. F. (2005). Impairment of blood-cerebrospinal fluid barrier properties by retrovirus-activated T lymphocytes: reduction in cere- brospinal fluid-to-blood efflux of prostaglandin E2. *J. Neurochem.* 94, 1580–1593. doi: 10.1111/j.1471- 4159.2005.03309.x

Kirk, J., Plumb, J., Mirakhur, M., and Mcquaid, S. (2003). Tight junctional abnormality in multiple sclerosis white matter affects all calibres of vessel and is associated with blood-brain barrier leakage and active demyelination. *J. Pathol.* 201, 319–327. doi: 10.1002/path.1434

Klosovskii, B. N., and Zhukova, T. P. (1963). Effect of colchicine on remote phases of growing capillaries inthebrain. *Arkh. Patol.* 35, 38–44.

Knott, G. W., Dziegielewska, K. M., Habgood, M. D., Li, Z. S., and Saunders, N. R. (1997). Albumin transfer across the choroid plexus of South American opossum (*Monodelphis domestica*). *J. Physiol.* 499(Pt1), 179–194.

Kooij, G., Van Horssen, J., De Lange, C., Reijerkerk, A., Van Der Pol, S. M., Van Het Hof, B., et al. (2010). T lymphocytes impair P-glycoprotein function during neuroinflamma- tion. *J. Autoimmun.* 34, 416–425. doi: 10.1016/j.jaut.2009.10.006

Kortekaas, R., Leenders, K. L., Van Oostrom, J. C., Vaalburg, W., Bart, J., Willemsen, A. T., et al. (2005). Blood-brain barrier dysfunction in parkinsonian midbrain *in vivo*. *Ann. Neurol.* 57, 176–179. doi: 10.1002/ana.20369

Kratzer, I., Liddelow, S. A., Saunders, N. R., Strazielle, N., and Ghersi-Egea, J. (2013). Transcriptomic profile of neuroprotective genes in the devel- oping rat choroid plexus. *Fluids Barriers CNS* 10:25. doi: 10.1186/ 2045-8118-10-25

Kratzer, I., Vasiljevic, A., Rey, C., Fevre-Montange, M., Saunders, N., Strazielle, N., et al. (2012). Complexity and developmental changes in the expression pattern of claudins at the blood-CSF barrier. *Histochem. Cell Biol.* 138, 861–879. doi: 10.1007/s00418-012-1001-9

Lathia, J. D., Okun, E., Tang, S. C., Griffioen, K., Cheng, A., Mughal, M. R., et al. (2008). Toll-like recep- tor 3 is a negative regulator of embryonic neural progenitor cell proliferation. *J. Neurosci.* 28, 13978–13984. doi: 10.1523/JNEUROSCI.2140-08.2008

Lefauconnier, J. M., and Trouve, R. (1983). Developmental changes in the pattern of amino acid transport at the blood-brain barrier in rats. *Brain Res.* 282, 175–182.

Lehtinen, M. K., Zappaterra, M. W., Chen, X., Yang, Y. J., Hill, A. D., Lun, M., et al. (2011). The cere- brospinal fluid provides a prolif- erative niche for neural progeni- tor cells. *Neuron* 69, 893–905. doi: 10.1016/j.neuron.2011.01.023

Liddelow, S. A., Dziegielewska, K. M., Ek, C. J., Habgood, M. D., Bauer, H., Bauer, H. C., et al. (2013). Mechanisms that determine the internal environment of the developing brain: a transcriptomic, functional and ultrastructural approach. *PLoS ONE* 8:e65629. doi: 10.1371/journal.pone.0065629

Liddelow, S. A., Dziegielewska, K. M., Ek, C. J., Johansson, P. A., Potter, A. M., and Saunders, N. R. (2009). Cellular transfer of macromolecules across the developing choroid plexus of *Monodelphis domestica*. *Eur. J. Neurosci.* 29, 253–266. doi: 10.1111/j.1460-9568.2008.06571.x

Liddelow, S. A., Temple, S., Møllgård, K., Gehwolf, R., Wagner, A., Bauer, H., et al. (2012). Molecular charac- terisation of transport mechanisms at the developing mouse blood- CSF interface: a transcriptome approach. *PLoS ONE* 7:e33554. doi: 10.1371/journal.pone.0033554

Marques, F., Sousa, J. C., Coppola, G., Falcao, A. M., Rodrigues, A. J., Geschwind, D. H., et al. (2009). Kinetic profile of the transcriptome changes induced in the choroid plexus by peripheral inflamma- tion. *J. Cereb. Blood Flow Metab.* 29, 921–932. doi: 10.1038/jcbfm. 2009.15

Matyszak, M. K., and Perry, V. H. (1998). Bacillus Calmette- Guerin sequestered in the brain parenchyma escapes immune recognition. *J. Neuroimmunol.* 82, 73–80. doi: 10.1016/S0165-5728 (97)00190-2

Mcclure, M. M., Riddle, A., Manese, M., Luo, N. L., Rorvik, D. A., Kelly, K. A., et al. (2008). Cerebral blood flow heterogeneity in preterm sheep: lack of physiologic support for vascular boundary zones in fetal cerebral white matter. *J. Cereb. Blood Flow Metab.* 28, 995–1008. doi: 10.1038/sj.jcbfm.9600597

Mcmahon, E. J., Bailey, S. L., Castenada, V., Waldner, H., and Miller, S. (2005). Epitope spreading ini- tiates in the CNS in two mouse models of multiple sclerosis. *Nat. Med.* 11, 335–339. doi: 10.1038/nm1202

Meager, A. (1999). Cytokine regula- tion of cellular adhesion molecule expression in inflammation. *Cytokine Growth Factor Rev.* 10, 27–39. doi: 10.1016/S1359-6101 (98)00024-0

Minagar, A., and Alexander, J. S. (2003). Blood-brain barrier disrup- tion in multiple sclerosis. *Mult. Scler.* 9, 540–549. doi: 10.1191/1352 458503ms965oa

Møllgård, K., Balslev, Y., Lauritzen, B., and Saunders, N. R. (1987). Cell junctions and membrane spe- cializations in the ventricular zone (germinal matrix) of the develop- ing sheep brain: a CSF-brain bar- rier. *J. Neurocytol.* 16, 433–444. doi: 10.1007/BF01668498

Møllgård, K., Dziegielewska, K. M., Saunders, N. R., Zakut, H., and Soreq, H. (1988). Synthesis and localization of plasma pro- teins in the developing human brain. Integrity of the fetal blood-brain barrier to endoge- nous proteins of hepatic origin. *Dev. Biol.* 128, 207–221. doi: 10.1016/0012-1606(88)90283-7

Møllgård, K., Lauritzen, B., and Saunders, N. R. (1979). Double replica technique applied to choroid plexus from early foetal sheep: completeness and complexity of tight junctions. *J. Neurocytol.* 8, 139–149. doi: 10.1007/BF01175557

Morgan, E. H., and Moos, T. (2002). Mechanism and developmen- tal changes in iron transport across the blood-brain barrier. *Dev. Neurosci.* 24, 106–113. doi: 10.1159/000065699

Nordborg, C., Sokrab, T. E., and Johansson, B. B. (1991). The rela- tionship between plasma protein extravasation and remote tissue changes after experimental brain infarction. *Acta Neuropathol.* 82, 118–126. doi: 10.1007/BF00293954

Okun, E., Griffioen, K. J., Son, T. G., Lee, J. H., Roberts, N. J., Mughal, M. R., et al. (2010). TLR2 activation inhibits embryonic neural progeni- tor cell proliferation. *J. Neurochem.* 114, 462–474. doi: 10.1111/j.1471- 4159.2010.06778.x

Ousman, S. S., and Kubes, P. (2012). Immune surveillance in the central nervous system. *Nat. Neurosci.* 15, 1096–1101. doi: 10.1038/nn.3161

Pan, W., and Kastin, A. J. (2002). TNFalpha transport across the blood-brain barrier is abol- ished in receptor knockout mice. *Exp. Neurol.* 174, 193–200. doi: 10.1006/exnr.2002.7871

Peng, J., He, F., Zhang, C., Deng, X., and Yin, F. (2011). Protein kinase C-alpha signals P115RhoGEF phos- phorylation and RhoA activation in TNF-alpha-induced mouse brain microvascular endothe- lial cell barrier dysfunction. *J. Neuroinflammation* 8, 28. doi: 10.1186/1742-2094-8-28

Perry, V. H., Bell, M. D., Brown, H. C., and Matyszak, M. K. (1995). Inflammation in the nervous system. *Curr. Opin. Neurobiol.* 5, 636–641. doi: 10.1016/0959-4388(95)80069-7

Plumb, J., McQuaid, S., Mirakhur, M., and Kirk, J. (2002). Abnormal endothelial tight junctions in active lesions and normal- appearing white matter in multiple sclerosis. *Brain Pathol.* 12, 154–169. doi: 10.1111/j.1750-3639.2002.tb00430.x

Porterfield, S. P., and Hendrich, C. E. (1992). Tissue iodothyronine levels in fetuses of control and hypothy- roid rats at 13 and 16 days ges- tation. *Endocrinology* 131, 195–200. doi: 10.1210/en.131.1.195

Proebstl, D., Voisin, M. B., Woodfin, A., Whiteford, J., D'acquisto, F., Jones, G. E., et al. (2012). Pericytes support neutrophil subendothelial cell crawling and breaching of venular walls *in vivo*. *J. Exp. Med.* 209, 1219–1234. doi: 10.1084/jem.20111622

Quan, N., Stern, E. L., Whiteside, M. B., and Herkenham, M. (1999). Induction of pro- inflammatory cytokine mRNAs in the brain after peripheral injection of subseptic doses of lipopolysaccharide in the rat. *J. Neuroimmunol.* 93, 72–80. doi: 10.1016/S0165-5728(98)00193-3

Ransohoff, R. M., and Engelhardt, B. (2012). The anatomical and cellu- lar basis of immune surveillance in the central nervous system. *Nat. Rev. Immunol.* 12, 623–635. doi: 10.1038/nri3265

Reboldi, A., Coisne, C., Baumjohann, D., Benvenuto, F., Bottinelli, D., Lira, S., et al. (2009). C-C chemokine receptor 6-regulated entry of TH-17 cells into the CNS through the choroid plexus is required for the initiation of EAE. *Nat. Immunol.* 10, 514–523. doi: 10.1038/ni.1716

Rigor, R. R., Beard, R. S. Jr., Litovka, O. P., and Yuan, S. Y. (2012). Interleukin-1beta-induced barrier dysfunction is signaled through PKC-theta in human brain microvascular endothelium. *Am. J. Physiol. Cell Physiol.* 302, C1513–C1522. doi: 10.1152/ajpcell.00371.2011

Sagar, D., Lamontagne, A., Foss, C. A., Khan, Z. K., Pomper, M. G., and Jain, P. (2012). Dendritic cell CNS recruitment correlates with disease severity in EAE via CCL2 chemotaxis at the blood-brain barrier through paracellular trans- migration and ERK activation. *J. Neuroinflammation* 9, 245. doi: 10.1186/1742-2094-9-245

Saunders, N. R., Daneman, R., Dziegielewska, K. M., and Liddelow, S. A. (2013). Transporters of the blood-brain and blood-CSF interfaces in devel- opment and in the adult. *Mol. Aspects Med.* 34, 742–752. doi: 10.1016/j.mam.2012.11.006

Saunders, N. R., Liddelow, S. A., and Dziegielewska, K. M. (2012). Barrier mechanisms in the developing brain. *Front. Pharmacol.* 3:46. doi: 10.3389/fphar.2012.00046

Serres, S., Anthony, D. C., Jiang, Y., Broom, K. A., Campbell, S. J., Tyler, D. J., et al. (2009). Systemic inflammatory response reactivates immune-mediated lesions in rat brain. *J. Neurosci.* 29, 4820–4828. doi: 10.1523/JNEUROSCI.0406-09.2009

Stamatovic, S. M., Sladojevic, N., Keep, R. F., and Andjelkovic, A. V. (2012). Relocalization of junctional adhesion molecule A during inflammatory stimulation of brain endothelial cells. *Mol. Cell. Biol.* 32, 3414–3427. doi: 10.1128/MCB.06678-11

Stanimirovic, D., and Satoh, K. (2000). Inflammatory mediators of cere- bral endothelium: a role in ischemic brain inflammation. *Brain Pathol.* 10, 113–126. doi: 10.1111/j.1750-3639.2000.tb00248.x

Stolp, H. B. (2013). Neuropoietic cytokines in normal brain devel- opment and neurodevelopmental disorders. *Mol. Cell. Neurosci.* 53, 63–68. doi: 10.1016/j.mcn.2012. 08.009

Stolp, H. B., and Dziegielewska, K. M. (2009). Review: role of developmental inflammation and blood-brain barrier dysfunction in neurodevelopmental and neurode- generative diseases. *Neuropathol. Appl. Neurobiol.* 35, 132–146. doi: 10.1111/j.1365-2990.2008.01005.x

Stolp, H. B., Dziegielewska, K. M., Ek, C. J., Habgood, M. D., Lane, M. A., Potter, A. M., et al. (2005a). Breakdown of the blood-brain bar- rier to proteins in white matter of the developing brain following sys- temicinflammation. *Cell Tissue Res.* 320, 369–378. doi: 10.1007/s00441- 005-1088-6

Stolp, H. B., Dziegielewska, K. M., Ek, C. J., Potter, A. M., and Saunders, N. R. (2005b). Long-term changes in blood-brain barrier permeability and white matter following prolonged systemic inflammation in early development in the rat. *Eur. J. Neurosci.* 22, 2805–2816. doi: 10.1111/j.1460- 9568.2005.04483.x

Stolp, H. B., Ek, C. J., Johansson, P. A., Dziegielewska, K. M., Bethge, N., Wheaton, B. J., et al. (2009). Factors involved in inflammation-induced developmental white matter dam- age. *Neurosci. Lett.* 451, 232–236. doi: 10.1016/j.neulet.2009.01.021

Stolp, H. B., Turnquist, C., Dziegielewska, K. M., Saunders, N. R., Anthony, D. C., and Molnar, Z. (2011). Reduced ventricular proliferation in the foetal cortex following maternal inflammation in the mouse. *Brain* 134, 3236–3248. doi: 10.1093/brain/awr237

Supramaniam, V., Vontell, R., Srinivasan, L., Wyatt-Ashmead, J., Hagberg, H., and Rutherford, M. (2013). Microglia activation in the extremely preterm human brain. *Pediatr. Res.* 73, 301–309. doi: 10.1038/pr.2012.186

Tomkins, O., Feintuch, A., Benifla, M., Cohen, A., Friedman, A., and Shelef, I. (2011). Blood-brain bar- rier breakdown following traumatic brain injury: a possible role in posttraumatic epilepsy. *Cardiovasc. Psychiatry Neurol.* 2011, 765923. doi: 10.1155/2011/765923

Verney, C., Monier, A., Fallet-Bianco, C., and Gressens, P. (2010). Early microglial colonization of the human forebrain and possible involvement in periventricular white-matter injury of preterm infants. *J. Anat.* 217, 436–448. doi: 10.1111/j.1469-7580.2010. 01245.x

Verney, C., Pogledic, I., Biran, V., Adle- Biassette, H., Fallet-Bianco, C., and Gressens, P. (2012). Microglial reaction in axonal crossroads is a hallmark of noncystic periventric- ular white matter injury in very preterm infants. *J. Neuropathol. Exp. Neurol.* 71, 251–264. doi: 10.1097/NEN.0b013e3182496429

Vexler, Z. S., Tang, X. N., and Yenari, M. A. (2006). Inflammation in adult and neonatal stroke. *Clin. Neurosci. Res.* 6, 293–313. doi: 10.1016/j.cnr.2006.09.008

Virgintino, D., Errede, M., Robertson, D., Capobianco, C., Girolamo, F., Vimercati, A., et al. (2004). Immunolocalization of tight junction proteins in the adult and developing human brain. *Histochem. Cell Biol.* 122, 51–59. doi: 10.1007/s00418-004-0665-1

Von Wedel-Parlow, M., Wolte, P., and Galla, H. J. (2009). Regulation of major efflux transporters under inflammatory conditions at the blood-brain barrier *in vitro*. *J. Neurochem.* 111, 111–118. doi: 10.1111/j.1471-4159.2009.06305.x

Wagner, K. R., Packard, B. A., Hall, C. L., Smulian, A. G., Linke, M. J., De Courten-Myers, G. M., et al. (2002). Protein oxidation and heme oxygenase-1 induc- tion in porcine white matter following intracerebral infusions of whole blood or plasma. *Dev. Neurosci.* 24, 154–160. doi: 10.1159/000065703

Westerlund, M., Belin, A. C., Anvret, A., Hakansson, A., Nissbrandt, H., Lind, C., et al. (2009). Association of a polymor- phism in the ABCB1 gene with Parkinson's disease. *Parkinsonism Relat. Disord.* 15, 422–424. doi: 10.1016/j.parkreldis.2008.11.010

Wolburg, H., Wolburg-Buchholz, K., Kraus, J., Rascher-Eggstein, G., Liebner, S., Hamm, S., et al. (2003). Localization of claudin-3 in tight junctions of the blood-brain barrier is selec- tively lost during experimental autoimmune encephalomyeli- tis and human glioblastoma multiforme. *Acta Neuropathol.* 105, 586–592.

Wolburg, K., Gerhardt, H., Schulz, M., Wolburg, H., and Engelhardt, B. (1999). Ultrastructural local- ization of adhesion molecules in the healthy and inflamed choroid plexus of the mouse. *Cell Tissue Res.* 296, 259–269. doi: 10.1007/s004410051287

Yang, J., Goetz, D., Li, J. Y., Wang, W., Mori, K., Setlik, D., et al. (2002). An iron delivery pathway mediated by a lipocalin. *Mol. Cell* 10, 1045–1056. doi: 10.1016/ S1097-2765(02)00710-4

Zaguia, F., Saikali, P., Ludwin, S., Newcombe, J., Beauseigle, D., Mccrea, E., et al. (2013). Cytotoxic NKG2C+ CD4 T cells target oligodendrocytes in multi- ple sclerosis. *J. Immunol.* 190, 2510–2518. doi: 10.4049/jimmunol. 1202725

Zamanian, J. L., Xu, L., Foo, L. C., Nouri, N., Zhou, L., Giffard, R. G., et al. (2012). Genomic analysis of reactive astrogliosis. *J. Neurosci.* 32, 6391–6410. doi: 10.1523/JNEUROSCI.6221-11.2012

9

Calcitonin gene-related peptide is a key neurotransmitter in the neuro-immune axis

Bakri M. Assas[1,2]*, Joanne I. Pennock[1†] and Jaleel A. Miyan[3†]

[1] Translational Medicine, Faculty of Medical and Human Sciences, The University of Manchester, Manchester, UK
[2] Department of Immunology, Faculty of Applied Sciences, King Abdulaziz University, Jeddah, Saudi Arabia
[3] Neurosciences, Faculty of Life Sciences, The University of Manchester, Manchester, UK

Edited by:
Adam Denes, University of Manchester, UK

Reviewed by:
Krisztina J. Kovacs, Institute of Experimental Medicine, Hungary
Cynthia Detre, Independent Scientist, USA

***Correspondence:**
Bakri M. Assas, Translational Medicine, Faculty of Medical and Human Sciences, The University of Manchester, AV Hill Building, Oxford Road, Manchester M13 9PT, UK
e-mail: mushref.assas@manchester.ac.uk

† Joint last authors.

The question of how the neural and immune systems interact in host defense is important, integrating a system that senses the whole body with one that protects. Understanding the mechanisms and routes of control could produce novel and powerful ways of promoting and enhancing normal functions as well as preventing or treating abnormal functions. Fragmentation of biological research into specialities has resulted in some failures in recognizing and understanding interactions across different systems and this is most striking across immunology, hematology, and neuroscience. This reductionist approach does not allow understanding of the *in vivo* orchestrated response generated through integration of all systems. However, many factors make the understanding of multisystem cross-talk in response to a threat difficult, for instance the nervous and immune systems share communication molecules and receptors for a wide range of physiological signals. But, it is clear that physical, hard-wired connections exist between the two systems, with the key link involving sensory, unmyelinated nerve fibers (c fibers) containing the neuropeptide calcitonin gene-related peptide (CGRP), and modified macrophages, mast cells and other immune and host defense cells in various locations throughout the body. In this review we will therefore focus on the induction of CGRP and its key role in the neuroimmune axis.

Keywords: CGRP, TRPV1, neuroimmunology, TNF-alpha, C fibers, gut-brain axis

SENSORY NEUROTRANSMITTER CGRP

Sensory neurotransmitters have been extensively studied and their ability to affect different body functions has been shown in a range of studies. One of the main sensory neurotransmitters involved in immune function is CGRP. CGRP exemplifies a neuroimmune connector, since it is released at the site of stimulation, affecting immediate responses as well as mediating information flow to the rest of the nervous system. CGRP is a critical, highly expressed sensory signal, making it an important member of neuro-immune communication pathways. C fibers, the smallest diameter unmyelinated sensory neurons, are the main source of this neuropeptide. Their small diameter generates one of the lowest threshold response elements in the nervous system indicating their vital role. To date, this low threshold has placed them in the category of nociceptive neurons as they are the first to register damage/toxins through the pain pathway. This categorization is reinforced by the fact that c fibers express on their surface the transient receptor potential vanilloid 1 (TRPV1) which is a key responder to tissue damage. However, below the pain threshold, C fibers are likely to be playing a critical role in physiological systems and in particular, in host monitoring and activation of host defense and immune responses due to their low activation potential.

CGRP RELEASE *IN VIVO*

CGRP is released in response to activation of TRPV1 in both the nervous and immune systems. In the nervous system, TRPV1 is expressed along the entire length of the sensory c fiber neurons, from the periphery to the somata in the CNS (Szallasi, 1995). These neurons innervate every organ and tissue in the body (Buck and Burks, 1986; Holzer, 1991; Szallasi and Blumberg, 1999). Although a key exogenous ligand for TRPV1 is capsaicin, TRPV1 is also activated by a range of other endogenous agonists including heat (>43°C) (Caterina et al., 1997; Tominaga et al., 1998), protons (~pH 4.5) (Vyklicky et al., 1998; Jordt et al., 2000), lipids like anandamide (Olah et al., 2001), phosphatidylinositol(4,5)-biphosphate (PIP_2) (Chuang et al., 2001), and voltage (Gunthorpe et al., 2000) (summarized in **Figure 1**). Heat and low pH activate TRPV1 by distinct molecular recognition sites (Jordt et al., 2000). Additionally, TRPV1 has been suggested to be a mechanosensitive receptor in mediating nociceptive signals; for example TRPV1 deficient mice exhibit reduced sensitivity to post colorectal distension compared to controls (Jones et al., 2005) adding an interesting physiological element to TRPV1 activation. In rats, sensory vanilloid receptor-bearing nerves are classed as peptidergic and/or purinergic (Guo et al., 1999). Peptidergic nerves express TRPV1 and co-express neuropeptides whilst purinergic nerves express TRPV1 and co-express an adenosine triphosphate (ATP) gated ion-channel known as $P2X_3$ (Yiangou et al., 2001).

Besides the well documented role of TRPV1 in the nervous system, we now know that it is also expressed on immune cells, which has direct relevance to this review. Absence of TRPV1 signaling has been shown variously to exacerbate inflammation (Massa

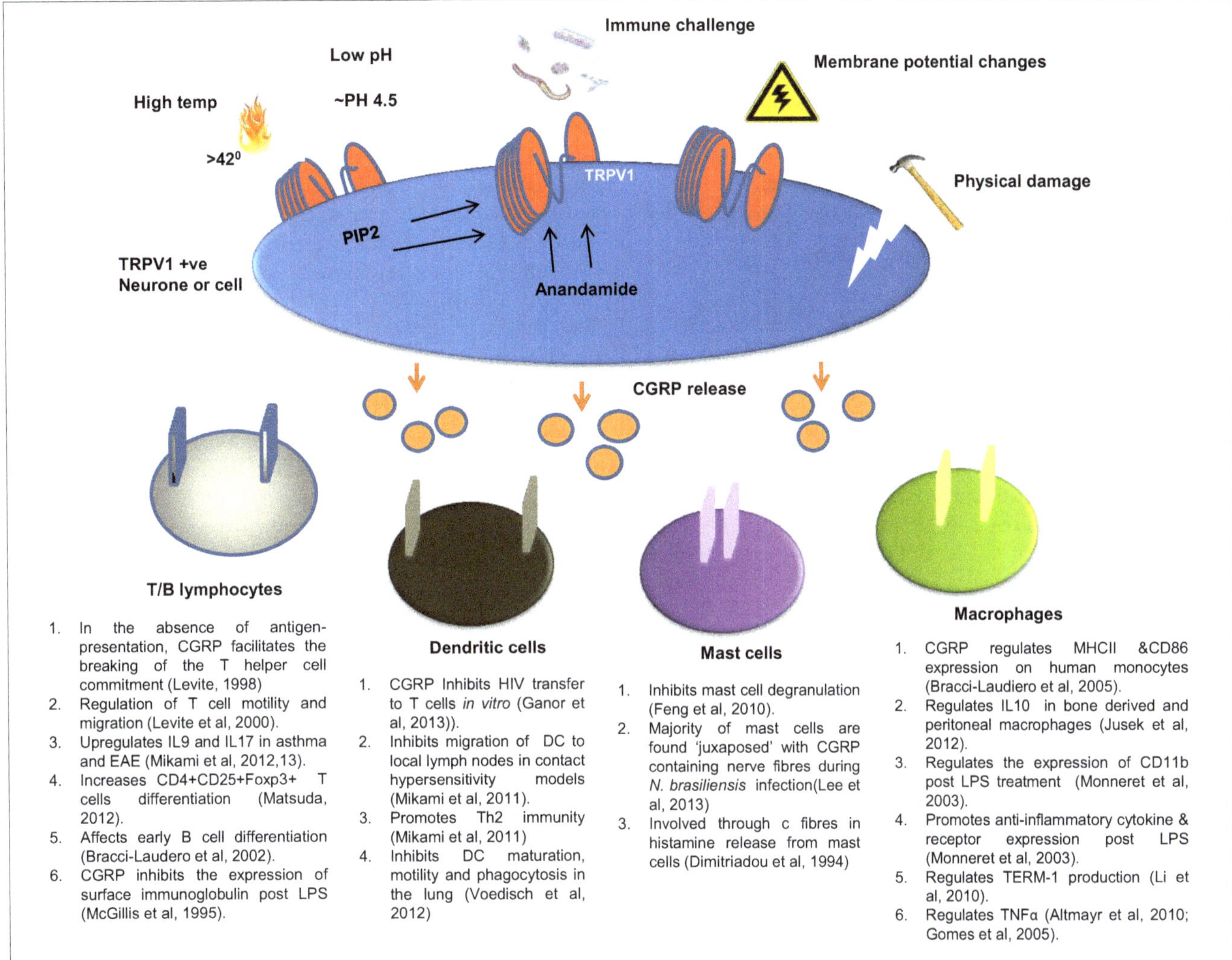

FIGURE 1 | Pathways of CGRP release via TRPV1 activation. TRPV1 is activated by many external factors associated with pain but also regular sensation below pain thresholds. These include the well characterized responses to heat, pH, and damage, as well as to toxins, immune challenges and membrane potential changes brought about by physiological and pathological processes. Endogenous and/or intracellular activation can also occur through the actions of PIP2 and Anandomide. Any activation of TRPV1 results in release of CGRP from the neuron. This released CGRP then acts on its specific receptor on cells immediately adjacent to the neuron, which in the case of sensory c fibers can be lymphocytes, DCs, mast cells, macrophages or cells within the hemopoietic microenvironment of the bone marrow (not shown). The range of activities stimulated by CGRP are listed below each cell type.

et al., 2006; Huang et al., 2009) and these effects can be attributed indirectly to the subsequent lack of CGRP. Similarly, agonism of TRPV1 with capsaicin has been shown to inhibit differentiation and cytokine secretion of human dendritic cells (Toth et al., 2009), thereby reducing early activation signals on challenge.

There are two isoforms of CGRP known: αCGRP and βCGRP. αCGRP has been shown to be a potent vasodilator and exhibits marked synergism with inflammatory mediators to induce local edema (Bernard and Shih, 1990). αCGRP's receptors are found on mouse bone marrow cells, providing strong evidence toward an eminent effect for αCGRP in modulating immune cell function and differentiation which in turn may affect the inflammatory cascade in response to a pathological threat (Mullins et al., 1993). αCGRP has also been identified as the predominant isotype in sensory neurons in the dorsal root ganglion (DRG) (Gibson et al., 1988). Unless stated otherwise, the observations discussed below refer to αCGRP only.

PHYSIOLOGICAL ROLE FOR CGRP

CGRP was first described as a vasodilator nearly 30 years ago (Brain et al., 1985). It is now well-established that CGRP regulates blood pressure (Brain and Grant, 2004), is associated with the onset of migraines when at high levels (Olesen, 2011a,b), promotes the maintenance of mucosal integrity in the gastrointestinal tract (GIT) (Szolcsanyi and Bartho, 2001), aids stem cell growth and maintenance *in vitro* (Dong et al., 2010) and modulates keratinocyte growth (Roggenkamp et al., 2013). CGRP plays a role in facilitating the absorption of intraluminal amino acids across the distal parts of the intestines (Mourad et al., 2009). In the lungs and elsewhere, CGRP promotes wound healing (Zhou et al., 2013). In the stomach, gastric acid stimulates the release of

CGRP via activation of local afferent neurons. CGRP itself orchestrates the secretion of chemical factors that inhibit gastric acid secretion and induce muscle repair (Aihara et al., 2005, 2006). Furthermore, CGRP and other neuropeptide containing nerve fibers extend all the way to the epithelial cell lining of the gut, suggesting a role in monitoring of the external (gut) environment. An association with immune cells present in gut epithelium also suggests an important role in the immune responses generated there (Engel et al., 2010, 2011).

CGRP AND IMMUNITY

CGRP is the main neurotransmitter of the nociceptive sensory c fibers, but is also present in other sensory nerve fibers i.e., type A and B medium-sized neurons. CGRP is released when these nerves are activated by specific agonists of TRPV1 usually during trauma or injury and therefore additionally associated with pain perception. However, c fibers have also been implicated in non-nociceptive activities including modulation of immune responses, through neuropeptide release (Beresford et al., 2004; Shepherd et al., 2005a,b). In fact CGRP is abundant in many immune organs. Nerve fibers containing CGRP have been identified in bone marrow, thymus, spleen, lymph nodes, skin, lungs, and gut and CGRP receptors are found on many hematopoietic cell types (Santambrogio et al., 1993; Petitto et al., 1994; Mach et al., 2002). In the bone marrow, these fibers accompany noradrenergic sympathetic fibers and are distributed throughout the marrow. The role of sensory neurotransmitters in the hematopoietic process has been examined for CGRP. Treatment with capsaicin, a potent neurotoxin to c fibers and activator of TRPV1, produced a dramatic change in bone marrow hematopoiesis when measured by *in vitro* colony-forming assays suggesting that CGRP has direct access to hematopoietic progenitors (Broome et al., 2000). CGRP positive nerves have also been detected in the cortical and vascular regions of lymph nodes. No evidence has been obtained/presented for the presence of parasympathetic nerves in lymph nodes or for the presence of the parasympathetic neurotransmitter acetyl choline (Schafer et al., 1998). However, non-neural sources for acetyl choline in lymphatic organs have been identified (Rosas-Ballina et al., 2011) where it is secreted by resident memory T cells in the spleen facilitating vagal anti-inflammatory functions, therefore, playing part in the vagal-immune pathways.

Many studies have demonstrated specific roles for CGRP and other peptides, including substance P, in the generation of both pro and anti-inflammatory immune responses. CGRP in particular has been the focus of many studies trying to unveil its involvement in a range of inflammatory models and immune conditions e.g., diabetes (Morrison et al., 2009), sepsis (De Winter et al., 2009), EAE (Mikami et al., 2012a) Crohn's Disease (Smith and Smid, 2005), and ulcerative colitis (Engel et al., 2012; Li et al., 2013a). In rats, dextran sulfate sodium (DSS)-induced colitis worsened when treated with a CGRP antagonist suggesting a protective role for CGRP in colitis (Engel et al., 2010).

Once released, CGRP plays multifunctional roles at different sites by binding to its receptor calcitonin receptor like receptor (CRLR) and its receptor activity-modifying protein 1 (RAMP1) found on T and B lymphocytes (Mikami et al., 2012a,b), macrophages (Fernandez et al., 2001), mast cells (Eftekhari et al., 2013), and dendritic cells (Mikami et al., 2011) among others (See **Figure 1**). CGRP is released from afferent fibers at the site of stimulation, presenting a motor-like mode of action conducted in parallel with afferent signaling to the DRG (Holzer and Maggi, 1998). However, it is well documented that cells of the immune system, i.e., lymphocytes (Wang et al., 1999), monocytes (Bracci-Laudiero et al., 2005), and macrophages (Linscheid et al., 2004; Lee and Zhang, 2012) also synthesize CGRP. It is thought that CGRP operates through the intracellular molecules Protein kinase C (PKC), PKA, and MAP kinase (MAPK) (Li et al., 2013b; Zhou et al., 2013) particularly in the lung and uterus (Bai et al., 2012; Mikami et al., 2013; Wong et al., 2013). In addition, CGRP influences NF-kappa-B activation and induction of cAMP suppressor genes in immune cells, particularly dendritic cells (Harzenetter et al., 2007) thereby regulating function.

CGRP REGULATES DENDRITIC CELL FUNCTIONS

Physiologically, CGRP was first found to be closely associated with dendritic cells (DC) in the skin (Hosoi et al., 1993). This study was the first to show a physical association between CGRP and Langerhans cells (LC) in the human epidermis. Functionally, it was one of the earliest publications to suggest an inhibitory function for CGRP on LC antigen presentation. So far, the majority of publications on the role of CGRP on DC suggest a predominant anti-inflammatory rather than pro-inflammatory effect. CGRP can modulate antigen presentation in DC (Mikami et al., 2011), and inhibit lipopolysaccharide induction of co-stimulatory signaling via the CD80 and CD28 receptors on dendritic cells and monocytes thereby affecting the function of T cells (Fox et al., 1997). Recently, Ganor et al. published a study on the role of CGRP during HIV-1 infection. Initially, CGRP plasma levels increased during the viral infection interfering with the induction of infection through LCs. CGRP inhibited the HIV-1 transfer to T cells, dampening the viral replication by 6 fold (Ganor et al., 2013). CGRP has also been shown to inhibit the migration of LC to local lymph nodes in contact hypersensitivity models, promoting Th2 type immunity in the process (Mikami et al., 2011). *In vitro* lung (DC) maturation was inhibited with CGRP (Rochlitzer et al., 2011). This correlated with a down regulation of the CGRP receptor on these DC during airway inflammation and these effects were reversed with the CGRP receptor antagonist $hCGRP_{8-37}$. CGRP continued to influence the antigen presenting functions of DCs in the lungs even when DCs were pre-treated with CGRP. DC phagocytosis and motility were modulated by CGRP (Voedisch et al., 2012) suggesting an important role for CGRP in maintaining immune integrity in the lungs via the control of DC functions. Similar to its effects on DCs in the skin and lungs, CGRP also inhibits the function of bone marrow-derived DCs. Through its receptor complex, CGRP inhibited the production of (Tumor necrosis factor) TNFα and IL12 post-LPS treatment highlighting its potent anti-inflammatory roles (Tsujikawa et al., 2007). CGRP has additionally been identified as a potent inhibitor of TLR induced inflammatory agents TNFα and CCL4 (Harzenetter et al., 2007). CGRP has also been shown to down regulate the surface expression of HLA-DR and CD86 on mature and immature human DC (Carucci et al., 2000), suggesting a mechanism whereby CGRP may dampen DC-T cell interaction.

CGRP REGULATES LYMPHOCYTE DIFFERENTIATION AND CYTOKINE PRODUCTION

CGRP shares aclose relationship with T cells. The interaction of T cell with DCs and macrophages, both of which express the CGRP receptor, is influenced by CGRP expression. (Ben-Horin and Chowers, 2008; Rochlitzer et al., 2011; Jusek et al., 2012; Holzmann, 2013). The capability of CGRP to regulate T cell function was proposed as early as 1988 (Umeda et al., 1988). In the last decade, studies have demonstrated a Th2 polarized T cell response after CGRP administration. Publications strongly suggest a TH2 preference by CGRP, through its influence on T cell differentiation (Levite, 2000; Ding et al., 2008). In more than one study, CGRP exposure to different DCs enhanced a TH2 type immunity increasing IL4 production while decreasing the TH1-associated cytokines interferon gamma (IFNγ) and IL2 (Wang et al., 1992; Tokoyoda et al., 2004; Mikami et al., 2011). The observed sensitization, according to Tokoyoda et al., occurs through the CGRP receptor activating cAMP/PKA pathways with the involvement of the conventional CD3/CD28 co-stimulation signal in T cells (Tokoyoda et al., 2004). CGRP has been shown to promote TH2 cytokine production *in vitro* and decrease TH1 cytokines (Levite, 1998, 2008). In 1998 and again in 2001, Levite et al., compared antigen-driven and neuropeptide-driven cytokine secretion from T helper cells (Levite, 1998; Levite and Chowers, 2001). They found that in a controlled *in vitro* environment TH0, TH1, and TH2 cells all produced "unconventional" cytokines respective to their phenotype when exposed to neuropeptide, with TH1 secreting IL4, TH2 secreting IFNγ, and TH0 secreting both. This suggests an ability to break the T helper line commitment and regulation of T cell functions. CGRP also up regulated IL9 and IL17 in both asthma and experimental autoimmune encephalomyelitis (EAE) models (Mikami et al., 2012a, 2013). IL17 has been attributed to a range of inflammatory functions and roles; however, its association with CGRP is still not understood. In an EAE model, IL17 levels dropped in RAMP-1$^{-/-}$ mice and TH17 functions were suppressed, suggesting a role for CGRP in the TH17 induced EAE (Mikami et al., 2012a). This has since been corroborated in models of psoriasis where TH17 cells are the dominant inflammatory phenotype (Ostrowski et al., 2011). In contrast, the association of CGRP with CD4+CD25+Foxp3+ cells has also been studied in a model of EAE (Matsuda et al., 2012). CGRP transfected DCs were able to increase differentiation of CD4+CD25+Foxp3+ regulatory cells (Matsuda et al., 2012). CGRP, is also produced by B lymphocytes in inflammatory conditions under the influence of nerve growth factor (NGF) (Bracci-Laudiero et al., 2002). The effect of CGRP on early B cell differentiation has been examined using a pre-B cell line population (70Z/3). CGRP inhibited the expression of surface immunoglobulin in response to LPS (McGillis et al., 1993, 1995). These studies suggest a crucial role for CGRP in early B cell differentiation, a finding supported by later studies (Fernandez et al., 2000; Schlomer et al., 2007).

CGRP AND IMMUNE MOTILITY, MIGRATION, AND ADHESION

In 1992, CGRP was described as a neuropeptide with "chemotactic" properties on human CD4 and CD8 T lymphocytes in the skin, inducing T cell trafficking (Foster et al., 1992). Ever since, T cells more than any other cell, have been the main targets for studies to understand the effect of CGRP on immune cell migration, adhesion, and motility. CGRP plays a key role in T cell adhesion to fibronectin (Levite, 1998; Levite et al., 1998) and beta integrin mediated T cell migration. Somatostatin, CGRP and neuropeptide Y all induced of freshly purified T cells to fibronectin coated plates (Springer et al., 2003). Deletion of CGRP results in a sustained decrease in leukocyte circulation and migration, highlighting its role in the bone marrow and in the mobilization of immune cells (Broome and Miyan, 2000; Broome et al., 2000). In the gut CGRP from c fibers stimulates T cell migration (Talme et al., 2008). *In vitro* studies showed that in contrast to other neuropeptides, CGRP can stimulate the migration of CD3 T cells into collagen matrix (Talme et al., 2008), an effect inhibited with CGRP receptor antagonist. In the absence of other immunological signals extracellular K(+) plays a critical role in stimulating T cell-integrin induced adhesion and migration. T cell voltage-gated K channels (Kv1.3) are targeted by a number of molecules to control T cell-integrin induced motility (Levite et al., 2000). CGRP binding to T cells, through its receptor, opens the voltage-gated K(+) channels, releasing K(+) from the intracellular matrix and activating β1 integrin. This facilitates T cell integrin-induced function highlighting a critical role for CGRP in alternative pathways for T cell adhesion, migration and motility. The effect of CGRP on macrophage and monocyte motility and chemotactic activity has also been studied. *In vitro*, inoculated promastigotes from cutaneous *Leishmania major,* demonstrated that CGRP, substance P, and somatstatin had regulatory effects on macrophage chemotactic activity (Ahmed et al., 1998; Han et al., 2010). CGRP was suggested to play an important role in human monocyte adhesion and migration (Linscheid et al., 2004). Human neutrophils cultured *in vitro* with CGRP and LPS secreted high levels of the chemokine IL8 (He et al., 2002), whilst CGRP has also been proposed to stimulate eosinophil migration (Dunzendorfer et al., 1998). CGRP increased the adhesion-related DC CD103+ ligand epithelial cadherin (E-cadherin) expression in human bronchial epithelial cells (Bai et al., 2012).

REGULATION OF OTHER IMMUNE CELLS

A wealth of literature can be found on the role of CGRP in the inhibition of mast cell degranulation. Many studies have reported mast cells and CGRP fibers "juxtaposed" in different models (Bienenstock et al., 1987; Lee et al., 2013). Controlled low dose capsaicin has been used to induce the release of CGRP from sensory nerves (Demirbilek et al., 2004). It has been estimated that nearly 60–70% of mast cells in the jejunum of rats infected with *Nippostrongylus brasiliensis* are juxtaposed to CGRP containing nerve fibers suggesting a role for this association in the immune response to this infection at least (Bienenstock et al., 1987; Dimitriadou et al., 1994) but no doubt in others also. Moreover, desensitization or deletion of c fibers with high doses of capsaicin severely impaired mast cell recruitment during *Schistosoma mansoni* infection in mice (De Jonge et al., 2003; Van Nassauw et al., 2007). Similarly, CGRP inhibited mast cell degranulation in a model of çerebral ischemia in rats (Feng et al., 2010) and in response to anti/IgE treatments, in comparison to other neuropeptides, in an *in vitro* assay with primary human mast cells (Kulka et al., 2008).

CGRP receptor is also expressed on human monocytes (Caviedes-Bucheli et al., 2008). Under the influence of NGF, CGRP has been shown to regulate the expression of MHCII, CD86 and the production of IL10 in human monocytes *in vitro* (Bracci-Laudiero et al., 2005). However, it seems that the role of CGRP in monocytes/macrophages seems to be less direct than that seen in other immune cells. CGRP is synthesized by monocytes/macrophages and can regulate immune functions of these cells (Ma et al., 2010). For instance CGRP can regulate CD11b expression after LPS exposure in human macrophages and neutrophils promoting anti-inflammatory functions (Monneret et al., 2003). Recently, macrophages have been studied in the context of pain induction and their involvement in pain pathways during inflammation (Hasegawa-Moriyama et al., 2013; Isami et al., 2013; Taves et al., 2013). In various studies, CGRP treatment increased IL10 from both peritoneal and bone marrow derived macrophages in response to LPS (Jusek et al., 2012). CGRP receptor absence resulted in the influx of neutrophils and inflammatory mediators into the peritoneal cavity (Jusek et al., 2012). CGRP was able to regulate the synthesis of triggering receptor expressed on myeloid cells-1 (TERM-1) in LPS-induced macrophages (Li et al., 2010). This effect was absent without LPS. However, the main contribution of CGRP to macrophage function is likely to incorporate its newly found links to the pro-inflammatory cytokine TNFα. This is the main cytokine released by macrophages in response to pathological challenges.

CGRP AND TNFα: A NEW CHAPTER

TNFα and CGRP are two important molecules that demonstrate a key bi-directional influence between the nervous and immune systems. TNFα functions through its receptors TNFRI and TNFRII. These receptors are found on glial cells in the spinal cord which, when activated, release prostaglandins, activating in turn nociceptive neurons and eliciting a pain response. Thus, the involvement of TNFα in peripheral and central pain is no longer a matter of doubt (Saito et al., 2010; Zhang et al., 2010a; Bressan et al., 2011; Gim et al., 2011; Teodorczyk-Injeyan et al., 2011). TNFα has been associated with the enhancement of trigeminal neuronal sensitivity to capsaicin in rats (Khan et al., 2008); exposure to TNFα for 5 min doubles the sensitivity of fura-loaded trigeminal neurons to capsaicin via TRPV1. Both TNFα receptors were present on capsaicin-sensitive trigeminal neurons co-expressed with TRPV1 (Khan et al., 2008). The presence of the TNFα receptors next to TRPV1 suggests that TNFα sensitizes TRPV1 positive neurons through its receptors. TNFRI plays a role in sensitizing tetrodotoxin (TTX)-resistant sodium channels (Jin and Gereau, 2006). It is likely that TNFRI has additional functions in immediate hyperalgesia and nociception to damage (Sommer et al., 1998), whileTNFRII is thought to have a role in nociception in persistent/chronic injurious conditions (Constantin et al., 2008; Schafers et al., 2008). A recent study has also linked TNFα to meningeal nociception (Zhang et al., 2010b), where it was suggested that TNFα functioned through TNFRI & TNFRII on nociceptive neurons and was associated with the "throbbing" sensation significant in migraines. Interestingly, neutralizing antibodies against TNFRI modulated thermal and mechanical hyperalgesia while antibodies against TNFRII had no affect (Sommer et al., 1998). Electrophysiological techniques showed that the local application of TNFα at the peripheral level of sensory neurons excites TRPV1 bearing sensory c fibers suggesting a specific role for TNFα in nociception (Sorkin and Doom, 2000). Additionally, TNFα increased CGRP release from sensitized capsaicin sensitive neurons when given 5 min prior to capsaicin treatment in comparison to vehicle treated rats (Khan et al., 2008). During LPS endotoxin treatment the increase in CGRP release was attributed to TNFα sensitizing afferent neurons in the presence of the prostaglandin sub types, prostanoids (Hua et al., 1996). These studies suggest that the nociceptive functions of TNFα occur via the specific capsaicin receptor TRPV1.

The activation of the specific capsaicin receptor TRPV1 located on c fibers or capsaicin sensitive neurons results in the release of sensory neuropeptides i.e., CGRP and SP (Helliwell et al., 1998; Bhave et al., 2002; Shepherd et al., 2005a; Ren et al., 2011). Additionally, reduction in CGRP tissue expression levels was seen in the dorsal root ganglia of rats injected with Entanercept (anti-TNFα treatment) (Horii et al., 2010). In both rats and humans with rheumatoid arthritis, CGRP and SP levels were reduced by 50% in the serum after treating with Etanercept (Origuchi et al., 2010). By contrast, TRPV1 activation via capsaicin and SA13353 (capsaicin analog) attenuated LPS-induced TNFα release in serum, and this effect was partially inhibited with CGRP antagonist treatment and in TRPV1$^{-/-}$ or sensory denervated mice (Tsuji et al., 2009) suggesting a regulatory function for CGRP on TNFα i.e., CGRP is able to downregulate TNFα *in vivo*. Both small doses (1 mg/kg) and large doses (150 mg/kg) of the TRPV1 agonist capsaicin have been found to downregulate serum levels of a range of pro-inflammatory cytokines including TNFα (Demirbilek et al., 2004), and the effects of capsaicin are attenuated in the presence of the antagonist for either TRPV1 or CGRP (Peng and Li, 2009).

In Toll-like receptor stimulated dendritic cells, CGRP causes a rapid up-regulation of inducible cAMP early repressor (ICER) which competes with ATF-2 for binding at the *Tnfα* promoter gene preventing gene expression of TNFα (Altmayr et al., 2010). In experiments using a non-irritating capsaicin analog (Vanillyl nonanoate) to examine the protective role capsaicin has on gastric mucosa (Luo et al., 2011), increased release of CGRP via TRPV1 activation had the ability to attenuate TNFα release in the serum post ethanol treatment. Blocking CGRP release from TRPV1 caused an increase in TNFα serum levels and increased gastric mucosal damage (Luo et al., 2011). Taken together all the findings suggest the presence of a TNFα-CGRP regulatory "loop" that is mediated via TRPV1 bearing sensory neurons releasing CGRP and/or through intracellular transcriptional interference of TNFα expression by immune cells.

CONCLUSION

CGRP has critical and wide-ranging control functions in various body systems and is particularly critical to normal hemopoietic and immune functions. CGRP-containing c nerve fibers are found everywhere in the body and are associated, in many locations, with specific immune cells including dendritic cells, mast cells and T cells. It appears to be the key mediator of neuro-immune communication with the c fibers acting as both sensory pathways, informing the nervous system of peripheral challenges, and as a local controller of immune functions. Knocking out this neural system results in major down-regulation of bone marrow hemopoietic output supporting a role for these nerve fibers in sensory feedback to immune control centers, already identified in the central nervous system by Denes et al. (2005). It is therefore becoming increasingly clear that this intimate connection between a specific subset of specialist sensory neurons and immune cells throughout the body, together with the connections to the brain and host defense control centers, is vital to the integrated, coordinated host defense response to any peripheral challenge. Moreover, it is clear that immune mediators, specifically pro-inflammatory cytokines IL-1a and TNFα, have direct effects on brain activity and whole body responses through the stimulation of specific circuits involved in so-called sickness behaviors (Dantzer and Kelley, 2007) that channel energy into host defense at the cost of social and other activities. A more complete understanding of this neural-immune interaction is vital to uncover key avenues for intervention to override abnormal functions and improve normal functions.

REFERENCES

Ahmed, A. A., Wahbi, A., Nordlind, K., Kharazmi, A., Sundqvist, K. G., Mutt, V., et al. (1998). *In vitro* Leishmania major promastigote-induced macrophage migration is modulated by sensory and autonomic neuropeptides. *Scand. J. Immunol.* 48, 79–85. doi: 10.1046/j.1365-3083.1998.00380.x

Aihara, E., Hayashi, M., Sasaki, Y., Kobata, A., and Takeuchi, K. (2005). Mechanisms underlying capsaicin-stimulated secretion in the stomach: comparison with mucosal acidification. *J. Pharmacol. Exp. Ther.* 315, 423–432. doi: 10.1124/jpet.105.087619

Aihara, E., Sasaki, Y., Ise, F., Kita, K., Nomura, Y., and Takeuchi, K. (2006). Distinct mechanisms of acid-induced HCO3- secretion in normal and slightly permeable stomachs. *Am. J. Physiol. Gastrointest. Liver Physiol.* 291, G464–G471. doi: 10.1152/ajpgi.00048.2006

Altmayr, F., Jusek, G., and Holzmann, B. (2010). The neuropeptide calcitonin gene-related peptide causes repression of tumor necrosis factor-alpha transcription and suppression of ATF-2 promoter recruitment in Toll-like receptor-stimulated dendritic cells. *J. Biol. Chem.* 285, 3525–3531. doi: 10.1074/jbc.M109.066787

Bai, H. B., Lu, Y. P., Duan, J. X., Zhou, Y., Sun, G. Y., and Guan, C. X. (2012). [Effects of CGRP on the E-cadherin expression in human bronchial epithelial cells]. *Zhongguo Ying Yong Sheng Li Xue Za Zhi* 28, 346–349.

Ben-Horin, S., and Chowers, Y. (2008). Neuroimmunology of the gut: physiology, pathology, and pharmacology. *Curr. Opin. Pharmacol.* 8, 490–495. doi: 10.1016/j.coph.2008.07.010

Beresford, L., Orange, O., Bell, E. B., and Miyan, J. A. (2004). Nerve fibres are required to evoke a contact sensitivity response in mice. *Immunology* 111, 118–125. doi: 10.1111/j.1365-2567.2004.01786.x

Bernard, G. W., and Shih, C. (1990). The osteogenic stimulating effect of neuroactive calcitonin gene-related peptide. *Peptides* 11, 625–632. doi: 10.1016/0196-9781(90)90171-Z

Bhave, G., Zhu, W., Wang, H., Brasier, D. J., Oxford, G. S., and Gereau, R. W. 4th. (2002). cAMP-dependent protein kinase regulates desensitization of the capsaicin receptor (VR1) by direct phosphorylation. *Neuron* 35, 721–731. doi: 10.1016/S0896-6273(02)00802-4

Bienenstock, J., Tomioka, M., Matsuda, H., Stead, R. H., Quinonez, G., Simon, G. T., et al. (1987). The role of mast cells in inflammatory processes: evidence for nerve/mast cell interactions. *Int. Arch. Allergy Appl. Immunol.* 82, 238–243. doi: 10.1159/000234197

Bracci-Laudiero, L., Aloe, L., Buanne, P., Finn, A., Stenfors, C., Vigneti, E., et al. (2002). NGF modulates CGRP synthesis in human B-lymphocytes: a possible anti-inflammatory action of NGF? *J. Neuroimmunol.* 123, 58–65. doi: 10.1016/S0165-5728(01)00475-1

Bracci-Laudiero, L., Aloe, L., Caroleo, M. C., Buanne, P., Costa, N., Starace, G., et al. (2005). Endogenous NGF regulates CGRP expression in human monocytes, and affects HLA-DR and CD86 expression and IL-10 production. *Blood* 106, 3507–3514. doi: 10.1182/blood-2004-10-4055

Brain, S. D., and Grant, A. D. (2004). Vascular actions of calcitonin gene-related peptide and adrenomedullin. *Physiol. Rev.* 84, 903–934. doi: 10.1152/physrev.00037.2003

Brain, W. T., S. D., Tippins, J. R., Morris, H. R., and MacIntyre, I. (1985). Calcitonin gene-related peptide is a potent vasodilator. *Nature* 313, 54–56. doi: 10.1038/313054a0

Bressan, E., Peres, K. C., and Tonussi, C. R. (2011). Evidence that LPS-reactive arthritis in rats depends on the glial activity and the fractalkine-TNF-alpha signaling in the spinal cord. *Neuropharmacology* 62, 947–958. doi: 10.1016/j.neuropharm.2011.09.028

Broome, C. S., and Miyan, J. A. (2000). Neuropeptide control of bone marrow neutrophil production. A key axis for neuroimmunomodulation. *Ann. N.Y. Acad. Sci.* 917, 424–434. doi: 10.1111/j.1749-6632.2000.tb05407.x

Broome, C. S., Whetton, A. D., and Miyan, J. A. (2000). Neuropeptide control of bone marrow neutrophil production is mediated by both direct and indirect effects on CFU-GM. *Br. J. Haematol.* 108, 140–150. doi: 10.1046/j.1365-2141.2000.01808.x

Buck, S. H., and Burks, T. F. (1986). The neuropharmacology of capsaicin: review of some recent observations. *Pharmacol. Rev.* 38, 179–226.

Carucci, J. A., Ignatius, R., Wei, Y., Cypess, A. M., Schaer, D. A., Pope, M., et al. (2000). Calcitonin gene-related peptide decreases expression of HLA-DR and CD86 by human dendritic cells and dampens dendritic cell-driven T cell-proliferative responses via the type I calcitonin gene-related peptide receptor. *J. Immunol.* 164, 3494–3499.

Caterina, M. J., Schumacher, M. A., Tominaga, M., Rosen, T. A., Levine, J. D., and Julius, D. (1997). The capsaicin receptor: a heat-activated ion channel in the pain pathway. *Nature* 389, 816–824. doi: 10.1038/39807

Caviedes-Bucheli, J., Moreno, G. C., Lopez, M. P., Bermeo-Noguera, A. M., Pacheco-Rodriguez, G., Cuellar, A., et al. (2008). Calcitonin gene-related peptide receptor expression in alternatively activated monocytes/macrophages during irreversible pulpitis. *J. Endod.* 34, 945–949. doi: 10.1016/j.joen.2008.05.011

Chuang, H. H., Prescott, E. D., Kong, H., Shields, S., Jordt, S. E., Basbaum, A. I., et al. (2001). Bradykinin and nerve growth factor release the capsaicin receptor from PtdIns(4, 5)P2-mediated inhibition. *Nature* 411, 957–962. doi: 10.1038/35082088

Constantin, C. E., Mair, N., Sailer, C. A., Andratsch, M., Xu, Z. Z., Blumer, M. J., et al. (2008). Endogenous tumor necrosis factor alpha (TNFalpha) requires TNF receptor type 2 to generate heat hyperalgesia in a mouse cancer model. *J. Neurosci.* 28, 5072–5081. doi: 10.1523/JNEUROSCI.4476-07.2008

Dantzer, R., and Kelley, K. W. (2007). Twenty years of research on cytokine-induced sickness behavior. *Brain Behav. Immun.* 21, 153–160. doi: 10.1016/j.bbi.2006.09.006

De Jonge, F., Van Nassauw, L., Adriaensen, D., Van Meir, F., Miller, H. R., Van Marck, E., et al. (2003). Effect of intestinal inflammation on capsaicin-sensitive afferents in the ileum of Schistosoma mansoni-infected mice. *Histochem. Cell Biol.* 119, 477–484. doi: 10.1007/s00418-003-0532-5

Demirbilek, S., Ersoy, M. O., Karaman, A., Gurbuz, N., Bayraktar, N., and Bayraktar, M. (2004). Small-dose capsaicin reduces systemic inflammatory responses in septic rats. *Anesth. Analg.* 99, 1501–1507. doi: 10.1213/01.ANE.0000132975.02854.65

Denes, A., Boldogkoi, Z., Uhereczky, G., Hornyak, A., Rusvai, M., Palkovits, M., et al. (2005). Central autonomic control of the bone marrow: multisynaptic tract tracing by recombinant pseudorabies virus. *Neuroscience* 134, 947–963. doi: 10.1016/j.neuroscience.2005.03.060

De Winter, B. Y., Bredenoord, A. J., Van Nassauw, L., De Man, J. G., De Schepper, H. U., Timmermans, J. P., et al. (2009). Involvement of afferent neurons in the pathogenesis of endotoxin-induced ileus in mice: role of CGRP and TRPV1 receptors. *Eur. J. Pharmacol.* 615, 177–184. doi: 10.1016/j.ejphar.2009.04.055

Dimitriadou, V., Rouleau, A., Dam Trung Tuong, M., Newlands, G. J., Miller, H. R., Luffau, G., et al. (1994). Functional relationship between mast cells and C-sensitive nerve fibres evidenced by histamine H3-receptor modulation in rat lung and spleen. *Clin. Sci.* 87, 151–163.

Ding, W., Stohl, L. L., Wagner, J. A., and Granstein, R. D. (2008). Calcitonin gene-related peptide biases Langerhans cells toward Th2-type immunity. *J. Immunol.* 181, 6020–6026.

Dong, J., He, Y., Zhang, X., Wang, L., Sun, T., Zhang, M., et al. (2010). Calcitonin gene-related peptide regulates the growth of epidermal stem cells *in vitro*. *Peptides* 31, 1860–1865. doi: 10.1016/j.peptides.2010.07.007

Dunzendorfer, S., Meierhofer, C., and Wiedermann, C. J. (1998). Signaling in neuropeptide-induced migration of human eosinophils. *J. Leukoc. Biol.* 64, 828–834.

Eftekhari, S., Warfvinge, K., Blixt, F. W., and Edvinsson, L. (2013). Differentiation of nerve fibers storing CGRP and CGRP receptors in the peripheral trigeminovascular system. *J. Pain* 14, 1289–1303. doi: 10.1016/j.jpain.2013.03.010

Engel, M. A., Becker, C., Reeh, P. W., and Neurath, M. F. (2010). Role of sensory neurons in colitis: increasing evidence for a neuroimmune link in the gut. *Inflamm. Bowel Dis.* 17, 1030–1033. doi: 10.1002/ibd.21422

Engel, M. A., Khalil, M., Mueller-Tribbensee, S. M., Becker, C., Neuhuber, W. L., Neurath, M. F., et al. (2012). The proximodistal aggravation of colitis depends on substance P released from TRPV1-expressing sensory neurons. *J. Gastroenterol.* 47, 256–265. doi: 10.1007/s00535-011-0495-6

Engel, M. A., Khalil, M., Siklosi, N., Mueller-Tribbensee, S. M., Neuhuber, W. L., Neurath, M. F., et al. (2011). Opposite effects of substance P and calcitonin gene-related peptide in oxazolone colitis. *Dig. Liver Dis.* 44, 24–29. doi: 10.1016/j.dld.2011.08.030

Feng, G., Xu, X., Wang, Q., Liu, Z., Li, Z., and Liu, G. (2010). The protective effects of calcitonin gene-related peptide on gastric mucosa injury after cerebral ischemia reperfusion in rats. *Regul. Pept.* 160, 121–128. doi: 10.1016/j.regpep.2009.11.008

Fernandez, S., Knopf, M. A., Bjork, S. K., and McGillis, J. P. (2001). Bone marrow-derived macrophages express functional CGRP receptors and respond to CGRP by increasing transcription of c-fos and IL-6 mRNA. *Cell. Immunol.* 209, 140–148. doi: 10.1006/cimm.2001.1795

Fernandez, S., Knopf, M. A., and McGillis, J. P. (2000). Calcitonin-gene related peptide (CGRP) inhibits interleukin-7-induced pre-B cell colony formation. *J. Leukoc. Biol.* 67, 669–676.

Foster, C. A., Mandak, B., Kromer, E., and Rot, A. (1992). Calcitonin gene-related peptide is chemotactic for human T lymphocytes. *Ann. N.Y. Acad. Sci.* 657, 397–404. doi: 10.1111/j.1749-6632.1992.tb22785.x

Fox, F. E., Kubin, M., Cassin, M., Niu, Z., Hosoi, J., Torii, H., et al. (1997). Calcitonin gene-related peptide inhibits proliferation and antigen presentation by human peripheral blood mononuclear cells: effects on B7, interleukin 10, and interleukin 12. *J. Invest. Dermatol.* 108, 43–48. doi: 10.1111/1523-1747.ep12285627

Ganor, Y., Drillet-Dangeard, A. S., Lopalco, L., Tudor, D., Tambussi, G., Delongchamps, N. B., et al. (2013). Calcitonin gene-related peptide inhibits Langerhans cell-mediated HIV-1 transmission. *J. Exp. Med.* 210, 2161–2170. doi: 10.1084/jem.20122349

Gibson, S. J., Polak, J. M., Giaid, A., Hamid, Q. A., Kar, S., Jones, P. M., et al. (1988). Calcitonin gene-related peptide messenger RNA is expressed in sensory neurones of the dorsal root ganglia and also in spinal motoneurones in man and rat. *Neurosci. Lett.* 91, 283–288. doi: 10.1016/0304-3940(88)90694-5

Gim, G. T., Lee, J. H., Park, E., Sung, Y. H., Kim, C. J., Hwang, W. W., et al. (2011). Electroacupuncture attenuates mechanical and warm allodynia through suppression of spinal glial activation in a rat model of neuropathic pain. *Brain Res. Bull.* 86, 403–411. doi: 10.1016/j.brainresbull.2011.09.010

Gomes, R. N., Castro-Faria-Neto, H. C., Bozza, P. T., Soares, M. B., Shoemaker, C. B., David, J. R., et al. (2005) Calcitonin gene-related peptide inhibits local acute inflammation and protects mice against lethal endotoxemia. *Shock* 24, 590–594. doi: 10.1097/01.shk.0000183395.29014.7c

Gunthorpe, M. J., Harries, M. H., Prinjha, R. K., Davis, J. B., and Randall, A. (2000). Voltage- and time-dependent properties of the recombinant rat vanilloid receptor (rVR1). *J. Physiol.* 525(Pt 3), 747–759. doi: 10.1111/j.1469-7793.2000.t01-1-00747.x

Guo, A., Vulchanova, L., Wang, J., Li, X., and Elde, R. (1999). Immunocytochemical localization of the vanilloid receptor 1 (VR1): relationship to neuropeptides, the P2X3 purinoceptor and IB4 binding sites. *Eur. J. Neurosci.* 11, 946–958. doi: 10.1046/j.1460-9568.1999.00503.x

Han, N., Zhang, D. Y., Wang, T. B., Zhang, P. X., and Jiang, B. G. (2010). Calcitonin gene-related peptide induces proliferation and monocyte chemoattractant protein-1 expression via extracellular signal-regulated kinase activation in rat osteoblasts. *Chin. Med. J. (Engl.)* 123, 1748–1753.

Harzenetter, M. D., Novotny, A. R., Gais, P., Molina, C. A., Altmayr, F., and Holzmann, B. (2007). Negative regulation of TLR responses by the neuropeptide CGRP is mediated by the transcriptional repressor ICER. *J. Immunol.* 179, 607–615.

Hasegawa-Moriyama, M., Kurimoto, T., Nakama, M., Godai, K., Kojima, M., Kuwaki, T., et al. (2013). Peroxisome proliferator-activated receptor-gamma agonist rosiglitazone attenuates inflammatory pain through the induction of heme oxygenase-1 in macrophages. *Pain* 154, 1402–1412. doi: 10.1016/j.pain.2013.04.039

He, Y., Ding, G., Xia, D., Zhu, T., and Fan, S. (2002). [Calcitonin gene-related peptide induces chemokine interleukine-8 synthesis in human monocytes]. *Zhonghua Yi Xue Za Zhi* 82, 131–134.

Helliwell, R. J., McLatchie, L. M., Clarke, M., Winter, J., Bevan, S., and McIntyre, P. (1998). Capsaicin sensitivity is associated with the expression of the vanilloid (capsaicin) receptor (VR1) mRNA in adult rat sensory ganglia. *Neurosci. Lett.* 250, 177–180. doi: 10.1016/S0304-3940(98)00475-3

Holzer, P. (1991). Capsaicin: cellular targets, mechanisms of action, and selectivity for thin sensory neurons. *Pharmacol. Rev.* 43, 143–201.

Holzer, P., and Maggi, C. A. (1998). Dissociation of dorsal root ganglion neurons into afferent and efferent-like neurons. *Neuroscience* 86, 389–398.

Holzmann, B. (2013). Antiinflammatory activities of CGRP modulating innate immune responses in health and disease. *Curr. Protein Pept. Sci.* 14, 268–274. doi: 10.2174/13892037113149990046

Horii, M., Orita, S., Nagata, M., Takaso, M., Yamauchi, K., Yamashita, M., et al. (2010). Direct application of the tumor necrosis factor-alpha inhibitor, etanercept, into a punctured intervertebral disc decreases calcitonin gene-related peptide expression in rat dorsal root ganglion neurons. *Spine (Phila Pa 1976)* 36, 80–85. doi: 10.1097/BRS.0b013e3181d4be3c

Hosoi, J., Murphy, G. F., Egan, C. L., Lerner, E. A., Grabbe, S., Asahina, A., et al. (1993). Regulation of Langerhans cell function by nerves containing calcitonin gene-related peptide. *Nature* 363, 159–163. doi: 10.1038/363159a0

Hua, X. Y., Chen, P., Fox, A., and Myers, R. R. (1996). Involvement of cytokines in lipopolysaccharide-induced facilitation of CGRP release from capsaicin-sensitive nerves in the trachea: studies with interleukin-1beta and tumor necrosis factor-alpha. *J. Neurosci.* 16, 4742–4748.

Huang, W., Rubinstein, J., Prieto, A. R., Thang, L. V., and Wang, D. H. (2009). Transient receptor potential vanilloid gene deletion exacerbates inflammation and atypical cardiac remodeling after myocardial infarction. *Hypertension* 53, 243–250. doi: 10.1161/HYPERTENSIONAHA.108.118349

Isami, K., Haraguchi, K., So, K., Asakura, K., Shirakawa, H., Mori, Y., et al. (2013). Involvement of TRPM2 in peripheral nerve injury-induced infiltration of peripheral immune cells into the spinal cord in mouse neuropathic pain model. *PLoS ONE* 8:e66410. doi: 10.1371/journal.pone.0066410

Jin, X., and Gereau, R. W. 4th. (2006). Acute p38-mediated modulation of tetrodotoxin-resistant sodium channels in mouse sensory neurons by tumor necrosis factor-alpha. *J. Neurosci.* 26, 246–255. doi: 10.1523/JNEUROSCI.3858-05.2006

Jones, R. C. 3rd, Xu, L., and Gebhart, G. F. (2005). The mechanosensitivity of mouse colon afferent fibers and their sensitization by inflammatory mediators require transient receptor potential vanilloid 1 and acid-sensing ion channel 3. *J. Neurosci.* 25, 10981–10989. doi: 10.1523/JNEUROSCI.0703-05.2005

Jordt, S. E., Tominaga, M., and Julius, D. (2000). Acid potentiation of the capsaicin receptor determined by a key extracellular site. *Proc. Natl. Acad. Sci. U.S.A.* 97, 8134–8139. doi: 10.1073/pnas.100129497

Jusek, G., Reim, D., Tsujikawa, K., and Holzmann, B. (2012). Deficiency of the CGRP receptor component RAMP1 attenuates immunosuppression during the early phase of septic peritonitis. *Immunobiology* 217, 761–767. doi: 10.1016/j.imbio.2012.04.009

Khan, A. A., Diogenes, A., Jeske, N. A., Henry, M. A., Akopian, A., and Hargreaves, K. M. (2008). Tumor necrosis factor alpha enhances the sensitivity of rat trigeminal neurons to capsaicin. *Neuroscience* 155, 503–509. doi: 10.1016/j.neuroscience.2008.05.036

Kulka, M., Sheen, C. H., Tancowny, B. P., Grammer, L. C., and Schleimer, R. P. (2008). Neuropeptides activate human mast cell degranulation and chemokine production. *Immunology* 123, 398–410. doi: 10.1111/j.1365-2567.2007.02705.x

Lee, J., Yamamoto, T., Hayashi, S., Kuramoto, H., and Kadowaki, M. (2013). Enhancement of CGRP sensory afferent innervation in the gut during the development of food allergy in an experimental murine model. *Biochem. Biophys. Res. Commun.* 430, 895–900. doi: 10.1016/j.bbrc.2012.12.058

Lee, S., and Zhang, J. (2012). Heterogeneity of macrophages in injured trigeminal nerves: cytokine/chemokine expressing vs. phagocytic macrophages. *Brain Behav. Immun.* 26, 891–903. doi: 10.1016/j.bbi.2012.03.004

Levite, M. (1998). Neuropeptides, by direct interaction with cells, T, induce cytokine secretion and break the commitment to a distinct T helper phenotype. *Proc. Natl. Acad. Sci. U.S.A.* 95, 12544–12549. doi: 10.1073/pnas.95.21.12544

Levite, M. (2000). Nerve-driven immunity. The direct effects of neurotransmitters on T-cell function. *Ann. N.Y. Acad. Sci.* 917, 307–321. doi: 10.1111/j.1749-6632.2000.tb05397.x

Levite, M. (2008). Neurotransmitters activate T-cells and elicit crucial functions via neurotransmitter receptors. *Curr. Opin. Pharmacol.* 8, 460–471. doi: 10.1016/j.coph.2008.05.001

Levite, M., Cahalon, L., Hershkoviz, R., Steinman, L., and Lider, O. (1998). Neuropeptides, via specific receptors, regulate T cell adhesion to fibronectin. *J. Immunol.* 160, 993–1000.

Levite, M., Cahalon, L., Peretz, A., Hershkoviz, R., Sobko, A., Ariel, A., et al. (2000). Extracellular K+ and opening of voltage-gated potassium channels activate T cell integrin function: physical and functional association between Kv1.3 channels and beta 1 integrins. *J. Exp. Med.* 191, 1167–1176. doi: 10.1084/jem.191.7.1167

Levite, M., and Chowers, Y. (2001). Nerve-driven immunity: neuropeptides regulate cytokine secretion of T cells and intestinal epithelial cells in a direct, powerful and contextual manner. *Ann. Oncol.* 12(Suppl. 2), S19–S25. doi: 10.1093/annonc/12.suppl_2.S19

Li, F. J., Zou, Y. Y., Cui, Y., Yin, Y., Guo, G., and Lu, F. G. (2013a). Calcitonin gene-related peptide is a promising marker in ulcerative colitis. *Dig. Dis. Sci.* 58, 686–693. doi: 10.1007/s10620-012-2406-y

Li, P., Sun, H. J., Han, Y., Wang, J. J., Zhang, F., Tang, C. S., et al. (2013b). Intermedin enhances sympathetic outflow via receptor-mediated cAMP/PKA signaling pathway in nucleus tractus solitarii of rats. *Peptides* 47, 1–6. doi: 10.1016/j.peptides.2013.05.002

Li, Y., Guan, C., Zhou, Y., Sun, G., Shi, M., Wu, J., et al. (2010). Effect of calcitonin gene-related peptide on the expression of triggering receptor expressed on myeloid cells-1 in lipopolysaccharide-induced macrophages. *Zhong Nan Da Xue Xue Bao Yi Xue Ban* 35, 100–106. doi: 10.3969/j.issn.1672-7347.2010.02.002

Linscheid, P., Seboek, D., Schaer, D. J., Zulewski, H., Keller, U., and Muller, B. (2004). Expression and secretion of procalcitonin and calcitonin gene-related peptide by adherent monocytes and by macrophage-activated adipocytes. *Crit. Care Med.* 32, 1715–1721. doi: 10.1097/01.CCM.0000134404.63292.71

Luo, X. J., Li, N. S., Zhang, Y. S., Liu, B., Yang, Z. C., Li, Y. J., et al. (2011). Vanillyl nonanoate protects rat gastric mucosa from ethanol-induced injury through a mechanism involving calcitonin gene-related peptide. *Eur. J. Pharmacol.* 666, 211–217. doi: 10.1016/j.ejphar.2011.05.032

Ma, W., Dumont, Y., Vercauteren, F., and Quirion, R. (2010). Lipopolysaccharide induces calcitonin gene-related peptide in the RAW264.7 macrophage cell line. *Immunology* 130, 399–409. doi: 10.1111/j.1365-2567.2009.03239.x

Mach, D. B., Rogers, S. D., Sabino, M. C., Luger, N. M., Schwei, M. J., Pomonis, J. D., et al. (2002). Origins of skeletal pain: sensory and sympathetic innervation of the mouse femur. *Neuroscience* 113, 155–166. doi: 10.1016/S0306-4522(02)00165-3

Massa, F., Sibaev, A., Marsicano, G., Blaudzun, H., Storr, M., and Lutz, B. (2006). Vanilloid receptor (TRPV1)-deficient mice show increased susceptibility to dinitrobenzene sulfonic acid induced colitis. *Mol. Med. J. (Berl.)* 84, 142–146. doi: 10.1007/s00109-005-0016-2

Matsuda, R., Kezuka, T., Nishiyama, C., Usui, Y., Matsunaga, Y., Okunuki, Y., et al. (2012). Suppression of murine experimental autoimmune optic neuritis by mature dendritic cells transfected with calcitonin gene-related Peptide gene. *Invest. Ophthalmol. Vis. Sci.* 53, 5475–5485. doi: 10.1167/iovs.12-9935

McGillis, J. P., Humphreys, S., Rangnekar, V., and Ciallella, J. (1993). Modulation of B lymphocyte differentiation by calcitonin gene-related peptide (CGRP). II. Inhibition of LPS-induced kappa light chain expression by CGRP. *Cell Immunol.* 150, 405–416. doi: 10.1006/cimm.1993.1208

McGillis, J. P., Rangnekar, V., and Ciallella, J. R. (1995). A role for calcitonin gene related peptide (CGRP) in the regulation of early B lymphocyte differentiation. *Can. J. Physiol. Pharmacol.* 73, 1057–1064. doi: 10.1139/y95-150

Mikami, N., Matsushita, H., Kato, T., Kawasaki, R., Sawazaki, T., Kishimoto, T., et al. (2011). Calcitonin gene-related peptide is an important regulator of cutaneous immunity: effect on dendritic cell and T cell functions. *J. Immunol.* 186, 6886–6893. doi: 10.4049/jimmunol.1100028

Mikami, N., Miyagi, Y., Sueda, K., Takatsuji, M., Fukada, S., Yamamoto, H., et al. (2013). Calcitonin gene-related peptide and cyclic adenosine 5'-monophosphate/protein kinase A pathway promote IL-9 production in Th9 differentiation process. *J. Immunol.* 190, 4046–4055. doi: 10.4049/jimmunol.1203102

Mikami, N., Fukada, S., Yamamoto, H., and Tsujikawa, K. (2012b). [The regulatory mechanisms of calcitonin gene-related peptide (CGRP) in skin inflammation]. *Yakugaku Zasshi* 132, 1211–1215. doi: 10.1248/yakushi.12-00232-1

Mikami, N., Watanabe, K., Hashimoto, N., Miyagi, Y., Sueda, K., Fukada, S., et al. (2012a). Calcitonin gene-related peptide enhances experimental autoimmune encephalomyelitis by promoting Th17-cell functions. *Int. Immunol.* 24, 681–691. doi: 10.1093/intimm/dxs075

Monneret, G., Arpin, M., Venet, F., Maghni, K., Debard, A. L., Pachot, A., et al. (2003). Calcitonin gene related peptide and N-procalcitonin modulate CD11b upregulation in lipopolysaccharide activated monocytes and neutrophils. *Intensive Care Med.* 29, 923–928.

Morrison, J. F., Dhanasekaran, S., and Howarth, F. C. (2009). Neuropeptides in the rat corpus cavernosum and seminal vesicle: effects of age and two types of diabetes. *Auton. Neurosci.* 146, 76–80. doi: 10.1016/j.autneu.2008.11.016

Mourad, F. H., Barada, K. A., Khoury, C., Hamdi, T., Saade, N. E., and Nassar, C. F. (2009). Amino acids in the rat intestinal lumen regulate their own absorption from a distant intestinal site. *Am. J. Physiol. Gastrointest. Liver Physiol.* 297, G292–G298. doi: 10.1152/ajpgi.00100.2009

Mullins, M. W., Ciallella, J., Rangnekar, V., and McGillis, J. P. (1993). Characterization of a calcitonin gene-related peptide (CGRP) receptor on mouse bone marrow cells. *Regul. Pept.* 49, 65–72. doi: 10.1016/0167-0115(93)90385-L

Olah, Z., Karai, L., and Iadarola, M. J. (2001). Anandamide activates vanilloid receptor 1 (VR1) at acidic pH in dorsal root ganglia neurons and cells ectopically expressing VR1. *J. Biol. Chem.* 276, 31163–31170. doi: 10.1074/jbc.M101607200

Olesen, J. (2011a). Calcitonin gene-related peptide (CGRP) in migraine. *Cephalalgia* 31, 510. doi: 10.1177/0333102410388438

Olesen, J. (2011b). CGRP in migraine. *Cephalalgia* 31, 638. doi: 10.1177/0333102410395790

Origuchi, T., Iwamoto, N., Kawashiri, S. Y., Fujikawa, K., Aramaki, T., Tamai, M., et al. (2010). Reduction in serum levels of substance P in patients with rheumatoid arthritis by etanercept, a tumor necrosis factor inhibitor. *Mod. Rheumatol.* 21, 244–250. doi: 10.1007/s10165-010-0384-5

Ostrowski, S. M., Belkadi, A., Loyd, C. M., Diaconu, D., and Ward, N. L. (2011). Cutaneous denervation of psoriasiform mouse skin improves acanthosis and inflammation in a sensory neuropeptide-dependent manner. *J. Invest. Dermatol.* 131, 1530–1538. doi: 10.1038/jid.2011.60

Peng, J., and Li, Y. J. (2009). The vanilloid receptor TRPV1, role in cardiovascular and gastrointestinal protection. *Eur. J. Pharmacol.* 627, 1–7. doi: 10.1016/j.ejphar.2009.10.053

Petitto, J. M., Huang, Z., and McCarthy, D. B. (1994). Molecular cloning of NPY-Y1 receptor cDNA from rat splenic lymphocytes: evidence of low levels of mRNA expression and [125I]NPY binding sites. *J. Neuroimmunol.* 54, 81–86. doi: 10.1016/0165-5728(94)90234-8

Ren, J. Y., Song, J. X., Lu, M. Y., and Chen, H. (2011). Cardioprotection by ischemic postconditioning is lost in isolated perfused heart from diabetic rats: involvement of transient receptor potential vanilloid 1, calcitonin gene-related peptide and substance P. *Regul. Pept.* 169, 49–57. doi: 10.1016/j.regpep.2011.04.004

Rochlitzer, S., Veres, T. Z., Kuhne, K., Prenzler, F., Pilzner, C., Knothe, S., et al. (2011). The neuropeptide calcitonin gene-related peptide affects allergic airway inflammation by modulating dendritic cell function. *Clin. Exp. Allergy* 41, 1609–1621. doi: 10.1111/j.1365-2222.2011.03822.x

Roggenkamp, D., Kopnick, S., Stab, F., Wenck, H., Schmelz, M., and Neufang, G. (2013). Epidermal nerve fibers modulate keratinocyte growth via neuropeptide signaling in an innervated skin model. *J. Invest. Dermatol.* 133, 1620–1628. doi: 10.1038/jid.2012.464

Rosas-Ballina, M., Olofsson, P. S., Ochani, M., Valdes-Ferrer, S. I., Levine, Y. A., Reardon, C., et al. (2011). Acetylcholine-synthesizing T Cells relay neural signals in a vagus nerve circuit. *Science* 334, 98–101. doi: 10.1126/science.1209985

Saito, O., Svensson, C. I., Buczynski, M. W., Wegner, K., Hua, X. Y., Codeluppi, S., et al. (2010). Spinal glial TLR4-mediated nociception and production of prostaglandin E(2) and TNF. *Br. J. Pharmacol.* 160, 1754–1764. doi: 10.1111/j.1476-5381.2010.00811.x

Santambrogio, L., Lipartiti, M., Bruni, A.,and Dal Toso, R. (1993). Dopamine receptors on human T- and B-lymphocytes. *J. Neuroimmunol.* 45, 113–119. doi: 10.1016/0165-5728(93)90170-4

Schafer, M. K., Eiden, L. E., and Weihe, E. (1998). Cholinergic neurons and terminal fields revealed by immunohistochemistry for the vesicular acetylcholine transporter. II. The peripheral nervous system. *Neuroscience* 84, 361–376. doi: 10.1016/S0306-4522(97)80196-0

Schafers, M., Sommer, C., Geis, C., Hagenacker, T., Vandenabeele, P., and Sorkin, L. S. (2008). Selective stimulation of either tumor necrosis factor receptor differentially induces pain behavior *in vivo* and ectopic activity in sensory neurons *in vitro*. *Neuroscience* 157, 414–423. doi: 10.1016/j.neuroscience.2008.08.067

Schlomer, J. J., Storey, B. B., Ciornei, R. T., and McGillis, J. P. (2007). Calcitonin gene-related peptide inhibits early B cell development *in vivo*. *J. Leukoc. Biol.* 81, 802–808. doi: 10.1189/jlb.0306229

Shepherd, A. J., Beresford, L. J., Bell, E. B., and Miyan, J. A. (2005a). Mobilisation of specific T cells from lymph nodes in contact sensitivity requires substance P. *J. Neuroimmunol.* 164, 115–123. doi: 10.1016/j.jneuroim.2005.04.008

Shepherd, A. J., Downing, J. E., and Miyan, J. A. (2005b). Without nerves, immunology remains incomplete -*in vivo* veritas. *Immunology* 116, 145–163. doi: 10.1111/j.1365-2567.2005.02223.x

Smith, A. S., and Smid, S. D. (2005). Impaired capsaicin and neurokinin-evoked colonic motility in inflammatory bowel disease. *J. Gastroenterol. Hepatol.* 20, 697–704. doi: 10.1111/j.1440-1746.2005.03759.x

Sommer, C., Schmidt, C., and George, A. (1998). Hyperalgesia in experimental neuropathy is dependent on the TNF receptor 1. *Exp. Neurol.* 151, 138–142. doi: 10.1006/exnr.1998.6797

Sorkin, L. S., and Doom, C. M. (2000). Epineurial application of TNF elicits an acute mechanical hyperalgesia in the awake rat. *J. Peripher. Nerv. Syst.* 5, 96–100. doi: 10.1046/j.1529-8027.2000.00012.x

Springer, J., Geppetti, P., Fischer, A., and Groneberg, D. A. (2003). Calcitonin gene-related peptide as inflammatory mediator. *Pulm. Pharmacol. Ther.* 16, 121–130. doi: 10.1016/S1094-5539(03)00049-X

Szallasi, A. (1995). Autoradiographic visualization and pharmacological characterization of vanilloid (capsaicin) receptors in several species, including man. *Acta Physiol. Scand. Suppl.* 629, 1–68.

Szallasi, A., and Blumberg, P. M. (1999). Vanilloid (Capsaicin) receptors and mechanisms. *Pharmacol. Rev.* 51, 159–212.

Szolcsanyi, J., and Bartho, L. (2001). Capsaicin-sensitive afferents and their role in gastroprotection: an update. *J. Physiol. Paris* 95, 181–188. doi: 10.1016/S0928-4257(01)00023-7

Talme, T., Liu, Z., and Sundqvist, K. G. (2008). The neuropeptide calcitonin gene-related peptide (CGRP) stimulates T cell migration into collagen matrices. *J. Neuroimmunol.* 196, 60–66. doi: 10.1016/j.jneuroim.2008.02.007

Taves, S., Berta, T., Chen, G., and Ji, R. R. (2013). Microglia and spinal cord synaptic plasticity in persistent pain. *Neural Plast.* 2013, 753656. doi: 10.1155/2013/753656

Teodorczyk-Injeyan, J. A., Triano, J. J., McGregor, M., Woodhouse, L., and Injeyan, H. S. (2011). Elevated production of inflammatory mediators including nociceptive chemokines in patients with neck pain: a cross-sectional evaluation. *J. Manipulative Physiol. Ther.* 34, 498–505. doi: 10.1016/j.jmpt.2011.08.010

Tokoyoda, K., Tsujikawa, K., Matsushita, H., Ono, Y., Hayashi, T., Harada, Y., et al. (2004). Up-regulation of IL-4 production by the activated cAMP/cAMP-dependent protein kinase (protein kinase A) pathway in CD3/CD28-stimulated naive T cells. *Int. Immunol.* 16, 643–653. doi: 10.1093/intimm/dxh072

Tominaga, M., Caterina, M. J., Malmberg, A. B., Rosen, T. A., Gilbert, H., Skinner, K., et al. (1998). The cloned capsaicin receptor integrates multiple pain-producing stimuli. *Neuron* 21, 531–543. doi: 10.1016/S0896-6273(00)80564-4

Toth, B. I., Benko, S., Szollosi, A. G., Kovacs, L., Rajnavolgyi, E., and Biro, T. (2009). Transient receptor potential vanilloid-1 signaling inhibits differentiation and activation of human dendritic cells. *FEBS Lett.* 583, 1619–1624. doi: 10.1016/j.febslet.2009.04.031

Tsuji, F., Murai, M., Oki, K., Seki, I., Ueda, K., Inoue, H., et al. (2009). Transient receptor potential vanilloid 1 agonists as candidates for anti-inflammatory and immunomodulatory agents. *Eur. J. Pharmacol.* 627, 332–339. doi: 10.1016/j.ejphar.2009.10.044

Tsujikawa, K., Yayama, K., Hayashi, T., Matsushita, H., Yamaguchi, T., Shigeno, T., et al. (2007). Hypertension and dysregulated proinflammatory cytokine production in receptor activity-modifying protein 1-deficient mice. *Proc. Natl. Acad. Sci. U.S.A.* 104, 16702–16707. doi: 10.1073/pnas.0705974104

Umeda, Y., Takamiya, M., Yoshizaki, H., and Arisawa, M. (1988). Inhibition of mitogen-stimulated T lymphocyte proliferation by calcitonin gene-related peptide. *Biochem. Biophys. Res. Commun.* 154, 227–235. doi: 10.1016/0006-291X(88)90674-2

Van Nassauw, L., Adriaensen, D., and Timmermans, J. P. (2007). The bidirectional communication between neurons and mast cells within the gastrointestinal tract. *Auton. Neurosci.* 133, 91–103. doi: 10.1016/j.autneu.2006.10.003

Voedisch, S., Rochlitzer, S., Veres, T. Z., Spies, E., and Braun, A. (2012). Neuropeptides control the dynamic behavior of airway mucosal dendritic cells. *PLoS ONE* 7:e45951. doi: 10.1371/journal.pone.0045951

Vyklicky, L., Knotkova-Urbancova, H., Vitaskova, Z., Vlachova, V., Kress, M., and Reeh, P. W. (1998). Inflammatory mediators at acidic pH activate capsaicin receptors in cultured sensory neurons from newborn rats. *J. Neurophysiol.* 79, 670–676.

Wang, F., Millet, I., Bottomly, K., and Vignery, A. (1992). Calcitonin gene-related peptide inhibits interleukin 2 production by murine T lymphocytes. *J. Biol. Chem.* 267, 21052–21057.

Wang, X., Xing, L., Xing, Y., Tang, Y., and Han, C. (1999). Identification and characterization of immunoreactive calcitonin gene-related peptide from lymphocytes of the rat. *J. Neuroimmunol.* 94, 95–102. doi: 10.1016/S0165-5728(98)00230-6

Wong, C. W., O, W. S., and Tang, F. (2013). Intermedin in rat uterus: changes in gene expression and peptide levels across the estrous cycle and its effects on uterine contraction. *Reprod. Biol. Endocrinol.* 11, 13. doi: 10.1186/1477-7827-11-13

Yiangou, Y., Facer, P., Ford, A., Brady, C., Wiseman, O., Fowler, C. J., et al. (2001). Capsaicin receptor VR1 and ATP-gated ion channel P2X3 in human urinary bladder. *BJU Int.* 87, 774–779. doi: 10.1046/j.1464-410x.2001.02190.x

Zhang, L., Berta, T., Xu, Z. Z., Liu, T., Park, J. Y., and Ji, R. R. (2010a). TNF-alpha contributes to spinal cord synaptic plasticity and inflammatory pain: distinct role of TNF receptor subtypes 1 and 2. *Pain* 152, 419–427. doi: 10.1016/j.pain.2010.11.014

Zhang, X. C., Kainz, V., Burstein, R., and Levy, D. (2010b). Tumor necrosis factor-alpha induces sensitization of meningeal nociceptors mediated via local COX and p38 MAP kinase actions. *Pain* 152, 140–149. doi: 10.1016/j.pain.2010.10.002

Zhou, Y., Zhang, M., Sun, G. Y., Liu, Y. P., Ran, W. Z., Peng, L., et al. (2013). Calcitonin gene-related peptide promotes the wound healing of human bronchial epithelial cells via PKC and MAPK pathways. *Regul. Pept.* 184, 22–29. doi: 10.1016/j.regpep.2013.03.020

10

Hormonal influences on neuroimmune responses in the CNS of females

Nela Monasterio[1], Edgar Vergara[2] and Teresa Morales[1] *

[1] *Departamento de Neurobiología Celular y Molecular, Instituto de Neurobiología, Universidad Nacional Autónoma de México, Santiago de Querétaro, México*
[2] *Departamento de Biología, Facultad de Química, Universidad Nacional Autónoma de México, Ciudad de México, México*

Edited by:
Beatriz Gomez-Gonzalez, Universidad Autónoma Metropolitana – Unidad Iztapalapa, Mexico

Reviewed by:
Beatriz Gomez-Gonzalez, Universidad Autónoma Metropolitana – Unidad Iztapalapa, Mexico
George Chrousos, National and Kapodistrian University of Athens, Greece

****Correspondence:***
Teresa Morales, Departamento de Neurobiología Celular y Molecular, Instituto de Neurobiología, Universidad Nacional Autónoma de México, Boulevard Juriquilla 3001, 76230, Santiago de Querétaro, México
e-mail: marter@unam.mx

Particular reproductive stages such as lactation impose demands on the female. To cope with these demands, her physiology goes through numerous adaptations, for example, attenuation of immune and stress responses. Hormonal fluctuation during lactation exerts a strong influence, inducing neuroplasticity in the hypothalamus and extrahypothalamic regions, and diminishing the stress and inflammatory responses. Thus, hormones confer decreased vulnerability to the female brain. This mini-review focuses on the adaptations of the immune and stress response during maternity, and on the neuroprotective actions of progesterone and prolactin and their effects on inflammation. The importance of pregnancy and lactation as experimental models to study immune responses and disease is also highlighted.

Keywords: stress, progesterone, prolactin, lactation, neuroimmune, HPA axis, female

INTRODUCTION

Reproduction is one of the most significant events in the life of a mammalian female. It can be described as a rich social and hormonal experience that begins by interacting and mating with a male, followed by pregnancy, parturition, and ultimately lactation, interaction with pups, and weaning (Mann and Bridges, 2001; Serafim and Felicio, 2002). Striking behavioral and neuroendocrine alterations due to motherhood have been reported in several mammalian species including mice, rats, rabbits, sheep, and humans. They are reflected by changes at almost all brain levels and are essential to protect the developing embryo, and for successful delivery, maternal behavior, and pup survival (Kinsley and Lambert, 2008). These neuroanatomical and functional changes observed during pregnancy and lactation are necessary to cope with the demands of reproduction and to protect the maternal organism against dramatic hormonal variations (Mann and Bridges, 2001; Kinsley and Lambert, 2008). They include a marked adaptation of the hypothalamus-pituitary-adrenal (HPA) axis, which results in hypo-responsiveness to stress, diminished inflammatory responses (Walker et al., 1992; Windle et al., 1997a; Lightman et al., 1998; Tilbrook and Clarke, 2006), and diminished sensitivity of the brain of the mother against excitotoxic damage (Morales, 2011).

MECHANISMS GOVERNING THE HYPO-RESPONSIVENESS TO STRESS DURING PREGNANCY AND LACTATION

One of the best-known examples of naturally attenuated stress response is seen in the female rat during late pregnancy and lactation (Tilbrook and Clarke, 2006). During these reproductive phases, the HPA axis maintains minimal responses necessary to cope with any situation that may threaten the homeostasis of the female. This axis comprises corticotropin-releasing hormone (CRH)- and vasopressin- neurons in the paraventricular nucleus of the hypothalamus (PVN), which when stimulated, release these peptides into the median eminence to stimulate pituitary cell production of adrenocorticotropic hormone (ACTH) that reaches the adrenal cortex to release cortisol or corticosterone. HPA axis activity is regulated by glucocorticoid negative feedback on the pituitary, the PVN, and higher brain centers.

The attenuation of the stress response during pregnancy and lactation has been documented in various different stress models (Lightman et al., 2001; Russell et al., 2008). Pregnancy in the rat is accompanied by a progressive decrease in HPA axis responses to a range of psychological (Neumann et al., 1998) and physical (Brunton et al., 2005; Douglas et al., 2005) stressors particularly in the last week of pregnancy, reflected by reduced ACTH and corticosterone secretion. This hypo-responsiveness persists through parturition (Wigger et al., 1999; Neumann et al., 2003) and lactation until weaning (Windle et al., 1997b). Suppressed responses to stress in pregnancy can be explained by adaptations in both the anterior pituitary and the hypothalamus (Brunton et al., 2005; Russell et al., 2008). Corticotrophs in the pituitary are less sensitive to secretagogs (Shanks et al., 1997; Neumann et al., 1998), and CRH mRNA expression induced by stress is attenuated (Brunton et al., 2005). Moreover, HPA axis responses to immune stress in early mid pregnancy are strong and similar to that in virgins, although activation of hypothalamic vasopressin neurons, rather than CRH neurons, may be more important in the stress response in pregnancy (Ma et al., 2005; Parker et al., 2011).

Studies in lactating rats have shown a flattening of the diurnal rhythm of corticosterone secretion (Walker et al., 1992; Atkinson and Waddell, 1995) during this phase, such that the nadir levels of corticosterone rise (Stern et al., 1973; Fischer et al., 1995) and the peak evening levels decrease (Windle et al., 2013). During lactation, basal plasma concentrations of both ACTH and corticosterone increased in lactating animals compared with those in virgin rats (Shanks et al., 1997, 1999). There is also an increased basal expression of CRH mRNA in the PVN in early lactation (day 3; da Costa et al., 1996), but low basal expression of CRH mRNA by the middle phase of the lactation period (days 7–10; Windle et al., 1997a; Walker et al., 2001). However, CRH expression in response to stress is diminished at either stage (Lightman and Young, 1989; Windle et al., 1997b), similar to findings in late pregnancy (Douglas et al., 2005).

The mechanisms for this altered neuroendocrine responses include diminished CNS excitatory signaling within stress-responsive systems like the catecholaminergic brainstem and limbic circuitry (Hoffman et al., 1994; da Costa et al., 1996; Wintrip et al., 1997) as well as an altered hypothalamic and adrenomedullary catecholamine function (Patel et al., 1993; Toufexis and Walker, 1996; Windle et al., 1997a; Toufexis et al., 1998). Attenuated noradrenergic tone also underlies stress hyporesponsiveness in lactation, and is clearly dependent upon suckling (Hoffman et al., 1994; Toufexis and Walker, 1996; Toufexis et al., 1998). Moreover, opioids switch to having a net inhibitory effect on HPA activity such that naloxone treatment enhances the ACTH response to IL-1β in late pregnant rats (Brunton et al., 2009). Growing evidence for an integrated participation of many other factors besides noradrenaline and opioids that underlie altered responses to stress, include CRH (Johnstone et al., 2000; da Costa et al., 2001), oxytocin (Neumann et al., 2003; Windle et al., 2004), prolactin (PRL; Torner and Neumann, 2002), steroids and neurosteroids (Douglas et al., 2000; Brunton and Russell, 2008, 2011; **Figure 1**).

Another mechanism for the attenuation of the stress response involves nitric oxide (NO) regulation of CRH expression within the PVN. NO is present in the PVN of female rats during lactation (Popeski et al., 1999; Otukonyong et al., 2000; Monasterio and Morales, 2011), as indicated by the NO markers NADPH-diaphorase and neuronal synthase (nNOS), and its synthesis dependent on suckling (Otukonyong et al., 2000) and PRL (Vega et al., 2010). These markers increase within the PVN in response to stress in male rats, but paradoxically, basal level of NO markers are present in the PVN of lactating females whose response to stress is attenuated. The activational c-fos response and an increase in NADPH-diaphorase- and nNOS-positive cells are clearly detected in the PVN of diestrus rats after an immune challenge, but not in lactating rats. Furthermore, the total concentration of nitrates in the hypothalamus and the circulating level of corticosterone and IL-6 increase significantly after stress in diestrus, but not in lactating rats, compared to their corresponding controls. Intracerebral administration of L-NAME, a general NOS inhibitor, reverses the attenuation of the activational response to stress in the lactating rats and increases CRH expression, suggesting that sustained NO production in the PVN during lactation contributes to attenuate the neuroendocrine response to stress (Monasterio and Morales, 2011; **Figure 1**).

HPA AXIS HORMONES, PROGESTERONE, AND PROLACTIN IN THE REGULATION OF THE IMMUNE RESPONSES DURING PREGNANCY AND LACTATION

HPA AXIS AND IMMUNE RESPONSES

Cytokines, peptide hormones, neurotransmitters, and their receptors are endogenous elements of the nervous, endocrine, and immune systems. These systems share ligands and receptors that serve to communicate (Haddad et al., 2002; Elenkov and

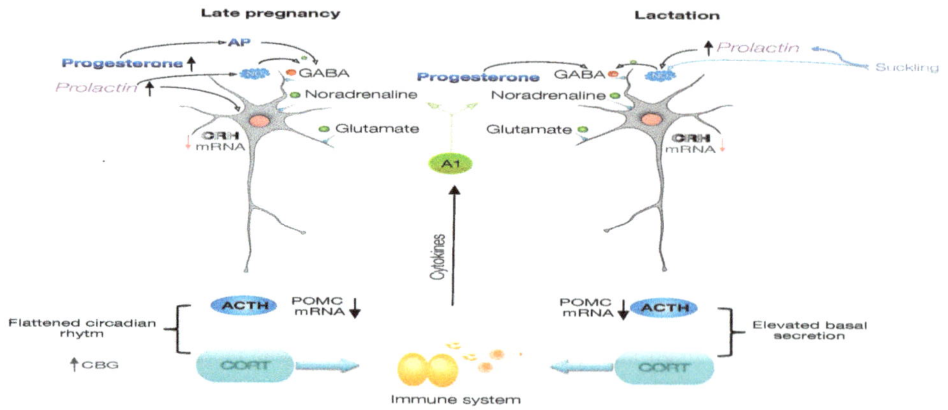

FIGURE 1 | Diagram illustrating the regulation of CRH expression in the parvocellular neurons of paraventricular nucleus of the hypothalamus. During late pregnancy and lactation, there is a diminished noradrenergic tone reaching CRH neurons, and progesterone, allopregnanolone, prolactin, and nitric oxide will contribute to the inhibitory regulation of the CRH neurons. The cascade of neuroendocrine responses, synthesis of ACTH and corticosteroids will also be modified. Neuroimmune interactions are represented by effects of glucocorticoids on cells of the immune system, and which molecules will affect CNS functions. ACTH, adrenocorticotropic hormone; AP, allopregnanolone; CRH, corticotropin-releasing hormone; CBG, corticosteroid-binding globulin; POMC, proopiomelanocortin.

Chrousos, 2006). In addition to altered endocrine responses during lactation, stress also changes immune function in comparison to non-lactating animals (Monasterio and Morales, 2011), suggesting that bi-directional communication between the immune and endocrine systems is also altered during lactation. Pregnancy and lactation represent interesting experimental models that illustrate how the elevated basal plasma level of corticosterone and the diminished stress responses, affect the immune system. It is established that dampened HPA responses are associated with increased vulnerability to inflammation (Shanks et al., 1997, 1999) and therefore, alterations in endocrine regulation of immune responses during lactation may predispose the animal to inflammatory disease. However, not all of the immune responses are dampened during pregnancy and lactation (Jaedicke et al., 2009).

Several reports have documented motherhood-induced adaptations of the immune system in female rats, showing that this is a not always an immune suppression condition (Jaedicke et al., 2009). Early pregnancy has been associated with an increased cell density in the thymus and spleen, whereas late pregnancy and lactation have been associated with a decreased cellularity despite the expansion of the thymus medulla (Kendall and Clarke, 2000). Lactation delays the return of the thymus medulla to the original pre-pregnancy state. In addition, the changes in the thymus can be attributed to the adaptation of the maternal immune system to the semi-allogeneic fetus (Kendall and Clarke, 2000). Hormonal and neural changes can partially explain these modifications. Progesterone, PRL, and estradiol levels in plasma fluctuate in early, mid, and late pregnancy (Neville et al., 2002; Brusco et al., 2008). Nerve growth factor, nearly absent in the medulla of the adult thymus, is high in the medulla of the thymus during late pregnancy (Aloe et al., 1997). Also, lactation is associated with an increased susceptibility to parasitic infections (Barger, 1993), but much controversy exists in the effects of pregnancy and lactation on the progression of autoimmune diseases as documented by studies in rodents and in humans (Elenkov et al., 2001; Buchel et al., 2002; Vukusic et al., 2004; Gregg, 2009).

The immune system of lactating rodents has been the focus of only a few studies, which have shown that some immune functions become suppressed in this phase, while others remain unaffected or are enhanced (Jaedicke et al., 2009). For example, antibody production after immunization, and IL-6 (Monasterio and Morales, 2011) and IL-2 production in the spleen (Shanks et al., 1997) were suppressed during lactation in rodents. Conversely, evidence of increased concentrations of plasma IL-6 or an enhanced proliferative response of lymphocytes from mesenteric lymph nodes suggests activation of other immune responses (Shanks et al., 1997). In male rats, activation of the HPA axis and glucocorticoid release occurs during bacterial lipopolysaccharide (LPS) exposure, triggering an elaborate inflammatory response that involves the release of the pro-inflammatory mediators IL-1β, IL-6, and tumor necrosis factor (TNF)-α (Grinevich et al., 2001), which stimulate cells to upregulate the inflammatory reaction, and systemically they activate the HPA axis (Chrousos, 1995). However, in lactating rats, LPS significantly elevates circulating levels of ACTH and corticosterone, but the magnitude of hormonal and hypothalamic responses to LPS are significantly reduced in lactating animals relative to virgin controls (Shanks et al., 1999). Despite this attenuated stress response, systemic immune responses to stressors are modulated during lactation indicating that the immune system is not generally suppressed but rather adjusted in this stage (Jaedicke et al., 2009).

In humans, the early postpartum period has been associated with up-regulated inflammatory responses and a relapse of autoimmune disorders such as rheumatoid arthritis and multiple sclerosis, often interpreted as a flare-up due to the rebound of the immune system after pregnancy (Elenkov et al., 2001; Buchel et al., 2002). However, long term-studies have shown that relapse rate of multiple sclerosis remains similar to pre-pregnancy level, after an increase in the first trimester postpartum (Vukusic et al., 2004). A broad state of immune activation is also characteristic of the early postpartum period, as measured by levels of neopterin, soluble IL-2 receptor, and soluble CD8 antigen (Burns et al., 1999). This may help women recover from the biological stress of parturition, but more studies about the magnitude and length of such a state are necessary. Immune and inflammatory activation in postpartum women may be factors leading to anxiety and depression in the early days after delivery (Maes et al., 2000). CD4 cell counts are reported to rise during postpartum, primarily due to γδ T cells (Watanabe et al., 1996). Natural killer (NK) subsets with weak cytotoxic activity (CD16+, CD57+) were found to increase during months 1–4 postpartum (Watanabe et al., 1997), and lymphocyte proliferation was higher than non-postpartum controls. Furthermore, the postpartum period is also associated with the onset of autoimmune thyroid syndrome (Muller et al., 2001). Thus, immune responses linked to reproduction can either be dampened or enhanced depending on the stimulus and hormonal status (De Bellis et al., 2005; Hughes, 2012; Shelly et al., 2012).

In summary, during both pregnancy and lactation the immune responses are altered, but instead of considering them to be immune-suppressed stages, they represent reproductive conditions in which either stress or immune responses can vary depending on the hormonal status (Mor and Cardenas, 2010). The immunology of reproduction is the result of the combination of signals and responses originating from the fetal-placental and the maternal immune systems. This last is under the regulation of the CNS through the hormonal (glucocorticoids) stress response, pituitary responses, and the autonomic nervous system.

PROGESTERONE ACTIONS ON CNS IMMUNE RESPONSES

Among the hormones that have been considered candidate inducers of pregnancy- and lactation-related adaptations in HPA axis and immune responses is progesterone. Progesterone is a steroid hormone synthesized by the corpus luteum in cycling females and by the placenta during pregnancy; it can enter the brain from the circulation and can also be synthesized in the brain by oligodendrocytes and excitatory neurons (Stein, 2011). During pregnancy, progesterone levels in plasma and brain are increased and are accompanied by elevated levels of its metabolite allopregnanolone (Brunton and Russell, 2008; Mostallino et al., 2009).

Progesterone (and its metabolite allopregnanolone) has important actions in the female's brain, such as the expression of maternal behavior (Bridges, 1984). During pregnancy, high levels of allopregnanolone suppress HPA -axis responses to stress: allopregnanolone may enhance the action of GABA in the PVN or on afferent inputs to the CRH neurons to suppress stress responses, and it also induces and maintains the endogenous inhibitory opioid mechanism in the nucleus of the solitary tract (Brunton et al., 2009). Blocking allopregnanolone restores HPA axis responses to systemically administered IL-1β in late pregnant rats (Brunton and Russell, 2008). Allopregnanolone acts as an agonist on the GABA receptor, exerting anxiolytic, sedative, and antiepileptic effects, and it enhances the myelination/remyelination process in the central and peripheral nervous system (Wang et al., 2008; Gangisetty and Reddy, 2010). These steroid hormones have been described as potent regulators of growth factor expression during pregnancy: epidermal growth factor (EGF), insulin-like growth factor (IGF), and transforming growth factor (TGF-β1) in particular are all up-regulated, promoting neural proliferation (Wang et al., 2008). Moreover, they increase neurogenesis within the subgranular zone of the dentate gyrus and subventricular zone (Pawluski et al., 2009), and induce regenerative responses in a mouse model of Alzheimer's disease (Pike et al., 2009; Borowicz et al., 2011). During lactation, progesterone participates in glial changes in brain areas such as the cingulate cortex (Salmaso et al., 2009) and the dentate gyrus of the hippocampus (Cabrera et al., 2013), and this steroid is part of the hormonal cocktail responsible for diminished responses of astrocyte and microglial cells in the hippocampus of lactating rats to damage induced by excitotoxic insults (Cabrera et al., 2013).

Progesterone and allopregnanolone attenuate traumatic brain injury, and diminish the elevation of pro-inflammatory cytokines in a time-dependent manner, suggesting that the protection occurs by limiting the overexpression of cytokines, when they peak at 3 h after a brain injury, rather than inhibiting their expression later in the post-injury cascade of toxic events (He et al., 2004). Both steroids prevent breakdown of the blood–brain barrier in edema and stroke (Ishrat et al., 2010). Progesterone exerts some of its actions through the intracellular, membrane-bound progesterone receptor, while allopregnanolone does not bind to the progesterone receptor (Ishrat et al., 2010). Also, progesterone can reduce the excessive excitotoxicity and inflammation by stimulating activation of the neuroprotective mitogen-activated protein kinase (MAPK) and PI3-K pathways (Kaur et al., 2007). Through use of calcium imaging, electrophysiology, and the measurement of changes in activity-dependent gene expression, progesterone was found to block calcium entry through voltage-gated calcium channels, leading to alterations in the signaling of the activity-dependent transcription factors nuclear factor of activated T-cells (NFAT) and cAMP response element-binding protein (CREB; Luoma et al., 2012). This effect of progesterone on calcium signaling provides a putative mechanism for its neuroprotective actions (Luoma et al., 2012). Furthermore, allopregnanolone is an allosteric modifier of the GABAA receptors expressed by oxytocin neurons (Koksma et al., 2003). Electrophysiological studies of hypothalamic oxytocin neurons showed that allopregnanolone acts via a G-protein mechanism involving protein kinase C to delay the closure of the Cl^- channel after activation (Brussaard and Koksma, 2003), enhancing both the tonic and phasic actions of GABA in oxytocin neurons. This modulatory action on GABA transmission represents an alternative candidate pathway for the protective actions of this steroid.

Progesterone also plays an important role in the periphery. Progesterone-dependent immunomodulation is one of the mechanisms that enable pregnancy to proceed to term, because it protects the fetus from immunological rejection. Recent evidence suggests that autocrine/paracrine factors such as cytokines play a crucial role, possible as effectors of steroid hormones (Agrawal et al., 2011). A growing body of evidence implicates progesterone in the establishment of an adequate immune response during pregnancy (Hirsch and Muhle, 2002; Aisemberg et al., 2013).

Thus, progesterone and its metabolite allopregnanolone are important modulators of the immune responses in the periphery and within the CNS. Such effects are aimed to diminish the impact of an acute lesion or degenerative process in the nervous system while in the periphery contributes to the regulation of immune response against the fetus (Aisemberg et al., 2013).

PROLACTIN ACTIONS ON CNS AND IMMUNE SYSTEM

Prolactin is a peptide hormone secreted from the anterior pituitary into the circulation; it is thought to cross the blood–brain barrier and is known to regulate a wide variety of physiological process (Bole-feysot et al., 1998; Grattan and Kokay, 2008). PRL is also produced in a broad spectrum of extrapituitary sites including cells of the nervous and the immune system (Montgomery, 2001; Torner et al., 2002; Ignacak et al., 2012), and it is an important mediator of the immunoneuroendocrine network. However, effects of PRL on the immune system are complex. Removal of PRL by hypophysectomy impairs thymus growth (Nagy and Berczi, 1978) and immune reaction to immunogenic factors (Bernton et al., 1988) in rats. On the other hand, hyperprolactinemia (HP), in mice injected with *Listeria monocytogenes* increases mortality associated with impaired lymphocyte proliferation and decreased macrophage-activating factor production by T lymphocytes (Bernton et al., 1988). Furthermore, a PRL-like mRNA and a secreted product have been detected in human B-lymphoblastoid cell lines (Bernton et al., 1988; Baglia et al., 1991). Peripheral blood mononuclear cells also secrete a PRL-like protein, suggesting that it binds to PRL receptors and migrates to the nucleus, where it serves as a co-mitogen and autocrine regulator of cell growth. But, there are several reports showing that PRL is not essential for the proper development and function of the mouse immune system. Using PRL-deficient animals it was shown that PRL is not required for normal hematopoiesis (Horseman et al., 1997), and that PRL receptor signaling is not required for normal immunity (Bouchard et al., 1999). PRL is known to have other contradictory actions on the immune system that depends upon the concentration: it inhibits lymphocyte proliferation at high concentrations, while having enhancing effects at lower concentrations (Matera et al., 1992).

During pregnancy in rats, PRL plasma levels are high in the first half, they decrease until term, and then rise again at postpartum and throughout lactation (Neville et al., 2002). PRL actions in early gestation are crucial to prepare the mammary gland for lactation and in the CNS to establish the appropriate adaptive behavioral responses of the mother (Grattan and Kokay, 2008) toward the pups. PRL has been related to behavioral and neuronal effects, such as maternal behavior (Mann and Bridges, 2001), attenuation of anxiety and hormonal and neuronal responses to various stressors (Lightman et al., 2001; Torner and Neumann, 2002; Donner et al., 2007), neurogenesis (Shingo et al., 2003; Torner et al., 2009; Larsen and Grattan, 2010; Walker et al., 2012), and neuroprotection (Torner et al., 2009; Tejadilla et al., 2010).

Inflammatory response after a brain injury, such as proliferation and activation of glia is enhanced by PRL (Möderscheim et al., 2007), and elevated levels of PRL stimulate mitogenesis in astrocyte and oligodendrocyte populations of the subventricular zone (Larsen and Grattan, 2010). PRL also increases oligodendrocyte precursor cell proliferation, which in turn enhances the capacity to generate new oligodendrocytes and myelination. This process is associated with the capacity to repair white matter damage in the maternal CNS by increasing myelin basic protein expression (Gregg, 2009). During lactation, a physiological hyperprolactinemic state, there is a reduced sensitivity to kainic acid-induced cell damage in the dorsal hippocampus of the dam, showing that lactation is a natural model of neuroprotection (Vanoye-Carlo et al., 2008; Cabrera et al., 2009) in which PRL can participate. PRL systemic administration has been reported to protect the dorsal hippocampus of female rats against excitotoxicity induced by kainic acid administration, blocking cell loss and neurodegeneration, and diminishing the progression of kainate-generated behavioral manifestation of seizures (Tejadilla et al., 2010). Overall, these studies on protective effects of PRL within the CNS draw attention to the importance of studying females, and the relevance of neuroendocrine–immune interactions when investigating effects of this hormone.

An interesting example of the neuroendocrine–immune interactions is seen in the HP occurring in patients with autoimmune diseases, such as rheumatoid arthritis and systemic lupus erythematosus, and with organ-specific autoimmune diseases, as celiac disease, type 1 diabetes mellitus, Addison's disease, autoimmune thyroid diseases (reviewed by, De Bellis et al., 2005). In these diseases PRL increases the synthesis of IFNγ and IL-2 by Th1 lymphocytes. Moreover, PRL activates Th2 lymphocytes with autoantibody production. The inhibitory effects of IL-1ß on the tuberoinfundibular dopaminergic neurons that inhibit PRL secretion could explain this HP. González et al. (2004), showed that i.c.v. injection of LPS in rats, produces a decrease in tyrosine hydroxylase (TH) activity in the medial eminence, an increase in the serum levels of PRL, and a decrease in the number of TH- and TH mRNA-positive cells in the arcuate nucleus, indicating that dopamine neurons of the hypothalamus are functionally susceptible to local inflammatory stimuli. Additionally, treatment with the dopamine-agonist, bromocriptine, inhibits both PRL secretion and the severity of acute experimental encephalomyelitis (Riskind et al., 1991). This is an example of how molecules of the immune system could affect the neurons in the hypothalamus increasing the secretion of PRL, which in its turn will enhance peripheral inflammatory responses.

CONCLUSION

In summary, during pregnancy and lactation, responses of the HPA axis and the immune system are altered and clearly regulated by suckling and hormone fluctuation. Pregnancy and lactation are the most important periods for the conservation of the species, and they represent fundamental stages at which both mother and offspring must be protected. The immune system is crucial to protect the mother and the product against the environment and there is evidence supporting the notion that immunity is suppressed during motherhood. In this sense, the immune responses of the mother should be adjusted to conserve defenses, but should be tuned to preserve the developing offspring (Mor and Cardenas, 2010). Therefore, pregnancy and lactation are unique conditions in which the immune system is modulated or adjusted, but not fully suppressed.

AUTHOR CONTRIBUTIONS

Nela Monasterio conceived the main premises that are the focus of this review and wrote the largest portion of the paper; Edgar Vergara wrote important subsections of the paper; and Teresa Morales conceived the main premises that are the focus of this review, designed the structure of the paper, wrote a large portion of the paper, and edited the final version.

ACKNOWLEDGMENTS

The authors thank Dr. Dorothy Pless for grammatical review. Cited work from our group was supported by PAPIIT-DGAPA, UNAM, and CONACYT, México. We are grateful to the reviewers whose comments help to improve this work.

REFERENCES

Agrawal, V., Jaiswal, M. K., and Jaiswal, Y. K. (2011). Lipopolysaccharide induces alterations in ovaries and serum level of progesterone and 17β-estradiol in the mouse. *Fertil. Steril.* 95, 1471–1474. doi: 10.1016/j.fertnstert.2010.08.046

Aisemberg, J., Vercelli, C. A., Bariani, M. V., Billi, S. C., Wolfson, M. L., and Franchi, A. M. (2013). Progesterone is essential for protecting against LPS-induced pregnancy loss. LIF as a potential mediator of the anti-inflammatory effect of progesterone. *PLoS ONE* 8:e56161. doi: 10.1371/ journal.pone.0056161

Aloe, L., Bracci-Laudiero, L., Bonini, S., and Manni, L. (1997). The expanding role of nerve growth factor: from neurotrophic activity to immunologic diseases. *Allergy* 52, 883–894. doi: 10.1111/j.1398-9995.1997.tb01247.x

Atkinson, H. C., and Waddell, B. J. (1995). The hypothalamic-pituitary-adrenal axis in rat pregnancy and lactation: circadian variation and interrelationship of plasma adrenocorticotropin and corticosterone. *Endocrinology* 136, 512–520. doi: 10.1210/en.136.2.512

Baglia, L. A., Cruz, D., and Shaw, J. E. (1991). An Epstein-Barr virus-negative Burkitt lymphoma cell line (sfRamos) secretes a prolactin-like protein during continuous growth in serum-free medium. *Endocrinology* 128, 2266–2272. doi: 10.1210/endo-128-5-2266

Barger, I. A. (1993). Influence of sex and reproductive status on susceptibility of ruminants to nematode parasitism. *Int. J. Parasitol.* 23, 463–469. doi: 10.1016/0020-7519(93)90034-V

Bernton, E. W., Meltzer, M. S., and Holaday, J. W. (1988). Suppression of macrophage activation and T-lymphocyte function in hypoprolactinemic mice. *Science* 239, 401–404. doi: 10.1126/science.3122324

Bole-feysot, C., Goffin, V., Edery, M., Binart, N., and Kelly, P. A. (1998). Prolactin (PRL) and its receptor: actions, signal transduction pathways and phenotypes observed in PRL receptor knockout mice. *Endocr. Rev.* 19, 225–268. doi: 10.1210/er.19.3.225

Borowicz, K. K., Piskorska, B., Banach, M., and Czuczwar, S. J. (2011). Neuroprotective actions of neurosteroids. *Front. Endocrinol.* 2:50. doi: 10.3389/fendo.2011.00050

Bouchard, B., Ormandy, C. J., Di Santo, J. P., and Kelly, P. A. (1999). Immune system development and function in prolactin receptor-deficient mice. *J. Immunol.* 163, 576–582.

Bridges, R. S. (1984). A quantitative analysis of the roles of dosage, sequence, and duration of estradiol and progesterone exposure in the regulation of maternal behavior in the rat. *Endocrinology* 114, 930–940. doi: 10.1210/endo-114-3-930

Brunton, P. J., McKay, A. J., Ochedalski, T., Piastowska, A., Rebas, E., Lachowicz, A., et al. (2009). Central opioid inhibition of neuroendocrine stress responses in pregnancy in the rat is induced by the neurosteroid allopregnanolone. *J. Neurosci.* 29, 6449–6460. doi: 10.1523/JNEUROSCI.0708-09.2009

Brunton, P. J., Meddle, S. L., Ma, S., Ochedalski, T., Douglas, A. J., and Russell, J. A. (2005). Endogenous opioids and attenuated hypothalamic-pituitary-adrenal axis responses to immune challenge in pregnant rats. *J. Neurosci.* 25, 5117–5126. doi: 10.1523/JNEUROSCI.0866-05.2005

Brunton, P. J., and Russell, J. A. (2008). Attenuated hypothalamo-pituitary-adrenal axis responses to immune challenge during pregnancy: the neurosteroid opioid connection. *J. Physiol.* 586, 369–375. doi: 10.1113/jphysiol.2007.146233

Brunton, P. J., and Russell, J. A. (2011). Allopregnanolone and suppressed hypothalamo-pituitary-adrenal axis stress responses in late pregnancy in the rat. *Stress* 14, 6–12. doi: 10.3109/10253890.2010.482628

Brusco, J., Wittmann, R., de Azevedo, M. S., Lucion, A. B., Franci, C. R., Giovenardi, M., et al. (2008). Plasma hormonal profiles and dendritic spine density and morphology in the hippocampal CA1 stratum radiatum, evidenced by light microscopy, of virgin and postpartum female rats. *Neurosci. Lett.* 438, 346–350. doi: 10.1016/j.neulet.2008.04.063

Brussaard, A. B., and Koksma, J.-J. (2003). Conditional regulation of neurosteroid sensitivity of GABAA receptors. *Ann. N. Y. Acad. Sci.* 1007, 29–36. doi: 10.1196/annals.1286.003

Buchel, E., Van Steenbergen, W., Nevens, F., and Fevery, J. (2002). Improvement of autoimmune hepatitis during pregnancy followed by flare-up after delivery. *Am. J. Gastroenterol.* 97, 3160–3165. doi: 10.1111/j.1572-0241.2002.07124.x

Burns, D. N., Nourjah, P., Wright, D. J., Minkoff, H., Landesman, S., Rubinstein, A., et al. (1999). Changes in immune activation markers during pregnancy and postpartum. *J. Reprod. Immunol.* 42, 147–165. doi: 10.1016/S0165-0378(98)00085-0

Cabrera, V., Cantú, D., Ramos, E., Vanoye-Carlo, A., Cerbón, M., and Morales, T. (2009). Lactation is a natural model of hippocampus neuroprotection against excitotoxicity. *Neurosci. Lett.* 461, 136–139. doi: 10.1016/j.neulet.2009.06.017

Cabrera, V., Ramos, E., González-Arenas, A., Cerbón, M., Camacho, I., and Morales, T. (2013). Lactation reduces glial activation induced by excitotoxicity in the rat hippocampus. *J. Neuroendocrinol.* 25, 519–527. doi: 10.1111/jne.12028

Chrousos, G. P. (1995). The hypothalamic-pituitary-adrenal axis and immune-mediated inflammation. *N. Engl. J. Med.* 332, 1351–1362. doi: 10.1056/NEJM199505183322008

da Costa, A. P., Ma, X., Ingram, C. D., Lightman, S. L., and Aguilera, G. (2001). Hypothalamic and amygdaloid corticotropin-releasing hormone (CRH) and CRH receptor-1 mRNA expression in the stress-hyporesponsive late pregnant and early lactating rat. *Brain Res. Mol. Brain Res.* 91, 119–130. doi: 10.1016/S0169-328X(01)00137-1

da Costa, A. P., Wood, S., Ingram, C. D., and Lightman, S. L. (1996). Region-specific reduction in stress-induced c-fos mRNA expression during pregnancy and lactation. *Brain Res.* 742, 177–184. doi: 10.1016/S0006-8993(96)00962-6

De Bellis, A., Bizzarro, A., Pivonello, R., Lombardi, G., and Bellastella, A. (2005). Prolactin and autoimmunity. *Pituitary* 8, 25–30. doi: 10.1007/s11102-005-5082-5

Donner, N., Bredewold, R., Maloumby, R., and Neumann, I. D. (2007). Chronic intracerebral prolactin attenuates neuronal stress circuitries in virgin rats. *Eur. J. Neurosci.* 25, 1804–1814. doi: 10.1111/j.1460-9568.2007.05416.x

Douglas, A. J., Johnstone, H., Brunton, P., and Russell, J. A. (2000). Sex-steroid induction of endogenous opioid inhibition on oxytocin secretory responses to stress. *J. Neuroendocrinol.* 12, 343–350. doi: 10.1046/j.1365-2826.2000.00460.x

Douglas, A. J., Meddle, S. L., Toschi, N., Bosch, O. J., and Neumann, I. D. (2005). Reduced activity of the noradrenergic system in the paraventricular nucleus at the end of pregnancy: implications for stress hyporesponsiveness. *J. Neuroendocrinol.* 17, 40–48. doi: 10.1111/j.1365-2826.2005.01272.x

Elenkov, I. J., and Chrousos, G. P. (2006). Stress system–organization, physiology and immunoregulation. *Neuroimmunomodulation* 13, 257–267. doi: 10.1159/000104853

Elenkov, I. J., Wilder, R. L., Bakalov, V. K., Link, A. A., Dimitrov, M. A., Fisher, S., et al. (2001). IL-12, TNF-alpha, and hormonal changes during late pregnancy and early postpartum: implications for autoimmune disease activity during these times. *J. Clin. Endocrinol. Metab.* 86, 4933–4938. doi: 10.1210/jc.86.10.4933

Fischer, D., Patchev, V. K., Hellbach, S., Hassan, A. H., and Almeida, O. F. (1995). Lactation as a model for naturally reversible hypercorticalism plasticity in the mechanisms governing hypothalamo-pituitary- adrenocortical activity in rats. *J. Clin. Invest.* 96, 1208–1215. doi: 10.1172/JCI118153

Gangisetty, O., and Reddy, D. S. (2010). Neurosteroid withdrawal regulates GABA-A receptor α4-subunit expression and seizure susceptibility by activation of progesterone receptor-independent early growth response factor-3 pathway. *Neuroscience* 170, 865–880. doi: 10.1016/j.neuroscience.2010.07.037

González, M. C., Abreu, P., Barroso-Chinea, P., Cruz-Muros, I., and González-Hernández, T. (2004). Effect of intracerebroventricular injection of lipopolysaccharide on the tuberoinfundibular dopaminergic system of the rat. *Neuroscience* 127, 251–259. doi: 10.1016/j.neuroscience.2004.04.057

Grattan, D. R., and Kokay, I. C. (2008). Prolactin: a pleiotropic neuroendocrine hormone. *J. Neuroendocrinol.* 20, 752–763. doi: 10.1111/j.1365-2826.2008.01736.x

Gregg, C. (2009). Pregnancy, prolactin and white matter regeneration. *J. Neurol. Sci.* 285, 22–27. doi: 10.1016/j.jns.2009.06.040

Grinevich, V., Ma, X. M., Herman, J. P., Jezova, D., Akmayev, I., and Aguilera, G. (2001). Effect of repeated lipopolysaccharide administration on tissue cytokine expression and hypothalamic-pituitary-adrenal axis activity in rats. *J. Neuroendocrinol.* 13, 711–723. doi: 10.1046/j.1365-2826.2001.00684.x

Haddad, J. J., Saadé, N. E., and Safieh-Garabedian, B. (2002). Cytokines and neuro-immune-endocrine interactions: a role for the hypothalamic-pituitary-adrenal revolving axis. *J. Neuroimmunol.* 133, 1–19. doi: 10.1016/S0165-5728(02)00357-0

He, J., Evans, C.-O., Hoffman, S. W., Oyesiku, N. M., and Stein, D. G. (2004). Progesterone and allopregnanolone reduce inflammatory cytokines after traumatic brain injury. *Exp. Neurol.* 189, 404–412. doi: 10.1016/j.expneurol.2004.06.008

Hirsch, E., and Muhle, R. (2002). Intrauterine bacterial inoculation induces labor in the mouse by mechanisms other than progesterone withdrawal. *Biol. Reprod.* 67, 1337–1341. doi: 10.1095/biolreprod67.4.1337

Hoffman, G. E., Le, W. W., Abbud, R., Lee, W. S., and Smith, M. S. (1994). Use of Fos-related antigens (FRAs) as markers of neuronal activity: FRA changes in dopamine neurons during proestrus, pregnancy and lactation. *Brain Res.* 654, 207–215. doi: 10.1016/0006-8993(94)90481-2

Horseman, N. D., Zhao, W., Montecino-Rodriguez, E., Tanaka, M., Nakashima, K., Engle, S. J., et al. (1997). Defective mammopoiesis, but normal hematopoiesis, in mice with a targeted disruption of the prolactin gene. *EMBO J.* 16, 6926–6935. doi: 10.1093/emboj/16.23.6926

Hughes, G. C. (2012). Progesterone and autoimmune disease. *Autoimmun. Rev.* 11, A502–A514. doi: 10.1016/j.autrev.2011.12.003

Ignacak, A., Kasztelnik, M., and Sliwa, T. (2012). Prolactin–not only lactotrophin. A "new" view of the "old" hormone. *J. Physiol. Pharmacol.* 63, 435–443.

Ishrat, T., Sayeed, I., Atif, F., Hua, F., and Stein, D. G. (2010). Progesterone and allopregnanolone attenuate blood-brain barrier dysfunction following permanent focal ischemia by regulating the expression of matrix metalloproteinases. *Exp. Neurol.* 226, 183–190. doi: 10.1016/j.expneurol.2010.08.023

Jaedicke, K. M., Fuhrmann, M. D., and Stefanski, V. (2009). Lactation modifies stress-induced immune changes in laboratory rats. *Brain. Behav. Immun.* 23, 700–708. doi: 10.1016/j.bbi.2009.02.005

Johnstone, H. A., Wigger, A., Douglas, A. J., Neumann, I. D., Landgraf, R., Seckl, J. R., et al. (2000). Attenuation of hypothalamic-pituitary-adrenal axis stress responses in late pregnancy: changes in feedforward and feedback mechanisms. *J. Neuroendocrinol.* 12, 811–822. doi: 10.1046/j.1365-2826.2000.00525.x

Kaur, P., Jodhka, P. K., Underwood, W. A., Bowles, C. A., de Fiebre, N. C., de Fiebre, C. M. et al. (2007). Progesterone increases brain-derived neuroptrophic factor expression and protects against glutamate toxicity in a mitogen-activated protein kinase- and phosphoinositide-3 kinase-dependent manner in cerebral cortical explants. *J. Neurosci. Res.* 85, 2441–2449. doi: 10.1002/jnr.21370

Kendall, M. D., and Clarke, A. G. (2000). The thymus in the mouse changes its activity during pregnancy: a study of the microenvironment. *J. Anat.* 197(Pt 3), 393–411. doi: 10.1046/j.1469-7580.2000.19730393.x

Kinsley, C. H., and Lambert, K. G. (2008). Reproduction-induced neuroplasticity: natural behavioural and neuronal alterations associated with the production and care of offspring. *J. Neuroendocrinol.* 20, 515–525. doi: 10.1111/j.1365-2826.2008.01667

Koksma, J.-J., van Kesteren, R. E., Rosahl, T. W., Zwart, R., Smit, A. B., Lüddens, H., et al. (2003). Oxytocin regulates neurosteroid modulation of GABA(A) receptors in supraoptic nucleus around parturition. *J. Neurosci.* 23, 788–797.

Larsen, C. M., and Grattan, D. R. (2010). Prolactin-induced mitogenesis in the subventricular zone of the maternal brain during early pregnancy is essential for normal postpartum behavioral responses in the mother. *Endocrinology* 151, 3805–3814. doi: 10.1210/en.20091385

Lightman, S. L., Windle, R., Da Costa, A., Shanks, N., and Ingram, C. (1998). "Lactation: a physiological model of stress hyporesponsiveness of the neuroendocrine system," in *New Frontiers in Stress Research. Modulation of Brain Function*, eds A. Levy, E. Grauer, D. Ben-Nathan, and E. R. de Kloet (Switzerland: Harwood Academic Publishers GmbH), 59–71.

Lightman, S. L., Windle, R. J., Wood, S. A., Kershaw, Y. M., Shanks, N., and Ingram, C. D. (2001). Peripartum plasticity within the hypothalamo-pituitary-adrenal axis. *Prog. Brain Res.* 133, 111–129. doi: 10.1016/S0079-6123(01)33009-1

Lightman, S. L., and Young, W. S. III. (1989). Lactation inhibits stress-mediated secretion of corticosterone and oxytocin and hypothalamic accumulation of corticotropin-releasing factor and enkephalin messenger ribonucleic acids. *Endocrinology* 124, 2358–2364. doi: 10.1210/endo-124-5-2358

Luoma, J. I., Stern, C. M., and Mermelstein, P. G. (2012). Progesterone inhibition of neuronal calcium signaling underlies aspects of progesterone-mediated neuroprotection. *J. Steroid Biochem. Mol. Biol.* 131, 30–36. doi: 10.1016/j.jsbmb.2011.11.002

Ma, S., Shipston, M. J., Morilak, D., and Russell, J. A. (2005). Reduced hypothalamic vasopressin secretion underlies attenuated adrenocorticotropin stress responses in pregnant rats. *Endocrinology* 146, 1626–1637. doi: 10.1210/en.2004-1368

Maes, M., Lin, A. H., Ombelet, W., Stevens, K., Kenis, G., De Jongh, R., et al. (2000). Immune activation in the early puerperium is related to postpartum anxiety and depressive symptoms. *Psychoneuroendocrinology* 25, 121–137. doi: 10.1016/S0306-4530(99)00043-8

Mann, P. E., and Bridges, R. S. (2001). Lactogenic hormone regulation of maternal behavior. *Prog. Brain Res.* 133, 251–262. doi: 10.1016/S0079-6123(01)33019-4

Matera, L., Cesano, A., Bellone, G., and Oberholtzer, E. (1992). Modulatory effect of prolactin on the resting and mitogen-induced activity of T, B, and NK lymphocytes. *Brain Behav. Immun.* 6, 409–417. doi: 10.1016/0889-1591(92)90039-Q

Möderscheim, T. A. E., Gorba, T., Pathipati, P., Kokay, I. C., Grattan, D. R., Williams, C. E., et al. (2007). Prolactin is involved in glial responses following a focal injury to the juvenile rat brain. *Neuroscience* 145, 963–973. doi: 10.1016/j.neuroscience.2006.12.053

Monasterio, N., and Morales, T. (2011). Nitric oxide has a role in attenuating the neuroendocrine response to anaphylactoid stress during lactation. *Brain Res.* 1402, 54–66. doi: 10.1016/j.brainres.2011.05.062

Montgomery, D. W. (2001). Prolactin production by immune cells. *Lupus* 10, 665–675. doi: 10.1191/096120301717164895

Mor, G., and Cardenas, I. (2010). The immune system in pregnancy: a unique complexity. *Am. J. Reprod. Immunol.* 63, 425–433. doi: 10.1111/j.1600-0897.2010.00836.x

Morales, T. (2011). Recent findings on neuroprotection against excitotoxicity in the hippocampus of female rats. *J. Neuroendocrinol.* 23, 994–1001. doi: 10.1111/j.1365-2826.2011.02141.x

Mostallino, M. C., Sanna, E., Concas, A., Biggio, G., and Follesa, P. (2009). Plasticity and function of extrasynaptic GABA(A) receptors during pregnancy and after delivery. *Psychoneuroendocrinology* 34(Suppl. 1), S74–S83. doi: 10.1016/j.psyneuen.2009.06.013

Muller, A. F., Drexhage, H. A., and Berghout, A. (2001). Postpartum thyroiditis and autoimmune thyroiditis in women of childbearing age: recent insights and consequences for antenatal and postnatal care. *Endocr. Rev.* 22, 605–630. doi: 10.1210/er.22.5.605

Nagy, E., and Berczi, I. (1978). Immunodeficiency in hypophysectomized rats. *Acta Endocrinol.* 89, 530–537. doi: 10.1530/acta.0.0890530

Neumann, I. D., Bosch, O. J., Toschi, N., Torner, L., and Douglas, A. J. (2003). No stress response of the hypothalamo-pituitary-adrenal axis in parturient rats: lack of involvement of brain oxytocin. *Endocrinology* 144, 2473–2479. doi: 10.1210/en.2003-0037

Neumann, I. D., Johnstone, H. A., Hatzinger, M., Liebsch, G., Shipston, M., Russell, J. A., et al. (1998). Attenuated neuroendocrine responses to emotional and physical stressors in pregnant rats involve adenohypophysial changes. *J. Physiol.* 508(Pt 1), 289–300. doi: 10.1111/j.1469-7793.1998.289br.x

Neville, M. C., McFadden, T. B., and Forsyth, I. (2002). Hormonal regulation of mammary differentiation and milk secretion. *J. Mammary Gland Biol. Neoplasia* 7, 49–66. doi: 10.1023/A:1015770423167

Otukonyong, E. E., Okere, C. O., Johnstone, L. E., Murata, T., Kaba, H., and Higuchi, T. (2000). Effect of suckling on NADPH-diaphorase (Nitric oxide synthase, NOS) reactivity and NOS gene expression in the paraventricular and supraoptic nuclei of lactating rats. *J. Neuroendocrinol.* 12, 1001–1008. doi: 10.1046/j.1365-2826.2000.00548.x

Parker, V. J., Menzies, J. R., and Douglas, A. J. (2011). Differential changes in the hypothalamic-pituitary-adrenal axis and prolactin responses to stress in early pregnant mice. *J. Neuroendocrinol.* 23, 1066–1078. doi: 10.1111/j.1365-2826.2011.02204.x

Patel, H., Chowdrey, H. S., Jessop, D. S., and Lightman, S. L. (1993). Hormonal responses to central alpha-1 receptor stimulation during lactation. *Ann. N. Y. Acad. Sci.* 689, 489–491. doi: 10.1111/j.1749-6632.1993.tb55577.x

Pawluski, J. L., Brummelte, S., Barha, C. K., Crozier, T. M., and Galea, L. A. (2009). Effects of steroid hormones on neurogenesis in the hippocampus of the adult female rodent during the estrous cycle, pregnancy, lactation and aging. *Front. Neuroendocrinol.* 30:343–357. doi: 10.1016/j.yfrne.2009.03.007

Pike, C. J., Carroll, J. C., Rosario, E. R., and Barron, A. M. (2009). Protective actions of sex steroid hormones in Alzheimer's disease. *Front. Neuroendocrinol.* 30:239–258. doi: 10.1016/j.yfrne.2009.04.015

Popeski, N., Amir, S., and Woodside, B. (1999). Changes in NADPH-d staining in the paraventricular and supraoptic nuclei during pregnancy and lactation in rats: role of ovarian steroids and oxytocin. *J. Neuroendocrinol.* 11, 53–61. doi: 10.1046/j.1365-2826.1999.00291.x

Riskind, P. N., Massacesi, L., Doolittle, T. H., and Hauser, S. L. (1991). The role of prolactin in autoimmune demyelination: suppression of experimental allergic encephalomyelitis by bromocriptine. *Ann. Neurol.* 29, 542–547. doi: 10.1002/ana.410290514

Russell, J. A., Douglas, A. J., and Brunton, P. J. (2008). Reduced hypothalamo-pituitary-adrenal axis stress responses in late pregnancy: central opioid inhibition and noradrenergic mechanisms. *Ann. N. Y. Acad. Sci.* 1148, 428–438. doi: 10.1196/annals.1410.032

Salmaso, N., Nadeau, J., and Woodside, B. (2009). Steroid hormones and maternal experience interact to induce glial plasticity in the cingulate cortex. *Eur. J. Neurosci.* 29, 786–794. doi: 10.1111/j.1460-9568.2009.06627.x

Serafim, A. P., and Felicio, L. F. (2002). Reproductive experience influences grooming behavior during pregnancy in rats. *Braz. J. Med. Biol. Res.* 35, 391–394. doi: 10.1590/S0100-879X2002000300016

Shanks, N., Kusnecov, A., Pezzone, M., Berkun, J., and Rabin, B. S. (1997). Lactation alters the effects of conditioned stress on immune function. *Am. J. Physiol.* 272, R16–R25.

Shanks, N., Windle, R. J., Perks, P., Wood, S., Ingram, C. D., and Lightman, S. L. (1999). The hypothalamic-pituitary-adrenal axis response to endotoxin is attenuated during lactation. *J. Neuroendocrinol.* 11, 857–865. doi: 10.1046/j.1365-2826.1999.00400.x

Shelly, S., Boaz, M., and Orbach, H. (2012). Prolactin and autoimmunity. *Autoimmun. Rev.* 11, A465–A470. doi: 10.1016/j.autrev.2011.11.009

Shingo, T., Gregg, C., Enwere, E., Fujikawa, H., Hassam, R., Geary, C., et al. (2003). Pregnancy-stimulated neurogenesis in the adult female forebrain mediated by prolactin. *Science* 299, 117–120. doi: 10.1126/science.1076647

Stein, D. G. (2011). Progesterone in the treatment of acute traumatic brain injury: a clinical perspective and update. *Neuroscience* 191, 101–106. doi: 10.1016/j.neuroscience.2011.04.013

Stern, J. M., Goldman, L., and Levine, S. (1973). Pituitary-adrenal responsiveness during lactation in rats. *Neuroendocrinology* 12, 179–191. doi: 10.1159/000122167

Tejadilla, D., Cerbón, M., and Morales, T. (2010). Prolactin reduces the damaging effects of excitotoxicity in the dorsal hippocampus of the female rat independently of ovarian hormones. *Neuroscience* 169, 1178–1185. doi: 10.1016/j.neuroscience.2010.05.074

Tilbrook, A. J., and Clarke, I. J. (2006). Neuroendocrine mechanisms of innate states of attenuated responsiveness of the hypothalamo-pituitary adrenal axis to stress. *Front. Neuroendocrinol.* 27:285–307. doi: 10.1016/j.yfrne.2006.06.002

Torner, L., Karg, S., Blume, A., Kandasamy, M., Kuhn, H.-G., Winkler, J., et al. (2009). Prolactin prevents chronic stress-induced decrease of adult hippocampal neurogenesis and promotes neuronal fate. *J. Neurosci.* 29, 1826–1833. doi: 10.1523/JNEUROSCI.3178-08.2009

Torner, L., and Neumann, I. D. (2002). The brain prolactin system: involvement in stress response adaptations in lactation. *Stress* 5, 249–257. doi: 10.1080/1025389021000048638

Torner, L., Toschi, N., Nava, G., Clapp, C., and Neumann, I. D. (2002). Increased hypothalamic expression of prolactin in lactation: involvement in behavioural and neuroendocrine stress responses. *Eur. J. Neurosci.* 15, 1381–1389. doi: 10.1046/j.1460-9568.2002.01965.x

Toufexis, D. J., Thrivikraman, K. V., Plotsky, P. M., Morilak, D. A., Huang, N., and Walker, C. D. (1998). Reduced noradrenergic tone to the hypothalamic paraventricular nucleus contributes to the stress hyporesponsiveness of lactation. *J. Neuroendocrinol.* 10, 417–427. doi: 10.1046/j.1365-2826.1998.00223.x

Toufexis, D. J., and Walker, C. D. (1996). Noradrenergic facilitation of the adrenocorticotropin response to stress is absent during lactation in the rat. *Brain Res.* 737, 71–77. doi: 10.1016/0006-8993(96)00627-0

Vanoye-Carlo, A., Morales, T., Ramos, E., Mendoza-Rodríguez, A., and Cerbón, M. (2008). Neuroprotective effects of lactation against kainic acid treatment in the dorsal hippocampus of the rat. *Horm. Behav.* 53, 112–123. doi: 10.1016/j.yhbeh.2007.09.004

Vega, C., Moreno-Carranza, B., Zamorano, M., Quintanar-Stéphano, A., Méndez, I., Thebault, S., et al. (2010). Prolactin promotes oxytocin and vasopressin release by activating neuronal nitric oxide synthase in the supraoptic and paraventricular nuclei. *Am. J. Physiol. Regul. Integr. Comp. Physiol.* 299, R1701–R1708. doi: 10.1152/ajpregu.00575.2010

Vukusic, S., Hutchinson, M., Hours, M., Moreau, T., Cortinovis-Tourniaire, P., Adeleine, P., et al. (2004). Pregnancy and multiple sclerosis (the PRIMS study): clinical predictors of post-partum relapse. *Brain* 127, 1353–1360. doi: 10.1093/brain/awh152

Walker, C. D., Lightman, S. L., Steele, M. K., and Dallman, M. F. (1992). Suckling is a persistent stimulus to the adrenocortical system of the rat. *Endocrinology* 130, 115–125. doi: 10.1210/en.130.1.115

Walker, C. D., Toufexis, D. J., and Burlet, A. (2001). Hypothalamic and limbic expression of CRF and vasopressin during lactation: implications for the control of ACTH secretion and stress hyporesponsiveness. *Prog. Brain Res.* 133, 99–110. doi: 10.1016/S0079-6123(01)33008-X

Walker, T. L., Vukovic, J., Koudijs, M. M., Blackmore, D. G., Mackay, E. W., Sykes, A. M., et al. (2012). Prolactin stimulates precursor cells in the adult mouse hippocampus. *PLoS ONE* 7:e44371. doi: 10.1371/journal.pone.0044371

Wang, J. M., Liu, L., Irwin, R. W., Chen, S., and Brinton, R. D. (2008). Regenerative potential of allopregnanolone. *Brain Res. Rev.* 57, 398–409. doi: 10.1016/j.brainresrev.2007.08.010

Watanabe, M., Iwatani, Y., Hidaka, Y., Mitsuda, N., and Amino, N. (1996). Changes in soluble CD4 and CD8 proteins in healthy pregnant and postpartum women. *Am. J. Reprod. Immunol.* 36, 220–227. doi: 10.1111/j.1600-0897.1996.tb00167.x

Watanabe, M., Iwatani, Y., Kaneda, T., Hidaka, Y., Mitsuda, N., Morimoto, Y., et al. (1997). Changes in T, B, and NK lymphocyte subsets during and after normal pregnancy. *Am. J. Reprod. Immunol.* 37, 368–377. doi: 10.1111/j.1600-0897.1997.tb00246.x

Wigger, A., Lörscher, P., Oehler, I., Keck, M. E., Naruo, T., and Neumann, I. D. (1999). Nonresponsiveness of the rat hypothalamo-pituitary-adrenocortical axis to parturition-related events: inhibitory action of endogenous opioids. *Endocrinology* 140, 2843–2849. doi: 10.1210/en.140.6.2843

Windle, R. J., Brady, M. M., Kunanandam, T., Da Costa, A. P., Wilson, B. C., Harbuz, M., et al. (1997a). Reduced response of the hypothalamo-pituitary-adrenal axis to alpha1-agonist stimulation during lactation. *Endocrinology* 138, 3741–3748. doi: 10.1210/en.138.9.3741

Windle, R. J., Wood, S., Shanks, N., Perks, P., Conde, G. L., da Costa, A. P., et al. (1997b). Endocrine and behavioural responses to noise stress: comparison of virgin and lactating female rats during non-disrupted maternal activity. *J. Neuroendocrinol.* 9, 407–414. doi: 10.1046/j.1365-2826.1997.00587.x

Windle, R. J., Kershaw, Y. M., Shanks, N., Wood, S. A., Lightman, S. L., and Ingram, C. D. (2004). Oxytocin attenuates stress-induced c-fos mRNA expression in specific forebrain regions associated with modulation of hypothalamo-pituitary-adrenal activity. *J. Neurosci.* 24, 2974–2982. doi: 10.1523/JNEUROSCI.3432-03.2004

Windle, R. J., Wood, S. A., Kershaw, Y. M., Lightman, S. L., and Ingram, C. D. (2013). Adaptive changes in basal and stress-induced HPA activity in lactating and post-lactating female rats. *Endocrinology* 154, 749–761. doi: 10.1210/en.2012-1779

Wintrip, N., Nance, D. M., and Wilkinson, M. (1997). The effect of lactation on induced Fos-like immunoreactivity in the rat hypothalamic paraventricular nucleus. *Brain Res.* 754, 113–120. doi: 10.1016/S0006-8993(97)00063-2

Conflict of Interest Statement: The authors declare that the research was conducted in the absence of any commercial or financial relationships that could be construed as a potential conflict of interest.

11

Kynurenines in CNS disease: regulation by inflammatory cytokines

Brian M. Campbell, Erik Charych, Anna W. Lee and Thomas Möller*

Neuroinflammation Disease Biology Unit, Lundbeck Research USA, Paramus, NJ, USA

Edited by:
Adam Denes, University of Manchester, UK

Reviewed by:
Robert Schwarcz, Maryland Psychiatric Research Center, USA
Robert Dantzer, MD Anderson Cancer Center, USA

***Correspondence:**
Thomas Möller, Neuroinflammation Disease Biology Unit, Lundbeck Research USA, 215 College Rd., Paramus, NJ 07652, USA
e-mail: tmoe@lundbeck.com

The kynurenine pathway (KP) metabolizes the essential amino acid tryptophan and generates a number of neuroactive metabolites collectively called the kynurenines. Segregated into at least two distinct branches, often termed the "neurotoxic" and "neuroprotective" arms of the KP, they are regulated by the two enzymes kynurenine 3-monooxygenase and kynurenine aminotransferase, respectively. Interestingly, several enzymes in the pathway are under tight control of inflammatory mediators. Recent years have seen a tremendous increase in our understanding of neuroinflammation in CNS disease. This review will focus on the regulation of the KP by inflammatory mediators as it pertains to neurodegenerative and psychiatric disorders.

Keywords: kynurenine, neuroinflammation, microglia, astrocytes, CNS disease, IDO, KMO, KAT

THE KYNURENINE PATHWAY

The metabolic fate of tryptophan (TRP), an essential amino acid, is conversion into a variety of neuroactive substances including the well-known neurotransmitters serotonin and melatonin, as well as a range of kynurenine metabolites such as kynurenic acid (KYNA), 3-hydroxykynurenine (3-HK), and quinolinic acid (QUIN). Enzymes involved in the metabolism of tryptophan along the kynurenine pathway (KP) are located thoughout the body and brain. Though the highest levels are found in the liver and kidney, all of the primary enzymes are also found within the brain. Kynurenine metabolism occurs in all cells within the brain, though various branches of the pathway appear segregated into specific cell types (Heyes et al., 1997; Amori et al., 2009). The first and rate-limiting enzyme into the KP is indole-2,3-dioxygenase (IDO), and to a lesser extent in the brain tryptophan-2,3-dioxygenase (TDO), which convert tryptophan to N-formylkynurenine (Shimizu et al., 1978; Takikawa et al., 1988) (for a schematic of the pathway see **Figure 1**). N-formylkynurenine is then metabolized to l-kynurenine (L-KYN) by kynurenine formamidase at which point the pathway bifurcates into at least two distinct branches regulated by kynurenine monooxygenase (KMO) and kynurenine aminotransferases (KATs I-IV). The majority of kynurenine metabolism within the brain takes place in glia. KMO, kynureninase (KYNU), and 3-hydroxyanthranillic acid oxidase (3-HAO) regulate production of a host of metabolites in microglia leading to formation of anthranillic acid (AA), 3-hydroxy anthranillic acid (3-HAA), 3-HK, and QUIN. QUIN is, an excitatory (excitotoxic) agent at NMDA-type glutamate receptors and synergizes with 3-HK to produce oxidative stress. Alternatively, L-KYN may be metabolized in astrocytes by KATs, with KAT II being the predominant brain subtype in humans and rats (Guidetti et al., 2007a). KATs convert L-KYN to KYNA, an inhibitor of glutamate neurotransmission and possibly an antagonist at nicotinic α_7 receptors. The endogenous function of kynurenine-derived neuroactive metabolites still requires further research since many have multiple receptor targets. In addition to NMDA and nicotinic a7 receptors, KYNA for example is reported to interact with GPR35 (Wang et al., 2006) and arylhydrocarbon receptors (Dinatale et al., 2010). A third possible pathway regulated by both KMO and KATs is the xanthurenic acid (XA) branch. Little is known about the endogenous function of XA, though recent literature indicates that it is a Group II metabotropic glutamate receptor agonist (Copeland et al., 2013) indicating that it could also regulate glutamate neurotransmission by impacting presynaptic release.

In recent years the regulation of kynurenine metabolism has been intensely evaluated as it relates to CNS disorders (Haroon et al., 2012; Schwarcz et al., 2012). Often termed the "neurotoxic" and "neuroprotective" branches of the KP, or alternatively the "excitatory" and "inhibitory" branches, KMO and KATs regulate the balance of QUIN:KYNA production which is important in both neurodegenerative and psychiatric disorders. Many kynurenine-derived metabolites poorly cross the blood brain barrier implying that CNS concentrations of kynurenine metabolites are largely regulated by local enzyme activity (Gal and Sherman, 1978). However, kynurenine itself is actively transported into the brain by the large neutral amino acid transporter (Fukui et al., 1991). Under normal physiological conditions much of the kynurenine which is converted to QUIN and KYNA in the brain is derived from peripheral sources (Kita et al., 2002). Following systemic inflammation, where IDO expression is greatly increased (Moreau et al., 2008; Macchiarulo et al., 2009), nearly all kynurenine in the CNS comes from the periphery. However, in contrast to this, direct induction of neuroinflammation causes >98% of the kynurenine available for metabolism in the brain to be derived from local production (Kita et al., 2002). The current review will evaluate this interplay between proinflammatory mediators and mechanisms by which they regulate the KP. It will then conclude with a review of the role of neuroinflammation-mediated kynurenine dysregulation in a range of neurodegenerative and psychiatric disorders.

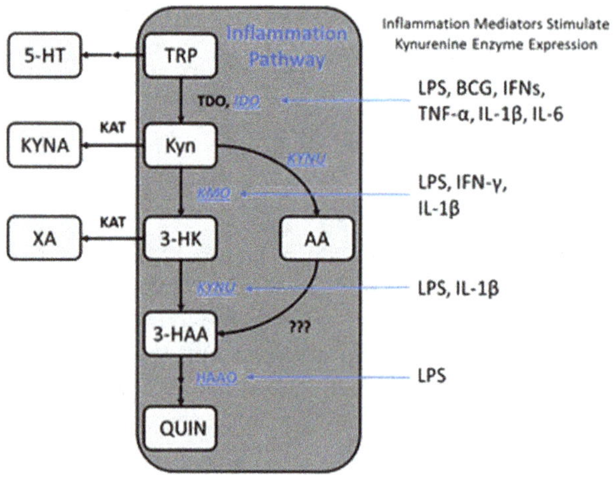

FIGURE 1 | Schematic representation of the kynurenine metabolic pathway. The kynurenine pathway is commonly segregated into two distinct branches that are regulated by KATs and KMO, as well as the availability of l-kynurenine within the brain. Additionally, kynurenine metabolism is regulated by a variety of proinflammatory mediators which impact enzyme expression levels, thereby altering substrate availability and metabolite formation favoring the KMO branch of the pathway under immune-related pathological conditions. TRP, tryptophan; 5-HT, serotonin; Kyn, kynurenine; KYNA, kynurenine acid; 3-HK, 3-hydroxykynurenine; AA, anthranilic acid; XA, xanthurenic acid; 3-HAA, 3-hydroxyanthranilic acid; QUIN, quinolinic acid; IDO, indoleamine-2,3-dioxygenase; KAT, kynurenine aminotransferase; KMO, kynurenine 3- monooxygenase; KYNU, kynureninase; HAAO, 3-hydroxyanthranilic acid oxidase; LPS, lipopolysaccharide; BCG, bacillus Calmette-Guerin; IFNs, interferons; TNF, tumor necrosis factor; IL, interleukin.

CYTOKINE-MEDIATED REGULATION OF KYNURENINE METABOLISM

IDO and TDO, which initiate the catabolism of tryptophan toward kynurenine, are generally thought to be regulated by different mechanisms. TDO is induced by corticosteroids and glucagon, while IDO is induced by proinflammatory cytokines during an immune response (Lestage et al., 2002). There is some evidence that TDO can also be induced by immune activation but this is suggested to be mediated indirectly by increased glucocorticoid receptor activation (Walker et al., 2013). While there is some evidence that other enzymes within the excitatory branch of the KP can also be induced by proinflammatory cytokines, the regulation of IDO, particularly by interferon (IFN)-γ, has been examined most extensively. In general, the body of work investigating the regulation of KP enzymes by inflammatory cytokine signaling is largely composed of expression studies and therefore must be interpreted with caution, since changes in mRNA or even protein expression are not necessarily indicative of functional changes in enzyme activity.

EFFECTS OF PROINFLAMMATORY MEDIATORS ON INDOLEAMINE 2,3-DIOXYGENASE (IDO)

IDO is expressed in various immune cells throughout the body, including dendritic cells, monocytes, macrophages, and, importantly in microglia, the resident CNS macrophage-like cell population (Mandi and Vecsei, 2012). IDO is preferentially induced by interferons and by IFN-inducers such as lipopolysaccharide (LPS) and viruses (Musso et al., 1994). IFN-γ, a type II interferon, is the predominant cytokine implicated in the induction of IDO, as has been shown in several myeloid cell types including dendritic cells, monocytes, immortalized murine macrophages, and microglia (Alberati-Giani et al., 1996; Fujigaki et al., 2006; Jung et al., 2007; O'connor et al., 2009a). In human macrophages, IDO expression and QUIN production can also be induced by the type 1 interferons, IFN-α and IFN-β, although to a lesser degree than with IFN-γ (Jansen and Reinhard, 1999; Guillemin et al., 2001). In the bacille Calmette-Guérin (BCG) mouse model of chronic inflammation, IDO induction closely parallels increased IFN-γ and tumor necrosis factor alpha (TNF-α) expression (Moreau et al., 2005, 2008). BCG-induced upregulation of IDO mRNA is completely inhibited in IFN-$\gamma R^{-/-}$ mice, along with an associated lack of IDO activity, demonstrating that IFN-γ receptor function is necessary for BCG-induced IDO activation (O'connor et al., 2009a).

Although IFN-γ is regarded as the primary inducer of IDO, there is some evidence that IDO expression can be induced independently of IFN-γ. Systemic LPS administration induces IDO expression in rat cortex and hippocampus accompanied by a robust increase in central TNF-α and interleukin (IL)-6 expression, but only modestly elevated IFN-γ (Connor et al., 2008). In the same paper, similar findings were reported in mixed glia cultures prepared from neonatal rat cortex suggesting that IFN-γ may not be necessary for LPS-induced IDO expression (Connor et al., 2008). Consistent with this finding, *in vitro* data with THP-1 cells, a human monocytic cell line, indicate that LPS-induced IDO activation can be mediated by an IFN-γ-independent mechanism involving synergistic effects of IL-1β, TNF-α, and IL-6 (Fujigaki et al., 2006). In human hippocampal progenitor cells, treatment with IL-1β greatly upregulated the transcript for IDO, but not TDO (Zunszain et al., 2012). The increase in IDO transcript was associated with a decrease in tryptophan and increase in kynurenine in the supernatant suggesting that IL-1β increased levels of functional IDO enzyme (Zunszain et al., 2012).

Studies examining the effects of anti-inflammatory cytokines on IDO expression are limited and often conflicting, likely due to differences in the cellular models used and experimental conditions applied. For example, the prototypical anti-inflammatory cytokine IL-10 dose-dependently decreased LPS-mediated IDO protein expression in mouse bone marrow-derived dendritic cells (BMDCs), whereas IL-10 enhanced IFN-γ-mediated IDO protein expression in these cells (Jung et al., 2009; Yanagawa et al., 2009). This discrepancy may point to the possibility that distinct mechanisms of IDO induction may be differentially regulated by anti-inflammatory cytokines such as IL-10, though whether this occurs in the CNS has not been determined. Interestingly, however, IL-10 suppressed IFN-γ-mediated IDO mRNA induction in GT1-7 cells, a transformed mouse hypothalamic neuronal cell line, contrary to that reported for mouse BMDCs treated with IFN-γ (Tu et al., 2005). In addition to the prototypical anti-inflammatory cytokine IL-10, studies with human monocytes and fibroblasts have demonstrated that IL-4 inhibits the induction of IDO mRNA and IDO activity by IFN-γ. In contrast, a study using the EOC13.31 mouse microglia cell line found that IL-4 enhanced, rather than suppressed, IFN-γ-induced IDO mRNA expression, which was abolished by the addition of IL-4 antiserum (Yadav et al., 2007). The potentiating effect of IL-4 on IFN-γ-induced IDO expression was also observed at the level of protein expression and enzymatic activity in these cells (Yadav et al., 2007). Furthermore, IL-4, as well as IL-13 which signals through the same receptor subunit, potentiated IFN-γ-mediated IDO expression in primary mouse microglia cultures (Yadav et al., 2007). These findings collectively suggest that microglia respond differently to anti-inflammatory cytokines compared to peripheral myeloid cells. Interestingly, central administration of IL-4 exacerbates the depressive-like behavioral effect of peripheral LPS, which is IDO-dependent, when both IL-4 and LPS are delivered simultaneously, but suppresses the depressive effect when administered 12 h before LPS, highlighting the complex relationship between IL-4 and IDO in the CNS (Bluthe et al., 2002).

IFN-γ-dependent mechanisms of IDO induction

The 5′-flanking region of the human gene encoding IDO (*INDO*) contains several regulatory elements including some that are essential for IFN-γ-mediated gene transcription. One of two identified IFN-γ-activated sites (GAS) and two interferon-sensitive response elements (ISREs), the latter highly homologous to that associated with IFN-α-inducible genes, are required for full induction of IDO by IFN-γ (Dai and Gupta, 1990; Hassanain et al., 1993; Chon et al., 1995, 1996; Konan and Taylor, 1996). As shown in **Figure 2**, canonical IFN-γ-mediated signal transduction leads to (1) tyrosine phosphorylation of STAT-1, triggering its dimerization and translocation to the nucleus where it binds the GAS sequence in the 5′-flanking region of *INDO*, and (2) NF-κB- and STAT-1-dependent synthesis of IFN-γ-regulated factor (IRF)-1, which binds to one or both of the ISREs found in the *INDO* 5′-flanking region (Darnell et al., 1994; Chon et al., 1995, 1996; Konan and Taylor, 1996). Thus, cooperative STAT-1 and IRF-1 binding to GAS and ISRE sequences, respectively, within the *INDO* 5′-flanking region are necessary for full IFN-γ-mediated induction of IDO transcription.

Synergistic mechanisms of IFN-γ-mediated IDO Induction

The regulatory mechanisms for IFN-γ-mediated IDO induction can be potentiated by other proinflammatory cytokines such as TNF-α and IL-1β, and toll-like receptor (TLR) agonists such as LPS, resulting in synergistic enhancement of IDO expression (Hu et al., 1995; Hissong and Carlin, 1997; Babcock and Carlin, 2000; Currier et al., 2000; Robinson et al., 2003). IL-1β and TNF-α can enhance the expression of IFN-γ receptor in an NF-κB-dependent manner, thereby lowering the threshold for IDO induction by IFN-γ (Krakauer and Oppenheim, 1993; Shirey et al., 2006). Moreover, together with IFN-γ, TNF-α synergistically induces IDO expression by increasing both STAT-1 activation and NF-κB-dependent IRF-1 expression (Krakauer and Oppenheim, 1993; Ohmori et al., 1997; Robinson et al., 2003, 2006; Shirey et al.,

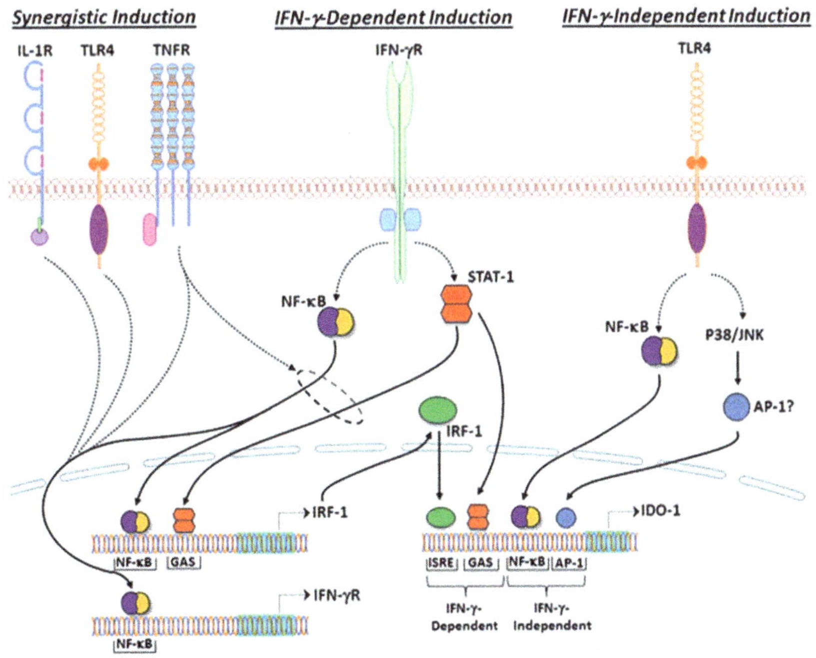

FIGURE 2 | Regulation of IDO1 transcription by inflammatory signaling. IFN-γ-dependent IDO1 induction (**middle**). Canonical IFN-γ receptor signal transduction leads to (1) NF-κB- and STAT-1-dependent transcription of IRF-1, and (2) IRF-1- and STAT-1-dependent transcription of IDO1. Synergistic IDO1 induction (**Left**). IL-1β, LPS, and TNF-α enhance transcription of IFN-γ receptor in an NF-κB-dependent manner. TNF-α has been shown to synergistically enhance IFN-γ-dependent IDO1 transcription by promoting NF-κB- and STAT-1-dependent IRF-1 transcription (within dashed circle). IFN-γ-Independent IDO induction (**Right**). TLR4 stimulation by LPS leads to transcription of IDO1 by a mechanism that requires NF-κB and either p38 or JNK, but not IFN-γ. The 5′-flanking region of *INDO*, the gene encoding IDO1, contains two IFN-γ-activated sites (GAS) and two interferon-sensitive response elements (ISREs). One of the two GAS sequences and both ISRE sequences are required for IFN-γ-mediated IDO1 induction. The 5′ flanking region of *INDO* also contains at least one NF-κB binding site and several AP-1 binding sites, which may be required for IFN-γ-independent mechanisms of IDO1 transcription.

2006). Given the requirement for both STAT-1 and IRF-1 binding to ISRE and GAS sequences, respectively, presumably other signaling mechanisms that increase both STAT-1 phosphorylation and NF-κB transactivation may also synergize with IFN-γ to enhance IDO induction, though these mechanisms have not yet been directly tested. Interestingly, the synergistic induction of IDO by IFN-γ and TNF-α occurs in primary murine microglia and, furthermore, *in vivo* studies suggest that this synergy participates in the IDO-mediated generation of depressive-like behavior in mice inoculated with BCG (O'connor et al., 2009a), a model of inflammation-related depression (Moreau et al., 2008).

IFN-γ-independent mechanisms of IDO induction

Studies using primary murine microglia demonstrated that LPS stimulates IDO transcription in an IFN-γ-independent manner, since IDO mRNA levels were enhanced but IFN-γ mRNA was undetectable following LPS stimulation in these cells (Connor et al., 2008; Wang et al., 2010). Furthermore, these studies showed that LPS-stimulated IDO induction was attenuated by an inhibitor of c-Jun-N-terminal kinase (JNK) (Wang et al., 2010). Similar studies using THP-1 cells, demonstrated that LPS-stimulated L-KYN production was not accompanied by STAT-1 or IRF-1 binding activities, but was attenuated by p38 and NF-κB inhibitors (Fujigaki et al., 2001, 2006). Collectively, these data suggest that LPS-stimulated IDO induction in monocyte/macrophage-like cells occurs in an IFN-γ-independent manner and involves NF-κB and stress-activated mitogen-activated protein (MAP) kinases such as p38 and JNK (Fujigaki et al., 2001, 2006, 2012; Wang et al., 2010). The downstream mechanisms leading from p38 or JNK activation to IDO induction in response to LPS stimulation have not been elucidated. However, the AP-1 transcription factors are conventional substrates of both p38 and JNK MAPKs and are important regulators of inflammation-related gene transcription (Huang et al., 2009; Wang et al., 2010). Supporting this possibility, a reanalysis of the 5′-flanking region of *INDO* has identified both NF-κB and several AP-1 recognition sequences, consistent with the participation of both NF-κB and stress-activated MAPK activity in LPS-stimulated IDO induction (Fujigaki et al., 2006; Wang et al., 2010).

In addition to TLR4 agonists such as LPS, the TLR3 agonist polyinosinic:polycytidylic acid (polyI:C) can induce IDO transcription in cultured human astrocytes in a manner dependent on IFN-β but not IFN-γ signaling, and requiring both NF-κB and IRF-3 (Suh et al., 2007). Though these signaling components have been shown to participate in astrocyte IDO induction, it is not yet clear whether the corresponding mechanism can be generalized to cell types other than astrocytes since the effect of TLR3 activation on IDO induction has not been demonstrated elsewhere.

Aryl hydrocarbon receptor-dependent IDO induction

Experiments using murine BMDCs have demonstrated that the TLR4 and TLR9 agonists LPS and CpG, respectively, induce expression of the aryl hydrocarbon receptor (AhR). The AhR is a ligand-gated transcription factor belonging to the basic helix-loop-helix Per-Arnt-Sim (PAS) family, widely known as the dioxin receptor (Vogel et al., 2008; Nguyen et al., 2010; Vondracek et al., 2011). Interestingly, these experiments suggested that LPS- or CpG-stimulated IDO induction was entirely dependent on the co-induction of AhR in these cells, since BMDCs derived from $AhR^{-/-}$ mice lost the ability to induce IDO expression in response to treatment with either LPS or CpG (Nguyen et al., 2010). Furthermore, dioxin, a potent agonist of the AhR, can also induce IDO expression in these cells, suggesting that AhR activation may positively regulate IDO transcription in response to TLR4 or TLR9 stimulation (Nguyen et al., 2010). Intriguingly, AhR-mediated IDO induction may act as a positive feedback mechanism further activating AhR since L-KYN and its metabolite KYNA are themselves potent AhR agonists (Dinatale et al., 2010; Opitz et al., 2011). The AhR exerts its effects on gene transcription through nuclear translocation and direct binding to dioxin response elements (DREs) in the promoter region of target genes. Curiously these elements have not been identified in the promotor region of *INDO*. Thus, it is not clear whether AhR can regulate IDO transcription directly or indirectly in these cells.

EFFECTS OF PROINFLAMMATORY MEDIATORS ON KYNURENINE-3-MONOOXYGENASE (KMO)

Aside from IDO, the regulation of other kynurenine enzymes by proinflammatory cytokines has not been studied extensively. However, studies are emerging indicating that, similar to IDO, enzymes within the KMO branch of the pathway may also be induced by proinflammatory stimuli. KMO expression is increased in rat brain after systemic LPS administration (Connor et al., 2008; Molteni et al., 2013). In a study that examined the effects of IFN-γ treatment on immortalized murine macrophage (MT2) and microglia (N11) cells, KMO was induced in both cells types, KYNU was induced only in MT2 macrophages, and 3-HAO was not effected (Alberati-Giani et al., 1996). Finally, in human hippocampal progenitor cells, IL-1β treatment upregulated the level of transcripts for KMO and KYNU, enzymes in the KMO branch of the pathway (Zunszain et al., 2012).

EFFECTS OF PROINFLAMMATORY MEDIATORS ON KYNURENINE AMINOTRANSFERASES (KATs)

While the expression of IDO and kynurenine enzymes in the excitatory branch of the KP are either elevated or not changed by proinflammatory stimuli, KAT expression is either unaffected or decreased. Systemic LPS administration had no effect on KAT II expression in rat brain (Connor et al., 2008; Molteni et al., 2013). In MT2 macrophage and N11 microglia cells, KAT appeared to be constitutively expressed, but there was no effect of IFN-γ treatment on KAT activity (Alberati-Giani et al., 1996). However, since in the CNS KATs are mainly expressed in astrocytes, further studies on the effects of proinflammatory stimuli on KAT expression and activity using relevant cell types are required. In human hippocampal progenitor cells, KAT I and KAT III, but not KAT II mRNA, were downregulated after IL-1β treatment (Zunszain et al., 2012).

DYSREGULATION OF THE KYNURENINE PATHWAY IN CNS DISEASES

In recent years dysregulation of kynurenine metabolism has been described in a wide range of CNS-related disorders. Several studies have demonstrated that altered cytokine levels and associated dysregulation of kynurenine metabolism plays as important role in the pathophysiology of neurodegenerative diseases and psychiatric disorders. Upregulation of kynurenines are observed in the serum, CSF and/or brain in neurodegenerative diseases (e.g., AD, PD, and HD), autoimmune diseases (e.g., MS), epilepsy, psychiatric diseases (e.g., MDD, schizophrenia, and ADHD) and infectious diseases (e.g., HIV-associated neurocognitive disorder). It is generally predicted that diseases where microglia are activated favor production of 3-HK and QUIN, whereas suppression of this branch or astrocyte activation may favor KYNA synthesis. The following sections will review the role of the kynurenine system and its regulation by cytokines in the pathophysiology of diseases, and discuss potential therapeutic interventions targeting the KP.

ALZHEIMER'S DISEASE

Alzheimer's disease (AD) is a progressive neurological disorder characterized by impaired memory, cognitive decline, and dementia. Currently there is still only a limited understanding of AD etiology, particularly in late onset AD. AD pathology hallmarks are the presence of β-amyloid (Aβ) plaques, neurofibrillary tangles, and gliosis. Multiple hypotheses exist regarding factors that contribute to the development and progression of AD including substantial evidence for neuroinflammatory processes. In fact, microglia activation states correlate with disease progression and levels of dementia (Arends et al., 2000; Cagnin et al., 2006). Analysis of serum samples and post-mortem brain tissue from AD patients demonstrate an imbalance in pro- and anti-inflammatory cytokines, as well as irregular tryptophan metabolism through activation of microglia and astrocytes.

(Neuro)inflammatory state in AD

Among the neurochemical changes in AD, IFN-γ, TNF-α, IL-1β, IL-2, and IL-8 are elevated along with lower levels of tryptophan and increased kynurenine levels in serum samples from AD patients (Widner et al., 1999; Alsadany et al., 2013; Niranjan, 2013). Similar changes are found in post-mortem brain tissue along with IL-6 also increased (Huell et al., 1995). Within the brains of AD patients, activated microglia and astrocytes are found in proximity to neuritic plaques. Treatment of human microglia and monocytes with $A\beta_{1-42}$ induces IDO expression (Guillemin et al., 2003) and primes the cells for synergistic induction of the KP by IFN-γ (Yamada et al., 2009). In astrocytes Aβ only modestly stimulated IL-6 and IL-8 secretion, but primed the cells to markedly respond to IL-1β with a 3–8 fold increase in IL-6 and IL-8 release (Gitter et al., 1995). Similarly, exposure of microglia cultures from AD patients to $A\beta_{1-42}$ induced TNF-α, pro-IL-1β, IL-6, and IL-8 (Lue et al., 2001). Thus, Aβ appears to alter the state of microglia to a more proinflammatory phenotype that may contribute to neuronal dysfunction and ultimately cell death through release of cytokines and free radical generating agents including NO and QUIN. In AD brains IDO was associated with senile plaques and was localized with neurofibrillary tangles (Bonda et al., 2010). Additionally, IDO and QUIN immunoreactivity were increased in microglia, astrocytes, and neurons within the hippocampus of AD patients (Guillemin et al., 2005) which is of particular interest since QUIN may cause tau hyperphosphorylation in human cortical neurons (Rahman et al., 2009).

Inflammation and kynurenine metabolism in animal models of AD

Studies in preclinical models support the hypothesis that induction of kynurenine metabolism by Aβ and/or cytokines may contribute to neural pathology in AD. Elevated $A\beta_{1-40}$ and $A\beta_{1-42}$ found in transgenic AD mice were associated with increased TNF-α, IL-6, and IL-1β (Patel et al., 2005). In Tg2576 mice, basal induction of IDO in activated microglia associated with Aβ plaques appears to be low, though robustly increased following stimulation with LPS suggesting that the cells are in a "primed" state ready to respond to immune challenges in a more durable way than WT controls (Akimoto et al., 2007). QUIN was strongly increased in the hippocampus, but not cerebellum, in a progressive and age dependent manner in triple transgenic mice (3×Tg: PS1M146V, APPSwe, and tauP301L) in line with data showing increased TDO and IDO-1 immunoreactivity in AD hippocampal tissue (Wu et al., 2013). Interestingly, modest but significant increases in TDO mRNA and protein, along with robust increases in 3-HAO were also found in the cerebellum of these mice, however, 3-HAA levels were unfortunately not reported. Furthermore, TDO was also colocalized with QUIN, neurofibrillary tangles, and amyloid deposits in 3×Tg mice. Recent studies using available pharmacological agents in AAPtg mice showed that chronic inhibition of KMO reduced synaptic loss as measured by synaptophysin, prevented spatial memory deficits in the Morris water maze, and reversed anxiogenic-like responses in the elevated plus maze (Zwilling et al., 2011). Together these data support the hypothesis that Aβ- and cytokine-mediated induction of kynurenine metabolism is an important link in the pathophysiological development of AD.

Induction of kynurenine metabolism, particularly along the KMO/QUIN branch of the pathway, appears likely in AD. The mechanism by which this happens, and the functional consequences, is still under investigation. To date, much of the data available is correlative indicating that Aβ is able to induce production of cytokines and kynurenine metabolizing enzymes which may both contribute to synaptic dysfunction and neuronal loss. Whether Aβ in AD brains independently induces cytokine production and kynurenine metabolism, activates cytokine release which in turn stimulates kynurenine production, or "primes" glia such that they are able to more robustly respond to cytokine signaling is currently not well-understood. Whichever the case, evidence is emerging that excess production of proinflammatory cytokines and QUIN by glia contribute to the progression, and perhaps etiology, of AD.

Preclinical evidence supports the use of IDO, TDO, KMO, and/or 3-HAO inhibitors to counteract the effects of neuroinflammation in AD. However, the contribution of peripheral vs. central inflammatory processes in any putative kynurenine-related AD pathology is not yet clear, and few of the tools available to test these hypotheses are able to directly target the brain. Association of IDO and TDO with plaques and tangles suggests that brain permeable drugs are needed, though peripheral inhibition of KMO was sufficient to produce a therapeutic effect in Tg2576 mice. Since the source of kynurenine feeding into the QUIN branch differs substantially under basal, systemic inflammation, or neuroinflammation conditions, understanding the contribution of central vs. peripheral (including endothelial cells at the blood brain barrier) kynurenine production will be important to help define an appropriate intervention strategy in AD.

PARKINSON'S DISEASE

Parkinson's disease (PD) is a chronic progressive neurodegenerative disorder characterized by loss of dopaminergic neurons in the midbrain and presence of protein inclusions called Lewy bodies (Zinger et al., 2011). The detailed pathogenesis of PD is not known, but several mechanisms have been proposed including mitochondrial dysfunction, neurotoxicity from excessive glutamatergic activity, and reactive oxygen species. Neuroinflammation, as measured by the presence of activated microglia in PD brain, as well as excessive production of cytokines and dysregulation of the KP have been suggested to be involved in these complex pathogenic events.

(Neuro)inflammatory state in PD

Many studies support the presence of widespread microglia activation in PD. In two such studies, MHC class II expression, a widely used marker of microglial activation, was assessed in PD post-mortem brain (McGeer et al., 1988; Imamura et al., 2003). The number of MHC class II-positive microglia was higher in the substantia nigra and putamen as well as in the hippocampus, transentorhinal cortex, cingulate cortex, and temporal cortex of PD brains, and frequently in association with α-synuclein-positive Lewy neurites and monoaminergic neurites (McGeer et al., 1988; Imamura et al., 2003). These activated microglia were also positive for TNF-α and IL-6 in the putamen of PD brain (Imamura et al., 2003). *In vivo* imaging of microglia activation with [^{11}C](R)-PK11195 PET in PD revealed widespread activation in brain regions including the pons, basal ganglia, and frontal and temporal cortex (Gerhard et al., 2006). Levels of several cytokines including TNF-α, IL-1β, IL-2, IL-4, IL-6, and transforming growth factor (TGF)-alpha have been shown to be elevated in the CSF and striatum of PD brain (Mogi et al., 1994a,b; Nagatsu et al., 2000). Some of these cytokines are known inducers or amplifiers of the KP and might contribute to the dysregulation of KPs in PD.

Dysregulation of kynurenine metabolites in PD

Changes in kynurenine metabolism have been reported in post-mortem PD brain and mouse models of PD. In mouse models of PD, mice injected with the dopaminergic neurotoxins 1-methyl-4-phenyl-1,2,3,6-tetrahydropyridine (MPTP) or 6-hydroxydopamine have diminished KAT-I immunoreactivity in the pars compacta of the substania nigra (Knyihar-Csillik et al., 2004, 2006). Treatment with the metabolite of MPTP, 1-methyl-4-phenylpyridinium ion (MPP$^+$), dose-dependently decreased KAT-II activity and KYNA concentration in rat cerebral cortical slices (Luchowski et al., 2002). Similar to the KYNA changes observed in rodent models of PD, KYNA levels were reported to be decreased in PD post-mortem brain (Ogawa et al., 1992). In contrast, levels of 3-HK were elevated in the frontal cortex, putamen, and pars compacta of the substantia nigra in PD brain (Ogawa et al., 1992). In terms of IDO activity, as measured by the K/T ratio, there were increases in both serum and CSF of PD patients compared to controls (Widner et al., 2002). Taken together, these studies suggest that there is an imbalance between the two main branches of the KP in PD, favoring kynurenine metabolism toward the KMO branch of the pathway.

Potential therapeutic intervention by modulation of kynurenine pathway

Numerous studies have been conducted demonstrating that modulation of the KP by enhancing KYNA and/or decreasing 3-HK and QUIN is a potential therapeutic strategy for PD. In an *in vitro* PD model, pretreatment with KYNA attenuated MPP$^+$-induced neurotoxicity in human neuroblastoma cell lines (Lee Do et al., 2008). In rats, KYNA injection into the brain prevented QUIN-induced reduction in striatal tyrosine hydroxylase activity, suggesting that KYNA can protect dopaminergic neurons against QUIN or NMDA-mediated excitotoxicity (Miranda et al., 1997). Since KYNA does not cross the blood brain barrier, investigators in one study attempted to increase KYNA levels in the brain with systemic injections of the substrate for KYNA, L-KYN, in combination with probenecid, an inhibitor of organic acid transport (Silva-Adaya et al., 2011). They reported that pretreatment with L-KYN and probenecid had a protective effect on 6-OHDA-induced locomotor asymmetry, striatal reactive gliosis and neurodegeneration, and changes in dopamine levels (Silva-Adaya et al., 2011). In another study, four synthetic kynurenine analogs were demonstrated to have beneficial effects in the MPTP model in mice (Acuna-Castroviejo et al., 2011). Finally, in MPTP-treated primates, intracerebral injections of KYNA alleviated symptoms of akinesia, tremor, and rigidity in MPTP-treated animals (Graham et al., 1990). Thus, KYNA or its analogs have been demonstrated to have neuroprotective effects in PD.

The effect of decreasing metabolites in the KMO branch of the KP and thereby increasing KYNA in the brain has been tested pharmacologically by several investigators. When nicotinylalanine, an inhibitor of both KMO and kynureninase, was administered intraventricularly in combination with systemic L-KYN and probenecid, there was an elevation in brain KYNA levels and protective effects against QUIN-induced toxicity in rats (Miranda et al., 1997). The effect of KMO inhibition has been tested in a variety of animal models of PD with the non-brain penetrant KMO inhibitor Ro 61-6048. Ro 61-6048 given either systemically or intrastriatally, reduced the severity of dystonia in dt^{sz} mutant hamsters, which are used as an animal model of paroxysmal dystonia with striatal dysfunctions (Richter and Hamann, 2003; Hamann et al., 2008). In non-human primates, chronic Ro 61-8048 administration reduced the development of levodopa-induced dyskinesia in MPTP-treated animals (Samadi et al., 2005; Gregoire et al., 2008; Ouattara et al., 2009; Tamim et al., 2010). Taken together, these studies indicate that drug development targeting the KP for PD may be a promising opportunity.

HUNTINGTON'S DISEASE

Huntington's disease (HD) is an adult-onset neurodegenerative disorder caused by expansion of a CAG repeat in the gene encoding the huntingtin (Htt) protein. Several mechanisms that are not mutually exclusive have been suggested to play a role in the pathogenesis of HD. These mechanisms include neuroinflammation, transcriptional dysregulation, excitotoxicity, and mitochondrial dysfunction. Damage of mutant Htt expressing neurons is suggested to lead to microglia activation, which includes secretion of cytokines as well as increased IDO transcription and generation of neuroactive kynurenine metabolites (Schwarcz and Pellicciari, 2002). Indeed, increased levels of metabolites have been reported in human post-mortem brain as well as in various animal models of HD as discussed below.

(Neuro)inflammatory state in HD

Several lines of evidence suggest both peripheral and central immune systems are activated in HD. Activation of the peripheral immune system is indicated by elevation in several plasma cytokines in HD patients including IL-6, IL-8, IL-4, IL-10, and TNF-α (Bjorkqvist et al., 2008). Interestingly, plasma levels of IL-6 were elevated on average 16 years prior to the predicted clinical onset of the disease in HD gene carriers, which is the earliest plasma abnormality identified in HD (Bjorkqvist et al., 2008). In a study that examined blood levels of kynurenine metabolites at different stages of HD, levels of IL-2 were found to be correlated with the K/T ratio, disease severity, and number of CAG repeats (Forrest et al., 2010).

Activation of the immune system in the CNS is evidenced by elevations in IL-6 and IL-8 in the CSF and increased expression of these inflammatory transcripts, as well as by increased TNF-α in post-mortem HD brain (Bjorkqvist et al., 2008; Silvestroni et al., 2009). There is ample evidence that microglia, the main mediators of neuroinflammation, contribute to the progressive neurodegeneration observed in HD (Möller, 2010). Interestingly they are also the main producers of 3-HK and QUIN in the CNS. Given the presence of IDO and KMO inducing enzymes and the data showing increased KP metabolism in HD and HD model brains, it is tempting to speculate that an increased flux through the microglial KMO metabolic pathway might be responsible for these observations.

Dysregulation of kynurenine metabolites in HD

Studies examining post-mortem HD brain found elevations in the levels of 3-HK and QUIN (Pearson and Reynolds, 1992; Guidetti et al., 2000, 2004). The activity of 3-HAO, the biosynthetic enzyme in the metabolism of 3-HAA, was increased in HD brains compared to controls, suggesting that the HD brain has the ability to produce elevated levels of QUIN (Schwarcz et al., 1988). On the other hand, levels of KYNA and the activity of its two biosynthetic enzymes (KAT I and KAT II) were reported to be reduced in HD brain and CSF compared to controls (Beal et al., 1990, 1992; Jauch et al., 1995) suggesting a dysregulation of the KP in the brain away from KYNA and toward QUIN.

R6/2 mice, a well-established model of HD, also have elevated 3-HK in the brain and have increased activity of the biosynthetic enzyme of 3-HK, KMO, which may account for the high levels (Guidetti et al., 2006; Sathyasaikumar et al., 2010). YAC128 transgenic mice, which have the full-length mutant Htt protein and show a similar degree of striatal neurodegeneration observed in early stage HD, have elevated 3-HK and QUIN in the brain (Guidetti et al., 2000, 2006). Intriguingly, QUIN injections into the striatum is commonly used as an experimental model of HD and produces cellular, neurochemical and behavioral changes resembling those observed in human HD (Beal et al., 1991; Huang et al., 1995).

Dysregulation of the KP, as measured by the K/T ratio, a marker of IDO activity, has been reported in the periphery as well (Stoy et al., 2005; Forrest et al., 2010). One study examined levels of kynurenine metabolites in the blood of patients at different stages of HD as well as the number of CAG repeats and found blood levels of K/T ratio were correlated with disease severity and the number of CAG trinucleotide repeats in HD patients (Forrest et al., 2010). In the same study, blood levels of anthranilic acid were correlated with the proinflammatory cytokine IL-23 (Forrest et al., 2010). Taken together, these studies suggest a role of dysregulation of the KP in HD which may be related to the degree of clinical disease severity.

Potential therapeutic intervention by modulation of kynurenine pathway in Huntington's disease

Studies in yeast, flies, and mice, have shown that blockade of the KMO branch of the KP, thus increasing KYNA in the brain, may protect against neurodegeneration. Genetic deletion of KMO in yeast cells engineered to over express mutated huntingtin protein reduced polyglutamine-mediated toxicity as well as generation of the neuroactive kynurenine metabolites 3HK and QUIN (Giorgini et al., 2005). Furthermore, when a high throughput screen was conducted on the yeast model an analog of the KMO inhibitor 3,4-dimethoxy-N-[4-(3-nitrophenyl)thiazol-2-yl]benzenesulfonamide (Ro61-8048) was identified that potently suppressed huntingtin-mediated toxicity (Giorgini et al., 2005). In transgenic *Drosophila melanogaster* flies that express mutant Htt protein, genetic or pharmacological blockade of KMO reduced neuronal cell loss (Campesan et al., 2011). In the R6/2 genetic mouse model of HD, peripheral blockade of KMO increased KYNA in the brain, reduced loss of synapses and microglia activation, and improved survival (Zwilling et al., 2011). In N171-82Q mice, another transgenic animal model of HD, a KYNA analog, N-(2-N,N-dimethylaminoethyl)-4-oxo-1H-quinoline2-carboxamide hydrochloride, was found to be neuroprotective as it prolonged survival, ameliorated hypolocomotion, prevented weight loss, and completely prevented the atrophy of the striatal neurons (Zadori et al., 2011). These investigations suggest that KMO inhibition and/or KYNA enhancement may be neuroprotective in HD and lend support for the KP as potential drug targets.

MULTIPLE SCLEROSIS

Multiple sclerosis (MS) is a chronic, demyelinating autoimmune disease of the CNS characterized by the presence of peripheral immune cells within sites of active demyelination (Carson, 2002). Based on human studies combined with experimental autoimmune encephalomyelitis (EAE), a widely-employed rodent model of MS, it is generally hypothesized that invading T-cells reactive to myelin-specific antigens are the principle effectors in MS pathogenesis (Lassmann and Ransohoff, 2004; Petermann and Korn,

2011; Fuvesi et al., 2012). Thus, a primary aim of MS research has been to define effector T-cell subpopulations relevant to disease pathogenesis and the mechanisms regulating their differentiation. As will be discussed below, accumulating evidence suggests that KP activity (1) is altered in a manner that is temporally related to the clinical course and treatment of the disease, (2) may play a role in autoimmunity by regulating T-cell differentiation, and (3) may influence the cross-talk of auto-reactive T-cells with resident microglia and infiltrating macrophages and dendritic cells.

Human studies implicating kynurenine pathway modulation in multiple sclerosis

Evidence for altered KP metabolism in MS first appeared in 1979 with the finding that TRP levels were significantly reduced in both plasma and CSF samples from MS patients compared with those of control subjects [Monaco et al., 1979; but see Ott et al. (1993)]. More recent studies have shown that, relative to control subjects, the downstream KP metabolite KYNA is significantly decreased in CSF of MS patients during remission, but elevated in the CSF and plasma of MS patients undergoing acute clinical exacerbation (Rejdak et al., 2002, 2007; Hartai et al., 2005). While this putative relationship between KYNA production and clinical phase has not been confirmed by single longitudinal studies, it has nevertheless collectively led to the speculation that such changes in KYNA levels during disease progression and remission reflect a compensatory protective mechanism against excitatory neurotoxicity. This hypothesis derives from the view that, as a putative NMDAR antagonist, the primary function of central KYNA is neuroprotective. However, this has not been directly tested in rodent models such as EAE as of yet. Nevertheless, these findings highlight the possibility that KP metabolism is related to the occurrence of MS and, importantly, to clinical phases of the disease.

A small number of studies have also related changes in KP metabolism to therapeutic intervention in MS patients. Therapeutically relevant concentrations of IFN-β, a standard fist-line immunomodulatory treatment for MS, leads to induction of IDO mRNA and a significant increase in the production of QUIN by human monocyte-derived macrophages (Guillemin et al., 2001). In MS patients, treatment with IFN-β leads to significant acute elevations in plasma or serum L-KYN levels and K/T ratio compared to baseline measurements, consistent with the induction of IDO in response to IFN-β (Amirkhani et al., 2005; Durastanti et al., 2011). Given the hypothesized role of KP metabolism in the mechanism underlying the depressive side-effects associated with IFN-α-based immunotherapy (Bonaccorso et al., 2002a), KP activation may be similarly involved in the depressive side-effects often reported for MS patients undergoing IFN-β treatment (Goeb et al., 2006). However, the precise relationship between IFN-β treatment and depressive symptoms in MS has not yet been definitively established, hindered in part by the partial overlap of MS symptoms with those of depression (Goeb et al., 2006). Moreover, in studies that have examined the occurrence of depressive symptoms in the context of IFN-β treatment for MS, the role that changes in KP metabolism may play has not been explored.

It has also been postulated that IFN-β-mediated IDO induction might contribute to the limited efficacy of IFN-β treatment in improving MS symptomatology (Vecsei et al., 2013). However, this idea is based on the *in vitro* finding that IFN-β leads to the production of QUIN in human monocyte-derived macrophages (Guillemin et al., 2001), incorporating the notion that QUIN is excitotoxic in the CNS (Vecsei et al., 2013). To date, though, there is no evidence that therapeutic IFN-β treatment in MS leads to central QUIN elevation as a result of IDO induction. In fact, it is not yet clear in which cell-type(s) the IFN-β-mediated IDO induction occurs in MS patients, nor which downstream KP branch is primarily affected.

Mechanistic insights into the role of the kynurenine pathway in multiple sclerosis: lessons from the EAE model

Since resident microglial activation and macrophage infiltration into the CNS are common features of both MS and EAE, initial interest in the role of KP metabolism in the pathogenesis of EAE arose from findings that cultured human macrophages can produce QUIN at neurotoxic levels in response to acute treatment with IFN-γ (Heyes et al., 1992; Chiarugi et al., 2001a). Indeed, in rats immunized with myelin basic protein (MBP) to induce EAE, the spinal cord concentration of QUIN is elevated compared to control rats with a time-course that closely follows the development of acute neurological symptoms, returning to control levels during remission (Flanagan et al., 1995). This presumably results from induction of IDO, but also of KMO, since anti-KMO immunoreactivity, KMO enzyme activity, as well as tissue levels of 3-HK and QUIN are enhanced in the spinal cords of EAE compared to control rats (Chiarugi et al., 2001b). Interestingly, treatment of EAE rats with the selective KMO inhibitor Ro 61-8048 significantly attenuates spinal cord 3-HK and QUIN and enhances L-KYN and KYNA, but does not alter the symptom severity in these animals (Chiarugi et al., 2001b). This observation seems to argue against a role of QUIN-mediated neurotoxicity and KYNA-mediated neuroprotection in acute clinical exacerbation and remission, respectively, in EAE and potentially MS. It does not, however, preclude a cumulative role for 3-HK and QUIN in the chronic neurodegeneration associated with secondary progressive MS.

Contrary to a contributing role in acute pathogenesis, mounting evidence from numerous EAE studies implicates IDO and specific KP metabolites in limiting autoimmunity and promoting immune tolerance, which might, in part, account for the periodic remissions observed in MS and EAE. In mice immunized with MBP or proteolipid protein 139–151 ($PLP_{139-151}$), brain and spinal cord K/T ratio, as well as IDO mRNA and protein expression within brain and spinal cord microglia/macrophages, progressively increases with the development of EAE compared to control mice (Sakurai et al., 2002; Kwidzinski et al., 2005). However, an opposing reduction in brain and spinal cord IFN-γ mRNA during the development of EAE (Sakurai et al., 2002) suggests that IDO activity may negatively regulate the survival of IFN-γ-producing T helper type 1 (Th1) cells, thought to be a primary pathogenic T-cell subset in both MS and EAE. Consistent with this hypothesis, inhibition of IDO enzymatic activity with 1-methyl- tryptophan (1-MT) was associated with earlier relapse phase onset, significantly greater maximum clinical score, and more extensive myelitis in spinal cords of EAE mice (Sakurai et al.,

2002). Similarly, EAE mice treated with 1-MT exhibit greater clinical scores during both relapse and remission phases, compared to EAE mice treated with vehicle control (Kwidzinski et al., 2005). Eliminating the possibility of off-target effects by 1-MT on exacerbation of EAE (Agaugue et al., 2006), $IDO^{-/-}$ EAE mice exhibit more severe clinical scores compared to wildtype EAE mice, beginning approximately 2 weeks post-immunization with myelin oligodendrocyte glycoprotein $(MOG)_{35-55}$ (Yan et al., 2010). Moreover, $IDO^{-/-}$ mice exhibit enhanced Th1/Th17-like cytokine profiles, two major T-cell phenotypes implicated in EAE-related autoimmunity, accompanying the exacerbation of clinical symptoms in these mutants (Yan et al., 2010). Thus, a model of IDO-mediated negative feedback in EAE is emerging. IFN-γ produced by accumulating autoreactive T-cells leads to IDO induction within local antigen presenting cells (APCs), such as microglia or infiltrating macrophages and dendritic cells. This, in turn, limits the survival of pathogenic T-cell phenotypes (i.e., Th1 and Th17) and/or promotes the expansion of immunoregulatory T-cell phenotypes (i.e., Th2 and regulatory T-cells [Treg]).

A firmly established mechanism by which IDO induction may limit the survival of pathogenic T-cells is by directly reducing local availability of TRP, since it has been shown that IDO induction in macrophages and dendritic cells suppresses T-cell proliferation by local TRP catabolism (Munn et al., 1998, 1999; Mellor et al., 2003). Thus, IFN-γ-mediated IDO induction within local APCs may provide an immunosuppressive environment to control self-tolerance during inflammation. In addition to the local reduction of TRP, KP metabolites 3-hydroxykynurenic acid (3-HKA, a.k.a. xanthurenic acid), N-(3,4-dimethoxycinnamoyl) anthranilic acid (3,4-DAA), the synthetic orally active 3-HAA derivative, and 3-HAA directly suppress the proliferation of myelin-specific T-cells, specifically inhibiting Th1 and/or Th17-like phenotypes, and improving EAE clinical symptoms (Platten et al., 2005; Yan et al., 2010). At least for Th17 suppression, 3-HAA enhances the expression of TGF-β in dendritic cells (DCs), stimulating the differentiation of Tregs from naïve T-cells (Tnaïve) (Yan et al., 2010). Thus, KP metabolism may suppress autoimmunity in EAE not only through local TRP depletion, but also through the influence of KP metabolites on DC-mediated T-cell differentiation.

Though the cellular sources of the 3-HAA that act on DCs to influence T-cell differentiation is not clear, it is likely that one source of 3-HAA, or other relevant KP metabolites, may be DCs themselves since bone marrow stem cell (BMSC)-induced down-regulation of EAE correlates with IDO induction in $CD11c^{+}$ DCs (Matysiak et al., 2008). Intriguingly, IDO induction in BMDCs and, as a consequence, Treg differentiation in BMDC/Tnaïve cocultures, requires AhR, the ligands of which include L-KYN, KYNA, and possibly other KP metabolites (Nguyen et al., 2010). In $AhR^{-/-}$ BMDCs cocultured with Tnaïve cells, the inability of these BMDCs to induce Treg differentiation is rescued by addition of L-KYN, though it cannot be excluded that the effect of L-KYN on Treg generation is not a direct effect on Tnaïve cells (Nguyen et al., 2010) since L-KYN can also lead to AhR-dependent Treg differentiation in isolated Tnaïve cells (Mezrich et al., 2010). This may nevertheless have implications for EAE since AhR can bidirectionally drive T-cell differentiation either toward Treg or Th17 phenotypes, ameliorating or worsening EAE, respectively, depending on the specific AhR ligand (Quintana et al., 2008, 2010; Veldhoen et al., 2008). Though the effects of specific KP metabolites on AhR-mediated T-cell differentiation has not been tested directly in EAE, it is still tempting to speculate that metabolites such as 3-HAA and L-KYN might ameliorate EAE through AhR-mediated Treg differentiation, either indirectly by stimulating DC TGF-β release, or directly within Tnaïve cells.

Potential therapeutic intervention by modulation of kynurenine pathway in multiple sclerosis

The emerging model of KP metabolism in the underlying biology of EAE and potentially MS suggests that IDO activity, enhanced by IFN-γ released from pathogenic T-cells, may in turn serve to limit their survival and/or facilitate the expansion of immunoregulatory T-cell phenotypes during inflammation. This is postulated to occur directly through the impact of TRP catabolism on Th1/Th17 cell survival and/or by the influence of downstream KP metabolites on T-cell differentiation toward immunoregulatory phenotypes. Given the compelling positive link between IDO activity and major depressive symptoms, highlighted by clinical studies examining the depressive side-effects of IFN-α-based immunotherapy (Bonaccorso et al., 2002a), a more favorable therapeutic entry-point for MS might be based on the hypothesis that selected downstream KP metabolites serve to limit autoimmunity by influencing T-cell differentiation toward regulatory phenotypes. This hypothesis has been tested in EAE with the synthetic 3-HAA derivative N-(3,4-dimethoxycinnamoyl) anthranilic acid (3,4-DAA), also known as Tranilast, currently approved in the U.S. for the treatment of allergic rhinitis, atopic dermatitis, and certain forms of asthma (Platten et al., 2005; Chen and Guillemin, 2009; Yan et al., 2010). However, Tranilast is also proposed to inhibit histamine release by mast cells, suppress TGF-β release, and inhibit angiogenesis (Chen and Guillemin, 2009). Thus, deeper investigation into the mechanism underlying the influence of KP metabolites on T-cell differentiation may further define novel and more selective therapeutic strategies for treating autoimmune diseases such as MS in this context. To the best of our knowledge, Tranilast is currently being developed by Nuon Therapeutics, Inc. (San Mateo, CA) for the treatment of autoimmune diseases including MS, though it has not entered clinical testing.

EPILEPSY

Research efforts to investigate the function and therapeutic potential of CNS KP metabolism was originally rooted in speculation about the pro- and anti-convulsant properties of endogenous QUIN and KYNA, respectively, in the etiology of human epilepsies (Perkins and Stone, 1985; Stone and Connick, 1985; Schwarcz et al., 1987). However, in over 25 years since these ideas surfaced, surprisingly little evidence has accumulated to date, neither clinical nor experimental, to solidify alterations in KP metabolism as a major etiological factor in human epilepsy. Furthermore, the therapeutic potential of experimental KP modulators such as Ro 61-8048 and various KYNA analogs in epilepsy treatment has not been fully explored (Vecsei et al., 2013). Given this, it is not surprising that even less is known about the regulation of KP metabolism by inflammatory mediators in this context. Though outside the scope of this review, it is becoming increasingly apparent that proinflammatory cytokine signaling plays a prominent role in the mechanisms underlying neuronal hyperexcitability and neurodegeneration in epilepsy, and has been extensively reviewed elsewhere (Devinsky et al., 2013; Vezzani et al., 2013a,b). Several studies suggest that the impact of epilepsy-related neuroinflammation on KP metabolism as a disease mechanism warrants deeper investigation.

A recent study analyzed serum K/T ratios in 271 classified epilepsy patients with 309 control subjects (Liimatainen et al., 2011). Results were consistent with elevated IDO activity in patients with idiopathic generalized epilepsy (Liimatainen et al., 2011). The central KP metabolites produced downstream of IDO activation in these patients may likely be biased toward the KMO branch since microglial activation is evident in surgical resections from several forms of epilepsy (Vezzani et al., 2013a). Furthermore, in mice inoculated with hamster neurotrophic measles virus, increases in microglial activation and brain levels of 3-HK and QUIN precede the onset of behavioral seizures in this model (Lehrmann et al., 2008). Consistent with the induction of microglial IDO and KMO by proinflammatory cytokine signaling in a mouse model of temporal lobe epilepsy, hippocampal elevations in mRNA encoding IL-1β, TNF-α, IFN-γ, CD11b, IDO, and KMO were detected 24 h after kainic acid injection (Gleeson et al., 2010). Though correlative, it is plausible that these elevations in proinflammatory cytokines underlie the induction of IDO and KMO in this model since IL-1β, TNF-α, and IFN-γ are all potent inducers of IDO and at least IFN-γ also induces KMO expression as well (Mandi and Vecsei, 2012). While it may be surmised that induction of IDO and KMO likely leads to central enhancement in 3-HK and QUIN production in this model, it is not at all clear what, if any, role these metabolites might play in either acute seizure activity or in epileptogenesis. It is reasonable to hypothesize that the pro-convulsant activity of QUIN may at least exacerbate neuronal hyperactivity and/or excitotoxicity. Furthermore, both QUIN and 3-HK may contribute to neuronal degeneration to further aggravate the neuroinflammatory responses that underlie or contribute to disease pathology. To answer such questions should be relatively straightforward with the availability of molecular, genetic, and pharmacological tools to dissect the relationship between inflammatory cytokine signaling and KP metabolism in the context of epilepsy.

Potential therapeutic intervention by modulation of kynurenine pathway in epilepsy

While there is little clinical evidence to date supporting the notion that KP metabolism is dysregulated in epilepsy, this possibility is strengthened by our emerging understanding of the role neuroinflammation may play in the precipitation and recurrence of epileptic seizure activity, combined with the regulation of KP activity by proinflammatory cytokine signaling. Based on this and recent pre-clinical data (Lehrmann et al., 2008; Gleeson et al., 2010), we may predict that the microglial branch is overactive with respect to the astrocytic branch of the KP in at least some forms of epilepsy, resulting in excessive accumulation of 3-HK and QUIN in the CNS. If 3-HK and QUIN-mediated excitotoxicity or neurodegeneration do indeed contribute to disease pathology, then chronic, adjunctive treatment with a centrally penetrant KMO inhibitor might improve long term outcome compared to treatment with standard anticonvulsants alone, since KMO inhibition is proposed to increase the production of KYNA while decreasing the production of 3-HK and QUIN in the CNS,

DEPRESSION AND MAJOR DEPRESSIVE DISORDER

Depression is the most prevalent neuropsychological disorder. Worldwide figures estimate that ~20% of people will experience a major depressive episode throughout the course of their lifetime (Kessler et al., 2005). Understanding the etiology of major depressive disorder (MDD) is complicated by sociodemographic factors and polygenetic contributions. Emerging data show that dysregulation of the immune system, over expression of proinflammatory cytokines, and aberrant tryptophan metabolism are contributing factors at least in a subset of MDD cases.

Role of inflammation and kynurenine metabolism in depression from clinical and human tissue studies

Clinical evidence for an inflammation component in MDD is quite strong. The most direct argument for a causative link stems from studies in which immune stimulating agents induce depressive symptoms in patients and/or healthy subjects. A common therapy for treating hepatitis C is the use of IFN-α. Up to 50% of these patients develop depressive symptoms that are maintained throughout the course of treatment but subside within a short period after completion (Bonaccorso et al., 2002a,b). Of interest within these patients, IFN-α treatment can enhance tryptophan metabolism through the KP pathway as measured by K/T ratios, an indicator of IDO activity (Capuron et al., 2003). Tryptophan was typically reduced in serum samples, though not always (Comai et al., 2011), and kynurenine levels increased during IFN-α treatment. The alteration in K/T ratios correlated with symptoms of depression and anxiety scores on the Montgomery–Åsberg Depression Rating Scale (MADRS), Beck Depression Inventory (BDI), and Hamilton Anxiety Rating Scale (HAM-A), respectively (Bonaccorso et al., 2002b). When evaluated using the BDI scale all hepatitis C patients treated with IFN-α showed worsening scores as well as increased K/T ratios. However, only a subset (26/45) reached the criteria to be considered depressed. Interestingly, this patient subset also showed the greatest disruption in tryptophan metabolism and highest K/T ratios.

Similar to the results reported in hepatitis C populations, cancer patients treated with IFN-α also increase production of kynurenine and often possess lower tryptophan levels. In these patients K/T ratios were elevated and appeared to correlate with worsening outcome of cancer as well as development of depressive symptoms (Kurz et al., 2011). However, Bannink et al. (2007) showed that cancer patients treated with IFN-α had higher K/T ratios but did not develop symptoms of depression. It is worth noting that patients with a history of depression were excluded from this trial and as such, they may have been measuring *de novo* depression in a symptom resistant population. This interpretation would seem in line with the findings in hepatitis C patients where only a subset of patients develop depression, potentially correlating with an underlying susceptibility (Comai et al., 2011). Furthermore, the relationship between K/T ratios and depressive symptoms in melanoma patients treated with IFN-α and paroxetine supports this hypothesis. IFN-α increased K/T ratios in melanoma patients and produced depressive symptoms (Capuron et al., 2003). Paroxetine reduced the depressive symptoms and increased tryptophan, without affecting kynurenine, resulting in only modestly elevated K/T ratios. Alternatively, in patients not receiving an antidepressant, tryptophan levels were lower and kynurenine levels higher in those who developed depression compared to more resilient patients.

In healthy volunteers, stimulation of the immune system causes increased proinflammatory cytokine production and increased kynurenine production associated with depressive symptoms (Eisenberger et al., 2010). Low doses of endotoxin (from *E. coli*) increased TNF-α, IL-6, and body temperature. Interestingly, induction of the immune response correlated with reduced ventral striatum activation in a monetary incentive task, suggesting reduced function of reward systems. In other studies, higher plasma K/T ratios correlated with anhedonia scores in adolescents with MDD (Gabbay et al., 2012). Furthermore, in children with melancholic MDD, K/T, kynurenine, and 3-HAA/L-KYN levels were associated with severity of depressive symptoms (Gabbay et al., 2010).

Though a broad range of clinical studies support a role for inflammation-mediated dysregulation of cytokine production and kynurenine metabolism in MDD, some studies demonstrate a lack of correlation between inflammation, K/T ratios, and depressive symptoms. In one case, plasma IL-6 levels were reported along with a minor increase in IFN-α in a depressed cohort (Hughes et al., 2012). No evidence of increased kynurenine metabolism was observed though tryptophan was decreased. These patients also possessed elevated C-reactive protein (CRP) levels (2.1 mg/L vs. 1.2 mg/L in controls), typically used as an indicator of underlying inflammation, though they remained within a normal range. These data support the hypothesis that tryptophan depletion occurs independent of kynurenine metabolism by IDO in patients with minimal inflammation. Indeed, anti-inflammatory therapies have been found to be effective at treating depression in patients with high levels of CRP (>5 mg/L) (Raison et al., 2013). Furthermore, where it has been evaluated, proinflammatory markers such as IL-1β, TNF-α, and macrophage migration inhibitory factor appear to predict lack of responsiveness to traditional antidepressant medications (Cattaneo et al., 2013). In addition, levels of tryptophan, kynurenine, and 3-HAA correlated to treatment response to fluoxetine across a broad range of clinical scales (Mackay et al., 2009). Together these data suggest that only a subset of MDD patients with high levels of underlying inflammation are associated with disruption in kynurenine metabolism that relates to depressive symptoms.

A genetic link between inflammation and kynurenine metabolism in MDD was reported in patients with IFN-γ (+874) T/A genotypes. Healthy women with the higher IFN-γ producing T allele were associated with increased IDO activity as measured by elevated plasma levels of K/T compared to the lower producing A allele (Raitala et al., 2005). In addition, TA carriers had a higher prevalence of depression than the AA genotype (Oxenkrug et al., 2011). More recently, an IFN-γ CA repeat polymorphism was identified that also conferred lower tryptophan levels along with higher kynurenine production (Myint et al., 2013), though the relationship between symptoms of depression and kynurenine metabolism have yet to be evaluated in these patients. Furthermore, a polymorphism in the promoter region of the gene for IDO correlated with increased depression in hepatitis C patients treated with IFN-α (Smith et al., 2012). In the Sequenced Treatment Alternatives to Relieve Depression (STAR*D) trial two common SNPs in the IDO1 gene were associated with treatment outcome for either citalopram or overall antidepressant treatment (Cutler et al., 2012).

Though upregulated kynurenine production in serum is a relatively common finding in MDD studies, fewer reports have evaluated neuroinflammation in this disorder. QUIN is elevated in the anterior cingulate cortex of depressed patients, but only in severely depressed individuals (Steiner et al., 2011). In addition, studies have now demonstrated that, along with increased plasma kynurenine (Sublette et al., 2011), QUIN and IL-6 are increased in the cerebrospinal fluid of suicide attempters (Erhardt et al., 2013). Intriguingly, the correlation between over activation of the QUIN branch of the KP in suicide attempters was confirmed in patients with a diagnosis other than MDD as well. These data suggest that in addition to inflammation-mediated IDO activation peripherally, and perhaps within the CNS, selective metabolism of kynurenine along the QUIN branch occurs in the brains of severely depressed patients.

Delineation of the role of inflammation on kynurenine metabolism and depressive symptoms in preclinical systems

Preclinical studies strongly support the link between immune stimulation, induction of kynurenine metabolism, and development of depressive-like symptoms (Dantzer et al., 2011; Leonard and Maes, 2012). Acute application of an immune stimulus such as LPS induces expression of IDO, IFN-γ, TNF-α, and IL-1β in animals (O'connor et al., 2009c) while also causing impairment in forced swim (FST) and tail suspension (TST) tests, assays measuring depressive-like behavior. Blockade of IDO with 1-MT prevented the induction of IDO, attenuated increased K/T in the brain and periphery, and alleviated behavioral impairments. Interestingly IFN-γ, TNF-α, and IL-1β remained elevated suggesting that these responses to LPS occurred upstream of IDO induction. Similarly, mice treated with LPS developed an anhedonic phenotype measured by sucrose or saccharine preference which was also blocked by IDO inhibition (Salazar et al., 2012). While LPS induces sickness-like behavior which may confound the measurement of depressive-like responses in animal models, most studies demonstrate that the sickness is more transient, allowing measurement of depressive-like behavior once sickness has subsided. In fractalkine-deficient mice ($CX3CR1^{-/-}$), chronic treatment with 1-MT prevented depressive symptoms precipitated by LPS for up to 72 h, though inhibiting IDO had no effect on sickness behavior which abated between 24 and 48 h (Corona et al., 2013).

Infusion of LPS intracerebroventricularly (icv) is used as a model of acute neuroinflammation to study the effects of cytokine regulation and depressive phenotypes in rodents. Local neuroinflammation increased kynurenine production and K/T ratios in both the CNS and in the periphery (Dobos et al., 2012). Furthermore, animals performed poorly in FST, though surprisingly no effect was observed in the elevated plus maze or in spontaneous alternation suggesting a lack of pro-anxiety responses or cognitive impairment. Inhibition of IDO with 1-MT prevented elevation of K/T as well as reduced immobility in the FST, suggesting that increased kynurenine production contributed to the depression-like phenotype. In addition to kynurenine dysregulation, icv LPS increased expression of IDO, TNF-α, IL-6, and iNOS mRNA in the brain (Fu et al., 2010). When tested acutely (4–8 h post-dose) animals also displayed significant reductions in social interaction, though it's worth noting that such an acute time period may be confounded by sickness behavior.

An alternative proinflammatory stimulus used to induce acute depressive-like responses is activation of TLR3 by Poly I:C, a synthetic dsRNA. Poly I:C induced a neuroinflammatory response characterized by transiently (<24 h) increased expression of TNF-α, IL-1β, and IL-6 with delayed increase in CD11b mRNA (24–28 h) in the frontal cortex and hippocampus of rats (Gibney et al., 2013). Depressive-like behaviors measured by saccharin preference and anxiogenic effects observed in the elevated plus maze after poly I:C treatment peaked at 48 h and persisted up to 72 h. Concurrent with the depressive phenotype, IDO expression along with tryptophan and kynurenine concentrations were elevated in the brain while no effect on 5-HT was observed. These data suggest that depressive phenotypes induced by viral-mimetic inflammation may be driven in part through dysregulation of the kynurenine system.

Chronic inflammatory stimuli also produce long-lasting depressive phenotypes associated with neuroinflammation and kynurenine dysregulation. BCG, an attenuated mycobacterium, induced an acute sickness period in mice lasting up to 5 days followed by a more prolonged depression-like phase that was sustained for weeks (Moreau et al., 2008). In this same model, kynurenine levels were increased for up to 3 weeks within the brain (Moreau et al., 2005). Dissection of the mechanism by which BCG regulates kynurenine metabolism and produces a depressive phenotype demonstrated that brain IDO, IFN-γ, and TNF-α are upregulated in concordance with depressive-like behavior. The depressive phenotype and kynurenine dysregulation produced by BCG inoculation was absent in IDO and IFN-γ KO mice (O'connor et al., 2009a,b). Furthermore, proinflammatory cytokines remained elevated in IDO KO mice, and to a lesser extent IFN-γ KO mice (e.g., IL-1β), suggesting that the impact on depression-like behaviors of cytokine induction subsequent to BCG treatment occurred through a downstream effect on kynurenine metabolism.

Both clinical and preclinical data support a link between neuroinflammation, kynurenine metabolism, and symptoms of depression. Induction of IDO, KMO, and KYNU by proinflammatory cytokines which cause disruption of normal physiological metabolism of tryptophan and/or kynurenine appears to be an important link in the cascade of events leading to certain forms of depression. Where tested in animal models, blockade of this induction has been beneficial in reversing or preventing development of depressive phenotypes. Though limited tools are available for testing the clinical benefit of manipulating the KP, it will be important for current (e.g., IDO inhibitors for the treatment of cancer) and future studies to evaluate the emotional status of patients in a systematic way to better understand the therapeutic potential of this system in MDD.

SCHIZOPHRENIA AND RELATED DISORDERS

Schizophrenia is a complex neuropsychiatric disorder affecting approximately 1% of the world population, characterized by positive (delusions, hallucinations, thought disorder), negative (anhedonia, alogia, asociality) and cognitive (deficits in attention, executive function, and memory) symptom clusters, attributed to disturbances in dopaminergic, glutamatergic, and GABAergic neurotransmission (Harrison and Weinberger, 2005; Lewis et al., 2005). A leading hypothesis posits that NMDAR hypofunction is a key neurobiological mechanism underlying the core features of the disease, initially inspired by the observation that NMDAR open channel blockers, such as phencyclidine and ketamine, recapitulate a wide spectrum of schizophrenia symptoms in healthy subjects, and exacerbate those of schizophrenic patients [for further review, see Coyle (2012), Moghaddam and Javitt (2012)]. This, combined with the notion that KYNA is proposed to function as an endogenous antagonist of the obligatory NMDAR co-agonist site, has stimulated intense interest in the involvement of KYNA in schizophrenia. Supporting this possibility, elevated KYNA levels have been detected in CSF (Erhardt et al., 2001; Nilsson et al., 2005; Linderholm et al., 2012) and post-mortem prefrontal cortex (Schwarcz et al., 2001) of schizophrenic patients compared to controls. While human or rodent brain tissue levels of KYNA (nM range) are below the reported IC_{50} for the NMDAR co-agonist site (μM range), emerging mechanistic and behavioral data from animal studies are consistent with an impact of fluctuations in endogenous brain KYNA on schizophrenia-related phenotypes (Erhardt et al., 2009; Wonodi and Schwarcz, 2010), suggesting that local synaptic or extrasynaptic concentrations of KYNA might be much higher than the reported global levels.

Putative mechanisms underlying kynurenic acid dysregulation in schizophrenia and related disorders

Elevation in the level of brain KYNA may result from increased availability of L-KYN for metabolism by KAT II, the predominant KYNA-synthesizing enzyme in human and rat brain (Guidetti et al., 1997). One mechanism by which this may occur is through astrocyte-specific enhancement of L-KYN production, since brain KAT II is predominantly expressed in astrocytes compared to other neural cell types (Kiss et al., 2003; Guidetti et al., 2007b). Indeed, protein expression of TDO2 is selectively upregulated in white matter astrocytes of post-mortem frontal cortex of schizophrenic patients compared to that from control subjects, coincident with a significant elevation of TDO2 but not IDO mRNA levels (Miller et al., 2004). Similar results were obtained for post-mortem anterior cingulate cortex of subjects with schizophrenia and bipolar disorder, accompanied by an increase in tissue levels of L-KYN compared to controls (Miller et al., 2006). Thus, selective upregulation of astrocytic TDO2-mediated L-KYN synthesis may partially account for the overproduction of KYNA in brain regions implicated in cognitive impairment associated with schizophrenia. Regulatory mechanisms governing astrocytic TDO2 expression are not well-understood, though it is worth noting that the regulatory region of the gene encoding both human and rat TDO2 contain at least two glucocorticoid response elements (GREs), and TDO2 mRNA is induced by dexamethasone in rat liver (Danesch et al., 1983, 1987; Comings et al., 1995). Given this, it is tempting to speculate that, unlike the microglial branch of the KP, activity of the KYNA-producing astrocytic branch may be positively regulated by anti-inflammatory, rather than by proinflammatory signaling. This is consistent with the enhancement of brain KYNA production following administration of the COX-2 inhibitor parecoxib in rat (Schwieler et al., 2006), though the mechanism underlying this effect is unknown.

Another mechanism by which L-KYN availability for KAT II-mediated metabolism may be increased is through suppression of KMO expression and/or enzyme activity. KMO exhibits a relatively high affinity for L-KYN compared to that of KAT II, and therefore exerts preferential control over the fate of L-KYN. Thus, reduction in KMO activity is expected to increase the availability of L-KYN for KAT II-mediated metabolism, an effect which has been demonstrated experimentally using the KMO inhibitor JM-6 (Zwilling et al., 2011). Recently it has been reported that a coding SNP within the human KMO gene is associated with reduced KMO mRNA expression and elevated CSF KYNA in bipolar patients with psychotic features during mania (Lavebratt et al., 2013). Moreover, an intronic SNP within the human KMO gene is associated with reduced KMO mRNA expression and impaired schizophrenia-related endophenotypes (Wonodi et al., 2011). Thus, disease-relevant genetic impairment of KMO expression/activity might play a contributing role in the overproduction of KYNA in schizophrenia and related psychiatric disorders. It remains to be seen, however, whether KMO expression/activity may be similarly influenced by dysregulated inflammatory signaling associated with these disorders. As discussed earlier, expression of both IDO and KMO is induced by proinflammatory cytokines such as IFN-γ. Conversely, IFN-γ-mediated IDO expression is inhibited by IL-4 and IL-13 (Musso et al., 1994; Chaves et al., 2001), though opposing results have been reported (Yadav et al., 2007). Since IDO and KMO expression appear to be positively regulated by similar mechanisms, it would be interesting to determine whether KMO expression is similarly inhibited by IL-4 and/or IL-13, and whether such inhibition leads to overproduction of central KYNA. Such a hypothesis might be relevant to a role of cytokine-mediated KP dysregulation in schizophrenia, since a recent study of 26 schizophrenic patients and 26 control subjects found that the ratios of serum IFN-γ/IL-4, IFN-γ/IL-10, IL-2/IL-4, and TNF-α/IL-4 were significantly reduced in schizophrenic patients compared to controls (Chiang et al., 2013). These data support an emerging, though controversial hypothesis which proposes that schizophrenia is associated with a subtle shift from the production of Th1 cytokines, such as IFN-γ, IL-2, and TNF-α, toward the production of Th2 cytokines, such as IL-4, IL-10, and IL-6 [reviewed in Muller et al. (2012)].

Potential therapeutic intervention by modulation of kynurenine pathway in schizophrenia

Given the hypothesis that excessive extracellular KYNA in the CNS, through its inhibitory action at NMDAR glycineB receptors and/or α7 nicotinic acetylcholine receptors, contributes to schizophrenia symptomatology, research efforts to evaluate the therapeutic potential of reducing KYNA have focused on inhibition of KAT II, the predominant KYNA synthesizing enzyme in human and rat brain (Guidetti et al., 1997). Mounting preclinical evidence suggest that KAT II-selective inhibitors produce a pro-cognitive effect in schizophrenia-relevant behavioral assays. Acute hippocampal application of S-ESBA, a first-generation, brain-impenetrant KAT II inhibitor, reduces extracellular KYNA by ~30% and leads to improved performance in the Morris water maze, an effect that was opposed by co-administration of a physiologically relevant concentration of KYNA (Pocivavsek et al., 2011). Acute systemic administration of second-generation KAT II-selective inhibitors, such as the brain-penetrant PF-04859989 (Dounay et al., 2013) reduce central KYNA concentrations by ~70%, improve performance in a rodent sustained attention task, and reverse ketamine-induced working memory deficits in rodent and monkeys (Abbott et al., 2010; Chapin et al., 2010; Horner et al., 2010). Thus, combined with clinical and post-mortem data indicating elevated brain KYNA levels associated with schizophrenia, these pre-clinical data support the therapeutic utility of KAT II inhibitors in treating cognitive impairments associated with schizophrenia, symptom domains that are poorly treated by current standards of care.

ATTENTION DEFICIT-HYPERACTIVITY DISORDER

Attention Deficit-Hyperactivity Disorder (ADHD) is the most commonly diagnosed psychiatric disorder in children and adolescents. Though estimates of prevalence vary widely, it is estimated that ~6–8% of school aged children suffer from this disorder (Larson et al., 2011; Willcutt, 2012). Patients show striking neuropsychological performance deficits compared to peers within their age-group which tend to diminish in severity over time. This may relate to a developmental delay of cortical maturation (Shaw and Rabin, 2009). The etiology of this delay is unknown but it has been hypothesized that impaired glial supply of energy to support neuronal activity could contribute. Recent developments in the study of ADHD suggest that patients may possess minor imbalances in their immunological systems, as measured by increased serum levels of IFN-γ and IL-13, while also having reduced levels of 3-HK though normal levels of kynurenine (Oades et al., 2010b). The altered levels of proinflammatory cytokine production and kynurenine metabolism trended toward normalizing in medicated subjects relative to medication naïve patients. These findings may be consistent with early hypotheses regarding an imbalance in tryptophan metabolism in ADHD which suggested that patients produce excess serotonin, at least in peripheral compartments (Irwin et al., 1981). An impaired production of 3-HK was predicted to reflect reduced activation of microglia and thus impaired neuronal pruning that could contribute to developmental delays.

While no study has looked directly at CNS cytokine and kynurenine profiles in ADHD, a few have attempted to define behavioral endophenotypes associated with these markers in serum. In one study it was demonstrated that levels of S100b were negatively correlated to oppositional and conduct disorder symptoms (Oades et al., 2010a). In this same study, an inverse relationship between S100b and IL-10/IL-16 was observed which was in contrast to findings in healthy children. A subsequent study reported that elevated IL-16 levels, along with reduced S100b, were strongly correlated with hyperactivity while IL-13 may be related to attentional capacity (Oades et al., 2010b). Tryptophan metabolism was not directly related to symptoms, though increased kynurenine as well as elevated IFN-γ (though reduced TNF-α) were associated with faster reaction times. Interestingly another study showed that shorter pregnancy and lower birth weight of ADHD patients, factors that are associated with severity of symptoms, have been linked to increased 3-HK and IFN-γ (Oades, 2011) which is only partially consistent with earlier reports of dysregulated cytokine production and kynurenine metabolism, where reduced 3-HK was found. While findings that alterations in peripheral cytokine and kynurenine systems are an interesting start, additional work to establish whether these results translate to changes in the CNS compartment are needed. Furthermore, a detailed analysis of cytokine levels and their relationship to kynurenine metabolism in the brain over the course of the disease may shed light on the contribution of this system to the developmental delay reported to occur in ADHD patients.

HIV-ASSOCIATED NEUROCOGNITIVE DISORDER

Human Immunodeficiency Virus (HIV) infection is a debilitating chronic disease that causes dramatic CD4$^+$ T-cell depletion resulting in immune response deficiency as well as chronic immune activation and inflammation responses. A strong case exists for an involvement of tryptophan metabolic disturbances in the pathology of HIV infection. Activation of tryptophan metabolism by IDO likely favors HIV persistence and exacerbation of disease progression through immune response suppression and generation of neurotoxic metabolites. Elevated circulating levels of IFN-γ and kynurenine metabolites are commonly found in HIV patients (Fuchs et al., 1990). QUIN is elevated in serum and CSF from HIV infected persons and levels are correlated with progression of neuropsychological impairment over the course of the disease (Heyes et al., 1991a). Indeed, patients with HIV-associated dementia were reported to possess levels of QUIN that are ~20-fold greater than non-infected controls. Similar increases in QUIN are observed in primate models after retroviral exposure indicating a causative link between HIV infection and activation of kynurenine metabolism (Heyes et al., 1990). However, the consequence of kynurenine dysregulation by HIV and its role in disease progression or symptomatology is unknown. Excessive activation of IDO may result in localized depletion of tryptophan availability leading to impaired T-cell differentiation, thereby suppressing immune function. In addition, inflammation-mediated induction of KMO and KYNU favors production of 3-HK and QUIN from kynurenine. 3-HK is involved in reactive oxygen species generation and also decreases the number of CD4$^+$ T-cells in corneal allograph studies (Zaher et al., 2011) suggesting this neuroactive metabolite could further impair immune function after HIV infection.

The mechanism by which HIV stimulates IDO expression is not entirely clear as it has been proposed to be mediated by both IFN-γ dependent (Brown et al., 1991) and independent (Boasso et al., 2009; Maneglier et al., 2009) mechanisms in human macrophages and T-cells. To be clear, both IFN-γ levels and IDO activity are increased in HIV patients, and though IFN-γ can induce IDO, the correlation that both pathways are engaged does not necessarily indicate a causative link between these effects. Thus, while IFN-γ production, particularly from opportunistic infections, may contribute to IDO expression and tryptophan metabolism, HIV also appears to be able to stimulate kynurenine production via an interaction with CD4 receptors independent of IFN-γ. Elevated CSF kynurenine metabolism occurs independent of macrophage infiltration in simian AIDs models (Heyes et al., 1991b), suggesting that elevated QUIN is synthesized by local CNS production, possibly by microglia in response to peripheral immune/inflammation signals. Further complicating this interaction is the fact that HIV replication is enhanced by TNF-α, IFN-γ, and IL-1β, all acting through NF-κB. Since NF-κB also stimulates IDO, KMO, and KYNU, it is possible that proinflammatory cytokine signaling underlies a vicious cycle that promotes viral replication, tryptophan/kynurenine metabolism, and progression of dementia symptoms. It can thus be hypothesized that HIV infects immune cells including macrophages, T-cells, and microglia causing activation and subsequent release of proinflammatory cytokines and induction of tryptophan metabolizing enzymes. The resulting impairment in immune response could allow for opportunistic infections which further increase proinflammatory cytokine production supporting generation of 3-HK and QUIN throughout the body and brain. While the precipitating factors behind viral replication and kynurenine dysregulation may be similar, the neurocognitive dysfunction observed in HIV-associated neurocognitive disorder or dementia may be mediated in part by aberrant kynurenine metabolism in microglia within the brain in response to chronic production of proinflammatory cytokines, which one might speculate could be treated by inhibition of IDO, KMO, or KYNU.

THERAPEUTIC POTENTIAL AND IMMUNE INTERACTIONS BY THE KYNURENINE PATHWAY

The KP is uniquely positioned to regulate both the nervous and immune systems in disease states, which presents an interesting potential for drug discovery efforts but also potential risks of immunological responses. A large number of ligands targeting inhibition of kynurenine-related enzymes are available, but none have thus far advanced to clinical studies with the exception of IDO inhibitors for cancer. Decreasing production of neurotoxic metabolites such as 3-HK and QUIN with IDO, KMO, or KYNU inhibitors may reduce neuronal loss or atrophy in diseases like AD, PD, and HD, and may also offer promising therapy for MDD and HIV-associated neurocognitive disorder where neuroinflammation may contribute to the pathophysiology. Unfortunately, most ligands currently available have poor drug-like properties and would require optimization in terms of their pharmacokinetic properties. Alternatively, elevating levels of KYNA, or delivering KYNA-mimetics to the brain, may offer a different option for neuroprotection. However, it's worth noting that while KYNA analogs would be predicted to reduce excitotoxicity, it is unclear whether they could reduce oxidative stress-mediated damage caused by excessive production of 3-HK and QUIN. Furthermore, increasing KYNA may lead to psychotomimetic effects including disruption of cognitive function, whereas decreasing KYNA may be a therapeutic option for treating schizophrenia. Manipulating kynurenine metabolism for MS should be approached cautiously because the direction of change in kynurenines seems to differ depending on the stage of the disease. Also, the variability in the time course of disease progression between individuals makes it difficult to predict the stage of disease.

Evidence is emerging suggesting that IDO and downstream tryptophan catabolites play an important role in modulating immune responses. Though a review of the impact of kynurenine metabolism on the peripheral immune system is beyond the scope of the current review, it is important to keep this function of the kynurenine system in mind when considering the therapeutic potential of this pathway. An important role of IDO in immunosuppression and tolerance has been demonstrated during pregnancy, autoimmunity, resistance to tumors, and tolerance to allografts (Mellor and Munn, 2004; Barth and Raghuraman, 2012; Ban et al., 2013). Thus, therapeutic interventions involving the KP must be approached cautiously to examine the potential consequence on immunomodulatory actions. Particular attention should be paid to patients with autoimmune diseases, given that IDO may act as a negative regulator of the immune system to counteract autoimmunity. Two non-mutually exclusive theories have been proposed about how IDO and/or the kynurenine metabolites regulate the immune system: (1) IDO catabolism of tryptophan depletes this critical amino acid which is important for T-cell proliferation and (2) downstream kynurenine metabolites themselves inhibit certain immune cells (Frumento et al., 2002). Elevated IDO expression and kynurenines can have immunosuppressive effects by inhibiting $CD4^+$ T-cell functions, inducing regulatory T-cells, and inhibiting Natural Killer (NK) cells (Mandi and Vecsei, 2012). Thus, the KP is directly implicated in excitatory and inhibitory neuronal communication, regulated by proinflammatory cytokines and immune signals, contributes to the production of oxidative stress, and regulates immune cell function/phenotypes, thereby positioning it to act as a key interface between the brain and immune systems. This dual role will be important to consider as the KP is mined for potential therapeutic agents to treat debilitating CNS disorders.

SUMMARY

Much has been learned in the thirty-some years since the first description of the KP in CNS disease. As detailed above, pathway dysregulations have been described in virtually all major CNS diseases. The pathway is sensitive to inflammatory signaling and its products have neuromodulatory properties. It has unique properties as an interface between the immune system and neuronal signaling. Inhibition of unique enzymes in this pathway has been employed to ameliorate symptomatologies in several animal models of CNS disease. Successful translation of these preclinical efforts into actual drugs might open the venue for novel therapeutic interventions in human CNS disease.

REFERENCES

Abbott, A., Roberts, B. M., Turner, L., Campbell, D. W., Schaffer, C. L., Campbell, B., et al. (2010). Inhibition of kynurenine aminotransferase II (KAT II) protects against ketamine-induced cognitive impairment and improves spatial working memory. *Soc. Neurosci. Abstr.* 472.18.

Acuna-Castroviejo, D., Tapias, V., Lopez, L. C., Doerrier, C., Camacho, E., Carrion, M. D., et al. (2011). Protective effects of synthetic kynurenines on 1-methyl-4-phenyl-1,2,3,6-tetrahydropyridine-induced parkinsonism in mice. *Brain Res. Bull.* 85, 133–140. doi: 10.1016/j.brainresbull.2011.03.008

Agaugue, S., Perrin-Cocon, L., Coutant, F., Andre, P., and Lotteau, V. (2006). 1-Methyl-tryptophan can interfere with TLR signaling in dendritic cells independently of IDO activity. *J. Immunol.* 177, 2061–2071.

Akimoto, H., Yamada, A., and Takikawa, O. (2007). Up-regulation of the brain indoleamine 2,3-dioxygenase activity in a mouse model of Alzheimer's disease by systemic endotoxin challenge. *Int. Cong.* 1304, 357–361. doi: 10.1016/j.ics.2007.07.026

Alberati-Giani, D., Ricciardi-Castagnoli, P., Kohler, C., and Cesura, A. M. (1996). Regulation of the kynurenine metabolic pathway by interferon-gamma in murine cloned macrophages and microglial cells. *J. Neurochem.* 66, 996–1004. doi: 10.1046/j.1471-4159.1996.66030996.x

Alsadany, M. A., Shehata, H. H., Mohamad, M. I., and Mahfouz, R. G. (2013). Histone deacetylases enzyme, copper, and IL-8 levels in patients with Alzheimer's disease. *Am. J. Alzheimers. Dis. Other Demen.* 28, 54–61. doi: 10.1177/1533317512467680

Amirkhani, A., Rajda, C., Arvidsson, B., Bencsik, K., Boda, K., Seres, E., et al. (2005). Interferon-beta affects the tryptophan metabolism in multiple sclerosis patients. *Eur. J. Neurol.* 12, 625–631. doi: 10.1111/j.1468-1331.2005.01041.x

Amori, L., Guidetti, P., Pellicciari, R., Kajii, Y., and Schwarcz, R. (2009). On the relationship between the two branches of the kynurenine pathway in the rat brain *in vivo*. *J. Neurochem.* 109, 316–325. doi: 10.1111/j.1471-4159.2009.05893.x

Arends, Y. M., Duyckaerts, C., Rozemuller, J. M., Eikelenboom, P., and Hauw, J. J. (2000). Microglia, amyloid and dementia in alzheimer disease. A correlative study. *Neurobiol. Aging* 21, 39–47. doi: 10.1016/S0197-4580(00)00094-4

Babcock, T. A., and Carlin, J. M. (2000). Transcriptional activation of indoleamine dioxygenase by interleukin 1 and tumor necrosis factor alpha in interferon-treated epithelial cells. *Cytokine* 12, 588–594. doi: 10.1006/cyto.1999.0661

Ban, Y., Chang, Y., Dong, B., Kong, B., and Qu, X. (2013). Indoleamine 2,3-dioxygenase levels at the normal and recurrent spontaneous abortion fetal-maternal interface. *J. Int. Med. Res.* 41, 1135–1149. doi: 10.1177/0300060513487642

Bannink, M., Fekkes, D., Van Gool, A. R., Kruit, W. H., Sleijfer, S., Van Der Holt, B., et al. (2007). Interferon-alpha influences tryptophan metabolism without inducing psychiatric side effects. *Neuropsychobiology* 55, 225–231. doi: 10.1159/000108382

Barth, H., and Raghuraman, S. (2012). Persistent infectious diseases say - IDO. Role of indoleamine-2,3-dioxygenase in disease pathogenesis and implications for therapy. *Crit. Rev. Microbiol.* 40, 360–368. doi: 10.3109/1040841X.2012.742037

Beal, M. F., Ferrante, R. J., Swartz, K. J., and Kowall, N. W. (1991). Chronic quinolinic acid lesions in rats closely resemble Huntington's disease. *J. Neurosci.* 11, 1649–1659.

Beal, M. F., Matson, W. R., Storey, E., Milbury, P., Ryan, E. A., Ogawa, T., et al. (1992). Kynurenic acid concentrations are reduced in Huntington's disease cerebral cortex. *J. Neurol. Sci.* 108, 80–87. doi: 10.1016/0022-510X(92)90191-M

Beal, M. F., Matson, W. R., Swartz, K. J., Gamache, P. H., and Bird, E. D. (1990). Kynurenine pathway measurements in Huntington's disease striatum: evidence for reduced formation of kynurenic acid. *J. Neurochem.* 55, 1327–1339. doi: 10.1111/j.1471-4159.1990.tb03143.x

Bjorkqvist, M., Wild, E. J., Thiele, J., Silvestroni, A., Andre, R., Lahiri, N., et al. (2008). A novel pathogenic pathway of immune activation detectable before clinical onset in Huntington's disease. *J. Exp. Med.* 205, 1869–1877. doi: 10.1084/jem.20080178

Bluthe, R. M., Lestage, J., Rees, G., Bristow, A., and Dantzer, R. (2002). Dual effect of central injection of recombinant rat interleukin-4 on lipopolysaccharide-induced sickness behavior in rats. *Neuropsychopharmacology* 26, 86–93. doi: 10.1016/S0893-133X(01)00305-0

Boasso, A., Vaccari, M., Fuchs, D., Hardy, A. W., Tsai, W. P., Tryniszewska, E., et al. (2009). Combined effect of antiretroviral therapy and blockade of IDO in SIV-infected rhesus macaques. *J. Immunol.* 182, 4313–4320. doi: 10.4049/jimmunol.0803314

Bonaccorso, S., Marino, V., Biondi, M., Grimaldi, F., Ippoliti, F., and Maes, M. (2002a). Depression induced by treatment with interferon-alpha in patients affected by hepatitis C virus. *J. Affect. Disord.* 72, 237–241. doi: 10.1016/S0165-0327(02)00264-1

Bonaccorso, S., Marino, V., Puzella, A., Pasquini, M., Biondi, M., Artini, M., et al. (2002b). Increased depressive ratings in patients with hepatitis C receiving interferon-alpha-based immunotherapy are related to interferon-alpha-induced changes in the serotonergic system. *J. Clin. Psychopharmacol.* 22, 86–90. doi: 10.1097/00004714-200202000-00014

Bonda, D. J., Mailankot, M., Stone, J. G., Garrett, M. R., Staniszewska, M., Castellani, R. J., et al. (2010). Indoleamine 2,3-dioxygenase and 3-hydroxykynurenine modifications are found in the neuropathology of Alzheimer's disease. *Redox Rep.* 15, 161–168. doi: 10.1179/174329210X12650506623645

Brown, R. R., Ozaki, Y., Datta, S. P., Borden, E. C., Sondel, P. M., and Malone, D. G. (1991). Implications of interferon-induced tryptophan catabolism in cancer, auto-immune diseases and AIDS. *Adv. Exp. Med. Biol.* 294, 425–435. doi: 10.1007/978-1-4684-5952-4_39

Cagnin, A., Kassiou, M., Meikle, S. R., and Banati, R. B. (2006). *In vivo* evidence for microglial activation in neurodegenerative dementia. *Acta Neurol. Scand. Suppl.* 185, 107–114. doi: 10.1111/j.1600-0404.2006.00694.x

Campesan, S., Green, E. W., Breda, C., Sathyasaikumar, K. V., Muchowski, P. J., Schwarcz, R., et al. (2011). The kynurenine pathway modulates neurodegeneration in a Drosophila model of Huntington's disease. *Curr. Biol.* 21, 961–966. doi: 10.1016/j.cub.2011.04.028

Capuron, L., Neurauter, G., Musselman, D. L., Lawson, D. H., Nemeroff, C. B., Fuchs, D., et al. (2003). Interferon-alpha-induced changes in tryptophan metabolism. Relationship to depression and paroxetine treatment. *Biol. Psychiatry* 54, 906–914. doi: 10.1016/S0006-3223(03)00173-2

Carson, M. J. (2002). Microglia as liaisons between the immune and central nervous systems: functional implications for multiple sclerosis. *Glia* 40, 218–231. doi: 10.1002/glia.10145

Cattaneo, A., Gennarelli, M., Uher, R., Breen, G., Farmer, A., Aitchison, K. J., et al. (2013). Candidate genes expression profile associated with antidepressants response in the GENDEP study: differentiating between baseline 'predictors' and longitudinal 'targets'. *Neuropsychopharmacology* 38, 377–385. doi: 10.1038/npp.2012.191

Chapin, D. S., Campbell, B., Strick, C., and Kozak, R. (2010). The impact of a KATII inhibitor on performance in the rat sustained attention task and conditioned avoidance responding. *Soc. Neurosci. Abstr.* 472.16.

Chaves, A. C., Ceravolo, I. P., Gomes, J. A., Zani, C. L., Romanha, A. J., and Gazzinelli, R. T. (2001). IL-4 and IL-13 regulate the induction of indoleamine 2,3-dioxygenase activity and the control of Toxoplasma gondii replication in human fibroblasts activated with IFN-gamma. *Eur. J. Immunol.* 31, 333–344. doi: 10.1002/1521-4141(200102)31:2<333::AID-IMMU333>3.0.CO;2-X

Chen, Y., and Guillemin, G. J. (2009). Kynurenine pathway metabolites in humans: disease and healthy states. *Int. J. Tryptophan Res.* 2, 1–19.

Chiang, S. S., Riedel, M., Schwarz, M., and Mueller, N. (2013). Is T-helper type 2 shift schizophrenia-specific? primary results from a comparison of related psychiatric disorders and healthy controls. *Psychiatry Clin. Neurosci.* 67, 228–236. doi: 10.1111/pcn.12040

Chiarugi, A., Calvani, M., Meli, E., Traggiai, E., and Moroni, F. (2001a). Synthesis and release of neurotoxic kynurenine metabolites by human monocyte-derived macrophages. *J. Neuroimmunol.* 120, 190–198. doi: 10.1016/S0165-5728(01)00418-0

Chiarugi, A., Cozzi, A., Ballerini, C., Massacesi, L., and Moroni, F. (2001b). Kynurenine 3-mono-oxygenase activity and neurotoxic kynurenine metabolites increase in the spinal cord of rats with experimental allergic encephalomyelitis. *Neuroscience* 102, 687–695. doi: 10.1016/S0306-4522(00)00504-2

Chon, S. Y., Hassanain, H. H., and Gupta, S. L. (1996). Cooperative role of interferon regulatory factor 1 and p91 (STAT1) response elements in interferon-gamma-inducible expression of human indoleamine 2,3-dioxygenase gene. *J. Biol. Chem.* 271, 17247–17252. doi: 10.1074/jbc.271.29.17247

Chon, S. Y., Hassanain, H. H., Pine, R., and Gupta, S. L. (1995). Involvement of two regulatory elements in interferon-gamma-regulated expression of human indoleamine 2,3-dioxygenase gene. *J. Interferon Cytokine Res.* 15, 517–526. doi: 10.1089/jir.1995.15.517

Comai, S., Cavalletto, L., Chemello, L., Bernardinello, E., Ragazzi, E., Costa, C. V., et al. (2011). Effects of PEG-interferon alpha plus ribavirin on tryptophan metabolism in patients with chronic hepatitis C. *Pharmacol. Res.* 63, 85–92. doi: 10.1016/j.phrs.2010.10.009

Comings, D. E., Muhleman, D., Dietz, G., Sherman, M., and Forest, G. L. (1995). Sequence of human tryptophan 2,3-dioxygenase (TDO2): presence of a glucocorticoid response-like element composed of a GTT repeat and an intronic CCCCT repeat. *Genomics* 29, 390–396. doi: 10.1006/geno.1995.9990

Connor, T. J., Starr, N., O'sullivan, J. B., and Harkin, A. (2008). Induction of indolamine 2,3-dioxygenase and kynurenine 3-monooxygenase in rat brain following a systemic inflammatory challenge: a role for IFN-gamma? *Neurosci. Lett.* 441, 29–34. doi: 10.1016/j.neulet.2008.06.007

Copeland, C. S., Neale, S. A., and Salt, T. E. (2013). Actions of Xanthurenic acid, a putative endogenous Group II metabotropic glutamate receptor agonist, on sensory transmission in the thalamus. *Neuropharmacology* 66, 133–142. doi: 10.1016/j.neuropharm.2012.03.009

Corona, A. W., Norden, D. M., Skendelas, J. P., Huang, Y., O'connor, J. C., Lawson, M., et al. (2013). Indoleamine 2,3-dioxygenase inhibition attenuates lipopolysaccharide induced persistent microglial activation and depressive-like complications in fractalkine receptor (CX(3)CR1)-deficient mice. *Brain Behav. Immun.* 31, 134–142. doi: 10.1016/j.bbi.2012.08.008

Coyle, J. T. (2012). NMDA receptor and schizophrenia: a brief history. *Schizophr. Bull.* 38, 920–926. doi: 10.1093/schbul/sbs076

Currier, A. R., Ziegler, M. H., Riley, M. M., Babcock, T. A., Telbis, V. P., and Carlin, J. M. (2000). Tumor necrosis factor-alpha and lipopolysaccharide enhance interferon-induced antichlamydial indoleamine dioxygenase activity independently. *J. Interferon Cytokine Res.* 20, 369–376. doi: 10.1089/107999000312306

Cutler, J. A., Rush, A. J., McMahon, F. J., and Laje, G. (2012). Common genetic variation in the indoleamine-2,3-dioxygenase genes and antidepressant treatment outcome in major depressive disorder. *J. Psychopharmacol.* 26, 360–367. doi: 10.1177/0269881111434622

Dai, W., and Gupta, S. L. (1990). Regulation of indoleamine 2,3-dioxygenase gene expression in human fibroblasts by interferon-gamma. Upstream control region discriminates between interferon-gamma and interferon-alpha. *J. Biol. Chem.* 265, 19871–19877.

Danesch, U., Gloss, B., Schmid, W., Schutz, G., Schule, R., and Renkawitz, R. (1987). Glucocorticoid induction of the rat tryptophan oxygenase gene is mediated by two widely separated glucocorticoid-responsive elements. *EMBO J.* 6, 625–630.

Danesch, U., Hashimoto, S., Renkawitz, R., and Schutz, G. (1983). Transcriptional regulation of the tryptophan oxygenase gene in rat liver by glucocorticoids. *J. Biol. Chem.* 258, 4750–4753.

Dantzer, R., O'connor, J. C., Lawson, M. A., and Kelley, K. W. (2011). Inflammation-associated depression: from serotonin to kynurenine. *Psychoneuroendocrinology* 36, 426–436. doi: 10.1016/j.psyneuen.2010.09.012

Darnell, J. E. Jr., Kerr, I. M., and Stark, G. R. (1994). Jak-STAT pathways and transcriptional activation in response to IFNs and other extracellular signaling proteins. *Science* 264, 1415–1421. doi: 10.1126/science.8197455

Devinsky, O., Vezzani, A., Najjar, S., De Lanerolle, N. C., and Rogawski, M. A. (2013). Glia and epilepsy: excitability and inflammation. *Trends Neurosci.* 36, 174–184. doi: 10.1016/j.tins.2012.11.008

Dinatale, B. C., Murray, I. A., Schroeder, J. C., Flaveny, C. A., Lahoti, T. S., Laurenzana, E. M., et al. (2010). Kynurenic acid is a potent endogenous aryl hydrocarbon receptor ligand that synergistically induces interleukin-6 in the presence of inflammatory signaling. *Toxicol. Sci.* 115, 89–97. doi: 10.1093/toxsci/kfq024

Dobos, N., De Vries, E. F., Kema, I. P., Patas, K., Prins, M., Nijholt, I. M., et al. (2012). The role of indoleamine 2,3-dioxygenase in a mouse model of neuroinflammation-induced depression. *J. Alzheimers. Dis.* 28, 905–915. doi: 10.3233/JAD-2011-111097

Dounay, A. B., Anderson, M., Bechle, B. M., Evrard, E., Gan, X., Kim, J. Y., et al. (2013). PF-04859989 as a template for structure-based drug design:

identification of new pyrazole series of irreversible KAT II inhibitors with improved lipophilic efficiency. *Bioorg. Med. Chem. Lett.* 23, 1961–1966. doi: 10.1016/j.bmcl.2013.02.039

Durastanti, V., Lugaresi, A., Bramanti, P., Amato, M., Bellantonio, P., De Luca, G., et al. (2011). Neopterin production and tryptophan degradation during 24-months therapy with interferon beta-1a in multiple sclerosis patients. *J. Transl. Med.* 9:42. doi: 10.1186/1479-5876-9-42

Eisenberger, N. I., Inagaki, T. K., Mashal, N. M., and Irwin, M. R. (2010). Inflammation and social experience: an inflammatory challenge induces feelings of social disconnection in addition to depressed mood. *Brain Behav. Immun.* 24, 558–563. doi: 10.1016/j.bbi.2009.12.009

Erhardt, S., Blennow, K., Nordin, C., Skogh, E., Lindstrom, L. H., and Engberg, G. (2001). Kynurenic acid levels are elevated in the cerebrospinal fluid of patients with schizophrenia. *Neurosci. Lett.* 313, 96–98. doi: 10.1016/S0304-3940(01)02242-X

Erhardt, S., Lim, C. K., Linderholm, K. R., Janelidze, S., Lindqvist, D., Samuelsson, M., et al. (2013). Connecting inflammation with glutamate agonism in suicidality. *Neuropsychopharmacology* 38, 743–752. doi: 10.1038/npp.2012.248

Erhardt, S., Olsson, S. K., and Engberg, G. (2009). Pharmacological manipulation of kynurenic acid: potential in the treatment of psychiatric disorders. *CNS Drugs* 23, 91–101. doi: 10.2165/00023210-200923020-00001

Flanagan, E. M., Erickson, J. B., Viveros, O. H., Chang, S. Y., and Reinhard, J. F. Jr. (1995). Neurotoxin quinolinic acid is selectively elevated in spinal cords of rats with experimental allergic encephalomyelitis. *J. Neurochem.* 64, 1192–1196. doi: 10.1046/j.1471-4159.1995.64031192.x

Forrest, C. M., Mackay, G. M., Stoy, N., Spiden, S. L., Taylor, R., Stone, T. W., et al. (2010). Blood levels of kynurenines, interleukin-23 and soluble human leucocyte antigen-G at different stages of Huntington's disease. *J. Neurochem.* 112, 112–122. doi: 10.1111/j.1471-4159.2009.06442.x

Frumento, G., Rotondo, R., Tonetti, M., Damonte, G., Benatti, U., and Ferrara, G. B. (2002). Tryptophan-derived catabolites are responsible for inhibition of T and natural killer cell proliferation induced by indoleamine 2,3-dioxygenase. *J. Exp. Med.* 196, 459–468. doi: 10.1084/jem.20020121

Fu, X., Zunich, S. M., O'connor, J. C., Kavelaars, A., Dantzer, R., and Kelley, K. W. (2010). Central administration of lipopolysaccharide induces depressive-like behavior *in vivo* and activates brain indoleamine 2,3 dioxygenase in murine organotypic hippocampal slice cultures. *J. Neuroinflammation* 7:43. doi: 10.1186/1742-2094-7-43

Fuchs, D., Moller, A. A., Reibnegger, G., Stockle, E., Werner, E. R., and Wachter, H. (1990). Decreased serum tryptophan in patients with HIV-1 infection correlates with increased serum neopterin and with neurologic/psychiatric symptoms. *J. Acquir. Immune Defic. Syndr.* 3, 873–876.

Fujigaki, H., Saito, K., Fujigaki, S., Takemura, M., Sudo, K., Ishiguro, H., et al. (2006). The signal transducer and activator of transcription 1alpha and interferon regulatory factor 1 are not essential for the induction of indoleamine 2,3-dioxygenase by lipopolysaccharide: involvement of p38 mitogen-activated protein kinase and nuclear factor-kappaB pathways, and synergistic effect of several proinflammatory cytokines. *J. Biochem.* 139, 655–662. doi: 10.1093/jb/mvj072

Fujigaki, H., Seishima, M., and Saito, K. (2012). Posttranslational modification of indoleamine 2,3-dioxygenase. *Anal. Bioanal. Chem.* 403, 1777–1782. doi: 10.1007/s00216-012-5946-2

Fujigaki, S., Saito, K., Sekikawa, K., Tone, S., Takikawa, O., Fujii, H., et al. (2001). Lipopolysaccharide induction of indoleamine 2,3-dioxygenase is mediated dominantly by an IFN-gamma-independent mechanism. *Eur. J. Immunol.* 31, 2313–2318. doi: 10.1002/1521-4141(200108)31:8%3C2313::AID-IMMU2313%3E3.0.CO;2-S

Fukui, S., Schwarcz, R., Rapoport, S. I., Takada, Y., and Smith, Q. R. (1991). Blood-brain barrier transport of kynurenines: implications for brain synthesis and metabolism. *J. Neurochem.* 56, 2007–2017. doi: 10.1111/j.1471-4159.1991.tb03460.x

Fuvesi, J., Rajda, C., Bencsik, K., Toldi, J., and Vecsei, L. (2012). The role of kynurenines in the pathomechanism of amyotrophic lateral sclerosis and multiple sclerosis: therapeutic implications. *J. Neural Transm.* 119, 225–234. doi: 10.1007/s00702-012-0765-3

Gabbay, V., Ely, B. A., Babb, J., and Liebes, L. (2012). The possible role of the kynurenine pathway in anhedonia in adolescents. *J. Neural Transm.* 119, 253–260. doi: 10.1007/s00702-011-0685-7

Gabbay, V., Liebes, L., Katz, Y., Liu, S., Mendoza, S., Babb, J. S., et al. (2010). The kynurenine pathway in adolescent depression: preliminary findings from a proton MR spectroscopy study. *Prog. Neuropsychopharmacol. Biol. Psychiatry* 34, 37–44. doi: 10.1016/j.pnpbp.2009.09.015

Gal, E. M., and Sherman, A. D. (1978). Synthesis and metabolism of L-kynurenine in rat brain. *J. Neurochem.* 30, 607–613. doi: 10.1111/j.1471-4159.1978.tb07815.x

Gerhard, A., Pavese, N., Hotton, G., Turkheimer, F., Es, M., Hammers, A., et al. (2006). *In vivo* imaging of microglial activation with [11C](R)-PK11195 PET in idiopathic Parkinson's disease. *Neurobiol. Dis.* 21, 404–412. doi: 10.1016/j.nbd.2005.08.002

Gibney, S. M., McGuinness, B., Prendergast, C., Harkin, A., and Connor, T. J. (2013). Poly I:C-induced activation of the immune response is accompanied by depression and anxiety-like behaviours, kynurenine pathway activation and reduced BDNF expression. *Brain Behav. Immun.* 28, 170–181. doi: 10.1016/j.bbi.2012.11.010

Giorgini, F., Guidetti, P., Nguyen, Q., Bennett, S. C., and Muchowski, P. J. (2005). A genomic screen in yeast implicates kynurenine 3-monooxygenase as a therapeutic target for Huntington disease. *Nat. Genet.* 37, 526–531. doi: 10.1038/ng1542

Gitter, B. D., Cox, L. M., Rydel, R. E., and May, P. C. (1995). Amyloid beta peptide potentiates cytokine secretion by interleukin-1 beta-activated human astrocytoma cells. *Proc. Natl. Acad. Sci. U.S.A.* 92, 10738–10741. doi: 10.1073/pnas.92.23.10738

Gleeson, L. C., Ryan, K. J., Griffin, E. W., Connor, T. J., and Harkin, A. (2010). The beta2-adrenoceptor agonist clenbuterol elicits neuroprotective, anti-inflammatory and neurotrophic actions in the kainic acid model of excitotoxicity. *Brain Behav. Immun.* 24, 1354–1361. doi: 10.1016/j.bbi.2010.06.015

Goeb, J. L., Even, C., Nicolas, G., Gohier, B., Dubas, F., and Garre, J. B. (2006). Psychiatric side effects of interferon-beta in multiple sclerosis. *Eur. Psychiatry* 21, 186–193. doi: 10.1016/j.eurpsy.2005.09.013

Graham, W. C., Robertson, R. G., Sambrook, M. A., and Crossman, A. R. (1990). Injection of excitatory amino acid antagonists into the medial pallidal segment of a 1-methyl-4-phenyl-1,2,3,6-tetrahydropyridine (MPTP) treated primate reverses motor symptoms of parkinsonism. *Life Sci.* 47, PL91–PL97. doi: 10.1016/0024-3205(90)90376-3

Gregoire, L., Rassoulpour, A., Guidetti, P., Samadi, P., Bedard, P. J., Izzo, E., et al. (2008). Prolonged kynurenine 3-hydroxylase inhibition reduces development of levodopa-induced dyskinesias in parkinsonian monkeys. *Behav. Brain Res.* 186, 161–167. doi: 10.1016/j.bbr.2007.08.007

Guidetti, P., Amori, L., Sapko, M. T., Okuno, E., and Schwarcz, R. (2007a). Mitochondrial aspartate aminotransferase: a third kynurenate-producing enzyme in the mammalian brain. *J. Neurochem.* 102, 103–111. doi: 10.1111/j.1471-4159.2007.04556.x

Guidetti, P., Hoffman, G. E., Melendez-Ferro, M., Albuquerque, E. X., and Schwarcz, R. (2007b). Astrocytic localization of kynurenine aminotransferase II in the rat brain visualized by immunocytochemistry. *Glia* 55, 78–92. doi: 10.1002/glia.20432

Guidetti, P., Bates, G. P., Graham, R. K., Hayden, M. R., Leavitt, B. R., Macdonald, M. E., et al. (2006). Elevated brain 3-hydroxykynurenine and quinolinate levels in Huntington disease mice. *Neurobiol. Dis.* 23, 190–197. doi: 10.1016/j.nbd.2006.02.011

Guidetti, P., Luthi-Carter, R. E., Augood, S. J., and Schwarcz, R. (2004). Neostriatal and cortical quinolinate levels are increased in early grade Huntington's disease. *Neurobiol. Dis.* 17, 455–461. doi: 10.1016/j.nbd.2004.07.006

Guidetti, P., Okuno, E., and Schwarcz, R. (1997). Characterization of rat brain kynurenine aminotransferases I and II. *J. Neurosci. Res.* 50, 457–465. doi: 10.1002/(SICI)1097-4547(19971101)50:3<457::AID-JNR12>3.0.CO;2-3

Guidetti, P., Reddy, P. H., Tagle, D. A., and Schwarcz, R. (2000). Early kynurenergic impairment in Huntington's disease and in a transgenic animal model. *Neurosci. Lett.* 283, 233–235. doi: 10.1016/S0304-3940(00)00956-3

Guillemin, G. J., Kerr, S. J., Pemberton, L. A., Smith, D. G., Smythe, G. A., Armati, P. J., et al. (2001). IFN-beta1b induces kynurenine pathway metabolism in human macrophages: potential implications for multiple sclerosis treatment. *J. Interferon Cytokine Res.* 21, 1097–1101. doi: 10.1089/107999001317205231

Guillemin, G. J., Smythe, G. A., Veas, L. A., Takikawa, O., and Brew, B. J. (2003). A beta 1-42 induces production of quinolinic acid by human macrophages and microglia. *Neuroreport* 14, 2311–2315. doi: 10.1097/00001756-200312190-00005

Guillemin, G. J., Smythe, G., Takikawa, O., and Brew, B. J. (2005). Expression of indoleamine 2,3-dioxygenase and production of quinolinic acid by human microglia, astrocytes, and neurons. *Glia* 49, 15–23. doi: 10.1002/glia.20090

Hamann, M., Sander, S. E., and Richter, A. (2008). Effects of the kynurenine 3-hydroxylase inhibitor Ro 61-8048 after intrastriatal injections on the severity of dystonia in the dt sz mutant. *Eur. J. Pharmacol.* 586, 156–159. doi: 10.1016/j.ejphar.2008.02.052

Haroon, E., Raison, C. L., and Miller, A. H. (2012). Psychoneuroimmunology meets neuropsychopharmacology: translational implications of the impact of inflammation on behavior. *Neuropsychopharmacology* 37, 137–162. doi: 10.1038/npp.2011.205

Harrison, P. J., and Weinberger, D. R. (2005). Schizophrenia genes, gene expression, and neuropathology: on the matter of their convergence. *Mol. Psychiatry* 10, 40–68; image 45. doi: 10.1038/sj.mp.4001558

Hartai, Z., Klivenyi, P., Janaky, T., Penke, B., Dux, L., and Vecsei, L. (2005). Kynurenine metabolism in multiple sclerosis. *Acta Neurol. Scand.* 112, 93–96. doi: 10.1111/j.1600-0404.2005.00442.x

Hassanain, H. H., Chon, S. Y., and Gupta, S. L. (1993). Differential regulation of human indoleamine 2,3-dioxygenase gene expression by interferons-gamma and -alpha. Analysis of the regulatory region of the gene and identification of an interferon-gamma-inducible DNA-binding factor. *J. Biol. Chem.* 268, 5077–5084.

Heyes, M. P., Brew, B. J., Martin, A., Price, R. W., Salazar, A. M., Sidtis, J. J., et al. (1991a). Quinolinic acid in cerebrospinal fluid and serum in HIV-1 infection: relationship to clinical and neurological status. *Ann. Neurol.* 29, 202–209. doi: 10.1002/ana.410290215

Heyes, M. P., Lackner, A., Kaufman, S., and Milstien, S. (1991b). Cerebrospinal fluid and serum neopterin and biopterin in D-retrovirus-infected rhesus macaques (*Macaca mulatta*): relationship to clinical and viral status. *AIDS* 5, 555–560. doi: 10.1097/00002030-199105000-00012

Heyes, M. P., Chen, C. Y., Major, E. O., and Saito, K. (1997). Different kynurenine pathway enzymes limit quinolinic acid formation by various human cell types. *Biochem. J.* 326(Pt 2), 351–356.

Heyes, M. P., Mefford, I. N., Quearry, B. J., Dedhia, M., and Lackner, A. (1990). Increased ratio of quinolinic acid to kynurenic acid in cerebrospinal fluid of D retrovirus-infected rhesus macaques: relationship to clinical and viral status. *Ann. Neurol.* 27, 666–675. doi: 10.1002/ana.410270614

Heyes, M. P., Saito, K., and Markey, S. P. (1992). Human macrophages convert L-tryptophan into the neurotoxin quinolinic acid. *Biochem. J.* 283(Pt 3), 633–635.

Hissong, B. D., and Carlin, J. M. (1997). Potentiation of interferon-induced indoleamine 2,3-dioxygenase mRNA in human mononuclear phagocytes by lipopolysaccharide and interleukin-1. *J. Interferon Cytokine Res.* 17, 387–393. doi: 10.1089/jir.1997.17.387

Horner, W., Gorczyca, R. R., Hughes, Z., Campbell, B., Fonseca, K., and Verhoest, P. (2010). *In vivo* characterization of a potent, selective KATII inhibitor as a regulator of kynurenic acid production in rat brain: a microdialysis study in freely moving rats. *Soc. Neurosci. Abstr.* 472.4.

Hu, B., Hissong, B. D., and Carlin, J. M. (1995). Interleukin-1 enhances indoleamine 2,3-dioxygenase activity by increasing specific mRNA expression in human mononuclear phagocytes. *J. Interferon Cytokine Res.* 15, 617–624. doi: 10.1089/jir.1995.15.617

Huang, G., Shi, L. Z., and Chi, H. (2009). Regulation of JNK and p38 MAPK in the immune system: signal integration, propagation and termination. *Cytokine* 48, 161–169. doi: 10.1016/j.cyto.2009.08.002

Huang, Q., Zhou, D., Sapp, E., Aizawa, H., Ge, P., Bird, E. D., et al. (1995). Quinolinic acid-induced increases in calbindin D28k immunoreactivity in rat striatal neurons *in vivo* and *in vitro* mimic the pattern seen in Huntington's disease. *Neuroscience* 65, 397–407. doi: 10.1016/0306-4522(94) 00494-P

Huell, M., Strauss, S., Volk, B., Berger, M., and Bauer, J. (1995). Interleukin-6 is present in early stages of plaque formation and is restricted to the brains of Alzheimer's disease patients. *Acta Neuropathol.* 89, 544–551. doi: 10.1007/BF00571510

Hughes, M. M., Carballedo, A., McLoughlin, D. M., Amico, F., Harkin, A., Frodl, T., et al. (2012). Tryptophan depletion in depressed patients occurs independent of kynurenine pathway activation. *Brain Behav. Immun.* 26, 979–987. doi: 10.1016/j.bbi.2012.05.010

Imamura, K., Hishikawa, N., Sawada, M., Nagatsu, T., Yoshida, M., and Hashizume, Y. (2003). Distribution of major histocompatibility complex class II-positive microglia and cytokine profile of Parkinson's disease brains. *Acta Neuropathol.* 106, 518–526. doi: 10.1007/s00401-003-0766-2

Irwin, M., Belendiuk, K., McCloskey, K., and Freedman, D. X. (1981). Tryptophan metabolism in children with attentional deficit disorder. *Am. J. Psychiatry* 138, 1082–1085.

Jansen, M., and Reinhard, J. F. Jr. (1999). Interferon response heterogeneity: activation of a proinflammatory response by interferon alpha and beta. A possible basis for diverse responses to interferon beta in MS. *J. Leukoc. Biol.* 65, 439–443.

Jauch, D., Urbanska, E. M., Guidetti, P., Bird, E. D., Vonsattel, J. P., Whetsell, W. O., et al. (1995). Dysfunction of brain kynurenic acid metabolism in Huntington's disease: focus on kynurenine aminotransferases. *J. Neurol. Sci.* 130, 39–47. doi: 10.1016/0022-510X(94)00280-2

Jung, I. D., Lee, C. M., Jeong, Y. I., Lee, J. S., Park, W. S., Han, J., et al. (2007). Differential regulation of indoleamine 2,3-dioxygenase by lipopolysaccharide and interferon gamma in murine bone marrow derived dendritic cells. *FEBS Lett.* 581, 1449–1456. doi: 10.1016/j.febslet.2007.02.073

Jung, I. D., Lee, M. G., Chang, J. H., Lee, J. S., Jeong, Y. I., Lee, C. M., et al. (2009). Blockade of indoleamine 2,3-dioxygenase protects mice against lipopolysaccharide-induced endotoxin shock. *J. Immunol.* 182, 3146–3154. doi: 10.4049/jimmunol.0803104

Kessler, R. C., Chiu, W. T., Demler, O., Merikangas, K. R., and Walters, E. E. (2005). Prevalence, severity, and comorbidity of 12-month DSM-IV disorders in the National Comorbidity Survey Replication. *Arch. Gen. Psychiatry* 62, 617–627. doi: 10.1001/archpsyc.62.6.617

Kiss, C., Ceresoli-Borroni, G., Guidetti, P., Zielke, C. L., Zielke, H. R., and Schwarcz, R. (2003). Kynurenate production by cultured human astrocytes. *J. Neural Transm.* 110, 1–14.

Kita, T., Morrison, P. F., Heyes, M. P., and Markey, S. P. (2002). Effects of systemic and central nervous system localized inflammation on the contributions of metabolic precursors to the L-kynurenine and quinolinic acid pools in brain. *J. Neurochem.* 82, 258–268. doi: 10.1046/j.1471-4159.2002.00955.x

Knyihar-Csillik, E., Chadaide, Z., Mihaly, A., Krisztin-Peva, B., Fenyo, R., and Vecsei, L. (2006). Effect of 6-hydroxydopamine treatment on kynurenine aminotransferase-I (KAT-I) immunoreactivity of neurons and glial cells in the rat substantia nigra. *Acta Neuropathol.* 112, 127–137. doi: 10.1007/s00401-006-0086-4

Knyihar-Csillik, E., Csillik, B., Pakaski, M., Krisztin-Peva, B., Dobo, E., Okuno, E., et al. (2004). Decreased expression of kynurenine aminotransferase-I (KAT-I) in the substantia nigra of mice after 1-methyl-4-phenyl-1,2,3,6-tetrahydropyridine (MPTP) treatment. *Neuroscience* 126, 899–914. doi: 10.1016/j.neuroscience.2004.04.043

Konan, K. V., and Taylor, M. W. (1996). Importance of the two interferon-stimulated response element (ISRE) sequences in the regulation of the human indoleamine 2,3-dioxygenase gene. *J. Biol. Chem.* 271, 19140–19145. doi: 10.1074/jbc.271.32.19140

Krakauer, T., and Oppenheim, J. J. (1993). IL-1 and tumor necrosis factor-alpha each up-regulate both the expression of IFN-gamma receptors and enhance IFN-gamma-induced HLA-DR expression on human monocytes and a human monocytic cell line (THP-1). *J. Immunol.* 150, 1205–1211.

Kurz, K., Schroecksnadel, S., Weiss, G., and Fuchs, D. (2011). Association between increased tryptophan degradation and depression in cancer patients. *Curr. Opin. Clin. Nutr. Metab. Care* 14, 49–56. doi: 10.1097/MCO.0b013e328340d849

Kwidzinski, E., Bunse, J., Aktas, O., Richter, D., Mutlu, L., Zipp, F., et al. (2005). Indolamine 2,3-dioxygenase is expressed in the CNS and down-regulates autoimmune inflammation. *FASEB J.* 19, 1347–1349. doi: 10.1096/fj.04-3228fje

Larson, K., Russ, S. A., Kahn, R. S., and Halfon, N. (2011). Patterns of comorbidity, functioning, and service use for US children with ADHD, 2007. *Pediatrics* 127, 462–470. doi: 10.1542/peds.2010-0165

Lassmann, H., and Ransohoff, R. M. (2004). The CD4-Th1 model for multiple sclerosis: a critical [correction of crucial] re-appraisal. *Trends Immunol.* 25, 132–137. doi: 10.1016/j.it.2004.01.007

Lavebratt, C., Olsson, S., Backlund, L., Frisen, L., Sellgren, C., Priebe, L., et al. (2013). The KMO allele encoding Arg is associated with psychotic features in bipolar disorder type 1, and with increased CSF KYNA level and reduced KMO expression. *Mol. Psychiatry*. doi: 10.1038/mp.2013.11. [Epub ahead of print].

Lee Do, Y., Lee, K. S., Lee, H. J., Noh, Y. H., Kim Do, H., Lee, J. Y., et al. (2008). Kynurenic acid attenuates MPP(+)-induced dopaminergic neuronal cell death via a Bax-mediated mitochondrial pathway. *Eur. J. Cell Biol.* 87, 389–397. doi: 10.1016/j.ejcb.2008.03.003

Lehrmann, E., Guidetti, P., Love, A., Williamson, J., Bertram, E. H., and Schwarcz, R. (2008). Glial activation precedes seizures and hippocampal neurodegeneration in measles virus-infected mice. *Epilepsia* 49(Suppl. 2), 13–23. doi: 10.1111/j.1528-1167.2008.01489.x

Leonard, B., and Maes, M. (2012). Mechanistic explanations how cell-mediated immune activation, inflammation and oxidative and nitrosative stress pathways and their sequels and concomitants play a role in the pathophysiology of unipolar depression. *Neurosci. Biobehav. Rev.* 36, 764–785. doi: 10.1016/j.neubiorev.2011.12.005

Lestage, J., Verrier, D., Palin, K., and Dantzer, R. (2002). The enzyme indoleamine 2,3-dioxygenase is induced in the mouse brain in response to peripheral administration of lipopolysaccharide and superantigen. *Brain Behav. Immun.* 16, 596–601. doi: 10.1016/S0889-1591(02)00014-4

Lewis, D. A., Hashimoto, T., and Volk, D. W. (2005). Cortical inhibitory neurons and schizophrenia. *Nat. Rev. Neurosci.* 6, 312–324. doi: 10.1038/nrn1648

Liimatainen, S., Lehtimaki, K., Raitala, A., Peltola, M., Oja, S. S., Peltola, J., et al. (2011). Increased indoleamine 2,3-dioxygenase (IDO) activity in idiopathic generalized epilepsy. *Epilepsy Res.* 94, 206–212. doi: 10.1016/j.eplepsyres.2011.02.003

Linderholm, K. R., Skogh, E., Olsson, S. K., Dahl, M. L., Holtze, M., Engberg, G., et al. (2012). Increased levels of kynurenine and kynurenic acid in the CSF of patients with schizophrenia. *Schizophr. Bull.* 38, 426–432. doi: 10.1093/schbul/sbq086

Luchowski, P., Luchowska, E., Turski, W. A., and Urbanska, E. M. (2002). 1-Methyl-4-phenylpyridinium and 3-nitropropionic acid diminish cortical synthesis of kynurenic acid via interference with kynurenine aminotransferases in rats. *Neurosci. Lett.* 330, 49–52. doi: 10.1016/S0304-3940(02)00735-8

Lue, L. F., Rydel, R., Brigham, E. F., Yang, L. B., Hampel, H., Murphy, G. M., et al. (2001). Inflammatory repertoire of Alzheimer's disease and nondemented elderly microglia *in vitro*. *Glia* 35, 72–79. doi: 10.1002/glia.1072

Macchiarulo, A., Camaioni, E., Nuti, R., and Pellicciari, R. (2009). Highlights at the gate of tryptophan catabolism: a review on the mechanisms of activation and regulation of indoleamine 2,3-dioxygenase (IDO), a novel target in cancer disease. *Amino Acids* 37, 219–229. doi: 10.1007/s00726-008-0137-3

Mackay, G. M., Forrest, C. M., Christofides, J., Bridel, M. A., Mitchell, S., Cowlard, R., et al. (2009). Kynurenine metabolites and inflammation markers in depressed patients treated with fluoxetine or counselling. *Clin. Exp. Pharmacol. Physiol.* 36, 425–435. doi: 10.1111/j.1440-1681.2008.05077.x

Mandi, Y., and Vecsei, L. (2012). The kynurenine system and immunoregulation. *J. Neural Transm.* 119, 197–209. doi: 10.1007/s00702-011-0681-y

Maneglier, B., Malleret, B., Guillemin, G. J., Spreux-Varoquaux, O., Devillier, P., Rogez-Kreuz, C., et al. (2009). Modulation of indoleamine-2,3-dioxygenase expression and activity by HIV-1 in human macrophages. *Fundam. Clin. Pharmacol.* 23, 573–581. doi: 10.1111/j.1472-8206.2009.00703.x

Matysiak, M., Stasiolek, M., Orlowski, W., Jurewicz, A., Janczar, S., Raine, C. S., et al. (2008). Stem cells ameliorate EAE via an indoleamine 2,3-dioxygenase (IDO) mechanism. *J. Neuroimmunol.* 193, 12–23. doi: 10.1016/j.jneuroim.2007.07.025

McGeer, P. L., Itagaki, S., Boyes, B. E., and McGeer, E. G. (1988). Reactive microglia are positive for HLA-DR in the substantia nigra of Parkinson's and Alzheimer's disease brains. *Neurology* 38, 1285–1291. doi: 10.1212/WNL.38.8.1285

Mellor, A. L., Baban, B., Chandler, P., Marshall, B., Jhaver, K., Hansen, A., et al. (2003). Cutting edge: induced indoleamine 2,3 dioxygenase expression in dendritic cell subsets suppresses T cell clonal expansion. *J. Immunol.* 171, 1652–1655.

Mellor, A. L., and Munn, D. H. (2004). IDO expression by dendritic cells: tolerance and tryptophan catabolism. *Nat. Rev. Immunol.* 4, 762–774. doi: 10.1038/nri1457

Mezrich, J. D., Fechner, J. H., Zhang, X., Johnson, B. P., Burlingham, W. J., and Bradfield, C. A. (2010). An interaction between kynurenine and the aryl hydrocarbon receptor can generate regulatory T cells. *J. Immunol.* 185, 3190–3198. doi: 10.4049/jimmunol.0903670

Miller, C. L., Llenos, I. C., Dulay, J. R., Barillo, M. M., Yolken, R. H., and Weis, S. (2004). Expression of the kynurenine pathway enzyme tryptophan 2,3-dioxygenase is increased in the frontal cortex of individuals with schizophrenia. *Neurobiol. Dis.* 15, 618–629. doi: 10.1016/j.nbd.2003.12.015

Miller, C. L., Llenos, I. C., Dulay, J. R., and Weis, S. (2006). Upregulation of the initiating step of the kynurenine pathway in postmortem anterior cingulate cortex from individuals with schizophrenia and bipolar disorder. *Brain Res.* 1073–1074, 25–37. doi: 10.1016/j.brainres.2005.12.056

Miranda, A. F., Boegman, R. J., Beninger, R. J., and Jhamandas, K. (1997). Protection against quinolinic acid-mediated excitotoxicity in nigrostriatal dopaminergic neurons by endogenous kynurenic acid. *Neuroscience* 78, 967–975. doi: 10.1016/S0306-4522(96)00655-0

Moghaddam, B., and Javitt, D. (2012). From revolution to evolution: the glutamate hypothesis of schizophrenia and its implication for treatment. *Neuropsychopharmacology* 37, 4–15. doi: 10.1038/npp.2011.181

Mogi, M., Harada, M., Kondo, T., Riederer, P., Inagaki, H., Minami, M., et al. (1994a). Interleukin-1 beta, interleukin-6, epidermal growth factor and transforming growth factor-alpha are elevated in the brain from parkinsonian patients. *Neurosci. Lett.* 180, 147–150. doi: 10.1016/0304-3940(94)90508-8

Mogi, M., Harada, M., Riederer, P., Narabayashi, H., Fujita, K., and Nagatsu, T. (1994b). Tumor necrosis factor-alpha (TNF-alpha) increases both in the brain and in the cerebrospinal fluid from parkinsonian patients. *Neurosci. Lett.* 165, 208–210. doi: 10.1016/0304-3940(94)90746-3

Möller, T. (2010). Neuroinflammation in Huntington's disease. *J. Neural Transm.* 117, 1001–1008. doi: 10.1007/s00702-010-0430-7

Molteni, R., Macchi, F., Zecchillo, C., Dell'agli, M., Colombo, E., Calabrese, F., et al. (2013). Modulation of the inflammatory response in rats chronically treated with the antidepressant agomelatine. *Eur. Neuropsychopharmacol.* 23, 1645–1655. doi: 10.1016/j.euroneuro.2013.03.008

Monaco, F., Fumero, S., Mondino, A., and Mutani, R. (1979). Plasma and cerebrospinal fluid tryptophan in multiple sclerosis and degenerative diseases. *J. Neurol. Neurosurg. Psychiatr.* 42, 640–641. doi: 10.1136/jnnp.42.7.640

Moreau, M., Andre, C., O'connor, J. C., Dumich, S. A., Woods, J. A., Kelley, K. W., et al. (2008). Inoculation of Bacillus Calmette-Guerin to mice induces an acute episode of sickness behavior followed by chronic depressive-like behavior. *Brain Behav. Immun.* 22, 1087–1095. doi: 10.1016/j.bbi.2008.04.001

Moreau, M., Lestage, J., Verrier, D., Mormede, C., Kelley, K. W., Dantzer, R., et al. (2005). Bacille Calmette-Guerin inoculation induces chronic activation of peripheral and brain indoleamine 2,3-dioxygenase in mice. *J. Infect. Dis.* 192, 537–544. doi: 10.1086/431603

Muller, N., Myint, A. M., and Schwarz, M. J. (2012). Inflammation in schizophrenia. *Adv. Protein Chem. Struct. Biol.* 88, 49–68. doi: 10.1016/B978-0-12-398314-5.00003-9

Munn, D. H., Shafizadeh, E., Attwood, J. T., Bondarev, I., Pashine, A., and Mellor, A. L. (1999). Inhibition of T cell proliferation by macrophage tryptophan catabolism. *J. Exp. Med.* 189, 1363–1372. doi: 10.1084/jem.189.9.1363

Munn, D. H., Zhou, M., Attwood, J. T., Bondarev, I., Conway, S. J., Marshall, B., et al. (1998). Prevention of allogeneic fetal rejection by tryptophan catabolism. *Science* 281, 1191–1193. doi: 10.1126/science.281.5380.1191

Musso, T., Gusella, G. L., Brooks, A., Longo, D. L., and Varesio, L. (1994). Interleukin-4 inhibits indoleamine 2,3-dioxygenase expression in human monocytes. *Blood* 83, 1408–1411.

Myint, A. M., Bondy, B., Baghai, T. C., Eser, D., Nothdurfter, C., Schule, C., et al. (2013). Tryptophan metabolism and immunogenetics in major depression: a role for interferon-gamma gene. *Brain Behav. Immun.* 31, 128–133. doi: 10.1016/j.bbi.2013.04.003

Nagatsu, T., Mogi, M., Ichinose, H., and Togari, A. (2000). Cytokines in Parkinson's disease. *J. Neural Transm. Suppl.* 58, 143–151. doi: 10.1007/978-3-7091-6301-6_19

Nguyen, N. T., Kimura, A., Nakahama, T., Chinen, I., Masuda, K., Nohara, K., et al. (2010). Aryl hydrocarbon receptor negatively regulates dendritic cell immunogenicity via a kynurenine-dependent mechanism. *Proc. Natl. Acad. Sci. U.S.A.* 107, 19961–19966. doi: 10.1073/pnas.1014465107

Nilsson, L. K., Linderholm, K. R., Engberg, G., Paulson, L., Blennow, K., Lindstrom, L. H., et al. (2005). Elevated levels of kynurenic acid in the cerebrospinal fluid of male patients with schizophrenia. *Schizophr. Res.* 80, 315–322. doi: 10.1016/j.schres.2005.07.013

Niranjan, R. (2013). Molecular basis of etiological implications in Alzheimer's Disease: focus on neuroinflammation. *Mol. Neurobiol.* 48, 412–428. doi: 10.1007/s12035-013-8428-4

Oades, R. D. (2011). An exploration of the associations of pregnancy and perinatal features with cytokines and tryptophan/kynurenine metabolism in children with attention-deficit hyperactivity disorder (ADHD). *Atten. Defic. Hyperact. Disord.* 3, 301–318. doi: 10.1007/s12402-011-0062-2

Oades, R. D., Dauvermann, M. R., Schimmelmann, B. G., Schwarz, M. J., and Myint, A. M. (2010a). Attention-deficit hyperactivity disorder (ADHD) and glial integrity: S100B, cytokines and kynurenine metabolism–effects of medication. *Behav. Brain Funct.* 6:29. doi: 10.1186/1744-9081-6-29

Oades, R. D., Myint, A. M., Dauvermann, M. R., Schimmelmann, B. G., and Schwarz, M. J. (2010b). Attention-deficit hyperactivity disorder (ADHD) and glial integrity: an exploration of associations of cytokines and kynurenine metabolites with symptoms and attention. *Behav. Brain Funct.* 6:32. doi: 10.1186/1744-9081-6-32

O'connor, J. C., Andre, C., Wang, Y., Lawson, M. A., Szegedi, S. S., Lestage, J., et al. (2009a). Interferon-gamma and tumor necrosis factor-alpha mediate the upregulation of indoleamine 2,3-dioxygenase and the induction of depressive-like behavior in mice in response to bacillus Calmette-Guerin. *J. Neurosci.* 29, 4200–4209. doi: 10.1523/JNEUROSCI.5032-08.2009

O'connor, J. C., Lawson, M. A., Andre, C., Briley, E. M., Szegedi, S. S., Lestage, J., et al. (2009b). Induction of IDO by bacille Calmette-Guerin is responsible for development of murine depressive-like behavior. *J. Immunol.* 182, 3202–3212. doi: 10.4049/jimmunol.0802722

O'connor, J. C., Lawson, M. A., Andre, C., Moreau, M., Lestage, J., Castanon, N., et al. (2009c). Lipopolysaccharide-induced depressive-like behavior is mediated by indoleamine 2,3-dioxygenase activation in mice. *Mol. Psychiatry* 14, 511–522. doi: 10.1038/sj.mp.4002148

Ogawa, T., Matson, W. R., Beal, M. F., Myers, R. H., Bird, E. D., Milbury, P., et al. (1992). Kynurenine pathway abnormalities in Parkinson's disease. *Neurology* 42, 1702–1706. doi: 10.1212/WNL.42.9.1702

Ohmori, Y., Schreiber, R. D., and Hamilton, T. A. (1997). Synergy between interferon-gamma and tumor necrosis factor-alpha in transcriptional activation is mediated by cooperation between signal transducer and activator of transcription 1 and nuclear factor kappaB. *J. Biol. Chem.* 272, 14899–14907. doi: 10.1074/jbc.272.23.14899

Opitz, C. A., Litzenburger, U. M., Sahm, F., Ott, M., Tritschler, I., Trump, S., et al. (2011). An endogenous tumour-promoting ligand of the human aryl hydrocarbon receptor. *Nature* 478, 197–203. doi: 10.1038/nature10491

Ott, M., Demisch, L., Engelhardt, W., and Fischer, P. A. (1993). Interleukin-2, soluble interleukin-2-receptor, neopterin, L-tryptophan and beta 2-microglobulin levels in CSF and serum of patients with relapsing-remitting or chronic-progressive multiple sclerosis. *J. Neurol.* 241, 108–114. doi: 10.1007/BF00869773

Ouattara, B., Belkhir, S., Morissette, M., Dridi, M., Samadi, P., Gregoire, L., et al. (2009). Implication of NMDA receptors in the antidyskinetic activity of cabergoline, CI-1041, and Ro 61-8048 in MPTP monkeys with levodopa-induced dyskinesias. *J. Mol. Neurosci.* 38, 128–142. doi: 10.1007/s12031-008-9137-8

Oxenkrug, G., Perianayagam, M., Mikolich, D., Requintina, P., Shick, L., Ruthazer, R., et al. (2011). Interferon-gamma (+874) T/A genotypes and risk of IFN-alpha-induced depression. *J. Neural Transm.* 118, 271–274. doi: 10.1007/s00702-010-0525-1

Patel, N. S., Paris, D., Mathura, V., Quadros, A. N., Crawford, F. C., and Mullan, M. J. (2005). Inflammatory cytokine levels correlate with amyloid load in transgenic mouse models of Alzheimer's disease. *J. Neuroinflammation* 2:9. doi: 10.1186/1742-2094-2-9

Pearson, S. J., and Reynolds, G. P. (1992). Increased brain concentrations of a neurotoxin, 3-hydroxykynurenine, in Huntington's disease. *Neurosci. Lett.* 144, 199–201. doi: 10.1016/0304-3940(92)90749-W

Perkins, M. N., and Stone, T. W. (1985). Actions of kynurenic acid and quinolinic acid in the rat hippocampus *in vivo*. *Exp. Neurol.* 88, 570–579. doi: 10.1016/0014-4886(85)90072-X

Petermann, F., and Korn, T. (2011). Cytokines and effector T cell subsets causing autoimmune CNS disease. *FEBS Lett.* 585, 3747–3757. doi: 10.1016/j.febslet.2011.03.064

Platten, M., Ho, P. P., Youssef, S., Fontoura, P., Garren, H., Hur, E. M., et al. (2005). Treatment of autoimmune neuroinflammation with a synthetic tryptophan metabolite. *Science* 310, 850–855. doi: 10.1126/science.1117634

Pocivavsek, A., Wu, H. Q., Potter, M. C., Elmer, G. I., Pellicciari, R., and Schwarcz, R. (2011). Fluctuations in endogenous kynurenic acid control hippocampal glutamate and memory. *Neuropsychopharmacology* 36, 2357–2367. doi: 10.1038/npp.2011.127

Quintana, F. J., Basso, A. S., Iglesias, A. H., Korn, T., Farez, M. F., Bettelli, E., et al. (2008). Control of T(reg) and T(H)17 cell differentiation by the aryl hydrocarbon receptor. *Nature* 453, 65–71. doi: 10.1038/nature06880

Quintana, F. J., Murugaiyan, G., Farez, M. F., Mitsdoerffer, M., Tukpah, A. M., Burns, E. J., et al. (2010). An endogenous aryl hydrocarbon receptor ligand acts on dendritic cells and T cells to suppress experimental autoimmune encephalomyelitis. *Proc. Natl. Acad. Sci. U.S.A.* 107, 20768–20773. doi: 10.1073/pnas.1009201107

Rahman, A., Ting, K., Cullen, K. M., Braidy, N., Brew, B. J., and Guillemin, G. J. (2009). The excitotoxin quinolinic acid induces tau phosphorylation in human neurons. *PLoS ONE* 4:e6344. doi: 10.1371/journal.pone.0006344

Raison, C. L., Rutherford, R. E., Woolwine, B. J., Shuo, C., Schettler, P., Drake, D. F., et al. (2013). A randomized controlled trial of the tumor necrosis factor antagonist infliximab for treatment-resistant depression: the role of baseline inflammatory biomarkers. *JAMA psychiatry* 70, 31–41. doi: 10.1001/2013.jamapsychiatry.4

Raitala, A., Pertovaara, M., Karjalainen, J., Oja, S. S., and Hurme, M. (2005). Association of interferon-gamma +874(T/A) single nucleotide polymorphism with the rate of tryptophan catabolism in healthy individuals. *Scand. J. Immunol.* 61, 387–390. doi: 10.1111/j.1365-3083.2005.01586.x

Rejdak, K., Bartosik-Psujek, H., Dobosz, B., Kocki, T., Grieb, P., Giovannoni, G., et al. (2002). Decreased level of kynurenic acid in cerebrospinal fluid of relapsing-onset multiple sclerosis patients. *Neurosci. Lett.* 331, 63–65. doi: 10.1016/S0304-3940(02)00710-3

Rejdak, K., Petzold, A., Kocki, T., Kurzepa, J., Grieb, P., Turski, W. A., et al. (2007). Astrocytic activation in relation to inflammatory markers during clinical exacerbation of relapsing-remitting multiple sclerosis. *J. Neural Transm.* 114, 1011–1015. doi: 10.1007/s00702-007-0667-y

Richter, A., and Hamann, M. (2003). The kynurenine 3-hydroxylase inhibitor Ro 61-8048 improves dystonia in a genetic model of paroxysmal dyskinesia. *Eur. J. Pharmacol.* 478, 47–52. doi: 10.1016/j.ejphar.2003.08.038

Robinson, C. M., Hale, P. T., and Carlin, J. M. (2006). NF-kappa B activation contributes to indoleamine dioxygenase transcriptional synergy induced by IFN-gamma and tumor necrosis factor-alpha. *Cytokine* 35, 53–61. doi: 10.1016/j.cyto.2006.07.007

Robinson, C. M., Shirey, K. A., and Carlin, J. M. (2003). Synergistic transcriptional activation of indoleamine dioxygenase by IFN-gamma and tumor necrosis factor-alpha. *J. Interferon Cytokine Res.* 23, 413–421. doi: 10.1089/107999003322277829

Sakurai, K., Zou, J. P., Tschetter, J. R., Ward, J. M., and Shearer, G. M. (2002). Effect of indoleamine 2,3-dioxygenase on induction of experimental autoimmune encephalomyelitis. *J. Neuroimmunol.* 129, 186–196. doi: 10.1016/S0165-5728(02)00176-5

Salazar, A., Gonzalez-Rivera, B. L., Redus, L., Parrott, J. M., and O'connor, J. C. (2012). Indoleamine 2,3-dioxygenase mediates anhedonia and anxiety-like behaviors caused by peripheral lipopolysaccharide immune challenge. *Horm. Behav.* 62, 202–209. doi: 10.1016/j.yhbeh.2012.03.010

Samadi, P., Gregoire, L., Rassoulpour, A., Guidetti, P., Izzo, E., Schwarcz, R., et al. (2005). Effect of kynurenine 3-hydroxylase inhibition on the dyskinetic and antiparkinsonian responses to levodopa in Parkinsonian monkeys. *Mov. Disord.* 20, 792–802. doi: 10.1002/mds.20596

Sathyasaikumar, K. V., Stachowski, E. K., Amori, L., Guidetti, P., Muchowski, P. J., and Schwarcz, R. (2010). Dysfunctional kynurenine pathway metabolism in the R6/2 mouse model of Huntington's disease. *J. Neurochem.* 113, 1416–1425. doi: 10.1111/j.1471-4159.2010.06675.x

Schwarcz, R., Bruno, J. P., Muchowski, P. J., and Wu, H. Q. (2012). Kynurenines in the mammalian brain: when physiology meets pathology. *Nat. Rev. Neurosci.* 13, 465–477. doi: 10.1038/nrn3257

Schwarcz, R., Okuno, E., White, R. J., Bird, E. D., and Whetsell, W. O. Jr. (1988). 3-Hydroxyanthranilate oxygenase activity is increased in the brains of Huntington disease victims. *Proc. Natl. Acad. Sci. U.S.A.* 85, 4079–4081. doi: 10.1073/pnas.85.11.4079

Schwarcz, R., and Pellicciari, R. (2002). Manipulation of brain kynurenines: glial targets, neuronal effects, and clinical opportunities. *J. Pharmacol. Exp. Ther.* 303, 1–10. doi: 10.1124/jpet.102.034439

Schwarcz, R., Rassoulpour, A., Wu, H. Q., Medoff, D., Tamminga, C. A., and Roberts, R. C. (2001). Increased cortical kynurenate content in schizophrenia. *Biol. Psychiatry* 50, 521–530. doi: 10.1016/S0006-3223(01)01078-2

Schwarcz, R., Speciale, C., and French, E. D. (1987). Hippocampal kynurenines as etiological factors in seizure disorders. *Pol. J. Pharmacol. Pharm.* 39, 485–494.

Schwieler, L., Erhardt, S., Nilsson, L., Linderholm, K., and Engberg, G. (2006). Effects of COX-1 and COX-2 inhibitors on the firing of rat midbrain dopaminergic neurons–possible involvement of endogenous kynurenic acid. *Synapse* 59, 290–298. doi: 10.1002/syn.20241

Shaw, P., and Rabin, C. (2009). New insights into attention-deficit/hyperactivity disorder using structural neuroimaging. *Curr. Psychiatry Rep.* 11, 393–398. doi: 10.1007/s11920-009-0059-0

Shimizu, T., Nomiyama, S., Hirata, F., and Hayaishi, O. (1978). Indoleamine 2,3-dioxygenase. Purification and some properties. *J. Biol. Chem.* 253, 4700–4706.

Shirey, K. A., Jung, J. Y., Maeder, G. S., and Carlin, J. M. (2006). Upregulation of IFN-gamma receptor expression by proinflammatory cytokines influences IDO activation in epithelial cells. *J. Interferon Cytokine Res.* 26, 53–62. doi: 10.1089/jir.2006.26.53

Silva-Adaya, D., Perez-De La Cruz, V., Villeda-Hernandez, J., Carrillo-Mora, P., Gonzalez-Herrera, I. G., Garcia, E., et al. (2011). Protective effect of L-kynurenine and probenecid on 6-hydroxydopamine-induced striatal toxicity in rats: implications of modulating kynurenate as a protective strategy. *Neurotoxicol. Teratol.* 33, 303–312. doi: 10.1016/j.ntt.2010.10.002

Silvestroni, A., Faull, R. L., Strand, A. D., and Moller, T. (2009). Distinct neuroinflammatory profile in post-mortem human Huntington's disease. *Neuroreport* 20, 1098–1103. doi: 10.1097/WNR.0b013e32832e34ee

Smith, A. K., Simon, J. S., Gustafson, E. L., Noviello, S., Cubells, J. F., Epstein, M. P., et al. (2012). Association of a polymorphism in the indoleamine-2,3-dioxygenase gene and interferon-alpha-induced depression in patients with chronic hepatitis C. *Mol. Psychiatry* 17, 781–789. doi: 10.1038/mp.2011.67

Steiner, J., Walter, M., Gos, T., Guillemin, G. J., Bernstein, H. G., Sarnyai, Z., et al. (2011). Severe depression is associated with increased microglial quinolinic acid in subregions of the anterior cingulate gyrus: evidence for an immune-modulated glutamatergic neurotransmission? *J. Neuroinflammation* 8:94. doi: 10.1186/1742-2094-8-94

Stone, T. W., and Connick, J. H. (1985). Quinolinic acid and other kynurenines in the central nervous system. *Neuroscience* 15, 597–617. doi: 10.1016/0306-4522(85)90063-6

Stoy, N., Mackay, G. M., Forrest, C. M., Christofides, J., Egerton, M., Stone, T. W., et al. (2005). Tryptophan metabolism and oxidative stress in patients with Huntington's disease. *J. Neurochem.* 93, 611–623. doi: 10.1111/j.1471-4159.2005.03070.x

Sublette, M. E., Galfalvy, H. C., Fuchs, D., Lapidus, M., Grunebaum, M. F., Oquendo, M. A., et al. (2011). Plasma kynurenine levels are elevated in suicide attempters with major depressive disorder. *Brain Behav. Immun.* 25, 1272–1278. doi: 10.1016/j.bbi.2011.05.002

Suh, H. S., Zhao, M. L., Rivieccio, M., Choi, S., Connolly, E., Zhao, Y., et al. (2007). Astrocyte indoleamine 2,3-dioxygenase is induced by the TLR3 ligand poly(I:C): mechanism of induction and role in antiviral response. *J. Virol.* 81, 9838–9850. doi: 10.1128/JVI.00792-07

Takikawa, O., Kuroiwa, T., Yamazaki, F., and Kido, R. (1988). Mechanism of interferon-gamma action. Characterization of indoleamine 2,3-dioxygenase in cultured human cells induced by interferon-gamma and evaluation of the enzyme-mediated tryptophan degradation in its anticellular activity. *J. Biol. Chem.* 263, 2041–2048.

Tamim, M. K., Samadi, P., Morissette, M., Gregoire, L., Ouattara, B., Levesque, D., et al. (2010). Effect of non-dopaminergic drug treatment on Levodopa induced dyskinesias in MPTP monkeys: common implication of striatal neuropeptides. *Neuropharmacology* 58, 286–296. doi: 10.1016/j.neuropharm.2009.06.030

Tu, H., Rady, P. L., Juelich, T., Smith, E. M., Tyring, S. K., and Hughes, T. K. (2005). Cytokine regulation of tryptophan metabolism in the hypothalamic-pituitary-adrenal (HPA) axis: implications for protective and toxic consequences in neuroendocrine regulation. *Cell. Mol. Neurobiol.* 25, 673–680. doi: 10.1007/s10571-005-4007-1

Vecsei, L., Szalardy, L., Fulop, F., and Toldi, J. (2013). Kynurenines in the CNS: recent advances and new questions. *Nat. Rev. Drug Discov.* 12, 64–82. doi: 10.1038/nrd3793

Veldhoen, M., Hirota, K., Westendorf, A. M., Buer, J., Dumoutier, L., Renauld, J. C., et al. (2008). The aryl hydrocarbon receptor links TH17-cell-mediated autoimmunity to environmental toxins. *Nature* 453, 106–109. doi: 10.1038/nature06881

Vezzani, A., Aronica, E., Mazarati, A., and Pittman, Q. J. (2013a). Epilepsy and brain inflammation. *Exp. Neurol.* 244, 11–21. doi: 10.1016/j.expneurol.2011.09.033

Vezzani, A., Friedman, A., and Dingledine, R. J. (2013b). The role of inflammation in epileptogenesis. *Neuropharmacology* 69, 16–24. doi: 10.1016/j.neuropharm.2012.04.004

Vogel, C. F., Goth, S. R., Dong, B., Pessah, I. N., and Matsumura, F. (2008). Aryl hydrocarbon receptor signaling mediates expression of indoleamine 2,3-dioxygenase. *Biochem. Biophys. Res. Commun.* 375, 331–335. doi: 10.1016/j.bbrc.2008.07.156

Vondracek, J., Umannova, L., and Machala, M. (2011). Interactions of the aryl hydrocarbon receptor with inflammatory mediators: beyond CYP1A regulation. *Curr. Drug Metab* 12, 89–103. doi: 10.2174/138920011795016827

Walker, A. K., Budac, D. P., Bisulco, S., Lee, A. W., Smith, R. A., Beenders, B., et al. (2013). NMDA receptor blockade by ketamine abrogates lipopolysaccharide-induced depressive-like behavior in C57BL/6J mice. *Neuropsychopharmacology* 38, 1609–1616. doi: 10.1038/npp.2013.71

Wang, J., Simonavicius, N., Wu, X., Swaminath, G., Reagan, J., Tian, H., et al. (2006). Kynurenic acid as a ligand for orphan G protein-coupled receptor GPR35. *J. Biol. Chem.* 281, 22021–22028. doi: 10.1074/jbc.M603503200

Wang, Y., Lawson, M. A., Dantzer, R., and Kelley, K. W. (2010). LPS-induced indoleamine 2,3-dioxygenase is regulated in an interferon-gamma-independent manner by a JNK signaling pathway in primary murine microglia. *Brain Behav. Immun.* 24, 201–209. doi: 10.1016/j.bbi.2009.06.152

Widner, B., Leblhuber, F., and Fuchs, D. (2002). Increased neopterin production and tryptophan degradation in advanced Parkinson's disease. *J. Neural Transm.* 109, 181–189. doi: 10.1007/s007020200014

Widner, B., Sepp, N., Kowald, E., Kind, S., Schmuth, M., and Fuchs, D. (1999). Degradation of tryptophan in patients with systemic lupus erythematosus. *Adv. Exp. Med. Biol.* 467, 571–577. doi: 10.1007/978-1-4615-4709-9_71

Willcutt, E. G. (2012). The prevalence of DSM-IV attention-deficit/hyperactivity disorder: a meta-analytic review. *Neurotherapeutics* 9, 490–499. doi: 10.1007/s13311-012-0135-8

Wonodi, I., and Schwarcz, R. (2010). Cortical kynurenine pathway metabolism: a novel target for cognitive enhancement in Schizophrenia. *Schizophr. Bull.* 36, 211–218. doi: 10.1093/schbul/sbq002

Wonodi, I., Stine, O. C., Sathyasaikumar, K. V., Roberts, R. C., Mitchell, B. D., Hong, L. E., et al. (2011). Downregulated kynurenine 3-monooxygenase gene expression and enzyme activity in schizophrenia and genetic association with schizophrenia endophenotypes. *Arch. Gen. Psychiatry* 68, 665–674. doi: 10.1001/archgenpsychiatry.2011.71

Wu, W., Nicolazzo, J. A., Wen, L., Chung, R., Stankovic, R., Bao, S. S., et al. (2013). Expression of tryptophan 2,3-dioxygenase and production of kynurenine pathway metabolites in triple transgenic mice and human Alzheimer's disease brain. *PLoS ONE* 8:e59749. doi: 10.1371/journal.pone.0059749

Yadav, M. C., Burudi, E. M., Alirezaei, M., Flynn, C. C., Watry, D. D., Lanigan, C. M., et al. (2007). IFN-gamma-induced IDO and WRS expression in microglia is differentially regulated by IL-4. *Glia* 55, 1385–1396. doi: 10.1002/glia.20544

Yamada, A., Akimoto, H., Kagawa, S., Guillemin, G. J., and Takikawa, O. (2009). Proinflammatory cytokine interferon-gamma increases induction of indoleamine 2,3-dioxygenase in monocytic cells primed with amyloid beta peptide 1-42: implications for the pathogenesis of Alzheimer's disease. *J. Neurochem.* 110, 791–800. doi: 10.1111/j.1471-4159.2009.06175.x

Yan, Y., Zhang, G. X., Gran, B., Fallarino, F., Yu, S., Li, H., et al. (2010). IDO upregulates regulatory T cells via tryptophan catabolite and suppresses encephalitogenic T cell responses in experimental autoimmune encephalomyelitis. *J. Immunol.* 185, 5953–5961. doi: 10.4049/jimmunol.1001628

Yanagawa, Y., Iwabuchi, K., and Onoe, K. (2009). Co-operative action of interleukin-10 and interferon-gamma to regulate dendritic cell functions. *Immunology* 127, 345–353. doi: 10.1111/j.1365-2567.2008.02986.x

Zadori, D., Nyiri, G., Szonyi, A., Szatmari, I., Fulop, F., Toldi, J., et al. (2011). Neuroprotective effects of a novel kynurenic acid analogue in a transgenic mouse model of Huntington's disease. *J. Neural Transm.* 118, 865–875. doi: 10.1007/s00702-010-0573-6

Zaher, S. S., Germain, C., Fu, H., Larkin, D. F., and George, A. J. (2011). 3-hydroxykynurenine suppresses CD4+ T-cell proliferation, induces T-regulatory-cell development, and prolongs corneal allograft survival. *Invest. Ophthalmol. Vis. Sci.* 52, 2640–2648. doi: 10.1167/iovs.10-5793

Zinger, A., Barcia, C., Herrero, M. T., and Guillemin, G. J. (2011). The involvement of neuroinflammation and kynurenine pathway in Parkinson's disease. *Parkinsons. Dis.* 2011, 716859. doi: 10.4061/2011/716859

Zunszain, P. A., Anacker, C., Cattaneo, A., Choudhury, S., Musaelyan, K., Myint, A. M., et al. (2012). Interleukin-1beta: a new regulator of the kynurenine pathway affecting human hippocampal neurogenesis. *Neuropsychopharmacology* 37, 939–949. doi: 10.1038/npp.2011.277

Zwilling, D., Huang, S. Y., Sathyasaikumar, K. V., Notarangelo, F. M., Guidetti, P., Wu, H. Q., et al. (2011). Kynurenine 3-monooxygenase inhibition in blood ameliorates neurodegeneration. *Cell* 145, 863–874. doi: 10.1016/j.cell.2011.05.020

12

The microbiota–gut–brain axis: neurobehavioral correlates, health and sociality

Augusto J. Montiel-Castro[1,2]*, Rina M. González-Cervantes[2,3], Gabriela Bravo-Ruiseco[2] and Gustavo Pacheco-López[2]

[1] *Centro Darwin de Pensamiento Evolucionista and Philosophy Department, Social Sciences and Humanities Division, Universidad Autonoma Metropolitana Iztapalapa, Mexico City, Mexico*
[2] *Health Sciences Department, Biological and Health Sciences Division, Universidad Autonoma Metropolitana Lerma, Lerma, Mexico*
[3] *Biological Systems Department, Biological and Health Sciences Division, Universidad Autonoma Metropolitana Xochimilco, Mexico City, Mexico*

Edited by:
Javier Velázquez-Moctezuma, Universidad Autonoma Metropolitana, Mexico

Reviewed by:
Toemme Noesselt, Otto-von-Guericke-University, Germany
Richard Stevenson, Macquarie University, Australia

****Correspondence:***
Augusto J. Montiel-Castro, Health Sciences Department, Biological and Health Sciences Division, Lerma Campus, Universidad Autónoma Metropolitana, Av. de las Garzas No. 10, Col. El Panteón Lerma de Villada, Municipio de Lerma, Estado de México, C. P. 52005, Mexico
e-mail: a.j.montiel@centrodarwin-uam.mx

Recent data suggest that the human body is not such a neatly self-sufficient island after all. It is more like a super-complex ecosystem containing trillions of bacteria and other microorganisms that inhabit all our surfaces; skin, mouth, sexual organs, and specially intestines. It has recently become evident that such microbiota, specifically within the gut, can greatly influence many physiological parameters, including cognitive functions, such as learning, memory and decision making processes. Human microbiota is a diverse and dynamic ecosystem, which has evolved in a mutualistic relationship with its host. Ontogenetically, it is vertically inoculated from the mother during birth, established during the first year of life and during lifespan, horizontally transferred among relatives, mates or close community members. This micro-ecosystem serves the host by protecting it against pathogens, metabolizing complex lipids and polysaccharides that otherwise would be inaccessible nutrients, neutralizing drugs and carcinogens, modulating intestinal motility, and making visceral perception possible. It is now evident that the bidirectional signaling between the gastrointestinal tract and the brain, mainly through the vagus nerve, the so called "microbiota–gut–vagus–brain axis," is vital for maintaining homeostasis and it may be also involved in the etiology of several metabolic and mental dysfunctions/disorders. Here we review evidence on the ability of the gut microbiota to communicate with the brain and thus modulate behavior, and also elaborate on the ethological and cultural strategies of human and non-human primates to select, transfer and eliminate microorganisms for selecting the commensal profile.

Keywords: microbiota–gut–brain axis, neurobiology, psychoneuroimmunology, evolutionary psychology, social bonds, kissing

INTRODUCTION

There is hardly a place on earth without bacteria. They are found in every habitat imaginable: in every leaf in the lush Amazon forests; below scorching deserts' sands; within the coldest ice of the Antarctica; and even in the inhospitable environment of the ocean depths, under crushing pressures and in streams of boiling water. Not surprisingly, their realm includes the body surfaces and interior of animals, from minute crawlers to those with exceptional cognitive capacities like the human being. Recent genome sequencing projects suggest that most life forms share up to a third of their genes, and that those in humans show up to a 37% homology with those found in Bacteria and Archaea (McFall-Ngai et al., 2013). The sheer quantity of microorganisms inhabiting human bodies is enormous: more than 1000 different species have been found in a single sample (Relman, 2012). Such data have impacted our self-perception; From a viewpoint of the human body as a self-sufficient individual, to a perception of our bodies as super-complex ecosystems. This change of perspective has included a reappraisal of the role of microorganisms within our bodies (i.e., *endosymbionts*). While the popularly-held belief is that any microorganism found within the human body must have a detrimental effect on its health, emerging research has renewed an emphasis on the fact that many microorganisms have mutually beneficial relationships with their hosts (Archie and Theis, 2011), acting as a *probiotic*: a live microbe with a beneficial effect on the host via modifications of host-associated microbial communities, enhancing the host's response toward disease, its nutrient-exploitation capacity, or improving its environment (Verschuere et al., 2000). Recent research suggests how *microbiota*, i.e., a microbial community occupying a particular habitat (e.g., the *gut* microbiota), can serve its host by protecting it against pathogens, metabolizing complex lipids and polysaccharides that otherwise would be inaccessible nutrients, neutralizing drugs and carcinogens, modulating intestinal motility, and affecting visceral perception. Across evolution, endosymbionts have established important feedback channels with the central nervous system (CNS), some of which are crucial for maintaining homeostasis. For example, as microbial life was increasingly tolerated across generations of organisms, its presence has shaped the evolution of the immune system (Kelly and Mulder, 2012). The recognition that the gut microbiota influences several signaling pathways led to the suggestion of the concept of a microbiota–gut–brain

(MGB) axis, a topic covered by extensive reviews (Rhee et al., 2009; Cryan and Dinan, 2012; Forsythe et al., 2012). The proposal of a MGB axis suggests that through a dynamic alignment, microbiota inhabiting the intestinal lumen affects its host's CNS activity (including vegetative and cognitive functions), and *vice versa* brain activity impacts microbiota development and composition. Clinical and experimental evidence indicate that this is also the case of human subjects, with such relationship playing a pivotal role in the development of metabolic and mental diseases. According to the World Health Organization, metabolic and mental disorders lead the global burden of disease, urging researchers and clinicians to set research priorities, and to governments, public agencies and private funds to apply urgent actions and investment (Mathers et al., 2008). In this regard, understanding the bidirectional signaling between the microbiota, gut and brain, underlie potential and significant impacts on global health, opening new preventive and therapeutic opportunities. Based on the above, the first section of our work provides an overview of the neurobiology supporting such interactions, focusing on key experimental and clinical data of the MGB axis and its potential impact on relevant metabolic and mental human disorders.

While recent years have witnessed an increasing interest in proximate questions regarding different aspects of microbiota, the coevolutionary interactions of animals and bacteria have been relatively unattended. This, in spite of the possibility that a focus on the evolution of the MGB axis could provide new theoretical frameworks for understanding complex evolutionary relationships involved in mutualisms between hosts and commensal bacteria. This includes the possibility that such mutualisms could influence the evolution of immunological systems, shape higher cognitive functions at the individual level, and work as a selective force promoting socialization and social structures, with an influence on the psychobiological basis of gregariousness, social perception, mate choice, and sexual behavior (Archie and Theis, 2011; Neuberg et al., 2011; Schaller, 2011). Therefore, our review is also aimed at understanding the relationship between the exchange of microbial-life among individuals and sociality. Clear suggestions in this regard have been advanced by Troyer (1984a) and Lombardo (2008). They have championed the hypothesis that social interactions may "tip" the precarious but crucial balance between the costs and benefits of group-living by providing an important but surreptitious benefit in the form of an exchange of mutualistic endosymbiotic microbes (e.g., as a defense against pathogens: Dillon et al., 2005). Thus, the next section, on the relationship between microbial-life and sociality, assumes a comparative viewpoint for evaluating such hypothesis. First, it begins by providing an overview of the evidence of symbioses across different animal taxa. It includes studies that either: (a) focus on the social aspect of endosymbiont-transmission or (b) describe whether an experimental intervention was used to clarify the degree by which the impairment of the vertical or horizontal transmission of endosymbionts may affect an organism's survival and/or reproductive success. Second, we suggest that the premises of Lombardo (2008) and Troyer (1984a) can be tested by means of the hypothesis that *the similarity of microbial communities across individuals is an index of the strength of their social bonds.* In our opinion, testing this hypothesis may add an important analytical tool to research focused on how social bonds (a social relationship defined by the degree upon which the exchange of any kind of information -or lack of it- has the potential to affect the survival and/or reproductive success of the individuals involved) translate into cooperation and cohesion at the group-level, an approach that could ultimately shed light on the origin and evolution of sociality (Dunbar and Shultz, 2010). We do this via a focus on the association between sociality and direct and indirect means of microbial-transmission in primates, with particular attention to mouth-to-mouth interactions. Finally, by means of an integrative perspective, the last section provides an overview of the different topics covered.

MICROBIOTA–GUT–BRAIN AXIS AND ITS HEALTH IMPACT

Multiple direct and indirect pathways maintain intensive and extensive bidirectional interactions between the gut microbiota and the CNS; involving endocrine, immune and neural pathways (Grenham et al., 2011), and form the basis of the so called MGB axis (**Figure 1**). For instance, under stress, the brain may influence the composition of the gut microbiota (Bailey and Coe, 1999) via the hypothalamus–pituitary–adrenal (HPA) axis, which regulates cortisol secretion, affecting immune cells activity; both locally in the gut and systemically. When the organism suffers an injury, the first immunological reaction is characterized by redness, pain and heat. These responses are constrained by neuronal regulation of inflammation process, carried out by the HPA axis via catecholamine (Sternberg, 2006) production. The necessary communication processes are based on neurotransmitters, neuropeptides, cytokines, hormones, growth factors (among others), which mediate the relationship between the immune system and the CNS. A feedback process leading to homeostasis (Downing and Miyan, 2000). Yet, disorders like stress (Glaser and Kiecolt-Glaser, 2005)can impact such equilibrium, leading to disease, allergic reactions, inflammatory disease and predisposition to infection. Additionally, cortisol can alter gut permeability and barrier function, and thus contribute to variations in gut microbiota composition (O'Mahony et al., 2011). Vice versa, experimental evidence indicates that the gut microbiota, and pre- and probiotic agents can alter the levels of circulating cytokines, which in turn can have a marked effect on several brain functions (Duerkop et al., 2009; Forsythe and Bienenstock, 2010). Additionally, both the afferent branch of the vagus nerve (Bercik et al., 2011a; Bravo et al., 2011) and modulation of systemic tryptophan, precursor of the neurotransmitter serotonin (Desbonnet et al., 2009), are strongly implicated in relaying the influence of the gut microbiota to the brain.

Experimental approaches on elucidating the MGB axis have so far included, the use of germ-free animals, animals with pathogenic bacterial infections, and animals exposed to probiotic agents or to antibiotics. For instance, germ-free mice have been used to assess neurodevelopmental effects of microbiota loss. Additionally, the administration of probiotic bacteria strains in adult animals or humans has been used to assess the effects of these bacteria on the host. On the other hand, infection studies have been used to assess the effects of pathogenic bacteria on brain and behavior, which are mediated largely through activation of the immune system. Finally, administration of antibiotics can disturb

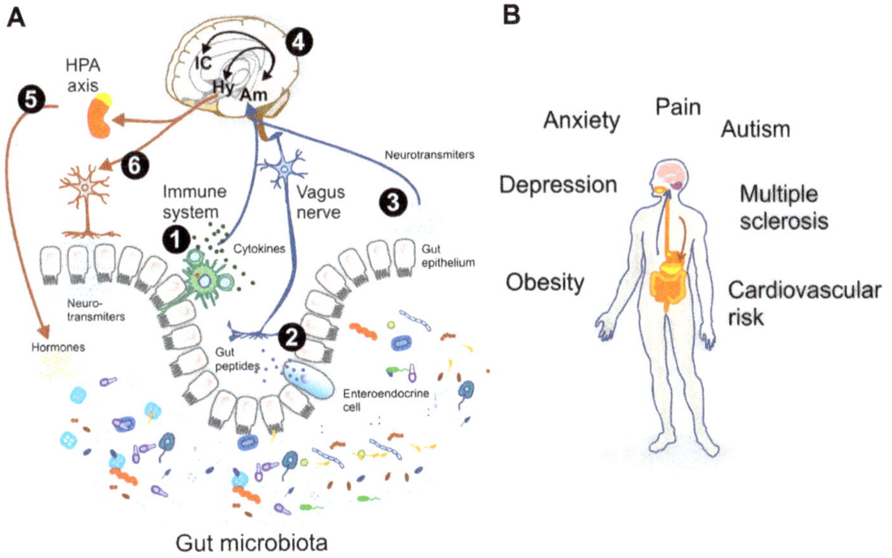

FIGURE 1 | (A) Microbiota–gut–brain (MGB) axis. Direct and indirect pathways support the bidirectional interactions between the gut microbiota and the central nervous system (CNS); involving endocrine, immune and neural pathways. On the afferent arm (blue arrows): (1) lymphocytes may sense the gut lumen and internally release cytokines which can have endocrine or paracrine actions, (2) Sensory neuronal terminals, such as on the vagus nerve may be activated by gut peptides released by enteroendocrine cells, (3) Neurotransmitters or its precursors produced as microbiota metabolites may reach the gut epithelium having endocrine or paracrine effects. (4) Centrally, after brainstem relays (e.g., nucleus *tractus solitarii*) a discrete neural network has been described consistently involving the amygdala (Am) and the insular cortex (IC) as main integrators of visceral inputs. Consistently hypothalamic (Hy) activation initiates the efferent arm (red arrows): (5) corticosteroids, release as results of the hypothalamic–pituitary–adrenal (HPA) axis activation, modulates gut microbiota composition. (6) Neuronal efferent activation may include the so called "anti-inflamatory cholinergic reflex" and/or sympathetic activation, both liberating classical neurotransmitters that may affect directly the gut microbiota composition. **(B)** Health conditions affected by the MGB axis. Recent and growing evidence suggests that several health conditions may be affected by intestinal microbiota, including: visceral pain (McKernan et al., 2010; Wang et al., 2010; Clarke et al., 2012), autism spectrum disorders (Adams et al., 2011; de Theije et al., 2011; Thomas et al., 2012; Wang et al., 2012), obesity (Turnbaugh and Gordon, 2009; Davey et al., 2012; Manco, 2012), cardiovascular risk (Tang et al., 2013), anxiety/depression (Bravo et al., 2011; Heijtz et al., 2011; Foster and McVey Neufeld, 2013), and multiple sclerosis (Berer et al., 2011; Lee et al., 2011).

microbiota composition in a temporally controlled and clinically realistic manner and has therefore been a powerful tool to assess the role of the gut microbiota on behavior.

To date, studies investigating the effects of intestinal microbiota composition on brain function predominantly involve animal models of behavioral disorders such as anxiety, depression and cognitive dysfunction; however, accumulating evidence suggests that the composition of the gut microbiota may also have a role in several other metabolic conditions that involve the CNS (**Figure 1**). In addition, recent data have revealed that MGB axis has multiple effects on emotions, motivation and other higher and complex cognitive functions; reviewed elsewhere (Mayer, 2011). Such evidence suggests that various forms of subliminal interoceptive inputs from the gut, including those generated by intestinal microbiota, may even influence memory formation, emotional arousal, affective behaviors and decision making processes (Craig, 2002; Berntson et al., 2003). The human insular cortex and related brain networks (including the anterior cingulate cortex, orbitofrontal cortex and amygdala), have emerged as the most plausible brain regions to support this integration (Craig, 2009).

MICROBIAL LIFE AND SOCIALITY

SYMBIOSES ACROSS ANIMAL TAXA

Symbioses have played a substantial role in the development of animal life. In their interaction with the geosphere, they shaped the ancient biosphere in which multicellularity and animal life emerged (Hickman, 2005). Multicellular organisms may have evolved as new conflict-mediation mechanisms (i.e., genetic codes) restricted lower-level individual fitness, increasing that of new individuals at higher levels of biological organization (Michod, 2003). From such humble beginnings and over extended periods of time, a diverse array of cooperative and organized groups of individuals (i.e., societies), have evolved. Since transmission vectors may originate across both the physical and the social environment, microbial communities found in an organism are dependent on its geoecology, physiology, and genotype, but also on the intensity of its social relationships (Archie and Theis, 2011). The following paragraphs provide an overview of selected research describing symbioses between microorganisms and different animal taxa.

Microbial endosymbionts have played an important role in the evolutionary and developmental modification of tissues and organs of several marine or *aquatic invertebrates*, for example in the construction of mineralized exoskeletons (Hickman, 2005). Hickman (2005) points out the example of sponges. This group acquires large symbiotic and diverse bacterial communities through vertical transmission, which perform functions like nutrient acquisition, stabilization of the sponge's skeleton, processing of metabolic waste, and production of important secondary metabolites. The phyla with the largest biomass (e.g., arthropods) are also those with more symbioses reported (McFall-Ngai, 2005). McFall-Ngai (2005) suggests that a crucial difference between vertebrates and invertebrates is based on the relationship between the immune system and its association with microbial life. On the one hand, invertebrates rely on an "innate immune system" consisting of a germline-encoded receptor system associated to cells like macrophages or epithelia. On the other hand, in addition to the innate immune system, vertebrates possess a "combinatorial" immune response (using T-cells and a major histocompatibility complex) which may have evolved as a more "permissive" form of association with long-term endosymbiont microbial consortia, but also as an improved capacity for distinguishing "friend from foe," leading to the identification of *specific* pathogens (McFall-Ngai, 2005). However, some recent studies suggest that these differences may be less clear-cut than previously thought. For instance, a study in *Daphnia magna* (an aquatic crustacean), found that, compared to those experimentally challenged with a different strain, individuals exposed to the specific strain of the pathogen to which their mothers had been exposed had better fitness, suggesting that some invertebrates may have some kind of specific adaptive immunity (Little et al., 2003). One of the best examples of a beneficial symbiotic-relationship in an aquatic invertebrate is the case of the mutualism between the squid *Euprymna scolopes* and the luminous, symbiotic bacteria *Vibrio fischeri*. This symbiosis is maintained by means of cyclic transmission, where the bacterial symbionts must be acquired from the environment each generation (McFall-Ngai, 1998). *V. fischeri* is first acquired directly from the environment, but then, the light organ of *E. scolopes* undergoes specific metamorphic changes that maintain the symbiosis (McFall-Ngai, 1994). Such relationship helps *E. scolopes* generating bioluminescence, camouflaging it from both prey and predators by eliminating the projection of its shadow (Ruby and McFall-Ngai, 1992). Finally, a study by Verschuere et al. (2000) suggests that *Artemia spp.* is protected from the pathogenic effects of *Vibrio proteolyticus* by specific bacterial strains.

Perhaps the best-studied examples of symbioses and transmission of microbiota is found among social *insects*. The phenomenon received close attention as a model for the study of the origins of sociality, permeating both scientific and popular accounts of the human society during the nineteenth and twentieth centuries (Sleigh, 2002). The niche of the hymenoptera, including a subterranean way of life, large biomass density at the nest, and frequent direct individual contact, can all make them particularly vulnerable to pathogens via a fast-spread of disease among conspecifics (Kaltenpoth and Engl, 2013). Therefore, based on selection at the individual and colony-level, social insects have developed different forms of prophylactic and active responses against some parasite-related costs of social-living, such as: environmental parasite uptake, parasite intrusion (i.e., into a colony), parasite establishment and spread within the colony, and transmission between colonies (Cremer et al., 2007). These responses are referred to as "collective" or "social immunity" by Cremer et al. (2007). Among them is also the possibility for the social-transmission of beneficial microbiota. Recently, Koch and Schmid-Hempel (2011) suggested that both honey and bumble bees present bacterial communities not found among solitary species which, importantly, protect them against a virulent and naturally occurring parasite (*Crithidia bombi*). In an experimental setting, they demonstrate that in order to observe the protective effect of microbiota, individuals had to be exposed to feces from nest mates after pupal eclosion, providing strong evidence for an important benefit of the transmission of microbiota between individuals. On the other hand, Evans and Lopez (2004) suggest that nonpathogenic bacteria may have a positive effect on honey bee immunity, helping them to survive pathogen-infection across different life-stages. In turn, McFrederick et al. (2012) suggested that beneficial *Lactobacillus* found in bees were acquired by both vertical transmission or by contact with flowers, and that the *Lactobacillus* strains associated to Sweet bees could suppress mold-growth and other spoilage organisms at the nest. Other species of eusocial insects feed each other by regurgitation of liquid secretions originating in the crop or alimentary tract (Wilson, 2000), a phenomenon named *trophallaxis* by Wheeler (1918). In termites, trophallaxis allows for the social transmission of protozooans, which they lose after periodic molting but are crucial for the digestion of cellulose (Wilson, 2000).

Experimental studies focused on the transmission of microbiota have been practiced in a few non-eusocial insects. For example, germ-free desert locusts (*Schistocerca gregaria*) were associated with up to three species of locust gut bacteria and then fed with a pathogen (*Serratia marcescens*) by Dillon et al. (2005). Results of this study showed a negative relationship between the density of *Serratia marcescens* and the number of gut bacterial species present, as well as a negative relationship between bacterial community-diversity and the proportion of locusts harboring *Serratia*. A more recent study (Wang and Aksoy, 2012) investigated the role of *Wigglesworthia glossinidia* as an endosymbiont associated to the nutrition, fecundity, and development of the immune system in Tsetse flies (Diptera: Glossinidae). The study describes how the peptidoglycan recognition protein (PGRP-LB) is found only in adult flies (as an important component of the milk that nourishes developing progeny), and how the experimental reduction of PGRP-LB decreases female fecundity by damaging the transmission of *Wigglesworthia* through induction of an antimicrobial peptide (Attacin). The conclusion of Wang and Aksoy (2012) is that the transmission of PGRP-LB has a major role in the fitness of Tsetse flies by means of protecting such symbiosis.

There are fewer but equally interesting studies on this subject in fishes, amphibians, and reptiles. Coldwater *fish* appear to acquire their microbiota from the environment after hatching (Hansen and Olafsen, 1999), and there is some indication that different types of probiotic bacteria may have beneficial effects as biological control agents in aquaculture, including immune system improvements (Gómez and Balcázar, 2008) or enhancement of water quality (Verschuere et al., 2000). In the freshwater zebrafish (*Danio rerio*), an experimentally induced lack of microbiota arrests the development of the species' gut at specific points of differentiation, an effect than can, nevertheless, be reversed by the introduction of bacteria (Bates et al., 2006). In the case of *amphibians*, Walke et al. (2011) found that innate immune defenses with a beneficial effect on the inhibition of the fungal pathogen *Batrachochytrium dendrobatidis* can be vertically transmitted. Their work found that both antimicrobial skin peptides and mutualistic microbiota found in the adult Panamanian "glass-frogs" of the species *Hyalinobatrachium colymbiphyllum*, could be transmitted to embryos, with a possible role of different types of physical contact as a means for this transmission, including female-eggs contact during deposition, and/or male urination on the egg-clutch. Another study by Troyer (1984b) focused on the horizontal acquisition of microbiota in *reptiles*. She investigated how green iguana (*Iguana iguana*) hatchlings employ a significant amount of time in acquiring microbiota before fully exploiting the food resources in their habitat. They do this in a three-step process. First, before having a fully functional digestive activity, they consume soil from within the nest chamber, by which they increase their hindgut microbial populations. Then, up to a week after hatching, they leave the nest and begin eating both plants and soil. Finally, between 2 and 3 weeks after hatching they leave the area around the nest, associate with other conspecifics and eat the feces of older individuals, gaining access to more complex microbial communities.

In comparison, Kohl (2012) presents a thorough review of the many aspects by which microbial communities influence nutrition, development, immunity, and processing of toxins in many species of *birds*. One interesting aspect observed by Kohl is that the symbiotic relationships between birds and microbiota can be, on some occasions, extraordinarily similar to those found in the relationship between mammals and their endosymbionts, while on other instances, they are just slightly distinguishable, by a few, nevertheless remarkable, aspects. A particularly interesting study (Kyle and Kyle, 1993) described by Lombardo (2008) observed that food-provisioning by itself was insufficient for enhancing the survival of orphan chimney swifts nestlings. To achieve this objective, food needed to be coated with the saliva of adults. While all nestlings younger than 6 days receiving food that was not covered by an adult's saliva died, a high proportion of those that received the saliva-covered food survived.

There is also a vast literature describing the influence of microbiota on a variety of *mammals* (a portion of it reviewed by Lombardo, 2008). Therefore, as a preface for the following subsection, next we focus solely on aspects of the relationship between kinship, lactation and microbiota in human and non-human primates. Several studies have examined the bacterial microbiota of breast-fed and bottle-fed human infants using both conventional plating and molecular techniques. These studies have shown that the large gut microbiota of breast-fed infants is generally dominated by bifidobacteria and lactic acid bacteria, both considered beneficial (Penders et al., 2006). In contrast, the gut microbiota of formula-fed infants is more diverse, but less stable, often containing more *Bacteroides*, *Clostridium* and *Enterobacteriaceae*. Early start of feeding formula milk changes the composition of the intestinal-microbiota, promoting colonization by obligate anaerobes such as the *Clostridium coccoides* group, the *Clostridium leptum* subgroup, *Prevotella* and *Atopobium* cluster during the 3 months after birth (Tsuji et al., 2012). Human milk is a complex bio-fluid containing mainly lactose, lipids, and protein. However, it is not widely recognized that, after lactose and lipids, oligosaccharides are the third largest solid component of human milk. The majority of this type of sugars is not digestible by human infants, instead, their main function may be related to their interaction or support of intestinal microbiota. Oligosaccharides in human milk encourage the growth of beneficial bifidobacteria in the colon, while they also bind competitively to cell adhesion receptors. This binding may prevent pathogen-binding to intestinal epithelial cells and thus pathogenesis. Analysis of the oligosaccharides in human milk resulted in 200 different molecules ranging in size from disaccharides up to approximately 22 residues (Ninonuevo et al., 2006). In this sense, through lactation, mothers provide food for both their infants and the bacteria helping assimilating milk's nutrients, allowing for the continued inoculation and establishment of infant's microbiota (Hinde and German, 2012). The importance of this "triangled" relationship is highlighted by the seminal work of Bailey and Coe (1999), who observed that due to strong emotional stress, the disruption of the mother-infant bond (i.e., by separation from the mother) in rhesus monkeys (*Macaca mulatta*) altered the composition of infants' gut microbiota, increasing their vulnerability to disease. The study of Bailey and Coe (1999) represents an important developmental piece of evidence of a health-related *cost* (i.e., increased vulnerability to disease) observed when the composition of microbiota is altered due to the interruption of microbial-transmission (i.e., by a disruption of the mother-infant bond).

Turnbaugh et al. (2009) found no significant correlations between separation of family members and the degree of similarity between their gut microbiota, as well as no significant differences in the composition of gut microbiota between monozygotic and dizygotic twins, suggesting a likely genetic factor underlying such commonalities. On the other hand, Yatsunenko et al. (2012), characterized bacterial species in fecal samples from 531 individuals from different nationalities. Groups included healthy children and adults from the Venezuelan Amazonas, rural areas of Malawi and US metropolitan areas, and included mono and dizygotic twins. An effect of kinship on gut microbiota was found across countries, focusing the discussion on how differences in social structures may influence the extent of vertical transmission of the microbiota and the flow of microbes among members of a group of people or family. Importantly, their results showed that the phylogeny of fecal microbiota of monozygotic twins was no more similar than the microbiota of dizygotic twins in all age groups tested. Likewise, there were no significant differences in the degree of similarity between the fecal microbiota of mothers and their teenage offspring, nor between teens and their biological fathers. Moreover, the microbiota of co-habiting couples was more similar to each other than to members of other households (Yatsunenko et al., 2012). These results, consistent across the populations studied, suggest that, as in other species, endosymbionts may have an important role in kin-recognition in humans.

THE ASSOCIATION BETWEEN MICROBIAL TRANSMISSION AND SOCIAL BONDING IN PRIMATES

In the case of primates, a behaviorally and cognitively complex social life has evolved across a range of group sizes and social structures as a prerequisite for individual's development, survival, and reproduction (Mitani et al., 2012). Either in the form of predator deterrence (e.g., Zuberbühler et al., 1997), cooperative breeding (e.g., Burkart and van Shaik, 2010) or group hunting (e.g., Watts and Mitani, 2002), primates use group-level cooperative strategies that in general enhance individual fitness. However, sociality also involves important costs, such as within-group competition for resources (van Schaik and van Noordwijk, 1986) or reduction of reproductive output due to socially induced stress (Dunbar, 1980; Altmann et al., 1988). Thus, a balance between the costs and benefits of social-life is by no means an easy task for primates. By increasing the frequency of contact and proximity between individuals, species living at higher densities, in larger groups, or with promiscuous mating are thought to be the most vulnerable to infection (Altizer et al., 2003). Nonetheless, primates exhibit cohesive and sometimes large groups with strong and long-lasting social bonds (Mitani, 2009) of a kind that, in other animal orders, are almost exclusively found among pair-bonded species (Shultz and Dunbar, 2007). These two observations are somewhat incompatible. However, this apparent paradox could be solved by recognizing the role of partner-choice mechanisms in the structuring of primate societies (Hinde, 1983a). Research suggests that endosymbionts are at the base of different mechanisms for individual recognition and partner selection (Archie and Theis, 2011) underlying social-bonding and the formation of cliques within larger social structures. When partner choice is exerted, not all subjects interact with all other group members, and thus, social bonds (or its absence) may act as a social barrier to pathogen transmission (Loehle, 1995). Hence, if endosymbionts' transmission is of any benefit to sociality, transmission should be facilitated as social bonds between individuals are stronger, and made more difficult as species use more frequent or more complex partner-selection mechanisms. As partner-choice limits the size of each individual's social network (Kudo and Dunbar, 2001), the increasing risk of pathogen transmission associated to large groups may set an upper limit to total group size (Freeland, 1976, 1979; Coté and Poulin, 1995; Bonds et al., 2005), leaving the beneficial link between endosymbionts and complex sociality (*sensu* Lombardo, 2008) intact in the form of bonded relationships. For example, the large social groups of the Hamadryas baboon (*Papio hamadryas*: Schreier and Swedell, 2009), classified as a multi-layered, fission-fusion society (Mitani et al., 2012), is a good example of the way social contact is less intense the larger a social-unit is, providing "borders" to microbial-transmission (**Figure 2**). Considering the role of social structure as a barrier against parasite transmission may explain why larger but more subdivided groups, tend to slow the spread of infectious diseases (Griffin and Nunn, 2011; Nunn, 2012), and connect the evolution of the MGB axis to primate sociality. This suggests that the *quality* of social relationships between subjects, but not necessarily the size of their social groups, should be associated to more frequent or direct mechanisms underlying endosymbionts' transmission between individuals.

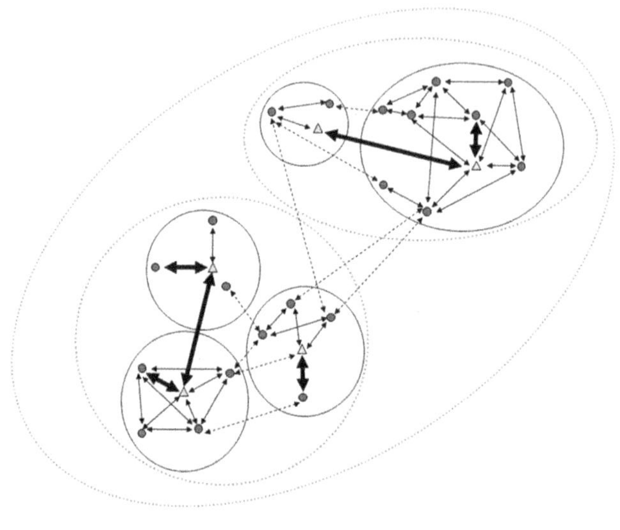

FIGURE 2 | The typical structure of the multi-layered Hamadryas baboon society. The smaller social unit (a "one-male-unit", OMU) in the Hamadryas society is that formed by an adult male (*triangles*), adult females (*circles*) and their offspring. In these units social relationships tend to be circumscribed to members of the same unit (expressed here by arrows, representing social relationships -within bold circles). These units are often formed when larger OMUs fission or when young bachelors sequester peripheral (usually young) females from a large OMU; retaining them in close proximity by force and aggression. Adult females in the same OMU are seldom kin. This produces that strong social relationships (*bold arrows*) are usually established between a female and her unit's male, not among females in the same OMU. While both sexes can have relatives in other OMUs, social contacts among females from different units are less common (*dotted arrows*), whereas adult males may in fact establish strong alliances with males from other units (which may actually be their kin) forming "clans" (*bold arrows across different* OMUs). Spatial association between individuals of different OMUs (e.g., foraging in relative proximity) can result in the third level of the Hamadryas society: a "band" (*medium-sized dotted ovals*). Finally, different bands congregate in the same cliffs to sleep, forming the largest identifiable group: the "troop" (*largest dotted oval*).

Indirect mechanisms

In indirect mechanisms of microbial transmission, inoculation is somehow mediated (e.g., by either a free-living pathogen, inanimate environmental features or by another infected host species; Cortez and Weitz, 2013). *Coprophagy* and *urine ingestion* are good examples of indirect mechanisms: often considered abnormal behaviors appearing due to stress (e.g., Baker and Easley, 1996; Nash et al., 1999), they promote beneficial mutualisms required for digestion of plant materials (as in colobus, howler monkeys and gorillas: Milton, 1981; Lambert, 1998; Graczyk and Cranfield, 2003). Even if they exacerbate exposure to parasites, risks can be circumvented by selectively ingesting excretes of relatives while avoiding those of parasitized conspecifics (Lombardo, 2008); two strategies made possible by the widespread individual-recognition capacities of primates (Langergraber, 2012).

Social *traditions* are behaviors maintained and transmitted by social learning that can distinguish between lineages, groups or populations (Avital and Jablonka, 2000). These traditions may represent an important horizontal mechanism for the transfer of microbiota in primates: on the one hand, they can help distinguishing between different chimpanzee communities (Whiten et al., 2001), while on the other, members of contiguous chimpanzee communities can be distinguished based on the contents of their gut microbiota (Degnan et al., 2012). Several social traditions involve the transfer of objects between individuals, such as that observed in *tool-sharing*. For instance, Pruetz and Lindshield (2012) describe how female chimpanzees retrieved tools directly from the mouth of other adults and later used them for their own termite-fishing. In another example, after naïve subjects or infants (both their offspring and other unrelated subjects) approached their tools with their mouths, adult chimpanzees offered them their *previously licked* tools, which were again used and licked (Hirata and Celli, 2003; Hirata, 2006).

Food itself can be another indirect vehicle for microbial transfer. In primates, *food sharing* occurs both among related and non-related individuals (Schaub, 1996; Stevens and Gilby, 2004). However, compared to social insects, food sharing among primates can be a highly selective process of partner choice. In a meta-analysis, Jaeggi and van Schaik (2011) recorded which variables predicted food-sharing among subjects of different primate species. Their results suggested, first, that as greater efforts were required to exploit a particular food-source (i.e., as in tool-use), food sharing between parents and offspring was more common; second, in species with a tendency to share food with infants, sharing between adults was also predicted, although diet-characteristics did not explain food sharing patterns among adults; third, instead, food sharing among *unrelated* adults was predicted by their propensity to exert partner choice, and patterns of *reciprocity* explained interchanges such as "food-for-sex" or "food-for-coalitionary-support." Particularly relevant for our argument is their observation of an indication that, within single-male species, food sharing between sexes was more common in monogamous species.

Direct mechanisms

Direct mechanisms of transmission of microbial life depend on physical contact between conspecifics (Cortez and Weitz, 2013). Among primates, social *grooming* is the most widespread example (**Figure 3**). During grooming, primates explore their own or other individual's body surface while removing ectoparasites or debris (e.g., food; Dunbar, 1991), which they often ingest. Primates select their social-partners carefully (Dunbar, 1998). They may exhibit "levels" (Zhou et al., 2005) of acquaintanceship, where those most closely bonded form each other's immediate "support clique" (Dunbar and Spoors, 1995; Crockford et al., 2008). However, when time available for sociality is scarce or during social instability, they can save social-time by reducing overall sociality, focusing grooming on a few primary partners (Dunbar and Dunbar, 1988; Wittig et al., 2008). Perhaps based on saliva's healing properties (Gröschl, 2009), different species practice *preening* or *licking* as another form of grooming (Mooring et al., 2004). In primates, this behavior is commonly observed between primate females and their offspring (e.g., apes: Lindburg and Hazell, 1972; *Colobus* sp.: Horwich and Manski, 1975; *Lemur catta*: Nakamichi and Koyama, 2000; *Alouatta palliata*: Duarte-Dias, 2005; *Macaca fuscata*: Turner et al., 2009). While other types of relationship develop through a mutually regulated process of acquaintanceship, as we have described above in detail, the strong bond between primate mothers and their infants is based on important physiological events like lactation (Hinde, 1983b; **Figure 3**).

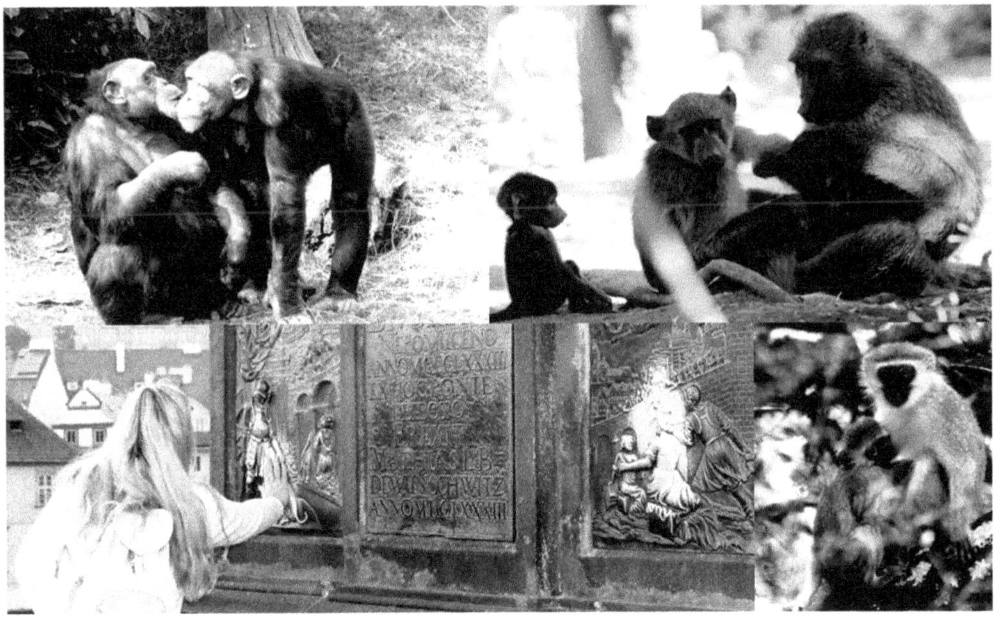

FIGURE 3 | Behaviors supporting an association between microbial-transmission and social bonding in primates. The intense sociality of primates provides several different *direct* (i.e., with contact between individuals) and *indirect* (i.e., mediated by any environmental feature) opportunities for the transmission of microbial-life associated to a social-bonding mechanism. Important examples (described in more detail in main text) include: (*upper-left*) mouth-to-mouth contact (in chimpanzees, *Pan troglodytes*): where microbial-life may be directly transmitted in saliva between individuals; (*upper-right*) social grooming (in savannah baboons, *Papio cynocephalus*): where groomers may feed on ectoparasites or food-debris, allowing for the transmission of microbiota; (*bottom-right*) lactation (in vervet monkeys, *Chlorocebus aethiops*): where microbiota directly acquired from the mother helps feeding bacterial communities which in turn help offspring assimilating milk's nutrients; and (*bottom-left*), indirect transmission of microbiota mediated by a social tradition (i.e., touching religious objects), a possible pathway for the homogenization of microbial-life across individuals of a culturally defined human group (all photos by Augusto J. Montiel-Castro).

Mouth-to-mouth interactions

Another means of direct microbial exchange is mouth-to-mouth contact (**Figure 3**). While this behavior has been reported for many primates (e.g.,: *Papio anubis*: Bolwig, 1978; *Pan paniscus*: Kuroda, 1980; *Cebus capuchinus*: Manson et al., 1997; *Cebus apella*: de Waal, 2000a; *Pan troglodytes*: Wittig and Boesch, 2003; *Callithrix jacchus:* Kasper et al., 2008; *Homosapiens*: Hughes et al., 2007; *Pongo abelii*: Hardus et al., 2012), different species perform it at different rates and in different contexts. For instance, the possible relationship between mouth-to-mouth exchange of microbiota and affiliative behavior can also be inferred from the *sociosexual* behavior of bonobos (*Pan paniscus*). Compared to that of common chimpanzees (*Pan troglodytes*) bonobo society is less aggressive, more relaxed or friendlier; sex can be used to repair social relationships, and among bonobos but not chimpanzees, reconciliation often involves sexual contact (Wrangham, 1993). Bonobos can mate several times per day; they manipulate other individuals' genitals with hands or mouth and have more varied forms of copulatory behavior than chimpanzees, including ventro-ventral copulation (i.e., partners facing each other), a sexual position used by bonobo females with their most-trusted partners (Wrangham, 1993). Moreover, bonobos use their tongues intensely (de Waal, 1989), in a way similar to humans, during mouth-to-mouth *kissing*. Being two concomitant forms of "face-to-face" interaction, ventro-ventral copulation and mouth-to-mouth contacts are particularly relevant for supporting the hypothesis that similarities in the composition of microbiota between individuals could be used as indices of bond-strength. This, given that: (1) they allow for the possibility that facial expression may act as a means for the communication of emotional states (Dobson, 2012), while (2) mutual body-contact can stimulate the production of oxytocin, vasopressin or endorphines: neuropeptide mechanisms underlying social-bonding processes in different species (Young and Wang, 2004; Dunbar, 2010); last but not least, (3) during ventro-ventral contact, mouth-to-mouth kissing can act as a means for the *concurrent* reciprocal exchange of microbiota between partners. Altogether, the process could provide the basis for the association of conditioned (e.g., mouth-to-mouth contact) and unconditioned stimuli (e.g., production of oxytocin), reinforcing such behavior through associative learning and thus producing a conditioned response (i.e., oxytocin release) even in the absence of copulation.

Kissing: differences across cultures

In humans, mouth-to-mouth kissing is frequently interpreted as the archetypal sign of a strong bond, an index of intimacy and relationship-satisfaction (Gulledge et al., 2003). Eibl-Eibesfeldt (1989, p.138) describes the behavior as follows: "the initiator presses his lips against the partner's and, when the behavior is fully executed, pushes his tongue between the partner's lips, while the recipient opens his lips and (in complete execution) begins suckling." From this archetypal form, some variations can be encountered. While it can be considered a (human) universal sign of affection, there are cultures where, when practiced *in public*, mouth-to-mouth kissing is considered a taboo (Eibl-Eibesfeldt, 1977). Yet, in the opinion of Eibl-Eibesfeldt (1989), as humans are capable of suppressing innate behaviors, this fact does not weaken the argument of its universality. Given that Eibl-Eibesfeldt (1975, 1989) offers an illustrative review of the homogeneity of this behavior across traditional cultures, the focus of the following paragraphs is on aspects of its cross-cultural variation.

Mouth-to-mouth kissing is certainly not found across all human cultures, nor it follows the same behavioral sequence where it is recorded (Eibl-Eibesfeldt, 1975). One occurs in some European traditional villages, where young men chew pine-resin and leave some pieces of it protruding from their mouths. Then, with this resin in their teeth, they playfully "dare" the girl of their romantic-interest to approach and try to pick it with their mouths (Eibl-Eibesfeldt, 1975). Another frequent variation is that observed among groups like Amerindians, Polynesians and Japanese, where, instead of a concurrent touching of lips, people smell (Mykytowycz, 1972) one another. Chamberlain (1906) recorded the observations of D'Enjoy (1897), who suggested that European kisses could be distinguished from Mongolian and Malayan ones given that the latter were forms of "sniffs" and "nose-rubbing," respectively. Similar observations on human groups from the artic regions (i.e., "Eskimos"), have been interpreted as indications that they sniff each other to check their health: not as a sign of affection, but as a preventive gesture against disease (Washburn Hopkins, 1907). Indeed, the term "Eskimo kiss" is still known and used in English, referring to a "touch of noses" but not of lips. Washburn Hopkins (1907) makes an encyclopedic argument with a detailed analysis of ancient Indian literature, based on which he suggests that ancient Indian words for "kissing" were functionally equivalent to those for "smelling," and thus that behaviors were similarly used. Another important source of cultural variation of the behavior revolves around who is, and who is not meant to be kissed. In a contemporary and empirical, cross-cultural study of jealousy, women reported being upset when their partner kissed someone else but not when they danced or hugged others, while men reported greater jealousy when their partners had sexual fantasies about other people, compared to when they hugged or danced with others (Buunk and Hupka, 1987). In a more recent study, significant ethnic differences were found among data on the age at which teenagers of different ethnic groups kissed for the first time. Compared to Asian Americans, more African Americans, Caucasians, and Latino/Hispanic subjects had kissed for the first time at earlier ages (Regan et al., 2004). Another cross-cultural study found no differences in the way Asians, versus American students expressed love: intimate behavior, including kissing, was an indicator of love in marriages but not in friendships (Kline et al., 2008). For Frijhoff (1991), regardless of intense historical and contemporary western influence, and the fact that the gesture *is* observed in these cultures, Africans and Asians consider the public performance of mouth-to-mouth kissing as disgusting or immoral, relegating it to the sphere of *intimacy*; not because the gesture is absent, but because it is not recognized as a "legitimate public rite." It is in these cultures, Frijhoff (1991) suggests, where greetings commonly involve the use of the "sniff-kiss" or/and a bow of the body, or a hand gesture. Chamberlain (1906) and Frijhoff (1991) also refer to contemporary cultural differences related to the greeting aspect of kissing: common (even among males) in Russia or France (where this gesture's underlying degree of affection may be indexed by its loudness), but rarer in England, the Netherlands or the USA.

The socio-religious aspect of kissing has been thoroughly analyzed by Frijhoff (1991), who makes interesting conclusions distinguishing the public and private aspects of kissing. On the one hand, he suggests, rituals may have adapted kissing and/or embracing as signals of group-membership, a sign of association and/or fraternity, ruled by cultural standards of public expression that provide a sense of group-identity (e.g., the rite of publicly kissing the feet of the statue of St. Peter in the Vatican, or touching a religious icon: **Figure 3**). On the other hand, Frijhoff (1991) suggests that, in the private sphere, both the experience of a religious person (e.g., when kissing a religious icon), and that of lovers during mouth-to-mouth kissing, appear to separate them from the group, creating a sense of psychological intimacy; a likely reason for why, in some cultures, kissing (i.e., mouth-to-mouth) in public is not considered polite.

Kissing: evolutionary perspective

In view of the previous analysis, it is somewhat surprising that while kissing is found across several cultures and is a topic of strong popular concern (Walter, 2008), its evolution is not yet fully understood. Hypotheses have certainly been suggested. For example, kissing is one of the many different behaviors observed during reconciliation in non-human primates (de Waal, 1989) suggesting its role as a means for appeasement. However, in spite of substantial evidence highlighting the role of kissing in the context of reconciliation (de Waal, 1989, 2000b), one could ask: if grooming can itself produce intrinsic positive reinforcement (i.e., beta-endorphins) in a primate's nervous system (Keverne et al., 1989), why would an additional behavior, one increasing the probability of pathogen-transmission, be used during reconciliation? This is an important consideration. Mouth-to-mouth contact and direct exchange of saliva expose individuals to pathogen transmission. In view of this probable cost and its role as an index of reconciliatory tendencies, one would expect it to provide some intrinsic benefit (Hendrie and Brewer, 2010) and to be a highly selective form of inter-individual interaction. Comparative evidence of mouth-to-mouth feeding in parent-offspring dyads across birds and mammals suggests that kissing could evolve as a form of mouth-to-mouth food exchange between offspring and progenitors (Eibl-Eibesfeldt, 1975). However, common marmosets (*Callithrix jacchus*: a new world monkey that exchanges food often) do not restrict these interactions to matting partners or offspring, and tolerate mouth-to-mouth exchanges with both dominants and subordinates (Kasper et al., 2008). Instead, since tolerating or rejecting a stressful event such as the transgression of personal space may provide information about the quality of a relationship, Kasper et al. (2008) suggest that these "up-close" exchanges may serve as tests of the quality of a relationship. For Nicholson (1984), kissing involves some form of social-bonding by means of semiochemical addiction: a direct and continued exchange of sebum and pheromones facilitating bonding and love. The possibility that chemo-signals have a role in communication, via body-secretions has been recently confirmed in humans by de Groot et al. (2012), observing that chemo-signals of fear and disgust can produce multimodal emotional synchronization between sender and receiver, and thus, that communication of emotional states is not restricted to language and visual stimuli. However, results showing that women prefer the scent of males' t-shirts with whom they have greater immunological dissimilarity (Wedekind et al., 1995), highlight the role of smell (Penn and Potts, 1998) as an alternative route for the development of a purported semiochemical-addiction.

The research of Hughes et al. (2007) on the relationship between pair bonding strategies and kissing in humans, points out other important aspects of this behavior. While men may use kissing for increasing the likelihood of sexual intercourse, women use it as a form of mate-assessment and a behavioral-monitor of the quality of long-term relationships (Hughes et al., 2007). This affiliative aspect of kissing may also be interpreted as a willingness to sustain close social bonds *at the risk of* contracting an illness (Hughes et al., 2007). Therefore, kissing has also been suggested as a strategy aimed at avoiding contagion by pathogens such as the human cytomegalovirus during infant's gestation, for which testing for such possibility before conception or before the onset of vulnerable periods of fetal development would be highly advantageous (Hendrie and Brewer, 2010). Moreover, since couples sharing previously used, food-related items "contaminated" by their partner (e.g., a licked spoon) are perceived as "more intimate" by third-parties (Alley, 2012), kissing may also function as a group-oriented "advert" or proxy of the strength of the bond between two individuals.

FINAL COMMENTS: INTEGRATIVE PERSPECTIVES

THE MICROBIOTA–GUT–BRAIN AXIS AND ITS IMPACT ON HEALTH

The excitement of emotion, the state of alertness and enhanced activation linking the viscera, in particular heart and gut, to the human mind, as well as the mechanisms for bidirectional signaling between these organs, was among the topics by which Charles Darwin himself advocated evolutionary continuity in *The Expression of Emotions in Man and Animals* (Darwin, 1872). With similar intentions, the present review has suggested how mutualistic endosymbionts may have a crucial role in these processes. Thus, the first integrating ideas emerging from our review are focused on the relevance of the different communication channels between the gut microbiota and the brain. For instance, the crucial relationship described in sections above, that between microbiota, cytokines, short-chain fatty acids, systemic tryptophan and their effect on brain function, signals interesting possibilities for fruitful research. For example, the recognition of the role of microbiota in the modulation of tryptophan and thus serotonin, could complement insights on the social and evolutionary basis of schizophrenia (Burns, 2004), while other fertile approaches should focus on the importance of probiotics as modifiers of health, behavior and mood. Such attempts should provide alternatives in clinical settings, and preventive aspects of some of the most prevalent mental and metabolic disorders of modern human societies, such as depression and obesity.

The reports on the role of gut microbiota as an influence in the formation of memories and emotional arousal suggest the existence of a crucial relationship between interoceptive stimuli and the evolution of higher cognitive processes, one that may be based on a system supporting *empathy*, or a capacity for understanding the feelings of other individuals. On the one hand, results showing how the anterior insular cortex can be activated by the images of other humans experiencing disgust (Wicker et al., 2003) suggest the action of a mechanism homologous to *mirror neurons* (Gallese, 1998). These neurons, first located in the ventral premotor cortex of macaque brains, activate both when subjects perform a particular action and when they observe similar actions performed by other individuals (Rizzolatti and Fogassi, 2007). Mirror neurons may be crucial for understanding the underlying intentions of actions, which has led some to suggest that they are part of the system upon which empathy is constructed (Ferrari et al., 2003). On the other hand, evidence suggests that another kind of cells, "*Von economo*" neurons or "spindle cells" in layer five of the anterior cingulate cortex are particularly involved in processes of self-experience, empathy and social bonding (Parr et al., 2005). For Parr et al. (2005), there are at least two important characteristics suggesting the role of such neurons as a neurological basis of sociality. First, these cells have been identified in humans and apes but not in monkeys, suggesting a recent evolutionary origin associated to higher cognition; second, since they seem to be reduced and abnormally located in autistic individuals, they may underlie the lack of empathy characterizing autism. Finally, such system of representation of emotions of others, may be complemented by the action of the vagus (i.e., the "pneumogastric" nerve, according to Darwin, 1872), as a means for activating responses and control of the metabolic output necessary for social interaction. In this regard, the Polyvagal theory (Porges, 2003) suggests that the myelienated branch of the vagus, found only in mammals, is a key for understanding the non-endocrine bases of social behavior. Given that this branch of the parasympathetic system controls facial expression, swallowing, breathing and vocalizing, and has an inhibitory effect upon the sympathetic system innerving the heart, it promotes the calmness and autonomic substrate of effective social interaction (Porges, 1997). Nonetheless, several details regarding such a system remain to be determined. For example, whether intuitive decision making is based on an interoceptive map of gut responses enabling the brain to make gut-based decisions based on interoceptive stimuli (Preuschoff et al., 2008).

MICROBIAL LIFE AND SOCIALITY

Lombardo (2008) has provided suggestions as to how to distinguish between the transmission of microorganisms as a causal benefit of social interactions versus a mere correlate, byproduct or cost of sociality. His first suggestion, primarily revised in the first section of this review, involves using antibiotics to modify microbial communities in an organism and then observing the effects of such intervention. Evidence across our review suggests that type of interventions can result in significant fitness effects in the experimental subjects. The second set of tests suggested by Lombardo (2008) are those impairing group-living individuals from horizontal transmission of microbial life but not from social contact. He suggests that by means of such intervention we would gain knowledge on how hosts may fail to thrive, not because of lack of social contact *per se*, but because of the impairment of endosymbiont-acquisition from conspecifics. In this sense, our review of the variety of symbioses found across different animal taxa was aimed at providing evidence describing the varied benefits due to such symbioses, and thus suggesting how an interruption of either vertical or horizontal transmission of microbial life could result in significant costs in terms of fitness. Then, based on evidence supporting the idea that "social immunity" is found among several animal taxa, the relationship between intense sociality and the exchange of microbiota was approached by examining the association between direct and indirect patterns of transmission of microbial-life and the intensity of social-partner selection in primates. For this purpose, we suggest that the hypothesis that more similar microbial communities would be found among subjects with stronger social bonds could be used for testing whether primates also obtain benefits associated to microbial transmission. Ultimately, as Dunbar and Shultz (2010) suggest, adding another operational index of sociality to previous, more orthodox, measures of bondedness (e.g., grooming or inter-individual distances), could help expanding our understanding of the evolution social complexity. Thus, we argue that, if endosymbionts' transmission is of any benefit to primate sociality, direct transmission of microbial life should be associated to stronger social bonds, but not to large group sizes. Such possibility, we suggest, allows for the beneficial exchange of endosymbionts across individuals, while at the same time, permits the necessary partner-choice mechanisms (associated to social-bonding processes) restricting group-size, leading to the formation of social-borders which limit the extent of microbial transmission. Indeed, research on primates suggests that greater modularity or greater structuring of social groups reduces parasite success (Griffin and Nunn, 2011). Moreover, indirect mechanisms of transmission allow subjects to exert at least three strategies for selection of the microbial load transmitted: first, one focused on the conditions or characteristics of the objects exchanged (i.e., the spoilage of food) allows subjects to decide whether a particular item deserves further processing or not (Laska et al., 2007); second, subjects may directly assess the phenotypical-characteristics of the interacting subjects, deciding whether to engage in social interaction or not. For example, by stressing immigrants in order to "test" whether they carry pathogens before allowing their full integration into a group (Freeland, 1976); third, certain species may apply *a posteriori* mechanisms for the elimination of pathogens like zoopharmacognosy (Huffman, 1997). In contrast, direct interaction restricts those mechanisms to the second and third strategies. Hence, individuals with stronger social bonds incur greater risks when interacting with their close associates compared to cases when they interact with "mere acquaintances," likely leading to an easier transmission of microbial life among strongly bonded subjects. In this sense, another suggestion stated above was that the transmission of microbial life would be increasingly difficult as primates would employ more complex partner selection mechanisms. From this perspective, since the Social Brain Hypothesis (Dunbar, 1998) is focused on the evolution of both sociality and primate neocortex by means of intense partner-selection due to increasing cognitive capacities, we can relate this hypothesis to the ideas of both Troyer (1984a) and Lombardo (2008) and hypothesize that, in primates: (i) other measures of the strength of social bonds will be positively correlated to the similarity of microbial species shared by members of a social group or reproductive pair; (ii) the number of microbial species shared by any two members of a social group will be positively correlated to that species relative neocortex size; (iii) the number of microbial species common to any two members of a social group and group size will be negatively correlated.

A particular point of concern emerging from this section is the apparent opposition of reports describing the relationship between microbiota and kinship in humans and apes. While both genetically and socially related humans show similar compositions of their gut microbiota (Degnan et al., 2012), the chimpanzees of Gombe showed similarities within sexes, as well as between members of different communities but not between individuals of the same community. This is remarkable, especially when taking into account evidence suggesting that primate females transmit necessary microbiota to their offspring. Such opposing results could imply that, while similarities in microbiota could be a useful index of the strength of social bonds for humans, the index would not be and adequate measure of prosocial tendencies in chimpanzees. In turn, this possibility would reduce the usefulness of the similarity of gut microbiota as a comparative index for examining the strength of social bonds in other species. However, these variations may be explained by pointing out important differences between the social behavior of apes and humans. Despite the fact that the social system of both chimpanzees and humans has been characterized as *fission-fusion* (Aureli et al., 2008), just like the slight differences observed between the socio-sexual behavior of *Pan troglodytes* and *Pan paniscus*, there are also important differences in the kind and degree of direct social contact observed among *Homo sapiens* and *Pan troglodytes*. The fission-fusion pattern of chimpanzee societies is substantially more fluid than that of humans: chimpanzee individuals within the same community can be alternatively found interacting within groups composed by different subjects at different points in time and in different locations (Aureli et al., 2008), whereas in humans, as bonds are stronger, they are generally more spatially, and socially stable. This observation, could explain why, compared to humans, most members of a chimpanzee community would show a similar composition of their gut microbiota (i.e., based on an incapacity to detect differences between its strongly interacting composing members). The second aspect of the discrepancy may be based on the fact that, while males remain within the same community, forming and strengthening their bonds with other relatives, females migrate between communities (Robinson and Janson, 1987).

Interesting lines of research relating social structure and composition of microbiota could develop from comparisons between the degree of similarity in the microbiota of humans (grouped, e.g., by pattern of social organization), and different non-human primate species (e.g., across different reproductive systems). If more frequent and direct contact promotes greater similarities in the composition of microbiota between individuals, we would expect that the most heavily bonded species (e.g., pair-bonded species), would show greater similarity to humans with stronger social bonds (e.g., couples), followed by the results of non-human primates across distinct reproductive patterns and humans in different types of groups. In this regard, Fincher et al. (2008), provide an important study suggesting an association between human group-level cohesion and pathogenicity. In this study, even after controlling for other confounding variables, human groups with a higher historical pathogen prevalence were also those with the strongest evidence of collectivism-prone *cultural* values, whereas those with a lower historical pathogen prevalence showed stronger cultural values supporting individualism. Therefore, we suggest that in the context of our proposal, this study provides strong evidence suggesting that, in humans, the more cohesive groups (e.g., indexed by more frequent cultural values favoring collectivism, and thus stronger social bonds between subjects) will show stronger similarities in the microbial communities of their individual members.

MOUTH-TO-MOUTH INTERACTIONS

Costly Signaling theory suggests that a possible function of seemingly "pointless" behaviors or traits, may be the conveyance of honest information that can benefit different interactants; both signalers and observers (Smith and Bird, 2005). In this context, direct means of microbial transmission have higher probabilities of involving potentially costly behaviors that could, nevertheless, provide valuable information to interactants, for example, in the case of mouth-to-mouth kissing (Hughes et al., 2007). In turn, these considerations suggest that the above accounts of the possible function of kissing may be reduced to a single one, in the form of kissing as a social signal or a means of communication. Here, communication may be defined as an action that alters the probability pattern of the behavior of another organism in a way adaptive to either one or both interactants (Wilson, 2000). Thus, either in the form of reconciliation, as a derivative of food sharing, and as a test of the quality of a relationship, kissing can be interpreted as a behavioral signal aimed at increasing the probability of future cooperation. In turn, in the case of the exchange of microbiota via mouth-to-mouth contact, or as a test for the risk of illness, kissing would represent an exchange of potentially costly information (*sensu* Smith and Bird, 2005), again, relating it to communication. The behavior may also be used by group members as an index of the strength of the relationship between two individuals: a group-oriented signal based upon which they can adjust their responses toward the individuals performing it. In the end, perhaps only cross-cultural research investigating the effects of kiss frequency relative to the composition of gut microbiota (to the best of our knowledge, not yet attempted), could bring significant light unto the matter. A comparative approach could focus in the sociosexual behavior of *Pan paniscus*, testing whether partners more often engaged in ventro-ventral copulation, mouth-to-mouth contact, and/or face-to-face interactions, compared to those engaging in other kinds of affiliative behavior, show greater similarities in their gut microbiota.

We cannot be blind to another alternative that may, nevertheless, still lend support to the hypothesis of an association between similar microbial communities and strong social bonds between individuals. Its main distinction lying in the suggestion that sociality does not represent the primary "medium" through which microbial communities across individuals are transmitted or homogenized. From this perspective, instead, given the beneficial effect of focused social contact upon glucocorticoid production (Crockford et al., 2008; Wittig et al., 2008), close social interaction will have a reducing effect on glucocorticoid production, which in turn will improve individual's capacity for sustaining an effective immune response. That "improved" resistance (e.g., byproduct of intense social support), would allow subjects to remain in close proximity without turning increasingly susceptible to the pathogens transmitted by the social-partner. Again, this possibility would still result in similarities in the microbial communities of closely bonded individuals. Further research should be focused into determining the effects of impairing microbial transmission between subjects while still allowing normal social interactions. For example, this suggestion could be approached by creating social groups where all but one of its members are kept under germ-free conditions by means of antibiotics and then evaluating the survival and reproductive success of the "non-germ free" individuals across groups. While such research design may be difficult, ethically and pragmatically, it could provide a way of discriminating between the alternatives at hand.

AUTHOR CONTRIBUTIONS

Augusto J. Montiel-Castro, conceived the main premises and relationships that are the focus of this review; wrote the largest portion of the paper; identified the theoretical relevance of the paper; edited the final version of the paper; designed **Figures 2** and **3**. Rina M. González-Cervantes, conceived some of the relationships that are discussed in the review; helped in the theoretical analysis of the premises of the review; wrote one important subsection of the paper; Gabriela Bravo-Ruiseco, wrote specific portions of the review; helped in the suggestion of specific relationships reviewed. Gustavo Pacheco-López, conceived the main premises and relationships that are the focus of this review; identified the theoretical relevance of the paper; designed the structure of the paper; wrote a large portion of the paper; edited the final version of the paper; designed **Figure 1**.

ACKNOWLEDGMENTS

This work was possible thanks to a postdoctoral scholarship, granted to Augusto J. Montiel-Castro by Iztapalapa Campus, Universidad Autonoma Metropolitana (UAM-I). Gustavo Pacheco-López was funded by a SEP-PROMEP grant No. 54510017 and by a Lerma Campus, Universidad Autonoma Metropolitana (UAM-L) institutional funding for publication. Authors would also like to thank the Centro Darwin de Pensamiento Evolucionista (CEDAR) for the support and efforts during the organization of the series of conferences and seminars between UAM-I and UAM-L that made this work possible. The suggestions of referees resulted in substantial improvements in the contents and clarity of the final version.

REFERENCES

Adams, J. B., Johansen, L. J., Powell, L. D., Quig, D., and Rubin, R. A. (2011). Gastrointestinal flora and gastrointestinal status in chil- dren with autism – comparisons to typical children and correlation with autism severity. *BMC Gastroen- terol.* 11:22.doi:10.1186/1471-230X- 11-22

Alley, T. R. (2012). Contaminated and uncontaminated feeding influ- ence perceived intimacy in mixed-sex dyads. *Appetite* 58, 1041–1045. doi: 10.1016/j.appet.2012.02.049

Altizer, S., Nunn, C. L., Thrall, P. H., Gittleman, J. L., Antonovics, J., Cunningham, A. A., et al. (2003). Social organization and parasite risk in mammals: integrating the- ory and empirical studies. *Annu. Rev. Ecol. Evol. Syst.* 34, 517–547. doi: 10.1146/annurev.ecolsys.34. 030102.151725

Altmann, J., Altmann, S., and Hausfater, G. (1988). "Determinants of repro- ductive success in Savannah baboons (*Papio cynocephalus*)," in *Reproduc- tive Success*, ed. T. H. Clutton-Brock (Chicago: University of Chicago Press), 403–418.

Archie, E. A., and Theis, K. R. (2011). Animal behavior meets microbial ecology. *Anim. Behav.* 82, 425– 436. doi: 10.1016/j.anbehav.2011.05.029

Aureli, F., Schaffner, C. M., Boesch, C., Bearder, S. K., Call, J., Chapman, A., et al. (2008). Fission-fusion dynamics. *Curr. Anthropol.* 49, 627– 654.doi:10.1086/586708

Avital, E., and Jablonka, E. (2000). *Ani- mal Traditions. Behavioral Inheritance in Evolution*. New York: Cambridge UniversityPress.

Bailey, M. T., and Coe, C. L. (1999). Maternal separation disrupts the integrity of the intestinal microflora in infant rhesus monkeys. *Dev. Psychobiol.* 35, 146–155. doi:10.1002/ (SICI)1098-2302(199909)35:2<146:: AID-DEV7>3.0.CO;2-G

Baker, K. C., and Easley, S. P. (1996). An analysis of regurgitation and reinges- tion in captive chimpanzees. *Appl. Anim. Behav. Sci.* 49, 403–415. doi: 10.1016/0168-1591(96)01061-1

Bates, J. M., Mittge, E., Kuhlman, J., Baden, K. N., Cheesman, S. E., and Guillemin, K. (2006). Distinct signals from the microbiota pro- mote different aspects of zebrafish gut differentiation. *Dev. Biol.* 297, 374–386. doi: 10.1016/j.ydbio.2006.05.006

Bercik, P., Park, A. J., SinclairKhoshdel, A., Lu J. Huang, X., Deng, Y., Belnnerhassett, P. A., et al. (2011a). The anxiolytic effect of *Bifidobacterium longum* NCC3001 involves vagal pathways for gut-brain communication. *Neu- rogastroenterol. Motil.* 23, 1132– 1139.doi:10.1111/j.1365-2982.2011. 01796.x

Berer, K., Mues, M., Koutrolos, M., Al Rasbi, Z., Boziki, M., Johner, C., et al. (2011). Commensal microbiota and myelin autoantigen cooperate to trigger autoimmune demyelina- tion. *Nature* 479, 538–541. doi: 10.1038/nature10554

Berntson, G. G., Sarter, M., and Cacioppo, J. T. (2003). Ascending visceral regulation of cortical affec- tive information processing. *Eur. J. Neurosci.* 18, 2103–2109. doi: 10.1046/j.1460-9568.2003.02967.x

Bolwig, N. (1978). Communicative signals and social behaviour of some African monkeys: a compar- ative study. *Brain* 19, 61–99. doi: 10.1007/BF02373227

Bonds, M. H., Keenan, D. C., Leid-ner, A. J., and Rohani, P. (2005). Higher disease prevalence can induce greater sociality: a game theo- retic coevolutionary model. *Evolution* 59, 1859–1866. doi: 10.1111/j.0014-3820.2005.tb01056.x

Bravo, J. A., Forsythe, P., Chew, M. V., Escaravage, E., Savignac, H. M., Dinan, T. G., et al. (2011). Ingestion of Lactobacillus strain regulates emotional behavior and central GABA receptor expression in a mouse via the vagus nerve. *Proc. Natl. Acad. Sci. U.S.A.* 108, 16050–16055. doi: 10.1073/pnas.1102999108

Buunk, B., and Hupka, R. B. (1987). Cross-cultural differences in the elicitation of sexual jeal- ousy. *J. Sex. Res.* 23, 12–22. doi: 10.1080/00224498709551338

Burkart, M. J., and van Shaik, C.P. (2010). Cognitive consequencesof cooperative breeding in pri- mates? *Anim. Cogn.* 13, 1–19. doi: 10.1007/s10071-009-0263-7

Burns, J. K. (2004). An evolu- tionary theory of schizophrenia: cortical connectivity, metarepresen- tation, and the social brain. *Behav. Brain Sci.* 27, 831–854. doi: 10.1017/S0140525X04000196

Chamberlain, A. F. (1906). Variation in early human culture. *J. Am. Folk.* 19, 177–190.doi:10.2307/534565

Clarke, G., Grenham, S., Scully, P., Fitzgerald, P., Moloney, R. D., Shanahan, F., et al. (2012). The microbiome-gut-brain axis during early life regulates the hippocam- pal serotonergic system in a sex- dependent manner. *Mol. Psychi- atry* 18, 666–673. doi: 10.1038/ mp.2012.77

Cortez, M. H., and Weitz, J. S. (2013). Distinguishing between indirect and direct modes of transmission using epidemiological time series. *Am. Nat.* 181, E43–E52. doi: 10.1086/668826

Coté, I. M., and Poulin, R. (1995). Parasitism and group size in social animals: a meta-analysis. *Behav. Ecol.* 6, 159–165. doi: 10.1093/beheco/6.2.159

Craig, A. D. (2002). How do you feel? Interoception: the sense of the physiological condition of the body. *Nat. Rev. Neurosci.* 3, 655–666. doi: 10.1038/nrn894

Craig, A. D. (2009). A rat is not a monkey is not a human: comment on Mogil (Nature Rev. Neurosci. 10,283–294 (2009)). *Nat. Rev. Neu-rosci.* 10, 466–466. doi: 10.1038/ nrn2606-c1

Cremer, S., Armitage, S. A., and Schmid- Hempel, P. (2007). Social immu- nity. *Curr. Biol.* 17, R693–R702. doi: 10.1016/j.cub.2007.06.008

Crockford, C., Wittig, R. M., Whitten, P. L., Seyfarth, R. M., and Cheney, L. (2008). Social stressors and coping mechanisms in wild female baboons (*Papio hamadryasursinus*). *Horm. Behav.* 53, 254–265. doi: 10.1016/j.yhbeh.2007.10.007

Cryan, J. F., and Dinan, T. G. (2012). Mind-altering microorganisms: the impact of the gut microbiota on brain andbehaviour. *Nat. Rev. Neurosci.* 13, 701–712. doi: 10.1038/nrn3346

Darwin, C. (1872). *The Expres- sion of Emotions in Man and Ani- mals*. London: John Murray. doi: 10.1037/10001-000

Davey, K. J., O'Mahony, S. M., Schellekens, H., O'Sullivan, O., Bienenstock, J., Cotter, P. D., et al. (2012). Gender-dependent conse- quences of chronic olanzapine in the rat: effects on body weight, inflammatory, metabolic and micro- biota parameters. *Psychopharmacol- ogy* 221, 155–169. doi: 10.1007/s00213-011-2555-2

Degnan, P. H., Pusey, A. E., Lons- dorf, E. V., Goodall, J., Wroblewski, E., Wilson, M. L., et al. (2012). Factors associated with the diversi- fication of the gut microbial com- munities within chimpanzees from Gombe National Park. *Proc. Natl. Acad. Sci. U.S.A.* 109, 13034–13039. doi: 10.1073/pnas.1110994109

de Groot, J. H. B., Smeets, M. A. M., Kaldewaij, A., Duijndam, M. J. A., and Semin, G. R. (2012). Chemosig- nals communicate human motions. *Psychol. Sci.* 23, 1417–1424. doi: 10.1177/0956797612445317

D'Enjoy, P. (1897). *Le baiser en Europe et en Chine*. Paris: Bulletin de la Soci- ete d'Anthropologie, 181–185. doi: 10.3406/bmsap.1897.5692

Desbonnet, L., Garrett, L., Clarke, G., Bienenstock, J., and Dinan, T. G. de Waal, F. B. M. (1989). *Peacemak- ing Among Primates*. USA: Harvard UniversityPress.

de Waal, F. B. M. (2000a). Attitu- dinal reciprocity in food sharing among brown capuchin monkeys. *Anim. Behav.* 60, 253–261. doi: 10.1006/anbe.2000.1471

de Waal, F. B. M. (2000b). Primates a natural heritage of conflict resolution. *Science* 289, 586–590. doi: 10.1126/science.289.5479.586

Dillon, R. J., Vennard, C. T., Buckling, A., and Charnley, A. K. (2005). Diver- sity of locust gut bacteria protects against pathogen invasion. *Ecol. Lett.* 8, 1291–1298. doi: 10.1111/j.1461- 0248.2005.00828.x

Dobson, S. (2012). Face to face with the social brain. *Philos. Trans. R. Soc. B Biol. Sci.* 367, 1901–1908. doi: 10.1098/rstb.2011.0224

Downing, J. E., and Miyan, J. A. (2000). Neural immunoregulation: emerging roles for nerves in immune home- ostasis and disease. *Immunol. Today* 21, 281–289. doi: 10.1016/S0167-5699(00)01635-2

Duarte-Dias, P. A. (2005). Observa- tion of parturition in the Mexican mantled howler monkeys (*Alouatta palliata*) on the Island of Agaltepec, Veracruz State, Mexico. *Am. J. Pri- matol.* 65, 93–98. doi: 10.1002/ajp.20100

Duerkop, B. A., Vaishnava, S., and Hooper, L. V. (2009). Immune responses to the microbiota at the intestinal mucosal surface. *Immu- nity* 31, 368–376. doi: 10.1016/j.immuni.2009.08.009

Dunbar, R. I. M. (1980). Deter- minants and evolutionary conse- quences of dominance among female gelada baboons. *Behav. Ecol. Socio- biol.* 7, 253–265. doi: 10.1007/ BF00300665

Dunbar, R. I. M. (1991). Functional sig- nificance of social grooming in pri- mates. *Folia Primatol.* 57, 121–131. doi: 10.1159/000156574

Dunbar, R. I. M. (1998). The social brain hypothesis. *Evol. Anthro*-Dunbar, R. I. M., and Shultz, S. (2010). Bondedness and social- ity. *Behaviour* 147, 775–803. doi: 10.1163/000579510X501151

Dunbar, R. I. M., and Spoors, M. (1995). Social networks, support cliques, and kinship. *Hum. Nat.* 6, 273–290. doi: 10.1007/BF02734142

Eibl-Eibesfeldt, I. (1975). *Ethology: The Biology of Behavior*. US: Holt, Rine- hart and Winston.

Eibl-Eibesfeldt, I. (1977). Thebiological unity of mankind: human ethology, concepts and implications. *Prospects* 7, 163–183. doi: 10.1007/BF02196076

Eibl-Eibesfeldt, I. (1989). *Human Ethol- ogy*. New York: Aldine De Gruyter. Evans, J. D., and Lopez, D. L. (2004). Bacterial probiotics induce an immune response in the honey bee (Hymenoptera: Apidae). *J. Econ. Entomol.* 97, 752–756. doi: 10.1603/0022-0493(2004)097[0752: BPIAIR]2.0.CO;2

Ferrari, P. F., Gallese, V., Rizzolatti, G., and Fogassi, L. (2003). Mirror neurons responding to the observa- tion of ingestive and communicative mouth actions in the monkey ven- tral premotor cortex. *Eur. J. Neurosci.* 17, 1703–1714. doi: 10.1046/j.1460-9568.2003.02601.x

Fincher, C. L., Thornhill, R., Mur- ray, D. R., and Schaller, M. (2008). Pathogen prevalence pre- dicts human cross-cultural variability in individualism/ collectivism. *Proc. Biol. Sci.* 275, 1279–1285. doi: 10.1098/rspb.2008.0094

Forsythe, P., and Bienenstock, J. (2010). Immunomodulation by commensal and probioticbacteria. *Immunol. Invest.* 39, 429–448. doi: 10.3109/08820131003667978

Forsythe, P., Kunze, W. A., and Bienenstock, J. (2012). On com- munication between gut microbes and the brain. *Curr. Opin. Gas- troenterol.* 28, 557–562. doi: 10.1097/MOG.0b013e3283572ffa

Foster, J. A., and McVey Neufeld, K. A. (2013). Gut–brain axis: how the microbiome influences anxiety and depression. *Trend. Neurosci.* 36, H. Roodenburg (Cambridge: Cam- bridge University Press), 210–236. Gallese, V. (1998). Mirror neurons: from graspingtolanguage. *Conscious. Bull.* 2,3–4.

Glaser, R., and Kiecolt-Glaser, J. K. (2005). Stress-induced immune dys- function: implications for health. *Nat. Rev. Immunol.* 5, 243–251. doi: 10.1038/nri1571

Gómez, G. D., and Balcázar, J. L. (2008). A review on the interac- tions between gut microbiota and innate immunity of fish. *FEMS. Immunol. Med. Microbiol.* 52, 145–154. doi: 10.1111/j.1574-695X.2007.00343.x

Graczyk, T. K., and Cranfield, M. R. (2003). Coprophagy and intesti- nal parasites: implications to human-habituated mountain goril- las (Gorilla gorilla beringei) of the Virunga Mountains and Bwindi impenetrable forest. *Prim. Conserv.* 19, 58–64.

Grenham, S., Clarke, G., Cryan, J. F., and Dinan, T. G. (2011). Brain–gut– microbe communication in health and disease. *Front. Physiol.* 2:1–15. doi: 10.3389/fphys.2011.00094

Griffin, R. H., and Nunn, C. L. (2011). Community structure and the spread of infectious disease in pri- mate social networks. *Evol. Ecol.* 26, 779–800. doi: 10.1007/s10682-011-9526-2

Gröschl, M. (2009). The physi- ological role of hormones in saliva. *BioEssays* 31, 843–852. doi: 10.1002/bies.200900013

Gulledge, A. K., Gulledge, M. H., and Stahmann, R. F. (2003). Roman- tic physical affection types and rela- tionship satisfaction. *Am. J. Fam. Ther.* 31, 233–242. doi: 10.1080/01926180390201936

Hansen, G. H., and Olafsen, J. A. (1999). Bacterial interactions in early life stages of marine cold water fish. *Microb. Ecol.* 38, 1–26. doi: 10.1007/s002489900158

Hardus, M. E., Lameira, A. R., and Wich, S. A. (2012). Behavioral, ecological, and evolutionary aspects of meat-eating bysumatranorangutans (Pongoabelii). Int.J.Primatol. 33, 287–304. doi:10.1007/s10764-011-9574-z

Heijtz, R.D., Wang, S.,Anuar,F., Qian, Y.,Björkholm,B.,Samuels-son, A.,etal.(2011). Normal gut microbiota modulates braindevel-opment andbehavior. Proc.Natl. Acad.Sci.U.S.A. 108, 3047–3052.doi:10.1073/pnas.1010529108

Hendrie, C.A., and Brewer, G. (2010). Kissing as an evolutionary adaptation to protect against human cytomegalovirus-like teratogenesis. Med.Hyp. 74, 222–224. doi: 10.1016/j.mehy.2009.09.033

Hickman, C. S. (2005). "How have bacteria contributed to the evolu- tion of multicellular animals?," in *The Influence of Cooperative Bacte- ria on Animal Host Biology*, eds M. J. McFall-Ngai, B. Henderson, andE. G. Ruby (New York: Cambridge University Press), 3–33.

Hinde, R. (1983a). "Description and proximate factors influencing social structure," in *Primate Social Relation- ships: An Integrated Approach*, ed. Robert Hinde (Oxford: Blackwell Sci- entific Publications), 65–120.

Hinde, R. (1983b). "Development and dynamics of relationships," in *Pri- mate Social Relationships: An Inte- grated Approach*, ed. R. Hinde (Oxford:Blackwell ScientificPublica- tions), 176–230.

Hinde, K., and German, J. B. (2012). Food in an evolutionary context: insights from mother's milk. *J. Sci. Food. Agric.* 92, 2219–2223. doi: 10.1002/jsfa.5720

Hirata, S. (2006). "Chimpanzee learn- ing and transmission of tool use to fish for honey," in *Cognitive Development in Chimpanzees*, edsT. Matsusawa, M. Tomonaga, andM. Tanaka (Tokyo: Springer Verlag), 201–213. doi: 10.1007/4-431-30248- 4_13

Hirata, S., and Celli, M. L. (2003). Role of mothers in the acquisition of tool-use behaviours by captive infant chimpanzees. *Anim. Cogn.* 6, 235–244.doi:10.1007/s10071-003-0187-6

Horwich, R. H., and Manski, D. (1975). Maternal care and infant transfer in two species of colobus monkeys. *Primates* 16, 49–73. doi: 10.1007/BF02381799

Huffman, M. A. (1997). Current evidence for self-medication in pri- mates: a multidisciplinary perspec- tive. *Am. J. Phys. Anthropol.* 200, 171–200. doi: 10.1002/(SICI)1096-8644(1997)25+<171::AID-AJPA7>3.0.CO;2-7

Hughes, S., Harrison, M., and Gallup, G. G. Jr. (2007). Sex differences in romantic kissing among college stu- dents: an evolutionary perspective. *Evol. Psychol.* 5, 612–631.

Jaeggi, A. V., and van Schaik, C. P. (2011). The evolution of food shar- ing in primates. *Behav. Ecol. Sociobiol.* 65, 2125–2140. doi: 10.1007/s00265-011-1221-3.

Kaltenpoth, M., and Engl, T. (2013). Defensive microbial symbionts in Hymenoptera. *Func. Ecol.* doi: 10.1111/1365-2435.12089 [Epubahead of print].

Kasper, C., Voelkl, B., and Huber, L. (2008). Tolerated mouth-to-mouth food transfers in common mar- mosets. *Anim. Behav.* 49, 153–156. doi: 10.1007/s10329-007-0069-7.

Kelly, D., and Mulder, I. E. (2012). Microbiome and immunological interactions. *Nutr. Rev.* 70, S18– S30. doi: 10.1111/j.1753-4887.2012. 00498.x

Keverne, E. B., Martensz, N., and Tuite, B. (1989). Beta-endorphin concentrations in cerebrospinal fluid of monkeys are influenced by grooming relationships. *Psychoneu- roendocrinology* 14, 155–161. doi: 10.1016/0306-4530(89)90065-6

Kline, S. L., Horton, B., and Zhang, S. (2008). Communicating love: com- parisons between American and East Asian university students. *Int. J. Intercult. Relat.* 32, 200–214. doi: 10.1016/j.ijintrel.2008.01.006

Koch, H., and Schmid-Hempel, P. (2011). Socially transmitted gut microbiota protect bumble bees against an intestinal parasite. *Proc. Natl. Acad. Sci. U.S.A.* 108, 19288–19292. doi: 10.1073/pnas.1110474108

Kohl, K. D. (2012). Diversity and func- tion of the avian gut microbiota. *J. Comp. Physiol. B* 182, 591–602. doi: 10.1007/s00360-012-0645-z

Kudo, H., and Dunbar, R. I. M. (2001). Neocortex size and social network size in primates. *Anim. Behav.* 61, 1–12. doi: 10.1006/anbe.2001.1808

Kuroda, S. (1980). Social behavior of the pygmy chimpanzees. *Primates* 21, 181–197. doi: 10.1007/BF02374032

Kyle, P. D., and Kyle, G. Z. (1993). An evaluation of the role of micro- bial flora in the salivary transfer technique for hand-rearing Chimney Swifts. *Wildl. Rehabil.* 8, 65–71.

Lambert, J. E. (1998). Primate digestion: interactions among anatomy, physiology, and feeding ecology. *Evol. Anthropol.* 7, 8–20. doi: 10.1002/(SI- CI)1520-6505(1998)7:1<8::AID-EV- AN3>3.0.CO;2-C

Langergraber, K. E. (2012). "Coopera- tion among kin," in *The Evolution of Primate Societies*, eds J. C. Mitani, J. Call, P. M. Kappeler, R. A. Palombit, and J. B. Silk (Chicago: The Univer- sity of Chicago Press), 491–513.

Laska, M., Bautista, R. M. R., Höfel- mann, D., Sterlemann, V., and Salazar, L. T. H. (2007). Olfac- tory sensitivity for putrefaction- associated thiols and indols in three species of non-human primate. *J. Exp. Biol.* 210, 4169–4178. doi: 10.1242/jeb.012237

Lee, Y. K., Menezes, J. S., Ume- saki, Y., and Masmanian, S. K. (2011). Protoinflammatory T- cell responses to gut microbiota promote experimental autoimmune encephalomyelitis. *Proc. Natl. Acad. Sci. U.S.A.* 108, 4615–4622. doi: 10.1073/pnas.1000082107

Lindburg, D. G., and Hazell, L. D. (1972). Licking of the neonate and duration of labor in great apes and man. *Am. Anthropol.* 74, 318–325. doi: 10.1525/aa.1972.74.3.02 a00040

Little, T. J., O'Connor, B., Cole- grave, N., Watt, K., and Read, A. F. (2003). Maternal transfer of strain-specific immunity in an inver- tebrate. *Curr. Biol.* 13, 489–492. doi: 10.1016/S0960-9822(03)00163-5

Loehle, C. (1995). Social barriers to pathogen transmission in wild ani- mal populations. *Ecology* 76, 326–335. doi: 10.2307/1941192

Lombardo, M. P. (2008). Access to mutualistic endosymbiotic microbes: an underappreciated benefit of group living. *Behav. Ecol. Sociobiol.* 62, 479–497. doi: 10.1007/s00265-007-0428-9

Manco, M. (2012). Gut micro- biota and developmental program- ming of the brain: from evidence in behavioral endophenotypes to novel perspective in obesity. *Front. Cell. Infect. Microbiol.* 2:109. doi: 10.3389/fcimb.2012.00109

Manson, J. H., Perry, S., and Parish, A. R. (1997). Nonconceptive sexual behavior in bonobos and capuchins. *Int. J. Primatol.* 18, 767–786. doi: 10.1023/A:1026395829818

Mathers, C., Fat, D. M., and Boerma, J. T. (2008). *The Global Burden of Disease: 2004 Update.* Geneva: World Health Organization.

Mayer, E. A. (2011). Gut feelings: the emerging biology of gut–brain com- munication. *Nat. Rev. Neurosci.* 12, 453–466. doi: 10.1038/nrn3071

McFall-Ngai, M. J. (1994). Animal- bacterial interactions in the early life history of marine invertebrates: the Euprymna scolopes/Vibrio fischeri symbiosis. *Am. Zool.* 34, 554–561. doi: 10.1093/icb/34.4.554

McFall-Ngai, M. J. (1998). The development of cooperative associ- ations between animals and bac- teria: establishing détente among domains. *Am. Zool.* 38, 593–608. doi: 10.1093/icb/38.4.593

McFall-Ngai, M. J. (2005). "The inter- face of microbiology and immunol- ogy: a comparative analysis of the animal kingdom," in *The Influence of Cooperative Bacteria on Animal Host Biology*, eds M. J. McFall-Ngai, B. Henderson, and E. G. Ruby (New York: Cambridge University Press), 35–56.

McFall-Ngai, M., Hadfield, M. G., Bosch, T. C. G., Carey, H. V., Domazet-Loso, T., Douglas, A. E., et al. (2013). Animals in a bacte- rial world, a new imperative for the life sciences. *Proc. Natl. Acad. Sci. USA.* 110, 3229–3236. doi: 10.1073/pnas.1218525110

McFrederick, Q. S., Wcislo, W. T., Tay- lor, D. R., Ishak, H. D., Dowd, S. E., and Mueller, U. G. (2012). Environ- ment or kin: whence do bees obtain acidophilic bacteria? *Mol. Ecol.* 21, 1754–1768. doi: 10.1111/j.1365-294X.2012.05496.x

McKernan, D. P., Fitzgerald, P., Dinan, T. G., and Cryan, J. F. (2010). The probiotic *Bifidobac- terium* infantis 35624 displays visceral antinociceptive effects in the rat. *Neurogastroenterol. Motil.* 22, 1029– 1035, e268. doi: 10.1111/j.1365-2982.2010.01520.x

Michod, R. E. (2003). "Cooperation and conflict mediation during the origin of multicellularity," in *Genetic and Cultural Evolution of Cooper- ation. Report of the 90th Dahlem Workshop on Genetic and Cultural Evolution of Cooperation, Berlin, June 23–28, 2002*, ed. P. Hammerstein (Cambridge, MA: MIT Press), 291– 308.

Milton, K. (1981). Food choice and digestive strategies of two sympatric primate species. *Am. Nat.* 117, 496–505. doi: 10.1086/283730

Mitani, J. C. (2009). Male chimpanzees form enduring and equitable social bonds. *Anim. Behav.* 77, 633–640. doi: 10.1016/j.anbehav.2008.11.021

Mitani, J. C., Call, J., Kappeler, P. M., Palombit, R. A., and Silk, J. B. (2012). *The Evolution of Primate Societies.* Chicago: The University of Chicago Press. doi: 10.7208/chicago/9780226531731.001. 0001

Mooring, M. S., Blumstein, D. T., and Stoner, C. J. (2004). The evolution of parasite-defence grooming in ungu- lates. *Biol. J. Linn. Soc.* 81, 17–37. doi: 10.1111/j.1095-8312.2004.00273.x

Mykytowycz, R. (1972). The behavioural role of the mammalian skin glans. *Naturwissenschaften* 59, 133–139. doi: 10.1007/BF00637350

Nakamichi, M., and Koyama, N. (2000). Intra-troop affiliative rela- tionships of females with newborn infants in wild ring-tailed lemurs (*Lemur catta*). *Am. J. Primatol.* 50, 187–203. doi: 10.1002/(SICI)1098-2345(200003)50:3<187::AID-AJP2>3.0.CO;2-Q

Nash, L. T., Fritz, J., Alford, P. A., and Brent, L. (1999). Variables influencing the origins of diverse abnormal behaviors in a large sam- ple of captive chimpanzees (*Pan troglodytes*). *Am. J. Primatol.* 48, 15–29. doi: 10.1002/(SICI)1098-2345(1999)48:1<15::AID-AJP2>3.0. CO;2-R

Neuberg, S. L., Kenrick, D. T., and Schaller, M. (2011). Human threat management systems: self-protection and disease avoidance. *Neurosci. Biobehav. Rev.* 35, 1042–1045. doi: 10.1016/j.neubiorev.2010.08.011

Nicholson, B. (1984). Does kissing aid human bonding by semiochem- ical addiction? *Br. J. Dermatol.* 111, 623–627. doi: 10.1111/j.1365-2133.1984.tb06635.x

Ninonuevo, M. R., Park, Y., Hongfeng, Y., Zhang, J., Ward, R. E., Clowers, B. H., et al. (2006). A strategy for annotating the human milk glycome. *J. Agric. Food. Chem.* 54, 7471–7480. doi: 10.1021/jf0615810

Nunn, C. L. (2012). Primate disease ecology in comparative and theo- retical perspective. *Am. J. Prima- tol.* 509, 497–509. doi: 10.1002/ajp.21986

O'Mahony, S. M., Hyland, N. P., Dinan, T. G., and Cryan, J. F. (2011). Mater- nal separation as a model of brain-gut axis dysfunction. *Psychopharmacol- ogy* 214, 71–88. doi: 10.1007/s00213- 010-2010-9

Parr, L. A., Waller, B. M., and Fugate, J. (2005). Emotional com- munication in primates: impli- cations for neurobiology. *Curr. Opin. Neurobiol.* 15, 716–720. doi: 10.1016/j.conb.2005.10.017

Penders, J., Thijs, C., Vink, C., Sterma, F. F., Snijdes, B., Kummeling, I., et al. (2006). Factors influencing the com- position of the intestinal microbiota in early infancy. *Pediatrics* 118, 511– 521. doi: 10.1542/peds.2005-2824

Penn, D., and Potts, W. K. (1998). Chemical signals and parasite- mediated sexual selection. *Tree* 13, 391–396. doi: 10.1016/S0169-5347(98)01473-6

Porges, S. W. (1997). Emotion: an evo- lutionary by-product of the neural regulation of the autonomic ner- vous system. *Ann. N. Y. Acad. Sci.* 807, 62–77. doi: 10.1111/j.1749-6632.1997.tb51913.x

Porges, S. W. (2003). The Polyva- gal theory: phylogenetic contribu- tions to social behavior. *Phys. Behav.* 79, 503–513. doi: 10.1016/S0031-9384(03)00156-2

Preuschoff, K., Quartz, S. R., and Bossaerts, P. (2008). Human insula activation reflects risk pre- diction errors as well as risk. *J. Neurosci.* 28, 2745–2752. doi: 10.1523/JNEUROSCI.4286-07.2008

Pruetz, J. D., and Lindshield, S. (2012). Plant-food and tool transfer among savanna chimpanzees at Fon- goli, Senegal. *Primates* 53, 133–145. doi: 10.1007/s10329-011-0287-x

Regan, P. C., Durvasula, R., Howell, L., Ureno, O., and Rea, M. (2004). Gen- der, ethnicity, and the developmental timing of first sexual and romantic experiences. *Soc. Behav. Pers.* 32, 667–676. doi: 10.2224/sbp.2004.32.7.667

Relman, D. A. (2012). The human microbiome: ecosystem resilience and health. *Nutr. Rev.* 70, S2–S9. doi: 10.1111/j.1753-4887.2012.00489.x

Rhee, S. H., Pothoulakis, C., and Mayer, E. A. (2009). Principles and clini- cal implications of the brain–gut– enteric microbiota axis. *Nat. Rev. Gastroenterol. Hepatol.* 6, 306–314. doi: 10.1038/nrgastro.2009.35

Rizzolatti, G., and Fogassi, L. (2007). "Mirror neurons and social cogni- tion", in *The Oxford Handbook of Evolutionary Psychology*, eds R. I.M. Dunbar and L. Barrett (Oxford: Oxford University Press), 179–195.

Robinson, J. G., and Janson, C. H. (1987). "Capuchins, squirrel mon- keys, and atelines: socioecological convergence with old world pri- mates," in *Primate Societies*, eds B. B. Smuts, D. L. Cheney, R. M. Seyfarth, W. Wrangham, and T. Struhsaker (Chicago: The University of Chicago Press), 69–82.

Ruby, E. G., and McFall-Ngai, M. J. (1992). A squid that glows in the night: development of an animal- bacterial mutualism. *J. Bacteriol.* 174, 4865–4870.

Schaller, M. (2011). The behavioural immune system and the psychology of human sociality. *Philos. Trans. R. Soc. B Biol. Sci.* 366, 3418–3426. doi: 10.1098/rstb.2011.0029

Schaub, H. (1996). Testing kin altru- ism in long-tailed macaques (*Macaca fascicularis*) in a food-sharing exper- iment. *Int. J. Primatol.* 17, 445–467. doi: 10.1007/BF02736631

Schreier, A. L., and Swedell, L. (2009). The fourth level of social structure in a multi-level society: ecologi- cal and social functions of clans in Hamadryas baboons. *Am. J. Primatol.* 71, 948–955. doi: 10.1002/ajp.20736

Shultz, S., and Dunbar, R. I. M. (2007). The evolution of the social brain: anthropoid primates con- trast with other vertebrates. *Proc. Biol. Sci.* 274, 2429–2436. doi: 10.1098/rspb.2007.0693

Sleigh, C. (2002). Brave new worlds: trophallaxis and the origin of soci- ety in the early twentieth century. *J. Hist. Behav. Sci.* 38, 133–156. doi: 10:1002/jhbs.10033

Smith, E. A., and Bird, B. (2005). "Costly signaling and cooperative behavior," in *Moral Sentiments and Material Interests: The Foundations of Cooper- ation in Economic Life*, eds H. Gintis, Bowles, R. Boyd, and E. Fehr (Cambridge, MA: The MIT Press), 115–148.

Sternberg, E. M. (2006). Neural regu- lation of innate immunity: a coor- dinated nonspecific host response to pathogens. *Nat. Rev. Immunol.* 6, 318–328. doi: 10.1038/nri1810

Stevens, J. R., and Gilby, I. C. (2004). A conceptual framework for nonkin food sharing: timing and currency of benefits. *Anim. Behav.* 67, 603–614. doi: 10.1016/j.anbehav.2003.04.012

Tang, W. W., Wang, Z., Levison, B. S., Koeth, R. A., Britt, E. B., Fu, X., et al. (2013). Intestinal micro- bial metabolism of phosphatidyl- choline and cardiovascular risk. *N. Engl. J. Med.* 368, 1575–1584. doi: 10.1056/NEJMoa1109400

Thomas, R. H., Meeking, M. M., Mepham, J. R., Tichenoff, L., Poss- mayer, F., Liu, S., et al. (2012). The enteric bacterial metabolite propi- onic acid alters brain and plasma phospholipid molecular species: fur- ther development of a rodent model of autism spectrum disorders. *J. Neuroinflammation* 9, 153. doi: 10.1186/1742-2094-9-153

Troyer, K. (1984a). Microbes, herbivory and the evolution of social behav- ior. *J. Theor. Biol.* 106, 157–169. doi: 10.1016/0022-5193(84)90016-X

Troyer, K. (1984b). Behavioral acqui- sition of the hindgut fermentation system by hatchling Iguana iguana. *Behav. Ecol. Sociobiol.* 14, 189–193. doi: 10.1007/BF00299618

Tsuji, H., Oozeer, R., Matsuda, K., Mat- suki, T., Ohta, T., Nomoto, K., et al. (2012). Molecular monitoring of the development of intestinal microbiota in Japanese infants. *Benef. Microbes* 3, 113–125. doi: 10.3920/BM2011.0038

Turnbaugh, P. J., and Gordon, J. I. (2009). The core gut microbiome, energy balance and obesity. *J. Physiol.* 587, 4153–4158. doi: 10.1113/jphys- iol.2009.174136

Turnbaugh, P. J., Hamady, M., Yat- sunenko, T., Cantarel, B. L., Duncan, A., Ley, R. E., et al. (2009). A core gut microbiome in obese and lean twins. *Nature* 457, 480–484. doi: 10.1038/nature07540

Turner, S. E., Fedigan, L. M., Nakamichi, M., Matthews, H. D., McKenna, K., Nobuhara, H., et al. (2009). Birth in free-ranging *Macaca fuscata*. *Int. J. Primatol.* 31, 15–37. doi: 10.1007/s10764-009-9376-8

van Schaik, C. P., and van Noord- wijk, M. A. (1986). The hidden costs of sociality: intra-group varia- tion in feeding strategies in Sumatran long-tailed macaques (*Macaca fascic- ularis*). *Behaviour* 99, 296–315. doi: 10.1163/156853986X00595

Verschuere, L., Heang, H., Criel, G., Dafnis, S., Sorgeloos, P., and Ver- straete, W. (2000). Selected bac- terial strains protect *Artemia* spp. from the pathogenic effects of *Vib- rio proteolyticus* CW8T2. *Appl. Env- iron. Microbiol.* 66, 1139–1146. doi: 10.1128/AEM.66.3.1139-1146.2000

Walke, J. B., Harris, R. N., Rein- ert, L. K., Rollins-Smith, L. A., and Woodhams, D. C. (2011). Social immunity in amphibians: evidence for vertical transmission of innate defenses. *Biotropica* 43, 396–400. doi: 10.1111/j.1744-7429.2011.00787.x

Walter, B. C. (2008). Affairs of the lips: why we kiss. *Sci. Am. Mind.* 19, 24–29. doi: 10.1038/scientificamericanmind0208-24 Wang, B., Mao, Y., Diorio, C., Wang, L., Huizinga, J. D., Bienenstock, J., et al. (2010). *Lactobacillus reuteri* inges- tion and IKCa channel blockade have similar effects on rat colon motility and myenteric neurones. *Neurogas- troenterol. Motil.* 22, 98–e33. doi: 10.1111/j.1365-2982.2009.01384.x

Wang, J., and Aksoy, S. (2012). PGRP-LB is a maternally transmit- ted immune milk protein that influ- ences symbiosis and parasitism in tsetse's offspring. *Proc. Natl. Acad. Sci. U.S.A.* 109, 10552–10557. doi: 10.1073/pnas.1116431109

Wang, L., Christophersen, C. T., Sorich, M. J., Gerber, J. P., Angley, M. T., and Conlon, M. A. (2012). Ele- vated faecal short chain fatty acid and ammonia concentrations in chil- dren with autism spectrum disorder. *Dig. Dis. Sci.* 57, 2096–2102. doi: 10.1007/s10620-012-2167-7

Washburn Hopkins, E. (1907). The Sniff-kiss in ancient India. *J. Am. Oriental Soc.* 28, 120–134. doi: 10.2307/592764

Watts, D. P., and Mitani, J. C. (2002). Hunting behavior of chimpanzees at Ngogo, Kibale National Park, Uganda. *Int. J. Primatol.* 23, 1–28. doi: 10.1023/A:1013270606320

Wedekind, C., Seebeck, T., Bet- tens, F., and Paepke, A. J. (1995). MHC-dependent mate preferences in humans. *Proc. Biol. Sci.* 260, 245–249. doi: 10.1098/rspb.1995.0087

Wheeler, W. (1918). A study of some young ant larvae with a considera- tion of the origin and meaning of social habits among insects. *Proc. Am. Philos. Soc.* 57, 293–343.

Whiten, A., Goodall, J., McGrew, W. C., Nishida, T., Reynolds, V., Sugiyama, Y., et al. (2001). Charting cultural variation in chimpanzees. *Behaviour* 138, 1481–1516. doi: 10.1163/156853901317367717

Wicker, B., Keysers, C., Plailly, J., Royet, J. P., Gallese, V., and Rizzolatti, G. (2003). Both of us disgusted in my insula: the common neural basis of seeing and feeling disgust. *Neuron* 40, 655–664. doi: 10.1016/S0896- 6273(03)00679-2

Wilson, E. O. (2000). *Sociobiology. The New Synthesis*, 25th anniversary Edn. Cambridge, MA: The Belknap Press of Harvard University Press.

Wittig, R. M., and Boesch, C. (2003). The choice of post-conflict inter- actions in wild chimpanzees (*Pan troglodytes*). *Behaviour* 140, 1527- 1559. doi: 10.1163/1568539037719 80701

Wittig, R. M., Crockford, C., Lehmann, J., Whitten, P. L., Seyfarth, R. M., and Cheney, D. L. (2008). Focused grooming networks and stress alleviation in wild female baboons. *Horm. Behav.* 54, 170–177. doi:10.1016/j.yhbeh.2008.02.009

Wrangham, R. W. (1993). The evolu- tion of sexuality in chimpanzees and bonobos. *Hum. Nat.* 4, 47–79. doi: 10.1007/BF02734089

Yatsunenko, T., Rey, F. E., Man- ary, M. J., Trehan, I., Dominguez- Bello, M. G., Contreras, M., et al. (2012). Human gut microbiome viewed across age and geography. *Nature* 486, 222–228. doi: 10.1038/ nature11053

Young, L. J., and Wang, Z. (2004). The neurobiology of pair bonding. *Nat. Neurosci.* 7, 1048–1054. doi: 10.1038/nn1327

Zhou, W., Sornette, D., Hill, R. A., and Dunbar, R. I. M. (2005). Discrete hierarchical organization of social group sizes. *Proc. Biol. Sci.* 272, 439- 444. doi: 10.1098/rspb.2004.2970

Zuberbühler, K., Noë, R., and Sey- farth, R. M. (1997). Diana mon- key long-distance calls: messages for conspecifics and predators. *Anim. Behav.* 53, 589–604. doi: 10.1006/ anbe.1996.0334

13

Surgical manipulation compromises leukocyte mobilization responses and inflammation after experimental cerebral ischemia in mice

Adam Denes[1,2]*, Jesus M. Pradillo[1], Caroline Drake[1], Hannah Buggey[1], Nancy J. Rothwell[1] and Stuart M. Allan[1]*

[1] *Faculty of Life Sciences, University of Manchester, Manchester, UK*
[2] *Laboratory of Molecular Neuroendocrinology, Institute of Experimental Medicine, Budapest, Hungary*

Edited by:
Eric W. Roubos, Radboud University Nijmegen, Netherlands

Reviewed by:
Jaleel A. Miyan, The University of Manchester, UK
James Downing, Liverpool John Moores University, UK
Eric W. Roubos, Radboud University Nijmegen, Netherlands

****Correspondence:***
Adam Denes, Laboratory of Molecular Neuroendocrinology, MTA KOKI, Szigony u. 43., 1083 Budapest, Hungary
e-mail: adam.denes@manchester.ac.uk; denesa@koki.hu;
Stuart M. Allan, Faculty of Life Sciences, University of Manchester, AV Hill Building, Oxford Road, Manchester M13 9PT, UK
e-mail: stuart.allan@manchester.ac.uk

Acute brain injury results in peripheral inflammatory changes, although the impact of these processes on neuronal death and neuroinflammation is currently unclear. To facilitate the translation of experimental studies to clinical benefit, it is vital to characterize the mechanisms by which acute brain injury induces peripheral inflammatory changes, and how these are affected by surgical manipulation in experimental models. Here we show that in mice, even mild surgical manipulation of extracranial tissues induced marked granulocyte mobilization (300%) and systemic induction of cytokines. However, intracranial changes induced by craniotomy, or subsequent induction of focal cerebral ischemia were required to induce egress of CXCR2-positive granulocytes from the bone marrow. CXCR2 blockade resulted in reduced mobilization of granulocytes from the bone marrow, caused an unexpected increase in circulating granulocytes, but failed to affect brain injury induced by cerebral ischemia. We also demonstrate that isoflurane anaesthesia interferes with circulating leukocyte responses, which could contribute to the reported vascular and neuroprotective effects of isoflurane. In addition, no immunosuppression develops in the bone marrow after experimental stroke. Thus, experimental models of cerebral ischemia are compromised by surgery and anaesthesia in proportion to the severity of surgical intervention and overall tissue injury. Understanding the inherent confounding effects of surgical manipulation and development of new models of cerebral ischemia with minimal surgical intervention could facilitate better understanding of interactions between inflammation and brain injury.

Keywords: experimental stroke, bone marrow, granulocyte, CXCR2, anaesthesia

INTRODUCTION

Brain injury due to cerebral ischemia, hemorrhage, or head trauma results in early activation of the immune system, followed later by immunosuppression (Dirnagl et al., 2007; Denes et al., 2010b). Activated immune cells and inflammatory mediators contribute to neuroinflammation and overall outcome after experimental brain injury. Blockade of toll-like receptors, proinflammatory mediators such as interleukin-1, and immune cells such as T cells, neutrophils, or mast cells, is protective in experimental models of brain injury (Iadecola and Anrather, 2011; Smith et al., 2013). However, oversuppression of the immune system in response to brain injury gives rise to opportunistic infections leading to impaired recovery and death of patients and experimental animals (Dirnagl et al., 2007; Murray et al., 2013). Therefore, understanding interactions between peripheral inflammatory responses and brain injury could pave the way for novel therapeutic interventions.

Lack of translation in stroke has triggered intense discussions, leading to improved preclinical guidelines on experimental modeling (Fisher et al., 2009). Yet, compared to the large number of clinical studies on peripheral inflammatory changes in stroke, studies on systemic inflammatory mechanisms in experimental animals remain relatively sparse.

We and others have shown that experimental stroke results in the activation of inflammatory responses in various immune organs such as the spleen, blood, or bone marrow (Offner et al., 2006a,b; Chapman et al., 2009; Denes et al., 2011). Using a filament model of transient, focal cerebral ischemia we also showed that anaesthesia and surgical intervention compromise stroke-induced inflammatory responses in the periphery (Denes et al., 2011). However, a systematic analysis of stroke-induced peripheral inflammatory actions, including the assessment of confounding effects of surgical manipulations has not yet been performed in experimental stroke that involves craniotomy. Such investigations could distinguish model-specific and ischemia-induced effects of experimental stroke on immune responses and yield important data for translation to patients.

Thus, we examined the effects of anaesthesia, surgical manipulation, and experimental stroke induced by transient, distal middle cerebral artery occlusion with craniotomy on peripheral inflammatory responses. We show that both isoflurane anaesthesia and surgical intervention induce changes in peripheral immune cell populations in the absence of stroke, and are likely to contribute to systemic inflammatory responses induced by experimental brain injury. These effects should be accounted for in experimental stroke modeling.

MATERIALS AND METHODS

MICE

Male 8–12 week-old C57BL/6 mice ($n = 58$) were kept at 21 ± 1°C and 65% humidity with a 12 h light-dark cycle and had free access to food and water. All animal procedures were performed under appropriate project license authority and adhered to the UK Animals (Scientific Procedures) Act (1986) and were in accordance with STAIR and ARRIVE (Fisher et al., 2009; Kilkenny et al., 2010) guidelines.

MIDDLE CEREBRAL ARTERY OCCLUSION (MCAo)

Distal, transient focal cerebral ischemia was induced as described earlier (Pradillo et al., 2009, 2012). Briefly, mice were anaesthetized with isoflurane and ischemia was induced by a transient ligature (60 min) of the left MCA trunk with a 10-0 suture (Prolene, Ethicon, Somerville, NJ, USA). Occlusion and reperfusion were confirmed visually under the surgical microscope. Core body temperature was maintained at 37.0 ± 0.5°C throughout the surgery by a heating blanket (Homeothermic Blanket Control Unit; Harvard Apparatus, Kent, UK) and monitored after recovery. After surgery, animals were returned to their cages and allowed free access to water and food. It was decided, *a priori*, to exclude from the study those animals that showed brain hemorrhage at any time of the surgery or with no reperfusion (2 mice). The survival rate was 100%.

SURGICAL CONTROLS

We investigated the effect of surgical manipulation and anaesthesia in the absence of MCAo on cellular and cytokine responses. To achieve this, three separate experimental conditions were used; the first involved only anaesthesia with no surgical manipulation (termed as "isoflurane"), the second exposure of the skull bone but no craniotomy (termed as "sham no cran.") and the third full craniotomy (termed as "sham"). Except for naive animals, all groups of mice were kept under isoflurane anaesthesia for the same time period (75 min for control experimental conditions and in the "MCAo" group).

BLOOD SAMPLING AND TISSUE PROCESSING

Blood samples were taken from the tail vein and from the right cardiac ventricle, using 3.8% sodium citrate 1:10 as an anticoagulant. Repeated tail vein samples were collected at various time points, with equal sampling times across different treatment groups: prior to surgery ("naïve"), 60 min after the onset of ischemia or corresponding control surgery ("0 min reperfusion"), and before transcardial perfusion (at 4 or 72 h reperfusion, not shown). Terminal cardiac blood samples were collected immediately prior to transcardial perfusion from naive mice, and from mice that had undergone surgical interventions, at 4 or 72 h reperfusion. Blood sample data from different vascular beds were analyzed separately. To avoid potential confounding effects of repeated tail vein samples at later time points, cardiac blood samples are presented throughout the manuscript, with the exception of **Figures 1A,B**. To isolate the bone marrow and the spleen, mice were perfused transcardially with saline under isoflurane anaesthesia. Brains were subsequently perfused with 4% paraformaldehyde, post-fixed for 24 h, cryoprotected in 20% sucrose/PBS, and sectioned (20 μm diameter) on a sledge microtome. Organs were homogenized as described previously (Denes et al., 2010a).

CXCR2 BLOCKADE

To prevent CXCR2-mediated release of granulocytes from the bone marrow, mice in the MCAo group were treated intraperitoneally with a selective CXCR2 antagonist (SB225002) or vehicle. SB225002 was dissolved in DMSO (stock), diluted in sterile saline 1:40 and injected as 2 mg/kg, 200 μl/mouse, 20 min prior to induction of anaesthesia for MCAo surgery.

In vitro STIMULATION OF BONE MARROW CELLS

Bone marrow cells were isolated 72 h after 60 min MCAo or the surgery control and stimulated *in vitro* with 1 μg/ml bacterial lipopolysaccharide (LPS, *E. coli* O26:B6), at a density of 7.5×10^6 cells/mL in RPMI medium, supplemented with 10% fetal calf serum and penicillin/streptomycin to investigate cytokine production. After 3 h incubation at 37°C, cells were pelleted with centrifugation at $400 \times g$, the supernatant was collected, and cells were lysed in lysis buffer.

CYTOMETRIC BEAD ARRAY

Circulating levels of IL-6 and KC (CXCL-1), and levels of IL-6 in bone marrow cell culture supernatants and lysates were measured by using CBA Flex Sets (BD Biosciences, UK) according to the manufacturers protocol. The detection limit for each cytokine was 5–10 pg/ml.

FLOW CYTOMETRY

Spleen, bone marrow, and blood cells were isolated and stained with appropriate combinations of CD45-PerCP-Cy5.5, Ly6c-PerCP-Cy5.5, CD4-PE-Cy7, CD8-PE, CD3-APC, CD19-PE-Cy7, MHCII-APC (eBioscience, UK), and Ly6G-PE (1A8, BD Biosciences, UK) following Fc receptor blockade (eBioscience). Contaminating red blood cells in bone marrow and spleen samples were removed by ACK solution, and FACS lysing solution (BD Biosciences) was used to remove red blood cells from blood samples. Total blood cell counts were calculated by using 15 μm polystyrene microbeads (Polysciences, 18328-5). Cells were acquired on an LSRII flow cytometer, using FACS Diva software (BD Biosciences, UK). Except for the 72 h time point, flow cytometric data have been pooled from three independent experiments, in which all experimental groups have been represented by at least one animal. Due to red blood cell contamination and cell labeling artifacts $n = 6$ blood samples, $n = 3$ bone marrow samples and $n = 4$ spleen samples have been excluded from analysis across experiments, *pre-hoc*.

RANDOMIZATION, QUANTIFICATION, AND STATISTICAL ANALYSIS

Animals were randomized for experiments and all quantitative analyses were performed in a blinded manner. Group sizes were determined based on our earlier *in vivo* experiments using

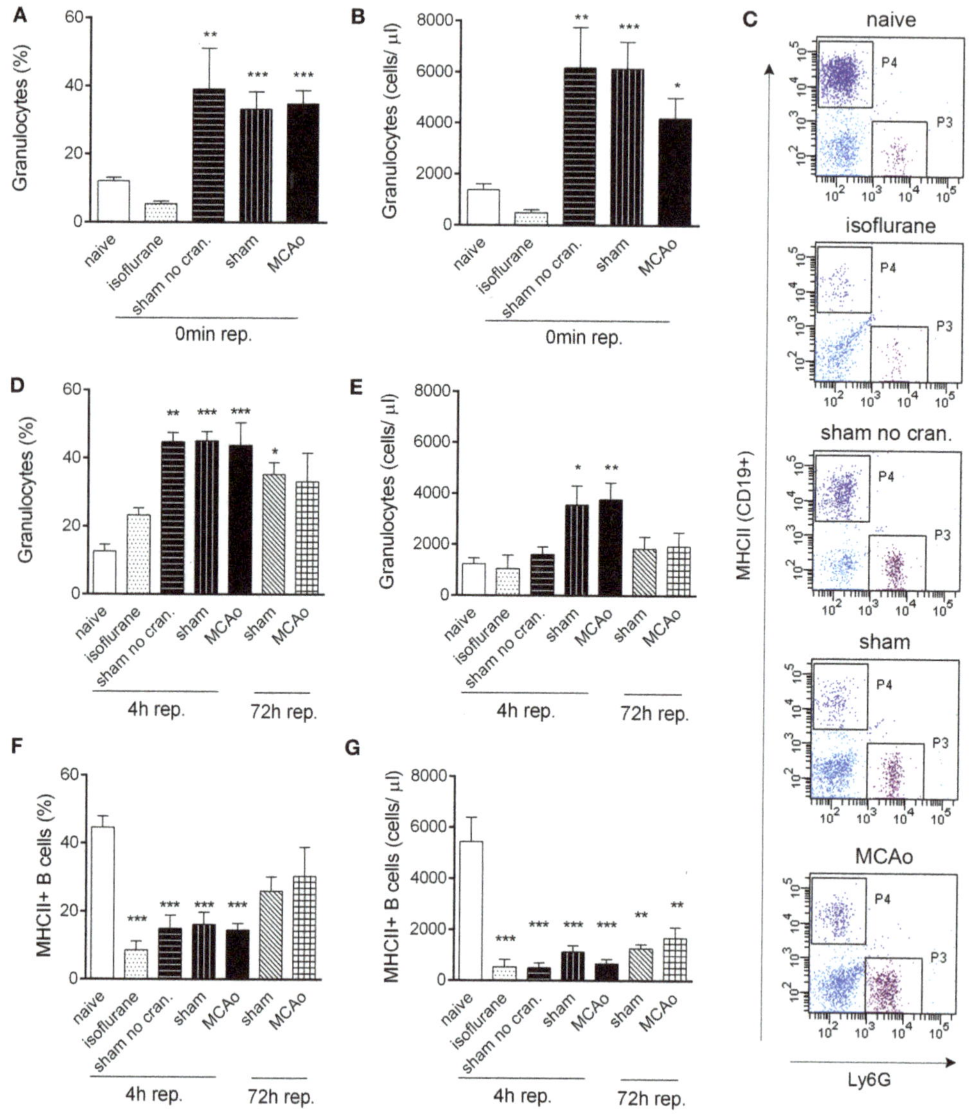

FIGURE 1 | Tissue injury, craniotomy, and anaesthesia result in rapid alteration of leukocyte responses. Extracranial tissue injury results in increased proportion **(A)** and cell numbers **(B)** of granulocytes in the circulation, which is indistinguishable from changes induced by sham surgery or MCAo. Blood samples taken from the tail vein prior to surgery and 60 min after the onset of MCAo/control surgery (0 min reperfusion) are shown. **(C)** Representative dot plots showing terminal cardiac blood samples at 4 h reperfusion for graphs **(D–G)**. P3 gate: Ly6G+ granulocytes, P4 gate: MHCII+ B cells (dark blue color indicates CD19+ positive cells). Proportion **(D)** and total cell numbers **(E)** of granulocytes in cardiac blood samples at 4 and 72 h reperfusion. Proportion **(F)** and total cell numbers **(G)** of MHCII+ B cells (CD19+) in cardiac blood samples at 4 and 72 h reperfusion. Sham no cran.—sham surgery without craniotomy. $n = 5, 4, 4, 5, 6–7, 3, 3$ in naïve, isoflurane, sham no cran., sham, MCAo, sham 72 h, and MCAo 72 h, respectively. $^{*}P < 0.05$, $^{**}P < 0.01$, $^{***}P < 0.001$ vs. naive. Light blue color indicates negative (unstained) population.

this experimental model. Normality of data sets was assessed using GraphPad Prism (KS normality test). Statistical analysis was performed by One-Way or Two-Way ANOVA followed by Tukey's or Bonferroni's *post-hoc* multiple-comparison, using GraphPad Prism 5 software. In case of non-parametric data, significance was confirmed by non-parametric *t*-test (Mann–Whitney *U*-test) or Kruskal–Wallis test followed by Dunn's multiple comparisons test. All data are expressed as mean ± standard error of the mean (s.e.m). $P < 0.05$ was considered statistically significant.

RESULTS

SURGICAL MANIPULATION AND ANAESTHESIA ALTER LEUKOCYTE RESPONSES IN THE BLOOD

Surgical manipulation of extracranial tissues was sufficient to induce rapid mobilization of granulocytes. In serial blood samples taken from the tail vein, the proportion of granulocytes (Ly6G+ CD11b+ SSC^{high} cells) increased from 12 to 40% within 70–80 min ("0 min reperfusion") in response surgery without craniotomy ("sham no cran.," **Figure 1A**), but not after isoflurane anaesthesia alone, representing a ~3-fold increase in total granulocyte numbers (**Figure 1B**). Granulocyte mobilization was not altered further by craniotomy or MCAo (**Figures 1A,B**). Granulocytosis was also evident 5–5.5 h after initiation of surgery in cardiac, terminal blood samples (termed as "4 h reperfusion," **Figures 1C,D**), although total granulocyte numbers were lower compared to the earlier time point and were significantly elevated only in response to craniotomy or MCAo (**Figure 1E**). An increased proportion of granulocytes in the sham and MCAo groups was observed up to 72 h after surgery (**Figure 1D**).

CD19+ MHCII+ B cells decreased profoundly (by 80–90%) in the blood in response to anaesthesia alone, which was apparent in all other groups of mice that underwent surgical manipulation or MCAo, at 4 h reperfusion (**Figures 1F,G**). Similarly, anaesthesia alone resulted in reduced circulating CD4+ and CD8+ T cell numbers within 4 h (**Figures 2A–C**). Interestingly, craniotomy and MCAo appeared to raise T cell numbers over levels after anaesthesia alone, which was more apparent in the case of CD4+ T cells (**Figures 2B,C**). Circulating B cells and CD8+ T cells remained significantly lower in number in surgery control groups and after MCAo compared to naïve mice at 72 h reperfusion (**Figures 1F,G, 2A,C**).

GRANULOCYTE RELEASE FROM THE BONE MARROW INCREASES PROPORTIONALLY TO THE LEVEL OF SURGICAL STRESS AND BRAIN INJURY

MCAo resulted in mobilization of granulocytes from the bone marrow at 4 h reperfusion (**Figure 3A**). Within the granulocyte population, CXCR2+ granulocytes (Ly6G+ CD11b+ SSC^{high} cells) showed a decrease in the bone marrow proportional to the level of surgical stress, reaching a significant 50% reduction after craniotomy and an over 60% reduction in response to MCAo (**Figure 3B**). Correspondingly, KC (CXCL-1) and IL-6 concentrations in the circulation increased by 20–40-fold after sham surgery and MCAo (**Figures 3C,D**). Circulating KC levels showed a significant ($P < 0.01$) negative correlation with numbers of CXCR2+ granulocytes in the bone marrow at 4 h reperfusion (not shown). Anaesthesia alone appeared to increase B cells and T cells in the bone marrow (**Figures 3E–G**) similarly to our earlier findings (Denes et al., 2011).

BONE MARROW CELLS DO NOT EXHIBIT A SUPPRESSED RESPONSE AFTER CEREBRAL ISCHEMIA

At 72 h reperfusion when systemic immunosuppression is apparent after cerebral ischemia (Prass et al., 2003), bone marrow cells showed no difference in LPS-induced IL-6 production *in vitro* as assessed in cell lysates (**Figure 4A**) and cell culture supernatants (**Figure 4B**), indicating that at this time point cells residing in the bone marrow maintain their ability to respond to endotoxin.

SURGICAL INTERVENTION AND CEREBRAL ISCHEMIA ALTER SPLENIC GRANULOCYTE RESPONSES

Surgical manipulation of extracranial tissues with or without craniotomy resulted in an early recruitment of granulocytes in

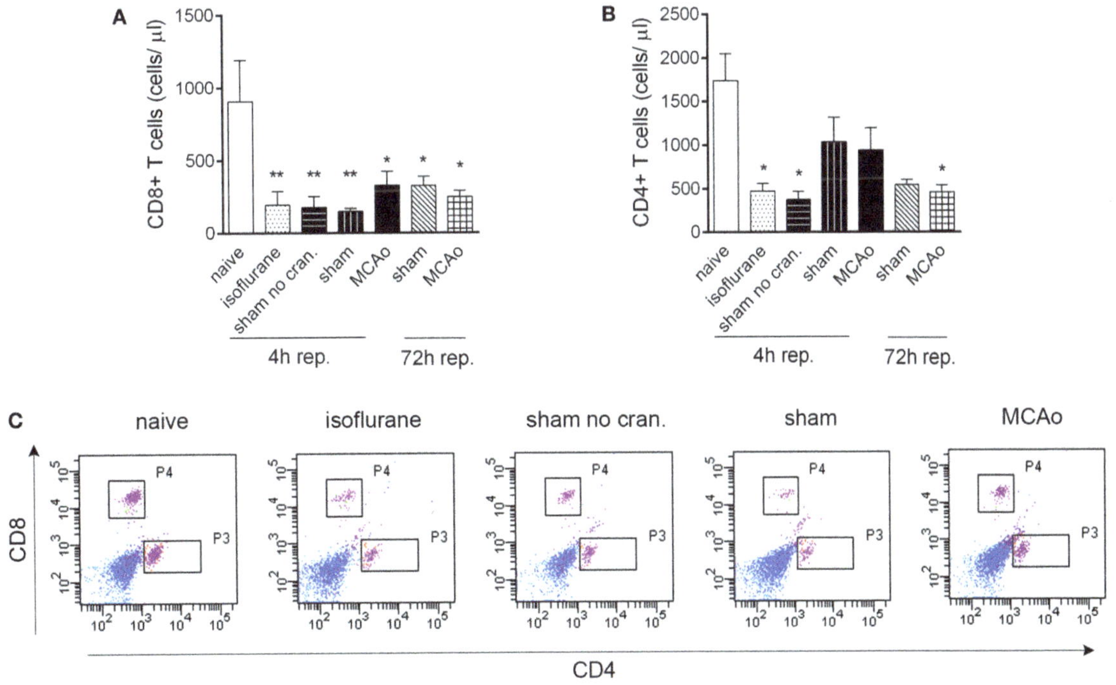

FIGURE 2 | Isoflurane anaesthesia results in reduced circulating T cell numbers. CD8+ T cells **(A)** and CD4+ T cells **(B)** are reduced in number in cardiac blood samples within 4 h following isoflurane anaesthesia. **(C)** Representative dot blots showing CD8+ and CD4+ T cells in cardiac blood samples 4 h after reperfusion, control surgeries, or anaesthesia. Purple color indicates cells gated on CD3. Sham no cran.—sham surgery without craniotomy. $n = 4, 4, 4, 5, 6, 3, 3$ in naïve, isoflurane, sham no cran., sham, MCAo, sham 72 h, and MCAo 72 h, respectively. $^{*}P < 0.05$, $^{**}P < 0.01$ vs. naive. Light blue color indicates negative (unstained) population.

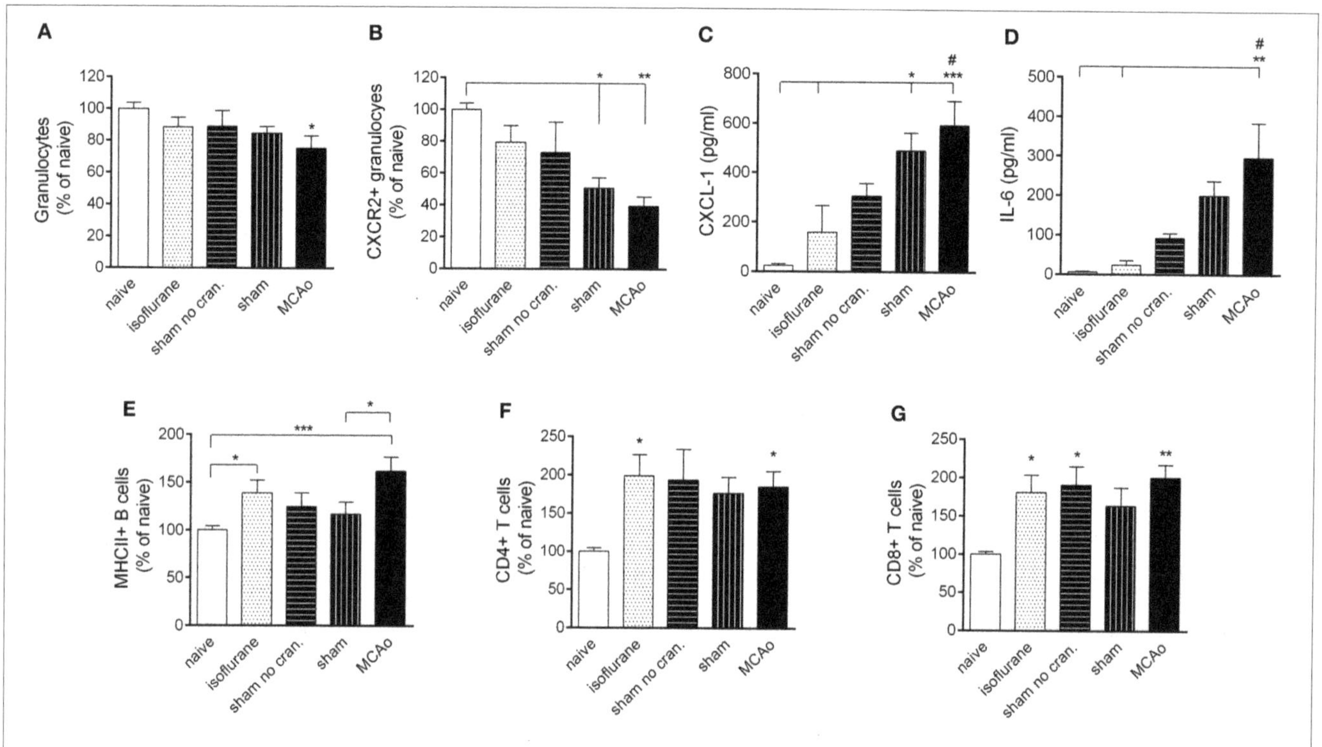

FIGURE 3 | Surgical intervention and anaesthesia result in altered leukocyte responses in the bone marrow. **(A)** Bone marrow granulocytes (Ly6G+, CD11b+, SSC^{high} cells) are reduced within 4 h after MCAo. **(B)** Both MCAo and craniotomy result in reduced CXCR2+ granulocytes in the bone marrow at 4 h reperfusion. KC (CXCL1, **C**) and IL-6 **(D)** levels increase in the circulation within 4 h proportionally to the amount of surgical stress. Anaesthesia results in increased MHCII+ B cells **(E)** CD4+ T cells **(F)** and CD8+ T cells **(G)** in the bone marrow within 4 h. Sham no cran.—sham surgery without craniotomy. $n = 7, 5, 6, 7, 7–8$ in naïve, isoflurane, sham no cran., sham, and MCAo, respectively. $*P < 0.05$, $**P < 0.01$, $***P < 0.001$ vs. naïve, unless indicated otherwise on the graphs; $^{\#}P < 0.05$ vs. isoflurane.

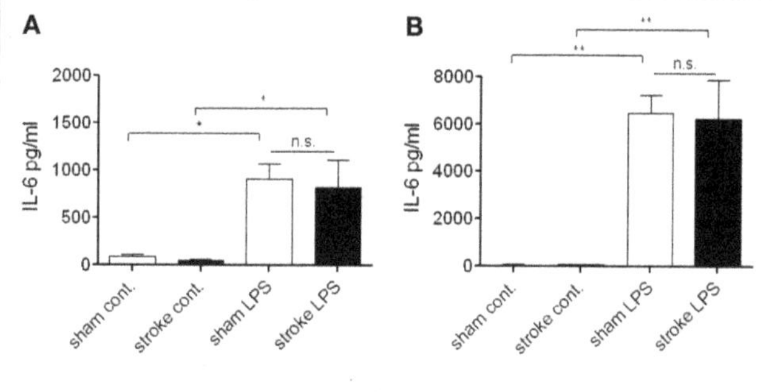

FIGURE 4 | Bone marrow cells do not exhibit a suppressed response to endotoxin after distal tMCAo. Bone marrow cells were isolated 72 h after MCAo and stimulated *in vitro* with bacterial lipopolysaccharide (LPS) to investigate cytokine production. Cell lysates **(A)** and supernatants **(B)** were measured for IL-6 production and release. n.s., not significant. $n = 3$. $*P < 0.05$, $**P < 0.01$ vs. control.

the spleen (**Figure 5A**). This effect was not apparent in the CXCR2+ granulocyte population (**Figure 5B**). MCAo significantly reduced splenic total granulocyte- and CXCR2+ granulocyte numbers (**Figures 5A,B**) compared to sham surgery at 4 h reperfusion. No changes were observed in B cell or T cell populations in the spleen in any of the surgical groups (**Figures 5C–E**).

CXCR2 BLOCKADE PREVENTS GRANULOCYTE MOBILIZATION FROM THE BONE MARROW BUT DOES NOT ALTER ISCHEMIC BRAIN INJURY

The selective CXCR2 inhibitor SB225002 (White et al., 1998) prevented granulocyte release from the bone marrow as confirmed by a significant reduction of granulocytes in the bone marrow in vehicle-treated mice 4 h after MCAo compared to mice treated with SB225002 (**Figures 6A,B**). Similarly to our earlier experiments using the intraluminal filament method to induce cerebral ischemia (Denes et al., 2011) bone marrow granulocyte numbers were stabilized by 24 h post MCAo (**Figure 6A**). To our surprise, CXCR2 blockade although reducing granulocyte release from the bone marrow, resulted in an increase in circulating granulocytes at 4 h reperfusion compared to vehicle (**Figure 6C**). We investigated whether CXCR2 blockade resulted in any changes in infarct size, but no difference between SB225002 treatment and vehicle was observed (**Figure 6D**), indicating that CXCR2-mediated signals do not contribute substantially to brain injury in the current experimental model of cerebral ischemia.

DISCUSSION

Here we present evidence that even mild surgical manipulation results in marked systemic granulocyte mobilization responses. Granulocyte mobilization is proportional to the level of surgical stress and is further augmented by brain injury. Granulocyte responses to cranial injury or cerebral ischemia involve primarily

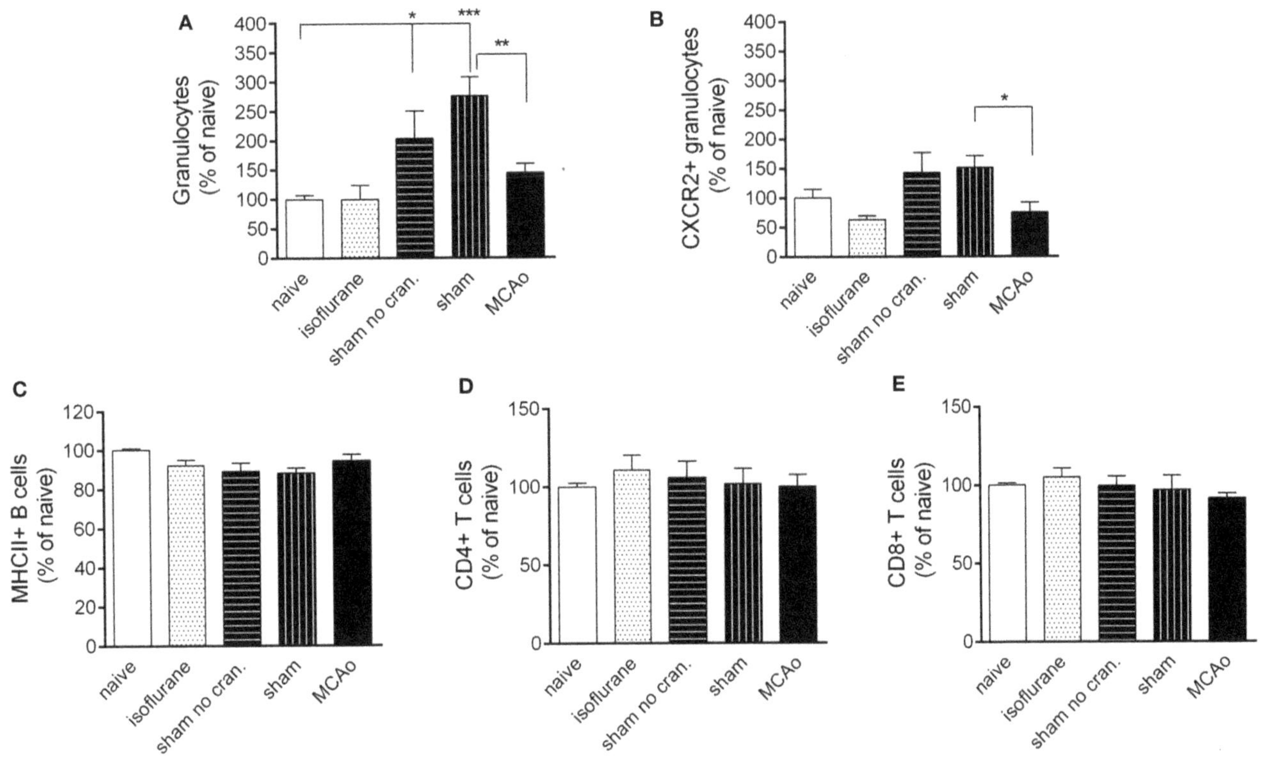

FIGURE 5 | Leukocyte responses in the spleen. Changes in total granulocytes (Ly6G+, CD11b+, SSC^{high} cells, **A**) and CXCR2+ granulocytes **(B)** in the spleen 4 h following reperfusion or control surgical interventions. No changes are observed in splenic MHCII+ B cells **(C)** CD4+ T cells **(D)** and CD8+ T cells **(E)** at 4 h reperfusion. Sham no cran.—sham surgery without craniotomy. $n = 6, 6, 6, 5, 6$ in naïve, isoflurane, sham no cran., sham, and MCAo, respectively. $^{*}P < 0.05$ and $^{***}P < 0.001$ vs. naïve; $^{**}P < 0.01$ **(A)** and $^{*}P < 0.05$ **(B)** sham vs. MCAo.

the mobilization of CXCR2-positive granulocytes, which is not seen after manipulation of extracranial tissues. In addition, we show that anaesthesia profoundly alters leukocyte responses, an effect that lasts for several hours or even days. Collectively, these data highlight the role of anaesthesia and surgical intervention in systemic inflammatory responses, which could have an impact on experimental models of cerebral ischemia, but could also serve important information for the management of patients subjected to various surgeries in the clinic.

In our previous study we revealed changes in the bone marrow in response to transient, focal cerebral ischemia induced by an intraluminal filament that is advanced through the internal carotid artery to occlude the MCA (Denes et al., 2011). Although we demonstrated changes induced by brain injury itself, we also showed that anaesthesia and surgical intervention could impact on bone marrow leukocyte responses (Denes et al., 2011). Since the filament MCAo model involves surgical manipulation around the neck including exposure of the salivary glands, the vagus nerve and other tissues around the trachea, in the present study we performed a systematic analysis of bone marrow, spleen, and blood responses, using a distal MCAo model, to reveal stroke-specific changes in leukocyte mobilization as well as the impact of surgical intervention and anaesthesia. Since the present model includes craniotomy, a potential confounder that disturbs the internal milieu of the brain, we also included control surgeries during which only extracranial tissues were manipulated. Extracranial manipulation consisting of an incision on the skin and temporary dislocation of small pericranial muscles was sufficient to generate a systemic inflammatory response evidenced by granulocyte mobilization and a 10-fold increase in circulating KC levels. Since these changes did not involve major alterations in CXCR2+ granulocytes, identification of the mechanisms involved (contribution of bone marrow-derived cells, signals that initiate and maintain systemic granulocyte responses, etc.) warrant further investigation. It is likely that activation of the HPA axis and the autonomic nervous system (Elenkov et al., 2000) could contribute to surgery-induced peripheral changes, however the exact signals mediating leukocyte responses need to be identified. In fact, we confirmed here our earlier findings showing an increased mobilization of CXCR2-positive granulocytes in response to brain injury, compared with other surgical manipulations (Denes et al., 2011).

We found that isoflurane anaesthesia alone resulted in a profound reduction in circulating lymphocytes within hours. Some effects of isoflurane on leukocyte activation have been reported earlier (Yuki et al., 2012; Carbo et al., 2013), and a decrease in Th1/Th2 ratio in the blood has been observed in patients undergoing craniotomy in response to isoflurane (Inada et al., 2004). However, the present study demonstrates a rapid and sustained reduction in circulating T cell numbers induced by isoflurane

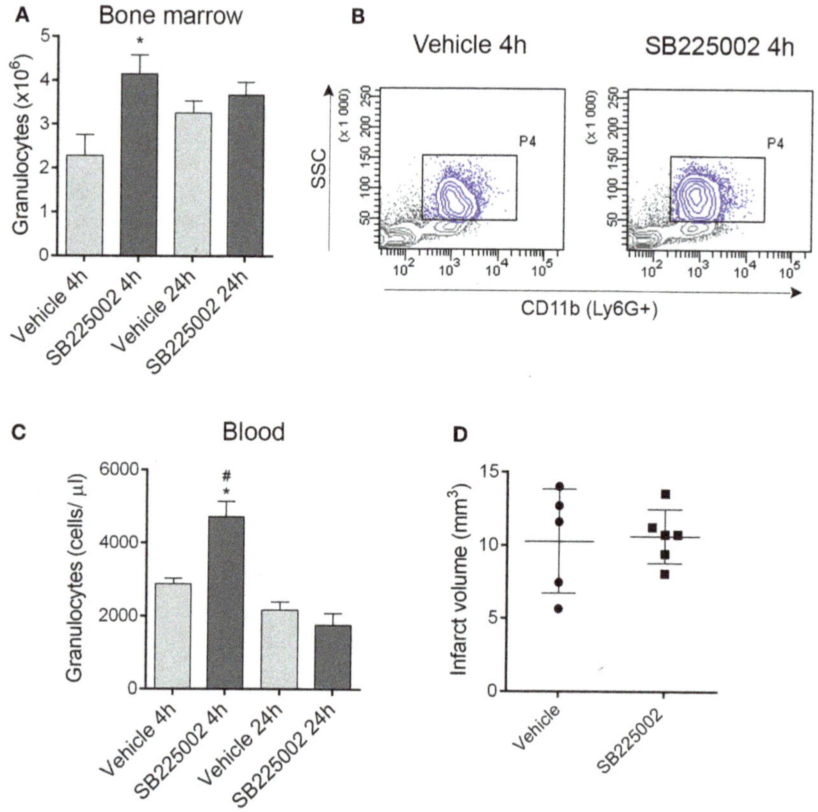

FIGURE 6 | Blockade of CXCR2-mediated granulocyte release from the bone marrow does not alter infarct size after experimental stroke. (A) Treatment with the selective CXCR2 antagonist SB225002 prevents granulocyte release from the bone marrow after MCAo compared to vehicle at 4 h reperfusion. Total granulocyte numbers recovered from 1 femur and 1 tibia are shown. **(B)** Representative density plots showing CD11b+ SSC^{high} granulocytes (gated also on Ly6G+, blue) in the bone marrow at 4 h reperfusion. **(C)** SB225002 increases granulocyte numbers in the cardiac blood at 4 h reperfusion after MCAo. **(D)** Infarct size is not altered in response to SB225002 treatment at 24 h reperfusion, after MCAo. **(A–C)** $n = 3, 3, 5, 5$ in vehicle 4 h, SB225002 4 h, vehicle 24 h, and SB225002 24 h samples, respectively, **(D)** $n = 5$–6. $^{*}P < 0.05$ vs. vehicle 4 h, $^{\#}P < 0.05$ vs. 24 h time points.

anaesthesia, which could have important implications clinically and also in models of experimental stroke. The contribution of T cells to the ischemic brain injury is well documented (Iadecola and Anrather, 2011). Since volatile anaesthetics can exert neuroprotective properties (Kawaguchi et al., 2005), it is possible that at least in part, these actions could be mediated via blunted T cell responses.

The spleen is profoundly affected by brain injury (Offner et al., 2006b), leading to loss of B cells and development of immunosuppression, however, much less is known about how cerebral ischemia contributes to responses of myeloid cells in the spleen. In fact, a population of splenic monocytes are released rapidly upon activation and contributes to ischemic processes in the heart (Swirski et al., 2009; Leuschner et al., 2012). We found that surgical manipulation results in increased granulocyte recruitment to the spleen whilst cerebral ischemia reduced surgery-induced increases in splenic granulocytes. Although the role and mechanisms of surgery-induced splenic granulocytosis requires further investigations, this scenario indicates that the effect of surgical manipulation on leukocyte responses in peripheral organs is likely to be a confounder in current experimental stroke models.

CXCR2 is the best characterized cell surface receptor on granulocytes involved in cell mobilization to stimuli mediated by CXCL1 (KC) and CXCL2/3 (MIP-2) (Matzer et al., 2004; Eash et al., 2010; Veenstra and Ransohoff, 2012). Although brain injury-induced granulocyte mobilization from the bone marrow was prevented by CXCR2 blockade, circulating granulocytes increased in response to SB225002 treatment. CXCR2 inhibition was found effective to reduce IL-8- or KC-induced granulocyte mobilization in the blood and block granulocyte egress from the bone marrow (White et al., 1998; Martin et al., 2003; Eash et al., 2010). We show here that very early granulocyte mobilization responses in response to brain injury are not dependent on CXCR2, and might not (or only in part) require the contribution of the bone marrow in the current experimental model. This could explain the lack of an effect by CXCR2 blockade on the size of ischemic brain injury, which has also been confirmed by another study (Brait et al., 2011). Brain injury in different experimental models might not be influenced by peripheral leukocyte actions to the same extent. For example, blockade of granulocyte responses or hematopoietic MyD88-dependent actions is not associated with reduced central inflammation or brain damage after cold-induced cortical injury (Koedel et al., 2007). In contrast, neutrophils contribute to brain injury when experimental stroke is preceded by systemic inflammation (McColl et al., 2007). Therefore, the source of neutrophils mobilized after brain injury and their contribution to the population that is recruited into the brain need to be investigated in further studies. Stroke in patients results in increased circulating granulocyte numbers and loss of T cells (Vogelgesang et al., 2008), which corresponds to the findings presented in our study. Surgical interventions and anaesthesia also influence leukocyte responses in patients (Inada et al., 2004). However, similarly to most experimental stroke models, the MCAo model is inherently confounded by effects of anaesthesia and surgical intervention, and we show that surgical interventions alone are capable of inducing profound changes in leukocyte responses. These changes might contribute to and/or alter brain injury in experimental models. Since circulating white blood cell- and blood cytokine data from stroke patients and from those undergoing anaesthesia or surgical interventions are widely available, blood cell responses and mechanisms of brain injury in experimental models should be investigated in a translational context.

In conclusion, our data indicate that anaesthesia- and surgery-induced leukocyte responses interact with those induced by experimental stroke, which needs to be accounted for in experimental models. Revealing the mechanisms of rapid, surgery- or brain injury-induced granulocyte responses could be fundamental for the development of new therapeutic regimen in a wide variety of diseases.

ACKNOWLEDGMENTS

We are grateful for funding provided by the Medical Research Council and European Union's Seventh Framework Program (FP7/2008–2013) under Grant agreements Nos. 201024 and 202213 (European Stroke Network) and TÁMOP-4.2.4.A/2-11/1-2012-0001 (Adam Denes).

REFERENCES

Brait, V. H., Rivera, J., Broughton, B. R., Lee, S., Drummond, G. R., and Sobey, C. G. (2011). Chemokine-related gene expression in the brain following ischemic stroke: no role for CXCR2 in outcome. *Brain Res.* 1372, 169–179. doi: 10.1016/j.brainres.2010.11.087

Carbo, C., Yuki, K., Demers, M., Wagner, D. D., and Shimaoka, M. (2013). Isoflurane inhibits neutrophil recruitment in the cutaneous Arthus reaction model. *J. Anesth.* 27, 261–268. doi: 10.1007/s00540-012-1508-1

Chapman, K. Z., Dale, V. Q., Denes, A., Bennett, G., Rothwell, N. J., Allan, S. M., et al. (2009). A rapid and transient peripheral inflammatory response precedes brain inflammation after experimental stroke. *J. Cereb. Blood Flow Metab.* 29, 1764–1768. doi: 10.1038/jcbfm.2009.113

Denes, A., Humphreys, N., Lane, T. E., Grencis, R., and Rothwell, N. (2010a). Chronic systemic infection exacerbates ischemic brain damage via a CCL5 (regulated on activation, normal T-cell expressed and secreted)-mediated proinflammatory response in mice. *J. Neurosci.* 30, 10086–10095. doi: 10.1523/JNEUROSCI.1227-10.2010

Denes, A., Thornton, P., Rothwell, N. J., and Allan, S. M. (2010b). Inflammation and brain injury: acute cerebral ischaemia, peripheral and central inflammation. *Brain Behav. Immun.* 24, 708–723. doi: 10.1016/j.bbi.2009.09.010

Denes, A., McColl, B. W., Leow-Dyke, S. F., Chapman, K. Z., Humphreys, N. E., Grencis, R. K., et al. (2011). Experimental stroke-induced changes in the bone marrow reveal complex regulation of leukocyte responses. *J. Cereb. Blood Flow Metab.* 31, 1036–1050. doi: 10.1038/jcbfm.2010.198

Dirnagl, U., Klehmet, J., Braun, J. S., Harms, H., Meisel, C., Ziemssen, T., et al. (2007). Stroke-induced immunodepression: experimental evidence and clinical relevance. *Stroke* 38, 770–773. doi: 10.1161/01.STR.0000251441.89665.bc

Eash, K. J., Greenbaum, A. M., Gopalan, P. K., and Link, D. C. (2010). CXCR2 and CXCR4 antagonistically regulate neutrophil trafficking from murine bone marrow. *J. Clin. Invest.* 120, 2423–2431. doi: 10.1172/JCI41649

Elenkov, I. J., Wilder, R. L., Chrousos, G. P., and Vizi, E. S. (2000). The sympathetic nerve–an integrative interface between two supersystems: the brain and the immune system. *Pharmacol. Rev.* 52, 595–638.

Fisher, M., Feuerstein, G., Howells, D. W., Hurn, P. D., Kent, T. A., Savitz, S. I., et al. (2009). Update of the stroke therapy academic industry roundtable preclinical recommendations. *Stroke* 40, 2244–2250. doi: 10.1161/STROKEAHA.108.541128

Iadecola, C., and Anrather, J. (2011). The immunology of stroke: from mechanisms to translation. *Nat. Med.* 17, 796–808. doi: 10.1038/nm.2399

Inada, T., Yamanouchi, Y., Jomura, S., Sakamoto, S., Takahashi, M., Kambara, T., et al. (2004). Effect of propofol and isoflurane anaesthesia on the immune response to surgery. *Anaesthesia* 59, 954–959. doi: 10.1111/j.1365-2044.2004.03837.x

Kawaguchi, M., Furuya, H., and Patel, P. M. (2005). Neuroprotective effects of anesthetic agents. *J. Anesth.* 19, 150–156. doi: 10.1007/s00540-005-0305-5

Kilkenny, C., Browne, W. J., Cuthill, I. C., Emerson, M., and Altman, D. G. (2010). Improving bioscience research reporting: the ARRIVE guidelines for reporting animal research. *PLoS Biol.* 8:e1000412. doi: 10.1371/journal.pbio.1000412

Koedel, U., Merbt, U. M., Schmidt, C., Angele, B., Popp, B., Wagner, H., et al. (2007). Acute brain injury triggers MyD88-dependent, TLR2/4-independent inflammatory responses. *Am. J. Pathol.* 171, 200–213. doi: 10.2353/ajpath.2007.060821

Leuschner, F., Rauch, P. J., Ueno, T., Gorbatov, R., Marinelli, B., Lee, W. W., et al. (2012). Rapid monocyte kinetics in acute myocardial infarction are sustained by extramedullary monocytopoiesis. *J. Exp. Med.* 209, 123–137. doi: 10.1084/jem.20111009

Martin, C., Burdon, P. C., Bridger, G., Gutierrez-Ramos, J. C., Williams, T. J., and Rankin, S. M. (2003). Chemokines acting via CXCR2 and CXCR4 control the release of neutrophils from the bone marrow and their return following senescence. *Immunity* 19, 583–593. doi: 10.1016/S1074-7613(03)00263-2

Matzer, S. P., Rodel, F., Strieter, R. M., Rollinghoff, M., and Beuscher, H. U. (2004). Constitutive expression of CXCL2/MIP-2 is restricted to a Gr-1high, CD11b+, CD62Lhigh subset of bone marrow derived granulocytes. *Int. Immunol.* 16, 1675–1683. doi: 10.1093/intimm/dxh169

McColl, B. W., Rothwell, N. J., and Allan, S. M. (2007). Systemic inflammatory stimulus potentiates the acute phase and CXC chemokine responses to experimental stroke and exacerbates brain damage via interleukin-1- and neutrophil-dependent mechanisms. *J. Neurosci.* 27, 4403–4412. doi: 10.1523/JNEUROSCI.5376-06.2007

Murray, K. N., Buggey, H. F., Denes, A., and Allan, S. M. (2013). Systemic immune activation shapes stroke outcome. *Mol. Cell. Neurosci.* 53, 14–25. doi: 10.1016/j.mcn.2012.09.004

Offner, H., Subramanian, S., Parker, S. M., Afentoulis, M. E., Vandenbark, A. A., and Hurn, P. D. (2006a). Experimental stroke induces massive, rapid activation of the peripheral immune system. *J. Cereb. Blood Flow Metab.* 26, 654–665. doi: 10.1038/sj.jcbfm.9600217

Offner, H., Subramanian, S., Parker, S. M., Wang, C., Afentoulis, M. E., Lewis, A., et al. (2006b). Splenic atrophy in experimental stroke is accompanied by increased regulatory T cells and circulating macrophages. *J. Immunol.* 176, 6523–6531.

Pradillo, J. M., Denes, A., Greenhalgh, A. D., Boutin, H., Drake, C., McColl, B. W., et al. (2012). Delayed administration of interleukin-1 receptor antagonist reduces ischemic brain damage and inflammation in comorbid rats. *J. Cereb. Blood Flow Metab.* 32, 1810–1819. doi: 10.1038/jcbfm.2012.101

Pradillo, J. M., Fernandez-Lopez, D., Garcia-Yebenes, I., Sobrado, M., Hurtado, O., Moro, M. A., et al. (2009). Toll-like receptor 4 is involved in neuroprotection afforded by ischemic preconditioning. *J. Neurochem.* 109, 287–294. doi: 10.1111/j.1471-4159.2009.05972.x

Prass, K., Meisel, C., Hoflich, C., Braun, J., Halle, E., Wolf, T., et al. (2003). Stroke-induced immunodeficiency promotes spontaneous bacterial infections and is mediated by sympathetic activation reversal by poststroke T helper cell type 1-like immunostimulation. *J. Exp. Med.* 198, 725–736. doi: 10.1084/jem.20021098

Smith, C. J., Lawrence, C. B., Rodriguez-Grande, B., Kovacs, K. J., Pradillo, J. M., and Denes, A. (2013). The immune system in stroke: clinical challenges and their translation to experimental research. *J. Neuroimmune Pharmacol.* 8, 867–887. doi: 10.1007/s11481-013-9469-1

Swirski, F. K., Nahrendorf, M., Etzrodt, M., Wildgruber, M., Cortez-Retamozo, V., Panizzi, P., et al. (2009). Identification of splenic reservoir monocytes and their deployment to inflammatory sites. *Science* 325, 612–616. doi: 10.1126/science.1175202

Veenstra, M., and Ransohoff, R. M. (2012). Chemokine receptor CXCR2: physiology regulator and neuroinflammation controller? *J. Neuroimmunol.* 246, 1–9. doi: 10.1016/j.jneuroim.2012.02.016

Vogelgesang, A., Grunwald, U., Langner, S., Jack, R., Broker, B. M., Kessler, C., et al. (2008). Analysis of lymphocyte subsets in patients with stroke and their influence on infection after stroke. *Stroke* 39, 237–241. doi: 10.1161/STROKEAHA.107.493635

White, J. R., Lee, J. M., Young, P. R., Hertzberg, R. P., Jurewicz, A. J., Chaikin, M. A., et al. (1998). Identification of a potent, selective non-peptide CXCR2 antagonist that inhibits interleukin-8-induced neutrophil migration. *J. Biol. Chem.* 273, 10095–10098. doi: 10.1074/jbc.273.17.10095

Yuki, K., Bu, W., Xi, J., Sen, M., Shimaoka, M., and Eckenhoff, R. G. (2012). Isoflurane binds and stabilizes a closed conformation of the leukocyte function-associated antigen-1. *FASEB J.* 26, 4408–4417. doi: 10.1096/fj.12-212746

14

Inflammatory process in Alzheimer's Disease

Marco A. Meraz-Ríos[1†], Danira Toral-Rios[2], Diana Franco-Bocanegra[3], Juana Villeda-Hernández[4] and Victoria Campos-Peña[5*]

[1] Departamento de Biomedicina Molecular, Centro de Investigación y de Estudios Avanzados, Mexico City, Mexico
[2] Departamento de Fisiología Biofísica y Neurociencias, Centro de Investigación y de Estudios Avanzados, Mexico City, Mexico
[3] Posgrado en Ciencias Biológicas, Universidad Nacional Autónoma de México, Mexico City, Mexico
[4] Departamento de Neuropatología Experimental, Instituto Nacional de Neurología y Neurocirugía, Mexico City, Mexico
[5] Laboratorio Experimental de Enfermedades Neurodegenerativas, Instituto Nacional de Neurología y Neurocirugía Manuel Velasco Suárez, Mexico City, Mexico

Edited by:
Beatriz Gomez-Gonzalez, Universidad Autonoma Metropolitana, Unidad Iztapalapa, Mexico

Reviewed by:
Benjamín Florán, Centro de Investigación y de Estudios Avanzados del IPN, Mexico
Clorinda Arias, Universidad Nacional Autónoma de México, Mexico
Abbas Mirshafiey, Tehran University of Medical Sciences, Iran

****Correspondence:***
Victoria Campos-Peña, Laboratorio Experimental de Enfermedades Neurodegenerativas, Instituto Nacional de Neurología y Neurocirugía Manuel Velasco Suárez, Insurgentes Sur 3877, ZIP 14269, Mexico City, Mexico
e-mail: neurovcp@ymail.com

†Present address:
Marco A. Meraz-Ríos, Departamento de Biomedicina Molecular, Centro de Investigación y de Estudios Avanzados, Av. Instituto Politécnico Nacional 2508, ZIP 07360, Mexico City, Mexico

Alzheimer Disease (AD) is a neurodegenerative disorder and the most common form of dementia. Histopathologically is characterized by the presence of two major hallmarks, the intracellular neurofibrillary tangles (NFTs) and extracellular neuritic plaques (NPs) surrounded by activated astrocytes and microglia. NFTs consist of paired helical filaments of truncated tau protein that is abnormally hyperphosphorylated. The main component in the NP is the amyloid-β peptide (Aβ), a small fragment of 40–42 amino acids with a molecular weight of 4 kD. It has been proposed that the amyloid aggregates and microglia activation are able to favor the neurodegenerative process observed in AD patients. However, the role of inflammation in AD is controversial, because in early stages the inflammation could have a beneficial role in the pathology, since it has been thought that the microglia and astrocytes activated could be involved in Aβ clearance. Nevertheless the chronic activation of the microglia has been related with an increase of Aβ and possibly with tau phosphorylation. Studies in AD brains have shown an upregulation of complement molecules, pro-inflammatory cytokines, acute phase reactants and other inflammatory mediators that could contribute with the neurodegenerative process. Clinical trials and animal models with non-steroidal anti-inflammatory drugs (NSAIDs) indicate that these drugs may decrease the risk of developing AD and apparently reduce Aβ deposition. Finally, further studies are needed to determine whether treatment with anti-inflammatory strategies, may decrease the neurodegenerative process that affects these patients.

Keywords: Alzheimer disease, amyloid-β, neurodegeneration, microglia, astrocyte, neuroinflammation, pro-inflammatory cytokine, anti-inflammatory strategies

INTRODUCTION

Alzheimer's disease (AD) is the most common cause of dementia in elderly adults. AD is clinically characterized by progressive loss of memory and other cognitive functions. Histopathologically is recognized by the presence of neuritic plaques (NPs) and neurofibrillary tangles (NFTs). The origin causes of AD can be classified as familial or sporadic. The incidence of familial cases is low (5–10%) and is related to the presence of mutations in three different genes: presenilin-1 (PS1), presenilin-2 (PS2), and amyloid-β precursor protein (APP-β) (Chartier-Harlin et al., 1991; Goate et al., 1991; Murrell et al., 1991; Levy-Lahad et al., 1995; Duff et al., 1996; Sisodia et al., 1999). Sporadic AD represents 90–95% of total cases, and although its etiology is multi-factorial, age is the main risk factor. Although there are different genetic and environmental causes, all patients have a similar clinical behavior and develop identical brain lesions: NFTs consisting of Tau (τ) protein and NPs consisting of amyloid-β (Aβ) peptides. These alterations are the final result of post-translational modifications and involve different genes and render AD as a complex multigenic neurodegenerative disorder.

In addition to this multi-genic complexity in AD, now we know that Aβ promotes an inflammatory response mediated by microglia and astrocytes, thus activating signaling pathways that could lead to neurodegeneration. It is currently unknown whether brain inflammation in AD patients is the cause of the disease or a secondary phenomenon. Although it was previously thought that the central nervous system (CNS) was an immune-privileged site, now is well known that certain features of inflammatory processes occur normally in response to an injury, infection or disease. The resident CNS cells generate inflammatory mediators, such as pro-inflammatory cytokines, prostaglandins (PGs), free radicals, complement factors, and simultaneously induce the production of adhesion molecules and chemokines, which could recruit peripheral immune cells. This review describes the cellular and molecular mediators involved in the inflammatory process associated with AD and several possible therapeutic approaches describe recently.

NPs AND Aβ IN THE NEURO-INFLAMMATORY PROCESS

NPs, are extracellular deposits structures that contain a highly insoluble fibrillar Aβ core formed by fragments of 39–42 amino acids surrounded by microglia, reactive astrocytes, and dystrophic neurites produced from degenerating neuronal processes (Iversen et al., 1995). Aβ normally originates from APP-β (Kang et al., 1987) through the sequential action of beta secretase and the multi-protein gamma-secretase complex.

Aβ accumulation in the brain, in one of the main pathological processes of AD patients. The formation of these deposits initiates a series of cellular events which are able to elicit an immune response where resident cells such as microglia and astrocytes could participate. Aβ accumulation in parenchyma and blood vessels causes microglial migration and promotes acute and chronic inflammatory responses against the aggregates, thus inducing the production of nitric oxide (NO), reactive oxygen species (ROS), pro-inflammatory cytokines (TNFα, IL-1β and IL-6), and PGs (PGE2), which eventually could promote neuronal death (**Figure 1**) (Akiyama et al., 2000; Kitazawa et al., 2004).

CELLULAR MEDIATORS

MICROGLIA

Microglia are resident brain cells, derived from monocyte precursors cells during embryogenesis, and are able to provide the initial response against any injury that occurs in the CNS. Although these cell were observed by Nissl over 100 years ago, their definitive identification and characterization was performed by Mrak (2012). Activated microglial association around NPs suggested that microglia participate in the accumulation of the Aβ observed in AD patients (Glenner et al., 1984); this hypothesis was supported by several studies (Rozemuller et al., 1986; Dickson et al., 1988).

Normally, microglia exists in an inactive state; morphologically, these cells have a small soma with branching processes. When activated by pathogens or injury, these cells suffer visible morphological changes, including decreased branching and soma growth, the acquisition of an amoeboid form and display a wide variety of specific cellular surface markers (Town et al., 2005). NPs in AD patients' brain activate the inflammatory response mediated by microglia and cause pro-inflammatory cytokine secretion, which may directly cause neuronal injury.

Microglia *in vitro* cell cultures are able to phagocyte the amyloid peptide. However, ultrastructural analysis of tissues from AD patients demonstrated that there is no presence of amyloid fibrils in the lysosomal compartments of local microglia cells (Frackowiak et al., 1992). Whereas microglia has the ability to phagocyte Aβ *in vitro*, its phagocytosis capacity is limited. An important observed feature was the abnormal presence of macrophages infiltrating from the periphery, which showed amyloid fibers in their lysosomal compartments (Wisniewski et al., 1991; Akiyama et al., 1996). Currently, we know that there are two types of phagocytic cells within the CNS that are able to initiate the innate immune response: microglia and peripheral macrophages (Rezai-Zadeh et al., 2009; Gate et al., 2010). These macrophages are recruited into the CNS by specific cytokines and

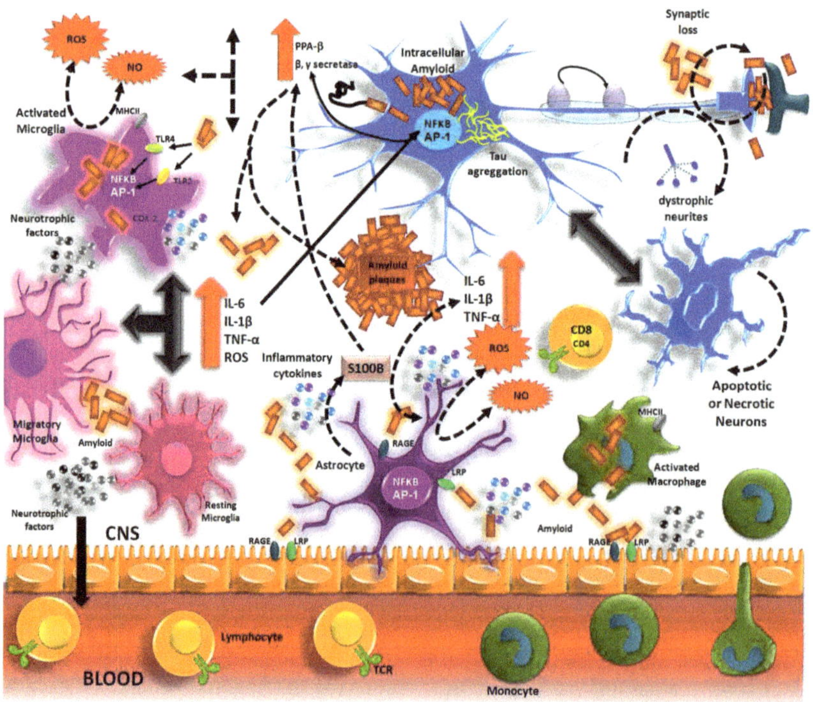

FIGURE 1 | Inflammation in Alzheimer's disease. The Aβ peptide produced by APP processing, form aggregates that activate microglia through TLRs and RAGE receptors. These receptors in turn, activate NF-κB and AP-1 transcription factors, which induce the reactive oxygen species (ROS) production and the expression of inflammatory cytokines (IL-1, IL-6, TNF). These inflammatory factors directly acting on the neurons and also stimulate the astrocytes, which amplify the pro-inflammatory signals, inducing a neurotoxic effects. The inflammatory mediators generate by resident CNS cells, induce the production of adhesion molecules and chemokines, which recruit peripheral immune cells.

chemokines, which are released during microglial and astrocytic activation and are able to cross the blood-brain barrier.

Similarly to macrophages, microglia recognizes pathogens through pattern recognition receptors (PRRs), which include specific toll-like receptors (TLRs), nucleotide-oligomerization binding domain (NOD) proteins, and C-type lectin receptors. These receptors interact with pathogen-associated molecular patterns (PAMPs) or damage-associated molecular patterns (DAMPs) to initiate the cellular defense mechanisms (Sterka and Marriott, 2006; Rubartelli and Lotze, 2007). Thus, the formation and release of ROS, pro-inflammatory cytokines (IL-1β, IL-6, TNF-α, and IFN-γ) (Lue et al., 2001), chemokines (MIP1α, MIP1β, RANTES, and MCP1), and growth factors such as macrophage colony-stimulating factor (MCSF) and complement factors (C1q, C3, C4, and C9) (Walker et al., 1995) begin. In addition to the before mentioned molecules, microglia is also able to express receptors for advanced glycosilation end products (RAGE), Fc receptors, CD40, FP receptors, and various scavenger-type receptors (El Khoury et al., 1998; Tan et al., 1999; Walker and Lue, 2005; Okun et al., 2010). Although microglia has the capacity to respond to various stimuli, the presence of Aβ is particularly important. Aβ induces a high accumulation of surface molecules of type I and II major histocompatibility complex (MHC) (McGeer et al., 1988).

Microglial cells primarily have an immunomodulatory role and express a large variety of immune response-related antigens and molecules; however, the specific role of microglia within the CNS remains controversial. Microglial activation is not a simple and unique phenomenon; instead, activation is a continuous series of events in which microglia awakens innate and adaptive phagocytic immune responses and consistently display activation through antigens on the cellular surface (Town et al., 2005). Under this principle, microglia displays a "variable" response, in which a mixture of the classical activation pathway and exacerbated increase of alternative activation can be observed in AD patients, which could leads to irreparable damage that result in persistent neurodegeneration.

ASTROCYTES

Astrocytes are the most abundant glial cells present in the CNS and have important functions in brain organization and maintenance (Sofroniew and Vinters, 2010). These cells interact with neurons and are involved in neurotransmitter secretion and recycling, ion homeostasis, energy metabolism regulation, synaptic remodeling and modulation of oxidative stress, information processing, and signal transmission (Halassa and Haydon, 2010; Henneberger et al., 2010).

In early stages of AD, activated astrocytes are located in two regions: the molecular layer of the cerebral cortex and near the amyloid deposits below the pyramidal cell layer. The mechanisms leading to the activation of these cells in response to the pathological changes produced by AD are not obvious, but it has been demonstrated that the presence of amyloid activates astrocytes. Activated astrocytes can phagocytose and degrade amyloid, which suggests that they importantly contribute to the removal of accumulated Aβ in parenchyma. Astrocytes and microglia are activated through TLRs and RAGE-dependent pathways, thus causing local inflammation that eventually could intensifies neuronal death.

Overall, the inflammatory process in AD patients is shown by changes in microglial morphology and astrogliosis, which is manifested by an increase in number, size and motility of astrocytes. Astrocyte activation is present in many neurodegenerative conditions, expressing high levels of glial fibrillary acidic protein (GFAP), vimentin, and nestin. Unfortunately, these changes cause a "disruption" of normal activities in astrocytes, which are essential for normal neuronal function. Maintenance of glutamate concentration in the extracellular space is among the normal physiological functions; altering homeostasis causes a local neuron depolarization, which leads to citotoxic damage. Thus, although astrocytic activation has a protective role in brain, intense activation exacerbates neuronal damage and accelerates disease progression.

Similarly to microglia, astrocytes quickly respond to injury; these cells are located near the fibrilar Aβ deposits, which are responsible for the astroglial activation observed in AD patients. Injection of Aβ oligomeric forms into the retrosplenial cortex of rats caused a significant astrocyte activation, as shown by transcription factor NF-κB activation and the presence of inflammatory mediators such as tumor necrosis factor (TNF-α), interleukin 1 (IL-1β), and cyclooxygenase-2 (COX-2)(Carrero et al., 2012). The activated astrocytes express on their cell surface, receptors that bind the Aβ peptides such as RAGE, receptor-like density lipoproteins, proteoglycans and various scavenger receptors (Wyss-Coray et al., 2003; Medeiros and Laferla, 2013). Thus, activated astrocytes are able to cause neurodegeneration and express inflammation-associated factors, such as S100β, consequently inducing neurite outgrowth. S100β expression correlates with the number of dystrophic neurites in AD patients (Mrak et al., 1996).

In astrocytes, NF-κB significantly controls chemokine and adhesion molecules secretion, favors peripheral lymphocyte infiltration and increases inflammatory response (Moynagh, 2005); this process becomes a self-regulating mechanism, which leads to neurodegeneration.

OLIGODENDROCYTES

Although oligodendroglia is important to maintain neuron morphology and function, little is known about how they are affected by Aβ deposits However, there are studies that indicate changes in white matter and abnormalities in myelin in AD patients (Kobayashi et al., 2002; Roth et al., 2005). Specifically, aberrations have been reported in the white matter of asymptomatic familial AD patients, particularly in patients with mutations in PS1 (Ringman et al., 2007). The presence of Aβ in oligodendrocyte cultures caused cell death. Although cell death can be prevented by the presence of anti-inflammatory agents, morphological alterations of the cells persist, suggesting that the damage cannot be completely reversed (Roth et al., 2005). Subsequently, oligodendrocyte differentiation and function is affected by the simultaneous presence of mutations in PS1 ($hPS1^{M146V}$) and Aβ accumulation, as demonstrated in a mouse model. These abnormalities can lead to the development of abnormal patterns of myelin basic protein (MBP) (Desai et al., 2011), which completely alters oligodendrocyte homeostasis. Finally, the loss of trophic support provided by these cells might lead to increased neuronal vulnerability and inflammation, thus favoring neurodegeneration.

MOLECULAR MEDIATORS OF INFLAMMATION IN AD

The Aβ deposition activates the acute immune response of microglial cells and astrocytes. At the same time, amyloid plaques are responsible for the production and the activation of inflammation-related proteins such as complement factors, acute-phase proteins, chemokines and cytokines like interleukin 1 (IL-1), interleukin 6 (IL-6), tumor necrosis factor α (TNF-α), and transforming growth factor β (TGF-β). These molecular mediators of inflammation have been linked with a series of concomitant deleterious and beneficial effects (**Figure 2**).

THE COMPLEMENT SYSTEM

The complement system is an important innate and adaptive immune response effector. This system is composed of a number of proteins and proteases that are activated in cascade (Forneris et al., 2012), and it appears to have a fundamental role in neurodegenerative diseases. Overall, the complement system uses the C1q molecule, mannose-binding protein or the interaction with the C3 multifunctional protein to recognize certain molecular patterns on pathogens. C3 activation recruits cells with phagocytic activity, and Membrane Attack Complex (MAC) is formed by binding C5–C9 (Ricklin et al., 2010). In adaptive immune response, the complement system is involved in T-cell response regulation and T-helper lymphocyte differentiation (Pekkarinen et al., 2011).

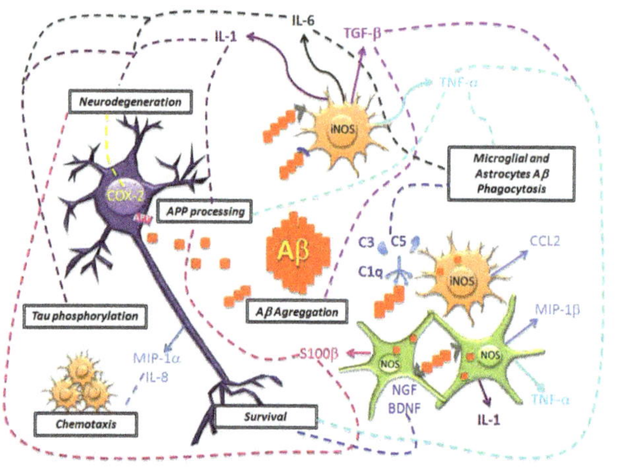

FIGURE 2 | Neuronal damage and Aβ deposition triggers microglial and astrocytes activation and the generation of inflammation molecular mediators. The acute production of molecules of the complement system (C1q, C3, and C5), pro-inflammatory cytokines (IL-1, IL-6, TNF-α), chemokines (CCL2, MIP-1α, MIP-1β, and IL-8) mediate the Aβ clearance. However, in a chronic stage these molecules could promote an increased expression and alteration of APP processing, Aβ deposition, Tau phosphorylation and neurodegeneration. Also, another effect of glial cells includes the generation of NO that promotes oxidative stress. The inflammatory microenvironment favors the production of COX-2 in neurons that leads to apoptosis. In contrast, it has been proposed that glial cells could mediate neuronal survival, by the production of TGF-β and neurotrophic factors (BDNF and NGF), but the disease progression results in failure to repair neurons.

In neurodegenerative diseases, there is a deregulation of the classical complement pathway. Studies in AD patient brains have revealed an increase in the immunoreactivity of C1q, C3b, C4d, C5b-9, and MAC surrounding senile plaques (McGeer et al., 1989; Rogers et al., 1992) and microglia surrounding the fibrillar aggregates of Aβ in the microvasculature (Fan et al., 2007). The co-existence of these molecules with the Aβ aggregates suggests a possible link between classical complement pathway activation, inflammation and pathological aggregation of Aβ. A decrease in C1q levels has been reported in cerebrospinal fluid (CSF) of AD patient and this result contrasts with an increase of C1q levels in the CNS (Smyth et al., 1994). *In vitro* studies revealed that C1q recognizes fibrillar and aggregated forms of Aβ1–42 and Aβ1–40, but not the monomeric forms. The C1q receptor is expressed in microglia, which contributed to the belief that the increase of this molecule in AD patient brains could affect the phagocytosis of Aβ. However, in primary microglia rat culture studies, exposure to Aβ1–42 and a nanomolar concentration of C1q caused a decrease in the phagocytosis of Aβ, compared to cultures exposed only to Aβ1–42 (Webster et al., 2000). A similar result was observed in a transgenic mouse model, which expressed mutated hAPP and an absence of C1q expression (APPQ$^{-/-}$). These mice showed no change in the amount of Aβ aggregates, but a decrease in glial cells activation was observed (Fonseca et al., 2004), thus establishing that C1q importantly contributes to microglial activation.

Microglia cells also produce C3. When these cells are exposed to Aβ synthetic peptides, their activation can be observed as well as an increase in C3 synthesis to 5-to 10 fold (Haga et al., 1993). When this molecule is inhibited, in the brain of an hAPP transgenic model, by the overexpression of the soluble form of the protein related to the complement receptor (sCrry), a 2- to 3-fold increase in Aβ deposits formation was observed in one-year-old hAPP/sCrry mice, which was accompanied by extensive neurodegeneration (Wyss-Coray et al., 2002). APP/C3$^{-/-}$ double transgenic generation confirmed that the molecule modulated the microglia phenotype, and promotes Aβ degradation (Maier et al., 2008).

Complement receptor 1 (CR1) is expressed in cells with phagocytic activity, C3b and C4b are CR1 ligands, and their binding facilitates phagocytosis. Genome-wide association studies (GWAS) in AD patients have shown a direct relationship between CR1 gene variants with cognitive impairment in patients and an increase in amyloid plaque formation (Chibnik et al., 2011).

The anaphylatoxin (C5) has been linked to excitotoxicity and apoptosis activation in the CNS, which is believed to play an important role in the development of neurodegenerative diseases. This molecule also promotes chemotaxis and glial cells activation. In AD animal models, the use of the C5a receptor antagonist (C5aR or CD88) reduces the amount of Aβ aggregates and hyperphosphorylated tau protein (Fonseca et al., 2009; Ager et al., 2010). It appears that the complement system activation in AD might have beneficial effects for Aβ clearance; however, this activation could eventually become deregulated and favor neurotoxic effects by promoting unwanted inflammation. For these reasons, more studies are required to understand the changes affecting the complement system in AD development.

CYTOKINES

Immune system cells are able to produce cytokines, which are soluble proteins that mediate inflammation. In the CNS, cytokines are produced by microglial cells and astrocytes and play a key role in CNS development during the embryonic stages. Cytokines are involved in the inflammatory processes of neurodegenerative diseases. In AD, these proteins may be important in the development of the pathology. Studies of AD patient tissues and CSF have shown elevated levels of pro-inflammatory cytokines such as IL-1β, IL-6, IL-10, TNF-α, and TGF-β (Blum-Degen et al., 1995; Tarkowski et al., 2002; Mrak and Griffin, 2005; Jiang et al., 2011). The increase of these cytokines is strongly related to microglia activation by exposure to Aβ aggregates (Meda et al., 1999). Animal models that overexpress the mutant hAPP protein have shown a direct relationship between the amount of Aβ aggregates and elevated levels of TNF-α, IL-6, IL-12, IL-1β, and IL-1α (Patel et al., 2005). In particular, studies have been performed seeking the relationship between each cytokine with AD.

IL-1

IL-1 is known to be able to induce APP-β mRNA expression in endothelial cells (Goldgaber et al., 1989), which suggests that IL-1 increasing in AD patients could be linked to Aβ formation. In a study with AD patients, it was also proposed that IL-1 was produced by microglial cells surrounding NPs and this cytokine could promote S100β synthesis in astrocytes (Griffin et al., 1989). Subsequently, it was discovered that IL-1 was a contributing factor to initiate dystrophic neurite formation in Aβ diffuse deposits (Griffin et al., 1995). Similarly, the exposure of primary cultures of rat cortical neurons to S100β promotes dystrophic neurite formation and APP-β mRNA expression (Li et al., 1998). Thus, IL-1 might promote the Aβ formation and neuronal degeneration through S100β present in reactive astrocytes. Additionally, the increase in IL-1 in AD patients might promote an increase in p38-MAP kinase activity, which could lead to Tau hyperphosphorilation (Sheng et al., 2000; Li et al., 2003). IL-1β signaling blockade decreases GSK-3β activity and Tau phosphorylation and promotes neurogenesis through the Wnt/β-catenin pathway (Kitazawa et al., 2011). However, it has been recently suggested that IL-1β could promote Aβ removal (Matousek et al., 2012).

IL-6

IL-6 is produced by microglial cells and is involved in the immunoreactivity present in patient tissues with clinical dementia (Hull et al., 1996). Similarly to IL-1, IL-6 promotes APP-β expression (Ringheim et al., 1998) and could also contribute to NFT formation by inducing Tau phosphorylation through cdk5/p35 pathway deregulation (Quintanilla et al., 2004). However, IL-6 overexpression has been observed in the brain of two hAPP transgenic models (TgCRND8 and Tg2576). This overexpression resulted in significant gliosis, a decrease in Aβ deposits in TgCRND8 mice brains due to phagocytic marker upregulation in glial cells and increasing microglial Aβ phagocytosis. IL-6-induced neuroinflammation, and has not any effect on APP-β processing in TgCRND8 mice, which suggests that reactive gliosis, could have a beneficial effect in early stages of disease by promoting Aβ elimination (Chakrabarty et al., 2010).

TNF-α

TNF-α is a cytokine that can have beneficial or harmful effects on different neurons. This cytokine stimulates NF-κB transcription factor which, induces the pro-inflammatory molecules expression, and promote the synthesis of neuronal survival factors such as calbindin, manganese superoxide dismutase enzyme, and anti-apoptotic Bcl-2 protein (Wajant et al., 2003; Kamata et al., 2005). This cytokine can stimulate microglia glutaminase to release glutamate, thus generating excitotoxicity (Takeuchi et al., 2006) and promoting the development of neurodegenerative diseases. In AD, the direct role of this cytokine remains uncertain; however, TNF-α could be associated with an increased β- and γ–secretase enzyme expression (Blasko et al., 2000; Liao et al., 2004). *In vitro* models have shown that TNF-α directly stimulates BACE1 expression, thus favoring APP processing (Yamamoto et al., 2007). The use of soluble TNF-α inhibitors had a protective effect on APP deregulation by decreasing amyloid aggregate formation and attenuating the cognitive impairment observed in 3xTgAD mice exposed to chronic peripheral inflammation (McAlpine et al., 2009). However, a long-term suppression of the TNF-α receptor signaling pathway can suppress the microglial ability to efficiently remove Aβ aggregates, thus favoring its aggregation at early stages (Montgomery et al., 2011).

TGF-β

TGF-β; is another cytokine with pleiotropic functions, which has an anti-apoptotic function and promotes neuronal survival. It is believed that this cytokine is involved in neurodegenerative diseases (Krieglstein et al., 2002; Konig et al., 2005). It has been reported an increase in TGF-β1 levels in the brain of AD patients (Flanders et al., 1995). Animal models (hAPP/TGF-β1) have shown that TGF-β1 overexpression promotes amyloidogenesis in the meninges and cerebral vasculature at early stages (2–3 months) (Wyss-Coray et al., 1997). By contrast, in hAPP/TGF-β1 transgenic mice parenchyma, there is a decrease in amyloid plaque formation, which correlates with microglial activation (Wyss-Coray et al., 2001). In AD patients, although TGF levels are elevated, there is a significant decrease in the expression of the TGF-β receptor type II (TβRII); this decrease may suggest that the signaling pathway mediated by this receptor has significant neuroprotective functions and could be altered during the development of the disease (Tesseur et al., 2006).

In summary, the role played by cytokines remains controversial. On one hand, cytokines might favor microglial and astrocytic activation to promote Aβ phagocytosis and neuronal survival. On the other hand, chronic cytokine production has been described as contributors of neurodegeneration.

CHEMOKINES

Chemokines are small proteins whose principal function is to attract monocytes, macrophages, lymphocytes, neutrophils, basophils, eosinophils, and dendritic cells toward sites in which an inflammatory response is required. Chemokines function through the activation of their G protein-coupled receptors and are divided into four families, CXC, CC, C, and CX_3C (Wells et al., 1998; Cyster, 1999).

Astrocytes and microglial cells, are the main producer of chemokines in the CNS, and their receptors are observed to be present in neurons. Chemokines and their receptors also participate in the CNS immune response and promote lymphocyte migration from the lymphoid organs in order to establish the inflammatory process (Ransohoff et al., 1996).

Evidence of the participation of chemokines in AD is the presence of monocyte chemotactic proteins (MCP-1 or CCL2) and chemokine receptors CCR3 and CCR5 in reactive microglia that surround senile plaques of AD patients. By contrast, the macrophage inflammatory protein 1α (MIP-1α) is located mainly in neurons, and MIP-1β is located primarily in astrocytes that surround the plaques (Ishizuka et al., 1997; Xia et al., 1998). The differential expression of chemokines and their receptors promotes glia-neuron communication to establish a local inflammatory response, which could favor Aβ phagocytosis in early stages of AD. Similarly, it is known that this inflammation contributes to Tau pathology and thereby accelerates the disease progression (Zilka et al., 2012).

Chronic inflammation in AD promotes the increased chemotaxis of phagocytic cells, thus favoring microglial recruitment around Aβ aggregates (Yamamoto et al., 2005). A recent study of CSF from AD patients revealed increased CCL2 levels, which correlated with cognitive decline (Westin et al., 2012). Moreover, because of Aβ aggregation, an increase in IL-8 production (CXCL8) is generated in neurons, which correlates with an increase in the formation of brain-derived neurotrophic factor (BDNF) (Ashutosh et al., 2011).

The presence of Aβ, in the microvasculature, promotes the release of IL-8, MCP-1, MIP-1 MIP-1α, and MIP-1β chemokines, and thereby promotes monocyte differentiation into macrophages and their migration through the blood-brain barrier (Fiala et al., 1998). CSF analysis from AD patients also showed an increase in MCP-1 and IL-8 chemokines levels (Galimberti et al., 2003; Correa et al., 2011). Similarly, *in vitro* models have demonstrated the migration ability of lymphocytes ($CD4^+$ and $CD8^+$) through the blood-brain barrier (Man et al., 2007) because of an increased MIP-1α level.

In conclusion, chemokines in the CNS are able to promote local and peripheral immune system cell migration in order to establish an immune response. In AD, it has been proposed that the chronic production of chemokines contributes to disease progression.

CYCLOOXYGENASES

Cyclooxygenases (COX) are enzymes responsible for converting arachidonic acid to H2 prostaglandin, which is a PG precursor. In general, these lipidic molecules are involved in inflammation because they cause vasodilation, thus allowing the immune system cell transport to operate at the target site (Williams, 1978). COX-1 and COX-2 isoforms are expressed in mammalian brain. COX-1 is expressed in microglia and neurons located in the pons and spinal cord that perform autonomous and sensory functions. COX-2 occurs in glutamatergic neurons of hippocampus and cortex and is thought to be involved in the modulation of plasticity processes and long-term potentiation (Yamagata et al., 1993; Breder et al., 1995); in pathological conditions, the presence of COX-1 in the CNS has been linked to inflammation development, whereas COX-2 is associated with neurotoxicity. Microglia surrounding the NPs in AD patient shows a high expression of COX-1, which suggests inflammation (Yermakova et al., 1999). On the other hand, COX-2 expression in the hippocampal CA3 region appears to be related with the quantity of NPs and NFTs and the observed cognitive impairment (Ho et al., 2001). COX-2 overexpression in a triple transgenic model (hAPP/PS1/hCOX-2) has resulted in an increase in active Caspase-3 immuoreactivity and retinoblastoma protein phosphorylation (S^{795}-pRb). The Rb protein regulates the G1 phase of the cell cycle, but S^{725} phosphorylation suppresses cell growth. *In vitro* studies revealed that hCOX-2 overexpression in primary cultures of cortical and hippocampal neurons derived from transgenic mice, accelerates the apoptotic damage induced by Aβ, causing cell cycle abnormalities (Xiang et al., 2002a). COX-2 also promotes amyloid plaque formation in parenchyma and increases prostaglandin E2 production. This increased plaque formation, correlates with an increase in amyloid peptide formation (Aβ1–40 and Aβ1–42) through the γ–secretase activation without affecting the APP expression levels (Xiang et al., 2002b). Studies performed in a mouse model using $COX\text{-}2^{-/-}$ deficient mice demonstrated that the inflammatory response mediated by Aβ was diminished, which suggested that COX-2 inhibition could be an important target to be use for therapy (Choi and Bosetti, 2009).

The analysis of post-mortem brain tissue from AD patients demonstrated that the maximum immunoreactivity for COX-2 and ppRb occurred in the early stages of the disease (Braak), before occur the maximum astrocytic and microglial activation. Contrary to *in vitro* observations, the post-mortem tissue analysis did not support the direct relationship between the microglial and astrocytic activation with the neuronal COX-2 and ppRb expression in AD (Hoozemans et al., 2005).

Currently, the cause of alterations in COX-2 levels during different stages of AD, remains unknown. However, it has been suggested that inflammation in the early stages of AD could promote such alterations, and IL-1β could promote an increase in COX-2 expression and PGs production (Hoozemans et al., 2001).

NITRIC OXIDE

NO is a molecule that contributes importantly in cell signaling. In the presence of oxygen, L-arginine, is converted to L-citrulline and release NO. Nitric oxide synthase (NOS) is the enzyme responsible for catalyzing this reaction, and it occurs in three isoforms. In the CNS, the neuronal isoform (nNOS) is widely distributed in neurons, astrocytes and blood vessels.

The endothelial isoform (eNOS) is located in the hippocampal pyramidal neurons, endothelial cells and some astrocytes. The expression of the inducible isoform (iNOS) is typically low but is increased in microglia and astrocytes during neuroinflammation. Under physiological conditions, it is believed that NO regulates the release of neurotransmitters and hormones and promotes cell survival and long-term potentiation. However, high levels of NO are generated in inflammatory conditions, which might contribute to synaptic transmission dysfunction, protein and lipid oxidative damage, excitotoxicity, and neuronal death (Liu et al., 2002; Bishop and Anderson, 2005; Calabrese et al., 2007).

Tissue and neuronal analyses of AD patients have revealed that Aβ is able to promote NOS expression and NO production in microglia cells and reactive astrocytes (Goodwin et al., 1997; Wallace et al., 1997; Akama et al., 1998). Aβ also promotes the pro-inflammatory cytokines IL-1β and TNF-α liberation which contribute to NO and peroxynitrite formation (Rossi and Bianchini, 1996; Combs et al., 2001) and cause protein and lipid modifications, mitochondrial damage, apoptosis and promote Aβ formation, increasing the γ-secretase complex activity (Torreilles et al., 1999; Keil et al., 2004; Guix et al., 2012). Under normal conditions, NO is synthesized in the microvasculature and regulates β-secretase activity which participate in APP processing (Austin et al., 2010). NOS2 also favors Aβ elimination by regulating MMP-9/TIMP-1 expression, which is a key enzyme that degrades amyloid (Ridnour et al., 2012). In addition, it has been shown that chronic NO formation may alter insulin-degrading enzyme activity (Kummer et al., 2012). NO synthesis during AD development could also contribute to NFT formation. In co-cultures of astrocytes and hippocampal neurons of rats, exposure to Aβ25–35 was found to increase NO levels, which correlated with increased hyperphosphorylated Tau protein. Interestingly, the use of a NOS inhibitors reduced Tau phosphorylation levels (Saez et al., 2004).

INFLAMMATION MODULATOR TREATMENTS: THERAPEUTICS IN AD

In the early 1990s, studies began to emerge relating the inflammation process with AD. Studies such as those of Fillit et al. (1991) showed that certain pro-inflammatory cytokines were elevated in AD patients.

Epidemiological studies (Li et al., 1992) indicates that subjects with arthritis have a lower prevalence of AD, after which it was proposed that this negative association could be related to the chronic use of anti-inflammatory drugs (Dickson and Rogers, 1992). From these and other results, these drugs began to be proposed as a new therapeutic approach for AD treatment. Currently, numerous epidemiological studies, experimental *in vitro* and *in vivo* models and clinical trials have been designed to elucidate the relationship between modulators of inflammation and AD.

Typically, anti-inflammatory agents are divided into non-steroidal anti-inflammatory drugs (NSAIDs) and glucocorticoids. This section will review the mechanisms of action of both types of anti-inflammatory agents and their role in AD and the results of some of the most relevant epidemiological and experimental studies. This section will also analyse the use of active and passive immunotherapy as a therapeutic strategy for AD (**Table 1**).

ANTI-INFLAMMATORY DRUGS

NSAIDs are a heterogeneous group of drugs that share a common mechanism of action, which involves COX-1 and COX-2 enzymes inhibition either selectively or non-selectively (Vane and Botting, 1987). These enzymes catalyze arachidonic acid conversion to prostaglandin H_2 (PGH_2), which is subsequently converted into various PGs (PGE_2, PGD_2, $PGF_{2\alpha}$, and PGI_2) and thromboxane (TX) (Dubois et al., 1998).

PG and TX synthesis increases in occurrence of tissue damage, acting as inflammation mediators, increasing blood flow and vasodilation in the damaged tissue and increasing microvascular permeability (Flower et al., 1976).

The results of several epidemiological studies designed to identify AD risk factors have shown that prolonged use of NSAID could reduce AD risk. The following are the results from some of the most representative studies conducted on different worldwide populations.

The *Sydney Old Persons Study* showed that NSAID use, is significantly lower in subjects who developed AD than in those who did not develop any type of dementia during the study period (Broe et al., 2000). Notably, NSAID use is not associated with any other type of dementia except AD. This result could suggest that NSAID use in AD may act through a different mechanism from their properties as cyclooxygenase inhibitors. The Rotterdam study (In'T Veld et al., 2001), Multi-Institutional Research Alzheimer's Genetic Epidemiology Study (Yip et al., 2005) and Canadian Study of Health and Aging (CSHA) (Coté et al., 2012) also observed an association between the NSAID use and a reduced AD risk. Szekely et al. conducted a meta-analysis of six studies (the Baltimore Longitudinal Study of Aging, Cache County Study, CSHA, Cardiovascular Health Study, Framingham Heart Study and Monongahela Valley Independent Elders Study) and reiterated the association between the NSAID use and a reduced AD risk (Szekely et al., 2008). However, some studies have failed to replicate this association. The Longitudinal Aging Study Amsterdam observed a reduction in AD risk associated with the use of aspirin alone and observed no association between AD risk and other NSAIDs (Jonker et al., 2003). Bendlin et al. also observed no significant differences in the results of neuropsychological memory and learning tests between NSAIDs users and non-users (Bendlin et al., 2010).

Other studies have observed controversial results, such as Fourrier et al. who observed an association between NSAIDs use and a decrease in Mini-Mental State Examination (MMSE) scores (Fourrier et al., 1996). Similarly, Breitner et al. reported a greater incidence of AD among NSAIDs users compared with controls (Breitner et al., 2009).

Martin et al. obtained equally unfavorable results when testing the effect of naproxen and celecoxib in older adults with a family history of AD (Martin et al., 2008). In this study, subjects treated with naproxen and those treated with celecoxib scored lower on the MMSE than subjects treated with placebo, which suggested a detrimental effect of the use of these drugs on cognitive performance. Aisen et al. tested the effect of rofecoxib and naproxen

Table 1 | Inflammation modulator treatments and their effects in animal models and clinical trials.

Therapy	Drug	Effects in animal models and clinical trials
NSAIDs	Naproxen	No beneficial effects reported. High frequency of adverse effects in drug-treated group, in clinical trials
	Celecoxib	Drug-treated group was found to score lower than placebo-treated group in cognitive tests, in clinical trials
	Rofecoxib	No beneficial effects reported. High frequency of adverse effects in drug-treated group, in clinical trials
	Indomethacin	In mice treated with this drug, lower Aβ levels in cortex and hippocampus were observed
	Mefenamic acid	Mice treated with this drug performed as well as healthy controls in cognitive tests
	Triflusal	In mice treated with this drug, a decrease in microglial and astrocytic activation, and a decrease in cytokine levels were observed
	Ibuprofen	Mice treated with this drug performed as well as healthy controls in cognitive tests. However, an increase in soluble Aβ levels and some behavior disturbances were observed in the drug-treated group
Glucocorticoids	Corticosterone/ Dexamethasone	Cortex, cerebellum and brainstem from mice treated with this drug showed increased expression of APP and beta-secretase, Aβ deposition, tau aggregation and caspase 3, cytochrome c, IL-1 and TNF-α levels. Drug-treated mice were found to score lower than placebo-treated mice in memory tasks
	Prednisone	No beneficial effects reported. Higher frequency of behavior disturbances was observed in the drug-treated group, in clinical trials
Immunotherapy	Aβ peptides	In mice, this therapy was able to prevent synaptic loss. Clinical trials have shown some beneficial effects in subjects who formed antibodies, but the incidence of meningoencephalitis as a side effect is notably high
	Anti-Aβ antibodies	In treated mice, a reduction in synaptic loss and number of dystrophic neurites and an increase in the number of dendritic spines have been reported. In clinical trials, no beneficial effects have been reported
	Tau peptides	Prevention of cognitive decline and a decrease in the number of NFTs has been reported in mouse model studies
	Anti-tau antibodies	A decrease in the number of NFTs has been reported in treated mice

Although most of these treatments have been successful in animal models, these beneficial results have not been reproduced in clinical trials, and even have been cause of detrimental effects.

on patients with mild to moderate AD (Aisen et al., 2003). The study, which lasted one year, showed no significant differences in the performance of subjects treated with rofecoxib or naproxen or placebo. In addition, subjects in NSAID-treated groups reported a high frequency of adverse effects such as fatigue and dizziness and had a significantly higher incidence of hypertension. Another study with rofecoxib, conducted in patients with mild cognitive impairment (MCI), suggested a deleterious effect of rofecoxib (Thal et al., 2005).

The results of AD animal model studies appear to support the hypothesis that the use of NSAID is beneficial, not only as a method of preventing the disease, but also as a therapeutic strategy. This support was observed in Tg2576 (Swe-APP) transgenic mice treated with indomethacin, which showed a marked decrease in Aβ levels ($A\beta_{1-40}$ and $A\beta_{1-42}$) in both cortex and hippocampus (Sung et al., 2004).

Subsequently, Joo et al. showed that mice treated with mefenamic acid for 3 weeks after being treated with Aβ1–42 or expressing Swe-APP, re-established their performance in the Morris water maze test in a comparable way to the vehicle-treated group (Joo et al., 2006). Coma et al. obtained similar results in Tg2576 transgenic mice treated with Triflusal (a NSAID from the salicylate family but a non-aspirin derivative), thus re-establishing transgenic mice (Tg+) performance in Morris test and a conditioning test (Coma et al., 2010). Although Triflusal had no effect on reducing NP size (NPS) or number, it reduced the amount of activated astrocytes and microglia and IL-1β and TNF-α levels in the hippocampal CA1 region and entorhinal cortex. Van Dam et al. observed similar results in TgAPP23 mice after treatment with Ibuprofen (Van Dam et al., 2010).

In the animal model (5XFAD), which overexpressed the Swedish double mutation (K670N, M671L), Florida mutation (I716V), London mutation (V717I), and double mutation in PS1 (M146L and L286V), treatment with ibuprofen for 3 months resulted in a reduction of the inflammatory response. However, it is notable that there was an increase in soluble Aβ42 levels and there was some changes in behavior, thus questioning whether anti-inflammatory drug use may actually be beneficial for AD treatment (Hillmann et al., 2012).

Whereas inflammation is a neuropathological feature always present in AD, and inflammatory processes significantly contribute to cell damage in this disease, previous studies performed *in vivo* and *in vitro* suggest that NSAIDs participation in AD occurs not only through an anti-inflammatory mechanism but also by modulating Aβ synthesis and removal in the CNS. Several studies have shown that NSAIDs stimulate the non-amyloidogenic APP-processing pathway (Avramovich et al., 2002), decrease β-secretase levels (Sastre et al., 2006), and reduce the Aβ formation (Hirohata et al., 2005).

Although animal models appear to show that NSAIDs are a promising therapeutic option, currently, no clinical trials conducted with these drugs have achieved favorable results in AD patients.

GLUCOCORTICOIDS

Similar to NSAIDs, glucocorticoids have potent anti-inflammatory effects, which have made them strong candidates for AD treatment. Basically, the mechanism of action of glucocorticoids is based on their ability to bind to its receptors (Glucocoticoid Receptor, GR), which is observed in the cytoplasm in its free form, which translocates into the nucleus after binding to one of its ligands. When GR locate at the nucleus, it binds to certain nucleotide sequences, glucocorticoid response elements (GREs), which are located in the promoter region of a variety of genes.

Depending on the type of GRE sequence to which it binds, GR will positively or negatively regulate gene expression (Beato et al., 1989). The importance of this binding in the inflammatory process is that some genes which GR binds to and activates, have anti-inflammatory effects such as annexin-1 (lipocortin-1), interleukin 10 and NF-κB inhibitor (IκB-α) (Barnes, 2006). In addition, it has also been suggested that glucocorticoids interact directly with Aβ.

The study of post-mortem AD brains showed a decrease in the presence of NPs in subjects under chronic treatment with corticosteroids. No significant differences were observed in the number of NFTs. This study also reported no association between chronic treatment with NSAIDs and the number of NPs (Beeri et al., 2012).

Despite its anti-inflammatory effect, the use of glucocorticoid as a therapeutic strategy in the treatment of AD is controversial, because numerous studies have associated increased levels of glucocorticoids (cortisol), to an increased AD risk. In 1994, Swaab et al. measured cortisol levels in post-mortem samples of CSF and observed an 83% increase in AD subjects compared to healthy controls (Swaab et al., 1994). These results coincide with the results of Laske who observed significantly higher levels of serum cortisol in AD patients compared with age-matched healthy controls (Laske et al., 2009).

The majority of animal model experiments does not support the use of corticosteroids as a therapeutic strategy for AD and suggests that these drugs promote the development of the neuropathological features of this disease.

The treatment of rats with glucocorticoids (corticosterone and dexamethasone) induces an increase in APP expression in cortex, cerebellum, and brain stem (Budas et al., 1999), thus suggesting an adverse effect. Additionally, there is an increase in Aβ formation because of the increased APP and β-secretase levels. These glucocorticoid levels also correlate with Tau accumulation (Green et al., 2006), memory, and learning impairment (Yao et al., 2007) and increased levels of caspase 3 and cytochrome c, which indicates the presence of a pro-apoptotic enviroment (Li et al., 2010). Finally, high levels of corticosterone in hippocampal cells have a pro-inflammatory effect, thus favoring IL-1 and TNF-α expression (Macpherson et al., 2005).

These studies indicates that the mechanisms that might associate glucocorticoids with an increase in AD risk are related with the increasing expression of proteins involved in Aβ synthesis (APP and β-secretase) or promoting apoptosis (Cotman and Anderson, 1995).

In humans, there is only one clinical trial investigating the effect of glucocorticoids in the treatment for AD, the trial investigate the used of a daily dose of prednisone or placebo for 1 year (Aisen et al., 2000). There were no significant differences in the cognitive performance of AD subjects treated with prednisone or placebo at the end of treatment; however, the prednisone-treated subjects showed a higher frequency of behavioral disturbances compared to controls.

In general, there is little evidence to suggest the neuroprotective or therapeutic role of glucocorticoids in AD; in contrast, there is extensive evidence of a possible neurotoxic role. Whereas it is possible that under certain conditions these substances are actually neuroprotective, details of their mechanism of action should be extensively evaluated in AD before a clinical testing protocol can be considered.

IMMUNOTHERAPY

Currently, there is no consensus among researchers regarding what triggers AD pathophysiology or which events are causes and which are bodily responses to counteract the damage caused by the disease. This problem has also been raised regarding inflammation.

Whereas therapies using NSAIDs and glucocorticoids were designed based on the idea that the immune response in AD has an adverse effect (Blasko et al., 2004) or may be a causal factor (McGeer and McGeer, 1995), there are other approaches which suggest that the immune response may be beneficial because it attempts to counteract the deleterious effects of Aβ oligomers and Tau aggregation.

Immunotherapy is one of the therapeutic strategies designed under these bases because it is underlying on promoting the immune response against the altered molecules that are present in the most distinctive histopathological lesions of the disease (NPs and NFTs) and destroy them. This section will review the types (anti-Aβ and anti-Tau immunotherapy) and some results of immunotherapeutic studies with AD patients.

ANTI-Aβ IMMUNOTHERAPY

Animal studies in which the anti-Aβ immunotherapy strategy has been tested have been promising. Buttini observed that either active (using four different Aβ sequence fragments) or passive immunotherapy (using 3D6 anti-Aβ and 12B4 antibodies) prevent the loss of synapses in PDAPP transgenic mice (Buttini et al., 2005).

The application of a single 3D6 anti-Aβ dose in Tg2576 mice demonstrated that there was no reduction in the number of NPs; nevertheless, there was a reduction in the number of dystrophic neurites (Rozkalne et al., 2009). On the other hand, the application of this antibody in PDAPP mice showed an increase in the number of dendritic spines, which suggests that this anti-Aβ immunotherapy approach, can increase neuronal plasticity and could contribute to the recovery of neural circuits. Subsequently, the effect of passive immunotherapy was studied with 7B6 anti-Aβ antibodies in Aβ APPswe/PS1dE9 mice (Spires-Jones et al., 2009; Liu et al., 2011). The authors observed that mice had a higher density of mono-aminergic axons in both the cortex and hippocampus. Immunotherapy using anti-Aβ CAD106 antibodies in different transgenic mouse models for APP (APP23 and APP24) showed a reduction in the presence of Aβ in both models (Wiessner et al., 2011).

In humans, some results suggest that anti-Aβ active immunotherapy could be beneficial; however, the frequency of adverse effects has been too high. In a study of active immunotherapy using $A\beta_{1-42}$ pre-aggregating (AN1792) in combination with immunogenic adjuvant QS-21 (a saponin of vegetable origin) observed a slower cognitive decline in subjects responding to the treatment (forming specific antibodies) (Hock et al., 2003; Orgogozo et al., 2003). However, 10% of the participants developed cases of aseptic meningoencephalitis. A similar result was obtained in an additional group of patients who were evaluated after stopping the treatment due to the adverse effects observed. The monitoring of these patients included cognitive testing and MRI scans to determine brain volume. Patients who were classified as antibody producers before the suspension of the study were tested for the presence of antibodies using ELISA; 89% of patients had antibodies at the time of investigation. These patients positive to antibodies production, performed better on cognitive tests than those treated with placebo, which suggests a possible beneficial effect of the treatment. However, brain volume loss was identical for both groups (Vellas et al., 2009).

The high incidence of aseptic meningoencephalitis among the subjects receiving active anti-Aβ immunotherapy could be attributed to an excessive pro-inflammatory response by T lymphocytes. Unfortunately, passive immunization with bapineuzumab, (a humanized murine monoclonal antibody), showed no differences in cognitive performance in subjects treated with bapineuzumab or placebo (Salloway et al., 2009).

ANTI-Tau IMMUNOTHERAPY

Most of the research efforts into AD immunotherapy have focused on anti-Aβ immunotherapy. However, some studies in animal models have also used anti-Tau immunization.

Boutajangout et al. showed that immunotherapy with the complete 441 amino acids peptides of the human Tau protein (hTau) prevented cognitive decline in an hTau transgenic mouse model, which expressed the hTau transgene (Boutajangout et al., 2010). Boimel et al. immunized the Tau transgenic mice presenting NFTs with phosphorylated Tau peptides. A 40% reduction in the number of NFTs was observed (Boimel et al., 2010). Chai et al. studied the effect of passive immunotherapy for Tau in JNPL3 and P301S transgenic mice. Using PHF1 and MC1 antibodies, the authors observed that the peripheral administration of both antibodies significantly reduced Tau pathology compared to controls (Chai et al., 2011). Although these results suggest that anti-Tau immunotherapy could provide favorable results, no clinical trial has been reported to date that evaluated the real effects on humans.

These results indicate that immunotherapy, particularly anti-Aβ active immunotherapy, could be advantageous when a strategy that minimizes its adverse effects is achieved. Further studies are also required with anti-Tau immunotherapy to evaluate whether this therapy could be functional in the future.

CONCLUSION

Currently, several genetic and epidemiological studies have provided an overview of the inflammatory mechanisms involved in AD. Although the molecular basis of the disease remains unknown, the inflammation induced by Aβ has an important role in the neurodegenerative process. The inflammatory process itself is driven by microglial and astrocytic activation through the induction of pro-inflammatory molecules and related signaling pathways, thus leading to synaptic damage, neuronal loss, and the activation of other inflammatory participants.

Although, the role of amyloid as a potential initiator of inflammation is not obvious, its accumulation exerts an indirect effect by activating caspases and transcription factors, such as NF-κB and AP-1, which produce numerous inflammation amplifiers (IL-1β, TNF-α, and IL-6). Pro-inflammatory cytokines, such as TNF-α and IL-1β and IL-6, could act directly on the neuron and induce apoptosis. Similarly, TNF-α and IL-1β can activate astrocytes, which could release factors that have the capacity to activate microglia.

Furthermore, APP, BACE1, and PSEN expression is governed by factors such as NF-κB. The genes encoding these proteins have sites in their promoter regions, which are recognized by NF-κB; in turn, the expression of these factors is upregulated by the presence of pro-inflammatory cytokines.

Inflammatory mediators acting on neurons contribute to an increase in amyloid production and activate microglia-mediated inflammation. The microglia-neuron communication amplifies the production of factors that contribute to AD-type pathology. However, the neural response is specific for the receptor type expressed in the different neuronal populations. For example, TNF-α binds TNFR1, which activates the cell survival pathway through NF-κB and the apoptotic pathway through the activation of caspases. Conversely, TNFRII signaling only activates NF-κB.

This cascade is primarily mediated by the pro-inflammatory cytokine IL-1β, which is expressed by microglia cells. IL-1β may cause neuronal death via various pathways, which activate microglia and consequently increase the release of IL-1β, thus generating a self-sustaining mechanism that is amplified by itself. This slow but steady inflammation state, generated for long periods in the brain eventually can destroy neurons and contribute to the clinical symptoms observed in the disease (**Figure 1**).

Finally, in accordance with all the above data, particularly because the results of the treatments used have been contradictory so far and there are no clinical trials that shown that anti-inflammatory treatments and the use of immunotherapy are completely safe or beneficial, it is necessary to develop and implement new strategies for AD immunological treatments.

ACKNOWLEDGMENTS

This work was supported by a grant from SEP/CONACYT (No. 157548).

REFERENCES

Ager, R. R., Fonseca, M. I., Chu, S. H., Sanderson, S. D., Taylor, S. M., Woodruff, T. M., et al. (2010). Microglial C5aR (CD88) expres- sion correlates with amyloid-beta deposition in murine models of Alzheimer's disease. *J. Neurochem.* 113, 389–401. doi: 10.1111/j.1471-4159.2010.06595. xAisen, P. S., Davis, K. L., Berg, J. D., Schafer, K., Campbell, K.,Thomas, R. G., et al. (2000). A randomized controlled trial of prednisone in Alzheimer's disease. Alzheimer's Disease Cooperative Study. *Neurology* 54, 588–593. doi: 10.1212/WNL.54.3.588

Aisen, P. S., Schaffer, K. A., Grundman, M., Pfeiffer, E., Sano, M., Davis,K. L., et al. (2003). Effects of rofecoxib or naproxen vs placebo on Alzheimer's Disease progres- sion. a randomized controlled trial. *JAMA* 289, 2819–2826. doi: 10.1001/jama.289.21.2819

Akama, K. T., Albanese, C., Pestell, R. G., and Van Eldik, L. J. (1998). Amyloid beta-peptide stimu- lates nitric oxide production in astrocytes through an NFkappaB- dependent mechanism. *Proc. Natl. Acad. Sci. U.S.A.* 95, 5795–5800. doi: 10.1073/pnas.95.10.5795 Akiyama, H., Barger, S., Barnum, S., Bradt, B., Bauer, J., Cole, G. M., et al. (2000). Inflammation and Alzheimer's disease. *Neurobiol. Aging* 21, 383–421. doi: 10.1016/S0197-4580(00)00124-X

Akiyama, H., Kondo, H., Mori, H., Kametani, F., Nishimura, T., Ikeda, K., et al. (1996). The amino- terminally truncated forms of amyloid beta-protein in brain macrophages in the ischemic lesions of Alzheimer's disease patients. *Neurosci. Lett.* 219, 115–118. doi: 10.1016/S0304-3940(96)13197-9

Ashutosh, Kou, W., Cotter, R., Borgmann, K., Wu, L., Persidsky, R., et al. (2011). CXCL8 protects human neurons from amyloid-beta-induced neuro-toxicity: relevance to Alzheimer's disease. *Biochem. Biophys. Res. Commun.* 412, 565–571. doi: 10.1016/j.bbrc.2011.07.127

Austin, S. A., Santhanam, A. V.,and Katusic, Z. S. (2010). Endothelial nitric oxide modu- lates expression and processing of amyloid precursor protein. *Circ. Res.* 107, 1498–1502. doi: 10.1161/CIRCRESAHA.110.233080

Avramovich, J., Amit, T., and Youdim, M. B. H. (2002). Non-steroidal anti-inflammatory drugs stimulate secretion of on-amyloidogenic precursor protein. *J. Biol. Chem.* 277, 31466–31473. doi: 10.1074/jbc.M201308200

Barnes, P. J. (2006). How corticos- teroids control inflammation: quintiles prize lecture 2005. *Br. J. Pharmacol.* 148, 245–254. doi: 10.1038/sj.bjp.0706736

Beato, M., Chalepakis, G., Schauer, M., and Slater, E. P. (1989). DNA regula-tory elements for steroid hormones. *J. Steroid Biochem.* 32, 737–747. doi: 10.1016/0022-4731(89)90521-9

Beeri, M. S., Schmeidler, J., Lesser, G. T., Maroukian, M., West, R., Leung, S., et al. (2012). Corticosteroids, but not NSAIDs, are associated with less Alzheimer neuropathology. *Neurobiol. Aging* 33, 1258–1264. doi: 10.1016/j. neurobiolaging. 2011.02.011

Bendlin, B. B., Newman, L. M., Ries, M. L., Puglielli, L., Carlsson, C. M., Sager, M. A., et al. (2010). NSAIDs may protect against age- related brain atrophy. *Front. Aging Neurosci.* 2, 1–8. doi: 10.3389/fnagi.2010.00035

Bishop, A., and Anderson, J. E. (2005). NO signaling in the CNS: from the physiological to the patholog- ical. *Toxicology* 208, 193–205. doi: 10.1016/j. tox.2004.11.034

Blasko, I., Stampfer-Kountchev, M., Robatscher, P., Veerhuis, R., Eikelenboom, P., and Grubeck- Loebenstein, B. (2004). How chronic inflammation can affect the brain and support the development of Alzheimer's disease in old age: the role of microglia and astro- cytes. *Aging Cell* 3, 169–176. doi: 10.1111/j.1474-9728.2004.00101.x

Blasko, I., Veerhuis, R., Stampfer- Kountchev, M., Saurwein-Teissl, M., Eikelenboom, P., and Grubeck-Loebenstein, B. (2000). Costimulatory effects of interferon- gamma and interleukin-1beta or tumor necrosis factor alpha on the synthesis of Abeta1-40 and Abeta1-42 by human astrocytes. *Neurobiol. Dis.* 7, 682–689. doi: 10.1006/nbdi.2000.0321

Blum-Degen, D., Muller, T., Kuhn, W., Gerlach, M., Przuntek, H., and Riederer, P. (1995). Interleukin-1 beta and interleukin-6 are elevated in the cerebrospinal fluid of Alzheimer's and *de novo* Parkinson's disease patients. *Neurosci. Lett.* 202, 17–20. doi: 10.1016/0304-3940(95)12192-7

Boimel, M., Grigoriadis, N., Lourbopoulos, A., Haber, E., Abramsky, O., and Rosenmann, H. (2010). Efficacy and safety of immunization with phosphorylated tau against neurofibrillary tangles in mice. *Exp. Neurol.* 224, 472–485. doi: 10.1016/j.expneurol.2010.05.010

Boutajangout, A., Quartermain, D., and Sigurdsson, E. M. (2010). Immunotherapy targeting pathological tau pre- vents cognitive decline in a new tangle mouse model. *J. Neurosci.* 30, 16559–16566. doi: 10.1523/ JNEUROSCI.4363-10.2010

Breder, C. D., Dewitt, D., and Kraig, R. P. (1995). Characterization of inducible cyclooxyge- nase in rat brain. *J. Comp. Neurol.* 355, 296–315. doi: 10.1002/ cne.903550208

an elderly community-based cohort. *Neurology* 72, 1899–1905. doi: 10.1212/ WNL.0b013e3181a18691

Broe, G. A., Grayson, D. A., Creasey,H. M., Waite, L. M., Casey, B. J., Bennett, H. P., et al. (2000). Anti- inflammatory drugs protect against Alzheimer's Disease at low doses. *Arch. Neurol.* 57, 1586–1591. doi: 10.1001/ archneur.57.11.1586

Budas, G., Coughlan, C. M., Seckl, J. R., and Breen, K. C. (1999). The effect of corticosteroids on amy- loid β precursor protein/amyloid precursor-like protein expres- sion and processing *in vivo*. *Neurosci. Lett.* 276, 61–64. doi: 10.1016/S0304-3940(99)00790-9.

Buttini, M., Masliah, E., Barbour, R., Grajeda, H., Motter, R., Johnson-Wood, K., et al. (2005). Beta-amyloid immunotherapy prevents synaptic degener- ation in a mouse model of Alzheimer's disease. *J. Neurosci.* 25, 9096–9101. doi: 10.1523/ JNEUROSCI.1697-05.2005

Calabrese, V., Mancuso, C., Calvani, M., Rizzarelli, E., Butterfield, D. A., and Stella, A. M. (2007). Nitric oxide in the central nervous system: neuroprotection versus neurotoxic- ity. *Nat. Rev. Neurosci.* 8, 766–775. doi: 10.1038/nrn2214

Carrero, I., Gonzalo, M. R., Martin, B., Sanz-Anquela, J. M., Arevalo- Serrano, J., and Gonzalo-Ruiz, A. (2012). Oligomers of beta-amyloid protein (Abeta1-42) induce the activation of cyclooxygenase-2 in astrocytes via an interac- tion with interleukin-1beta, tumour necrosis factor-alpha, and a nuclear factor kappa-B mechanism in the rat brain. *Exp. Neurol.* 236, 215–227. doi: 10.1016/j.expneurol.2012.05.004

Coma, M., Serenó, L., Da Rocha- Souto, B., Scotton, T. C., España, J., Sánchez, M. B., et al. (2010). Triflusal reduces dense-core plaque load, associated axonal alterations and inflammatory changes, and rescues cognition in a transgenic mouse model of Alzheimer's dis- ease. *Neurobiol. Dis.* 38, 482–491.

Combs, C. K., Karlo, J. C., Kao, S. C., and Landreth, G. E. (2001). beta-Amyloid stimulation of microglia and monocytes results in TNFalpha-dependent expression of inducible nitric oxide synthase and neuronal apoptosis. *J. Neurosci.* 21, 1179–1188.

Correa, J. D., Starling, D., Teixeira, A. L., Caramelli, P., and Silva, T. A. (2011). Chemokines in CSF of Alzheimer's disease patients. *Arq. Neuropsiquiatr.* 69, 455–459. doi: 10.1590/S0004- 282X2011000400009

Coté, S., Carmichael, P.-H., Verrault, R., Lindsay, J., Lefebvre, J., and Laurin, D. (2012). Nonsteroidal anti-inflammatory drug use and the risk of cognitive impair-ment and Alzheimer's disease. *Alzheimers Dement.* 8, 219–226. doi: 10.1016/j. jalz.2011.03.012

Cotman, C., and Anderson, A. (1995). A potential role for apoptosis in neurodegeneration and Alzheimer's disease. *Mol. Neurobiol.* 10, 19–45. doi: 10.1007/BF02740836

Cyster, J. G. (1999). Chemokines and cell migration in sec- ondary lymphoid organs. *Science* 286, 2098–2102. doi: 10.1126/science.286.5447.2098

Chai, X., Wu, S., Murray, T. K., Kinley, R., Cella, C. V., Sims, H., et al. (2011). Passive immuniza- tion with anti-tau antibodies in two transgenic models reduc- tion of tau pathology and delay of disease progression. *J. Biol. Chem.* 286, 34457–34467. doi: 10.1074/jbc.M111.229633

Chakrabarty, P., Jansen-West, K., Beccard, A., Ceballos-Diaz, C., Levites, Y., Verbeeck, C., et al. (2010). Massive gliosis induced by interleukin-6 suppresses Abeta deposition *in vivo*: evidence against inflammation as a driving force for amyloid deposition. *FASEB J.* 24, 548–559. doi: 10.1096/fj.09-141754

Chartier-Harlin, M. C., Crawford, F., Hamandi, K., Mullan, M., Goate, A., Hardy, J., et al. (1991). Screening for the beta-amyloid precursor pro- tein mutation (APP717: Val—Ile) in extended pedigrees with early onset Alzheimer's disease. *Neurosci. Lett.* 129, 134–135. doi: 10.1016/0304-3940(91)90738-F

Chibnik, L. B., Shulman, J. M., Leurgans, S. E., Schneider, J. A., Wilson, R. S., Tran, D., et al. (2011). CR1 is associated with amyloid plaque burden and age-related cognitive decline. *Ann. Neurol.* 69, 560–569. doi: 10.1002/ana.22277

Choi, S. H., and Bosetti, F. (2009). Cyclooxygenase-1 null mice show reduced neuroinflammation in response to beta-amyloid. *Aging* 1, 234–244.

Desai, M. K., Guercio, B. J., Narrow, W. C., and Bowers, W. J. (2011). An Alzheimer's disease-relevant presenilin-1 mutation augments amyloid-beta-induced oligodendro- cyte dysfunction. *Glia* 59, 627–640. doi: 10.1002/ glia.21131

Dickson, D. W., Farlo, J., Davies, P., Crystal, H., Fuld, P., and Yen, S. H. (1988). Alzheimer's disease. a double-labeling immuno- histochemical study of senile plaques. *Am. J. Pathol.* 132, 86–101.

Dickson, D. W., and Rogers, J. (1992). Neuroimmunology of Alzheimer's Disease: a conference report. *Neurobiol. Aging* 13, 793–798. doi: 10.1016/0197-4580(92)90104-6

Dubois, R. N., Abramson, S. B., Crofford, L., Gupta, R. A., Simon, L. S., Van De Putte, L. B. A.,et al. (1998). Cyclooxygenase in biology and disease. *FASEB J.* 12, 1063–1073.

presenilin 1. *Nature* 383, 710–713. doi: 10.1038/383710a0

El Khoury, J., Hickman, S. E., Thomas, C. A., Loike, J. D., and Silverstein, S. C. (1998). Microglia, scavenger receptors, and the pathogen- esis of Alzheimer's disease. *Neurobiol. Aging* 19, S81–S84. doi: 10.1016/S0197-4580(98)00036-0

Fan, R., Defilippis, K., and Van Nostrand, W. E. (2007). Induction of complement proteins in a mouse model for cerebral microvascular a beta deposition. *J. Neuroinflammation* 4, 22. doi: 10.1186/1742-2094-4-22

Fiala, M., Zhang, L., Gan, X., Sherry, ., Taub, D., Graves, M. C., et al. (1998). Amyloid-beta induces chemokine secretion and monocyte migration across a human blood– brain barrier model. *Mol. Med.* 4, 480–489.

Fillit, H., Ding, W., Buee, L., Kalman, J.,Alstiel, L., Lawlor, B., et al. (1991). Elevated circulating tumor necrosis factor levels in Alzheimer's disease. *Neurosci. Lett.* 129, 318–320. doi: 10.1016/0304-3940(91)90490-K

Flanders, K. C., Lippa, C. F., Smith, T. W., Pollen, D. A., and Sporn, M. B. (1995). Altered expres- sion of transforming growth factor-beta in Alzheimer's disease. *Neurology* 45, 1561–1569. doi: 10.1212/WNL.45.8.1561

Flower, R. J., Harvey, E.A and Kingston, W. P. (1976). Inflammatory effects of prostaglandin D2 in rat and human skin. *Br. J. Pharmacol.* 56, 229–233. doi: 10.1111/j.1476- 5381.1976.tb07446.x

Fonseca, M. I., Ager, R. R., Chu, S. H., Yazan, O., Sanderson, S. D., Laferla, F. M., et al. (2009). Treatment with a C5aR antagonist decreases pathology and enhances behavioral performance in murine models of Alzheimer's disease. *J. Immunol.* 183, 1375–1383. doi: 10.4049/jimmunol.0901005

Fonseca, M. I., Zhou, J., Botto, M., and Tenner, A. J. (2004). Absence of C1q leads to less neuropathology in transgenic mouse models of Alzheimer's disease. *J. Neurosci.* 24, 6457–6465. doi: 10.1523/ JNEUROSCI.0901-04.2004

Forneris, F., Wu, J., and Gros, P. (2012). The modular serine proteases of the complement cascade. *Curr. Opin. Struct. Biol.* 22, 333–341. doi: 10.1016/ j.sbi.2012.04.001

Fourrier, A., Letenneur, L., Bégaud, B., and Dartigues, J. F. (1996). Nonsteroidal anti-inflammatory drug use and cognitive func- tion in the elderly: inconclusive results from a population.based cohort study. *J. Clin. Epidmiol.* 49, 1201. doi: 10.1016/0895-4356(96) 00202-8

Frackowiak, J., Wisniewski, H. M., Wegiel, J., Merz, G. S., Iqbal, K., and Wang, K. C. (1992). Ultrastructure of the microglia that phagocy- tose amyloid and the microglia that produce beta-amyloid fibrils. *Acta Neuropathol.* 84, 225–233. doi: 10.1007/BF00227813

Galimberti, D., Schoonenboom, N., Scarpini, E., and Scheltens, P. (2003). Chemokines in serum and cerebrospinal fluid of Alzheimer's disease patients. *Ann. Neurol.* 53, 547–548. doi: 10.1002/ana.10531

Gate, D., Rezai-Zadeh, K., Jodry, D., Rentsendorj, A., and Town, T. (2010). Macrophages in Alzheimer's disease: the blood-borne identity. *J. Neural Transm.* 117, 961–970. doi: 10.1007/s00702-010-0422-7

Glenner, G. G., Wong, C. W., Quaranta, V., and Eanes, E. D. (1984). The amyloid deposits in Alzheimer's disease: their nature and pathogen- esis. *Appl. Pathol.* 2, 357–369.

Goate, A., Chartier-Harlin, M. C., Mullan, M., Brown, J., Crawford, F., Fidani, L., et al. (1991). Segregation of a missense mutation in the amyloid precursor protein gene with familial Alzheimer's dis- ease. *Nature* 349, 704–706. doi: 10.1038/349704a0

Goldgaber, D., Harris, H. W., Hla, T., Maciag, T., Donnelly, R. J., Jacobsen, J. S., et al. (1989). Interleukin 1 regulates synthesis of amyloid beta- protein precursor mRNA in human endothelial cells. *Proc. Natl. Acad. Sci. U.S.A.* 86, 7606–7610. doi: 10.1073/pnas.86.19.7606

Goodwin, J. L., Kehrli, M. E. Jr., and Uemura, E. (1997). Integrin Mac-1 and beta-amyloid in microglial release of nitric oxide. *Brain Res.* 768, 279–286. doi: 10.1016/S0006- 8993(97)00653-7

Green, K. N., Billings, L. M., Roozendaal, B., McGaugh, J. L., and Laferla, F. M. (2006). Glucocorticoids increase amyloid-beta and tau pathol- ogy in a mouse model of Alzheimer's disease. *J. Neurosci.* 26, 9047–9056. doi: 10.1523/ JNEUROSCI.2797-06.2006

Griffin, W. S., Sheng, J. G., Roberts, G. W., and Mrak, R. E. (1995). Interleukin-1 expression in differ- ent plaque types in Alzheimer's dis- ease: significance in plaque evolu- tion. *J. Neuropathol. Exp. Neurol.* 54, 276–281. doi: 10.1097/00005072- 199503000-00014

Griffin, W. S., Stanley, L. C., Ling, ., White, L., Macleod, V., Perrot, L. J., et al. (1989). Brain inter- leukin 1 and S-100 immunoreactiv- ity are elevated in Down syndrome and Alzheimer disease. *Proc. Natl. Acad. Sci. U.S.A.* 86, 7611–7615. doi: 10.1073/pnas.86.19.7611

Guix, F. X., Wahle, T., Vennekens, K., Snellinx, A., Chavez-Gutierrez, L., Ill-Raga, G., et al. (2012). Modification of gamma-secretase by nitrosative stress links neuronal ageing to sporadic Alzheimer's dis- ease. *EMBO Mol. Med.* 4, 660–673. doi: 10.1002/emmm.201200243

by cultured microglial cells. *Brain Res.* 601, 88–94. doi: 10.1016/0006-8993(93)91698-R

Halassa, M. M., and Haydon, P. G. (2010). Integrated brain circuits: astrocytic networks modulate neu- ronal activity and behavior. *Annu. Rev. Physiol.* 72, 335–355. doi: 10.1146/annurev-physiol-021909- 135843

Henneberger, C., Papouin, T., Oliet, S. H., and Rusakov, D. A. (2010). Long-term potentiation depends on release of D-serine from astro- cytes. *Nature* 463, 232–236. doi: 10.1038/nature08673

Hillmann, A., Hahn, S., Schilling, S., Hoffmann, T., Demuth, H.-U., Bulic, B., et al. (2012). No improvement after chronic ibupro- fen treatment in the 5XFAD mouse model of Alzheimer's disease. *Neurobiol. Aging* 33, 833. e39–833.e50. doi: 10.1016/j. neurobiolaging.2011.08.006 Hirohata, M., Ono, K., Naiki, H., and Yamada, M. (2005). Non- steroidal anti-inflammatory drugs have anti-amyloidogenic effects for Alzheimer's ß-amyloid fib- rils *in vitro*. *Neuropharmacology* 49, 1088–1099. doi: 10.1016/j.neuropharm.2005.07.004

Ho, L., Purohit, D., Haroutunian, V., Luterman, J. D., Willis, F., Naslund, J., et al. (2001). Neuronal cyclooxy- genase 2 expression in the hip- pocampal formation as a func- tion of the clinical progression of Alzheimer disease. *Arch. Neurol.* 58, 487–492. doi: 10.1001/archneur.58.3.487

Hock, C., Konietzko, U., Streffer, J. R., Tracy, J., Signorell, A., Muller-Tillmanns, B., et al. (2003). Antibodies against ß- amyloid slow cognitive decline in Alzheimer's disease. *Neuron* 38, 547–554. doi: 10.1016/ S0896-6273(03)00294-0

Hoozemans, J. J., Van Haastert, E. S., Veerhuis, R., Arendt, T., Scheper, W., Eikelenboom, P., et al. (2005). Maximal COX-2 and ppRb expres- sion in neurons occurs during early Braak stages prior to the maxi- mal activation of astrocytes and microglia in Alzheimer's disease. *J. Neuroinflammation* 2, 27. doi: 10.1186/1742-2094-2-27

Hoozemans, J. J., Veerhuis, R., Janssen, I., Rozemuller, A. J., and Eikelenboom, P. (2001). Interleukin-1beta induced cyclooxygenase 2 expression and prostaglandin E2 secretion by human neuroblastoma cells: impli- cations for Alzheimer's disease. *Exp. Gerontol.* 36, 559–570. doi: 10.1016/ S0531-5565(00)00226-6

Hull, M., Berger, M., Volk, B., and Bauer, J. (1996). Occurrence of interleukin-6 in cortical plaques of Alzheimer's disease patients may precede transformation of diffuse into neuritic plaques. *Ann. N.Y. Acad. Sci.* 777, 205–212. doi: 10.1111/j.1749-6632.1996. tb34420.x

In'T Veld, B. A., Ruitenberg, A., Hofman, A., Launer, L., Van Duijn, C. M., Stijnen, T., et al. (2001). Nonsteroidal anti- inflammatory drugs and the risk of Alzheimer's Disease. *N. Eng. J. Med.* 345, 1515–1521. doi: 10.1056/ NEJMoa010178

Ishizuka, K., Kimura, T., Igata-Yi, R., Katsuragi, S., Takamatsu, J., and Miyakawa, T. (1997). Identification of monocyte chemoattractant protein-1 in senile plaques and reactive microglia of Alzheimer's disease. *Psychiatry Clin. Neurosci.* 51, 135–138. doi: 10.1111/j.1440- 1819.1997.tb02375.x

Iversen, L. L., Mortishire-Smith, R. J., Pollack, S. J., and Shearman, M. S. (1995). The toxicity *in vitro* of beta- amyloid protein. *Biochem. J.* 311(Pt 1), 1–16.

Jiang, H., Hampel, H., Prvulovic, D., Wallin, A., Blennow, K., Li, R., et al. (2011). Elevated CSF levels of TACE activity and soluble TNF receptors in subjects with mild cognitive impairment and patients with Alzheimer's disease. *Mol. Neurodegener.* 6, 69. doi: 10.1186/1750-1326-6-69

Jonker, C., Comijs, H. C., and Smit, J. H. (2003). Does aspirin or other NSAIDs reduce the risk of cognitive decline in elderly persons? Results from a population- based study. *Neurobiol. Aging* 24, 583–588. doi: 10.1016/ S0197-4580(02)00188-4

Joo, Y., Kim, H.-S., Woo, R.-S., Park, C. H., Shin, K.-Y., Lee, J.-P., et al. (2006). Mefenamic acid shows neu- roprotective effects and improves cognitive impairment in *in vitro* and *in vivo* Alzheimer's Disease models. *Mol. Pharmacol.* 69, 76–84.

Kamata, H., Honda, S., Maeda, S., Chang, L., Hirata, H., and Karin, M. (2005). Reactive oxygen species promote TNFalpha-induced death and sustained JNK activation by inhibiting MAP kinase phos- phatases. *Cell* 120, 649–661. doi: 10.1016/j.cell.2004.12.041

Kang, J., Lemaire, H. G., Unterbeck, A., Salbaum, J. M., Masters, C. L., Grzeschik, K. H., et al. (1987). The precursor of Alzheimer's disease amyloid A4 protein resembles a cell-surface receptor. *Nature* 325, 733–736. doi: 10.1038/325733a0

Keil, U., Bonert, A., Marques, C. A., Scherping, I., Weyermann, J., Strosznajder, J. B., et al. (2004). Amyloid beta-induced changes in nitric oxide production and mito- chondrial activity lead to apopto- sis. *J. Biol. Chem.* 279, 50310–50320. doi: 10.1074/jbc.M405600200

Kitazawa, M., Yamasaki, T. R., and Laferla, F. M. (2004). Microglia as a potential bridge between the amy- loid beta-peptide and tau. *Ann. N.Y. Acad. Sci.* 1035, 85–103. doi: 10.1196/annals.1332.006

Kobayashi, K., Hayashi, M., Nakano, H., Fukutani, Y.,Sasaki, K., Shimazaki, M., et al. (2002). Apoptosis of astrocytes with enhanced lysosomal activity and oligodendrocytes in white matter lesions in Alzheimer's disease. *Neuropathol. Appl. Neurobiol.* 28, 238–251. doi: 10.1046/ j.1365-2990.2002.00390.x

Konig, H. G., Kogel, D., Rami, A., and Prehn, J. H. (2005). TGF-{beta}1 activates two distinct type I receptors in neurons: implications for neuronal NF-{kappa}B signal- ing. *J. Cell Biol.* 168, 1077–1086. doi: 10.1083/jcb.200407027

Krieglstein, K., Strelau, J., Schober, A., Sullivan, A., and Unsicker, K. (2002). TGF-beta and the regulation of neuron sur- vival and death. *J. Physiol. Paris* 96, 25–30. doi: 10.1016/ S0928-4257(01)00077-8

Kummer, M. P., Hulsmann, C., Hermes, M., Axt, D., and Heneka, M. T. (2012). Nitric oxide decreases the enzymatic activ- ity of insulin degrading enzyme in APP/PS1 mice. *J. Neuroimmune Pharmacol.* 7, 165–172. doi: 10.1007/ s11481-011-9339-7

Laske, C., Stransky, E., Fritsche, A., Eschweiler, G., and Leyhe, T. (2009). Inverse association of cortisol serum levels with T-tau, P-tau 181 and P- tau 231 peptide levels and T-tau/Aβ 1-42 ratios in CSF in patients with mild Alzheimer's disease dementia. *Eur. Arch. Psychiatry Clin. Neurosci.* 259, 80–85. doi: 10.1007/s00406- 008-0838-3

Levy-Lahad, E., Wijsman, E. M., Nemens, E., Anderson, L., Goddard, K. A., Weber, J. L., et al. (1995). A familial Alzheimer's disease locus on chromosome 1. *Science* 269, 970–973. doi: 10.1126/science.7638621

Li, G., Shen, Y. C., Li, Y. T., Chen, C. H., Zhau, Y. W., and Silverman, J. M. (1992). A case-control study of Alzheimer's disease in China. *Neurology* 42, 1481–1488. doi: 10.1212/WNL.42.8.1481

Li, W.-Z., Li, W.-P., Yao, Y.-Y., Zhang, W., Yin, Y.-Y., Wu, G.- C., et al. (2010). Glucocorticoids increase impairments in learn- ing and memory due to elevated amyloid precursor protein expres- sion and neuronal apoptosis in 12-month old mice. *Eur. J. Pharmacol.* 628, 108–115. doi: 10.1016/j. ejphar.2009.11.045

Li, Y., Liu, L., Barger, S. W., and Griffin, W. S. (2003). Interleukin-1 mediates pathological effects of microglia on tau phosphorylation and on synaptophysin synthesis in cortical neu- rons through a p38-MAPK pathway. *J. Neurosci.* 23, 1605–1611.

Li, Y., Wang, J., Sheng, J. G., Liu, L., Barger, S. W., Jones, R. A., et al. (1998). S100 beta increases lev- els of beta-amyloid precursor pro- tein and its encoding mRNA in rat neuronal cultures. *J. Neurochem.* 71, 1421–1428. doi: 10.1046/j.1471- 4159.1998.71041421.x

Liao, Y. F., Wang, B. J., Cheng, H. T., Kuo, L. H., and Wolfe, M. S. (2004). Tumor necrosis factor-alpha, interleukin- 1beta, and interferon-gamma stimulate gamma-secretase- mediated cleavage of amyloid precursor protein through a JNK- dependent MAPK pathway. *J. Biol. Chem.* 279, 49523–49532. doi: 10.1074/jbc.M402034200

Liu, B., Gao, H. M., Wang, J. Y., Jeohn, G. H., Cooper, C. L., and Hong, J. S. (2002). Role of nitric oxide in inflammation-mediated neurode- generation. *Ann. N.Y. Acad. Sci.* 962, 318–331. doi: 10.1111/j.1749- 6632.2002.tb04077.x

Liu, Y., Lee, M. K., James, M. M., Price, D. L., Borchelt, D. R., Troncoso, J. C., et al. (2011). Passive (Amyloid-β Immunotherapy Attenuates Monoaminergic Axonal Degeneration in the AβPPswe/PS1dE9 Mice. *J. Alzheimer's Dis.* 23, 271–279.

Lue, L. F., Rydel, R., Brigham, E. F., Yang, L. B., Hampel, H., Murphy, G. M. Jr., et al., (2001). Inflammatory repertoire of Alzheimer's disease and nondemented elderly microglia *in vitro*. Glia 35, 72–79. doi: 10.1002/glia.1072

Macpherson, A., Dinkel, K., and Sapolsky, R. (2005). Glucocorticoids worsen excitotoxin-induced expression of pro-inflammatory cytokines in hippocampal cultures. *Exp. Neurol.* 194, 376–383. doi: 10.1016/j.expneurol.2005.02.021

Maier, M., Peng, Y., Jiang, L., Seabrook, T. J., Carroll, M. C., and Lemere, C. A. (2008). Complement C3 deficiency leads to accelerated amyloid beta plaque deposition and neurodegeneration and modulation of the microglia/ macrophage phenotype in amyloid precur- sor protein transgenic mice. *J. Neurosci.* 28, 6333–6341. doi: 10.1523/JNEUROSCI.0829-08.2008

Man, S. M., Ma, Y. R., Shang, D. S., Zhao, W. D., Li, B., Guo, D. W., et al. (2007). Peripheral T cells overexpress MIP-1alpha to enhance its transendothelial migration in Alzheimer's disease. *Neurobiol. Aging* 28, 485–496. doi: 10.1016/j. neurobiolaging.2006.02.013

Martin, B., Szekely, C., Brandt, J., Piantadosi, S., Breitner, J., Craft, S., et al. (2008). Cognitive function over time in the Alzheimer's Disease Anti-inflammatory Prevention Trial (ADAPT): results of a ran- domized, controlled trial of naproxen and celecoxib. *Arch. Neurol.* 65, 896. doi: 10.1001/archneur.2008.65.7.nct70006

McAlpine, F. E., Lee, J. K., Harms, A. S., Ruhn, K. A., Blurton-Jones, M., Hong, J., et al. (2009). Inhibition of soluble TNF signaling in a mouse model of Alzheimer's disease prevents pre-plaque amyloid-associated neuropathol- ogy. *Neurobiol. Dis.* 34, 163–177. doi: 10.1016/j.nbd.2009.01.006

McGeer, P. L., Akiyama, H., Itagaki, S., and McGeer, E. G. (1989). Activation of the classical comple- ment pathway in brain tissue of Alzheimer patients. *Neurosci. Lett.* 107, 341–346. doi: 10.1016/0304-3940(89)90843-4

McGeer, P. L., Itagaki, S., and McGeer, E. G. (1988). Expression of the histocompatibility glycoprotein HLA-DR in neurological disease. *Acta Neuropathol.* 76, 550–557. doi: 10.1007/BF00689592

McGeer, P. L., and McGeer, E. G. (1995). The inflammatory response system of brain: implications for therapy of Alzheimer and other neurodegenerative diseases. *Brain Res. Rev.* 21, 195–218. doi: 10.1016/0165-0173(95)00011-9

Meda, L., Baron, P., Prat, E., Scarpini, E., Scarlato, G., Cassatella, M. A., et al. (1999). Proinflammatory profile of cytokine produc- tion by human monocytes and murine microglia stimu- lated with beta-amyloid[25-35]. *J. Neuroimmunol.* 93, 45–52. doi: 10.1016/S0165-5728(98)00188-X

Medeiros, R., and Laferla, F. M. (2013). Astrocytes: conduc- tors of the Alzheimer disease neuroinflammatory symphony. *Exp. Neurol.* 239, 133–138. doi: 10.1016/j.expneurol.2012.10.007

Montgomery, S. L., Mastrangelo, M. A., Habib, D., Narrow, W. C., Knowlden, S. A., Wright, T. W., et al. (2011). Ablation of TNF-RI/RII expression in Alzheimer's disease mice leads to an unexpected enhancement of pathology: implications for chronic pan-TNF-alpha suppressive therapeutic strategies in the brain. *Am. J. Pathol.* 179, 2053–2070. doi: 10.1016/j.ajpath.2011.07.001

Moynagh, P. N. (2005). The interleukin-1 signalling pathway in astrocytes: a key contrib- utor to inflammation in the brain. *J. Anat.* 207, 265–269. doi: 10.1111/j.1469-7580.2005.00445.x

Mrak, R. E. (2012). Microglia in Alzheimer brain: a neuropatholog- ical perspective. *Int. J. Alzheimers Dis.* 2012, 165021. doi: 10.1155/ 2012/165021

Mrak, R. E., and Griffin, W. S. (2005). Potential inflammatory biomarkers in Alzheimer'sdisease. *J. Alzheimers Dis.* 8, 369–375.

Mrak, R. E., Sheng, J. G., and Griffin, W. S. (1996). Correlation of astrocytic S100 beta expression with dystrophic neurites in amyloid plaques of Alzheimer's disease. *J. Neuropathol. Exp. Neurol.* 55, 273–279. doi: 10.1097/00005072- 199603000-00002

Murrell, J., Farlow, M., Ghetti, B., and Benson, M. D. (1991). A mutation in the amyloid pre- cursor protein associated with hereditary Alzheimer's dis- ease. *Science* 254, 97–99. doi: 10.1126/science.1925564

Okun, E., Mattson, M. P., and Arumugam, T. V. (2010). Involvement of Fc receptors in disorders of the central nervous sys- tem. *Neuromol. Med.* 12, 164–178. doi: 10.1007/s12017-009-8099-5

Orgogozo, J.-M., Gilman, S., Dartigues, J.-F., Laurent, B., Puel, M., Kirby, L., et al. (2003). Subacute menin- goencephalitis in a subset of patients with AD after Aβ42 immunization. *Neurology* 61, 46–54. doi: 10.1212/ 01.WNL.0000073623.84147.A8

Patel, N. S., Paris, D., Mathura, V., Quadros, A. N., Crawford, F. C., and Mullan, M. J. (2005). Inflammatory cytokine levels corre- late with amyloid load in transgenic mouse models of Alzheimer's dis- ease. *J. Neuroinflammation* 2, 9. doi: 10.1186/1742-2094-2-9

Pekkarinen, P. T., Vaali, K., Junnikkala, S., Rossi, L. H., Tuovinen, H., Meri, S., et al. (2011). A functional com- plement system is required for nor- mal T helper cell differentiation. *Immunobiology* 216, 737–743. doi: 10.1016/j. imbio.2010.10.004

Quintanilla, R. A., Orellana, D. I., Gonzalez-Billault, C., and Maccioni, B. (2004). Interleukin-6 induces Alzheimer-type phosphorylation of tau protein by deregulat- ing the cdk5/p35 pathway. *Exp. Cell Res.* 295, 245–257. doi: 10.1016/j.yexcr.2004.01.002

Ransohoff, R. M., Glabinski, A., and Tani, M. (1996). Chemokines in immune-mediated inflammation of the central nervous system. *Cytokine Growth Factor Rev.* 7, 35–46. doi: 10.1016/1359-6101(96)00003-2

Rezai-Zadeh, K., Gate, D., and Town, T. (2009). CNS infil- tration of peripheral immune cells: D-Day for neurodegener- ative disease? *J. Neuroimmune Pharmacol.* 4, 462–475. doi: 10.1007/s11481-009-9166-2

Ricklin, D., Hajishengallis, G., Yang, K., and Lambris, J. D. (2010). Complement: a key system for immune surveillance and home- ostasis. *Nat. Immunol.* 11, 785–797. doi: 10.1038/ni.1923

Ridnour, L. A., Barasch, K. M., Windhausen, A. N., Dorsey, T. H., Lizardo, M. M., Yfantis, H. G., et al. (2012). Nitric oxide synthase and breast cancer: role of TIMP-1 in NO-mediated Akt activation. *PLoS ONE* 7:e44081. doi: 10.1371/ journal.pone.0044081

Ringman, J. M., O'Neill, J., Geschwind, D., Medina, L., Apostolova, L. G., Rodriguez,

Y., et al. (2007). Diffusion tensor imaging in preclin- ical and presymptomatic carriers of familial Alzheimer's disease mutations. *Brain* 130, 1767–1776. doi: 10.1093/brain/awm102

Ringheim, G. E., Szczepanik, A. M., Petko, W., Burgher, K. L., Zhu, Z., and Chao, C. C. (1998). Enhancement of beta-amyloid precursor protein transcription and expression by the soluble interleukin-6 receptor/interleukin-6 complex. *Brain Res. Mol. Brain Res.* 55, 35–44. doi: 10.1016/S0169-328X(97)00356-2

Rogers, J., Cooper, N. R., Webster, S., Schultz, J., McGeer, P. L., Styren, S. D., et al. (1992). Complement activation by beta-amyloid in Alzheimer disease. *Proc. Natl. Acad. Sci. U.S.A.* 89, 10016–10020. doi: 10.1073/pnas.89.21.10016

Rossi, F., and Bianchini, E. (1996). Synergistic induction of nitric oxide by beta-amyloid and cytokines in astrocytes. *Biochem. Biophys. Res. Commun.* 225, 474–478. doi: 10.1006/bbrc.1996.1197

Roth, A. D., Ramirez, G., Alarcon, R., and Von Bernhardi, R. (2005). Oligodendrocytes damage in Alzheimer's disease: beta amyloid toxicity and inflammation. *Biol. Res.* 38, 381–387. doi: 10.4067/S0716- 97602005000400011

Rozemuller, J. M., Eikelenboom, P., and Stam, F. C. (1986). Role of microglia in plaque formation in senile dementia of the Alzheimer type. An immunohistochemical study. *Virchows Arch. B Cell Pathol. Incl. Mol. Pathol.* 51, 247–254. doi: 10.1007/BF02899034

Rozkalne, A., Spires-Jones, T. L., Stern, E. A., and Hyman, B. T. (2009). A single dose of passive immunotherapy has extended benefits on synapses and neurites in an Alzheimer's disease mouse model. *Brain Res.* 1280, 178–185. doi:10.1016/j.brainres.2009.05.045

Rubartelli, A., and Lotze, M. T. (2007). Inside, outside, upside down: damage-associated molecular- pattern molecules (DAMPs) and redox. *Trends Immunol.* 28, 429–436. doi: 10.1016/j.it.2007. 08.004

Saez, T. E., Pehar, M., Vargas, M., Barbeito, L., and Maccioni, R. B. (2004). Astrocytic nitric oxide trig- gers tau hyperphosphorylation in hippocampal neurons. *In Vivo* 18, 275–280.

Salloway, S., Sperling, R., Gilman, S., Fox, N., Blennow, K., Raskind, M., et al. (2009). A phase 2 multiple ascending dose trial of bapineuzumab in mild to moderate Alzheimer disease. *Neurology* 73, 2061–2070. doi: 10.1212/WNL.0b013e3181c67808

Sastre, M., Dewachter, I., Rossner, S., Bogdanovic, N., Rosen, E., Borghgraef, P., et al. (2006). Nonsteroidal anti-inflammatory drugs repress -secretase gene pro- moter activity by the activation of PPAR. *Proc. Natl. Acad. Sci. U.S.A.* 103,443–448.

Sheng, J. G., Zhu, S. G., Jones, R. A., Griffin, W. S., and Mrak, R. E. (2000). Interleukin-1 promotes expression and phosphorylation of neurofilament and tau proteins *in vivo*. *Exp. Neurol.* 163,388–391. doi: 10.1006/exnr.2000.7393

Sisodia, S. S., Kim, S. H., and Thinakaran, G. (1999). Function and dysfunction of the presenilins. *Am. J. Hum. Genet.* 65, 7–12. doi: 10.1086/302475

Smyth, M. D., Cribbs, D. H., Tenner, A. J., Shankle, W. R., Dick, M., Kesslak, J. P., et al. (1994). Decreased lev- els of C1q in cerebrospinal fluid of living Alzheimer patients correlate with disease state. *Neurobiol. Aging* 15, 609–614. doi: 10.1016/0197- 4580(94)00055-7

Sofroniew, M. V., and Vinters, H. V. (2010). Astrocytes: biology and pathology. *Acta Neuropathol.* 119, 7–35. doi: 10.1007/s00401-009- 0619-8

Spires-Jones, T. L., Mielke, M. L., Rozkalne, A., Meyer-Luehmann, M., De Calignon, A., Bacskai, B. J., et al. (2009). Passive immunother- apy rapidly increases structural plasticity in a mouse model of Alzheimer disease. *Neurobiol. Dis.* 33, 213–220. doi: 10.1016/j.nbd. 2008.10.011

Sterka, D. Jr., and Marriott, I. (2006). Characterization of nucleotide- binding oligomerization domain (NOD) protein expression in primary murine microglia. *J. Neuroimmunol.* 179, 65–75. doi: 10.1016/j.jneuroim.2006.06.009

Sung, S., Yang, H., Uryu, K., Lee, E. B., Zhao, L., Shineman, D., et al. (2004). Modulation of nuclear factor-κb activity by indomethacin influences aβ levels but not aβ precursor pro- tein metabolism in a model of alzheimer's disease. *Am. J. Pathol.* 165, 2197–2206. doi: 10.1016/ S0002-9440(10)63269-5

Swaab, D. F., Raadsheer, F. C., Endert, E., Hofman, M. A., Kamphorst, W., and Ravid, R. (1994). Increased cor- tisol levels in aging and Alzheimer's disease in postmortem cere- brospinal fluid. *J. Neuroendocrinol.* 6, 681–687. doi: 10.1111/j.1365-2826.1994.tb00635.x

Szekely, C. A., Green, R. C., Breitner, J. C. S., Ostbye, T., Beiser, A. S., Corrada, M. M., et al. (2008). No advantage of "Aβ42-lowering" NSAIDs for prevention of AD insix pooled cohort studies. *Neurology* 70,2291–2298. doi:10.1212/01.wnl. 0000313933.17796.f6

Takeuchi, H., Jin, S., Wang, J., Zhang, G., Kawanokuchi, J., Kuno, R., et al. (2006). Tumor necrosis factor-alpha induces neurotoxicity via glutamate release from hemichannels of acti- vated microglia in an autocrine manner. *J. Biol. Chem.* 281, 21362–21368. doi: 10.1074/jbc. M600504200

Tarkowski, E., Issa, R., Sjogren, M., Wallin, A., Blennow, K., Tarkowski, A., et al. (2002). Increased intrathecal levels of the angiogenic factors VEGF and TGF-beta in Alzheimer's disease and vascular dementia. *Neurobiol. Aging* 23, 237–243. doi: 10.1016/ S0197-4580(01)00285-8

Tesseur, I., Zou, K., Esposito, L., Bard, F., Berber, E., Can, J. V., et al. (2006). Deficiency in neuronal TGF-beta signaling promotes neurodegener- ation and Alzheimer's pathology. *J. Clin. Invest.* 116, 3060–3069. doi: 10.1172/JCI27341

Thal, L. J., Ferris, S. H., Kirby, L., Block, G. A., Lines, C. R., Yuen, E., et al. (2005). A randomized, double-blind, study of rofecoxib in patients with mild cognitive impair- ment. *Neuropsychopharmacology* 30, 1204–1215. doi: 10.1038/sj.npp. 1300690

Torreilles, F., Salman-Tabcheh, S., Guerin, M., and Torreilles, J. (1999). Neurodegenerative disorders: the role of peroxynitrite. *Brain Res. Brain Res. Rev.* 30, 153–163. doi: 10.1016/S0165-0173(99)00014-4

Town, T., Nikolic, V., and Tan, J. (2005). The microglial "activation" continuum: from innate to adaptive responses. *J. Neuroinflammation* 2, 24. doi: 10.1186/1742-2094-2-24

Van Dam, D., Coen, K., and De Deyn, P. P. (2010). Ibuprofen mod- ifies cognitive disease progression in an Alzheimer's mouse model. *J. Psychopharmacol.* 24, 383–388. doi: 10.1177/0269881108097630

Vane, J., and Botting, R. (1987). Inflammation and the mechanism of action of anti-inflammmatory drugs. *FASEB J.* 1,89–96.

Vellas, B., Black, R., Thal, L. J., Fox, N. C., Daniels, M., McLennan, G., et al. (2009). Long-term follow-up of patients immunized with AN1792: reduced functional decline in antibody responders. *Curr. Alzheimer Res.* 6, 144. doi: 10.2174/156720509787602852

Wajant, H., Pfizenmaier, K., and Scheurich, P. (2003). Tumor necrosis factor signaling. *Cell Death Differ.* 10, 45–65. doi: 10.1038/sj.cdd.4401189

Walker, D. G., Kim, S. U., and McGeer, P. L. (1995). Complement and cytokine gene expression in cul- tured microglial derived from postmortem human brains. *J. Neurosci. Res.* 40, 478–493. doi: 10.1002/jnr.490400407

Walker, D. G., and Lue, L. F. (2005). Investigations with cultured human microglia on pathogenic mecha- nisms of Alzheimer's disease and other neurodegenerative diseases. *J. Neurosci. Res.* 81, 412–425. doi: 10.1002/jnr.20484

Wallace, M. N., Geddes, J. G., Farquhar, D. A., and Masson, M. R. (1997). Nitric oxide synthase in reactive astrocytes adjacent to beta-amyloid plaques. *Exp. Neurol.* 144,266–272. doi: 10.1006/exnr.1996.6373

Webster, S. D., Yang, A. J., Margol, L., Garzon-Rodriguez, W., Glabe, C. G., and Tenner, A. J. (2000). Complement component C1q modulates the phagocy- tosis of Abeta by microglia. *Exp. Neurol.* 161, 127–138. doi: 10.1006/ exnr.1999.7260

Wells, T. N., Power, C. A., and Proudfoot, A. E. (1998). Definition, function and pathophysiolog- ical significance of chemokine receptors. *Trends Pharmacol. Sci.* 19, 376–380. doi: 10.1016/ S0165-6147(98)01247-4

Westin, K., Buchhave, P., Nielsen, H., Minthon, L., Janciauskiene, S., and Hansson, O. (2012). CCL2 is associated with a faster rate of cognitive decline during early stages of Alzheimer's disease. *PLoS ONE* 7:e30525. doi: 10.1371/ jour- nal.pone.0030525

Wiessner, C., Wiederhold, K. H., Tissot, A. C., Frey, P., Danner, S., Jacobson, L. H., et al. (2011). The second-generation active Abeta immunotherapy CAD106 reduces amyloid accumulation in APP transgenic mice while minimizing potential side effects. *J. Neurosci.* 31, 9323–9331. doi: 10.1523/ JNEUROSCI.0293-11.2011

Williams, T. J. (1978). The role of prostaglandins in inflammation. *Ann. R. Coll. Surg. Engl.* 60, 198–201.

Wisniewski, H. M., Barcikowska, M., and Kida, E. (1991). Phagocytosis of beta/ A4 amyloid fibrils of the neuritic neocortical plaques. *Acta Neuropathol.* 81, 588–590. doi: 10.1007/BF00310142

Wyss-Coray, T., Lin, C., Yan, F., Yu, G. Q., Rohde, M., McConlogue, L., et al. (2001). TGF-beta1 promotes microglial amyloid-beta clearance and reduces plaque burden in transgenic mice. *Nat. Med.* 7, 612–618. doi:10.1038/87945

Wyss-Coray, T., Loike, J. D., Brionne, T. C., Lu, E., Anankov, R., Yan, F., et al. (2003). Adult mouse astrocytes degrade amyloid-beta *in vitro* and *in situ*. *Nat. Med.* 9, 453–457. doi: 10.1038/nm838

Wyss-Coray, T., Masliah, E., Mallory, M., McConlogue, L., Johnson- Wood, K., Lin, C., et al. (1997). Amyloidogenic role of cytokine TGF-beta1 in transgenic mice and in Alzheimer's disease. *Nature* 389, 603–606. doi:10.1038/39321

Wyss-Coray, T., Yan, F., Lin, A. H., Lambris, J. D., Alexander, J. J., Quigg, R. J., et al. (2002). Prominent neurodegeneration and increased plaque forma- tion in complement-inhibited Alzheimer's mice. *Proc. Natl. Acad. Sci. U.S.A.* 99, 10837–10842. doi: 10.1073/pnas.162350199

Xiang, Z., Ho, L., Valdellon, J., Borchelt, D., Kelley, K., Spielman, L., et al. (2002a). Cyclooxygenase (COX)-2 and cell cycle activity in a transgenic mouse model of Alzheimer's disease neuropathology. *Neurobiol. Aging* 23, 327–334. doi: 10.1016/S0197- 4580(01)00282-2

Xiang, Z., Ho, L., Yemul, S., Zhao, Z., Qing, W., Pompl, P., et al. (2002b). Cyclooxygenase-2 promotes amy- loid plaque deposition in a mouse model of Alzheimer's disease neuropathology. *Gene Expr.* 10, 271–278.

Yamagata, K., Andreasson, K. I., Kaufmann, W. E., Barnes, C. A., and Worley, P. F. (1993). Expression of a mitogen-inducible cyclooxygenase in brain neurons: regulation by synaptic activity and glucocorti- coids. *Neuron* 11, 371–386. doi: 10.1016/0896-6273(93)90192-T

Yamamoto, M., Horiba, M., Buescher, J. L., Huang, D., Gendelman, H. E., Ransohoff, R. M., et al. (2005). Overexpression of monocyte chemotactic protein-1/CCL2 in beta-amyloid precursor protein transgenic mice show accel- erated diffuse beta-amyloid deposition. *Am. J. Pathol.* 166, 1475–1485. doi: 10.1016/S0002- 9440(10)62364-4

Yamamoto, M., Kiyota, T., Horiba, M., Buescher, J. L., Walsh, S. M., Gendelman, H. E., et al. (2007). Interferon-gamma and tumor necrosis factor-alpha regulate amyloid-beta plaque deposition and beta-secretase expression in Swedish mutant APP transgenic mice. *Am. J. Pathol.* 170, 680–692. doi: 10.2353/ajpath.2007.060378

Yao, Y.-Y., Liu, D.-M., Xu, D.-F., and Li, W.-P. (2007). Memory and learn- ing impairment induced by dex- amethasone in senescent but not young mice. *Eur. J. Pharmacol.* 574, 20–28. doi: 10.1016/j.ejphar.2007. 07.021

Yermakova, A. V., Rollins, J., Callahan, M., Rogers, J., and O'Banion, K. (1999). Cyclooxygenase-1 in human Alzheimer and con- trol brain: quantitative analysis of expression by microglia and CA3 hippocampal neurons. *J. Neuropathol. Exp. Neurol.* 58, 1135–1146. doi: 10.1097/00005072- 199911000-00003

Yip, A. G., Green, R. C., Huyck, M., Cupples, L. A., and Farrer, L. A. (2005). Nonsteroidal anti- inflammatory drug use and Alzheimer's disease risk: the MIRAGE Study. *BMC Geriatr.* 5:2. doi: 10.1186/1471-2318-5-2

Zilka, N., Kazmerova, Z., Jadhav, S., Neradil, P., Madari, A., Obetkova, D., et al. (2012). Who fans the flames of Alzheimer's disease brains? Misfolded tau on the crossroad of neurodegenera- tive and inflammatory pathways. *J. Neuroinflammation* 9, 47. doi: 10.1186/1742-2094-9-47

15

The gateway theory: bridging neural and immune interactions in the CNS

Daisuke Kamimura, Moe Yamada, Masaya Harada, Lavannya Sabharwal, Jie Meng, Hidenori Bando, Hideki Ogura, Toru Atsumi, Yasunobu Arima and Masaaki Murakami*

JST-CREST, WPI Immunology Frontier Research Center, Graduate School of Frontier Biosciences, Graduate School of Medicine, Osaka University, Suita, Osaka, Japan

Edited by:
Jaleel A. Miyan, The University of Manchester, UK

Reviewed by:
Synthia H. Mellon, University of California, San Francisco, USA
Emmanuel Pinteaux, The University of Manchester, UK

****Correspondence:***
Masaaki Murakami, Center for Advanced Science and Innovation, Building A, 4th floor, Office for University-Industory Collaboration, Room 401, 2-1, Yamada-oka, Suita, Osaka 565-0871, Japan
e-mail: murakami@molonc.med.osaka-u.ac.jp

The central nervous system (CNS) is considered an immune-privileged tissue protected by a specific vessel structure, the blood-brain barrier (BBB). Upon infection or traumatic injury in the CNS, the BBB is breached, and various immune cells are recruited to the affected area. In the case of autoimmune diseases in the CNS like multiple sclerosis (MS), autoreactive T cells against some CNS-specific antigens can theoretically attack neurons throughout the CNS. The affected CNS regions in MS patients can be detected as multiple focal plaques in the cerebrum, thoracic cord, and other regions. Vision problems are often associated with the initial phase of MS, suggesting a disturbance in the optic nerves. These observations raise the possibility that there exist specific signals that direct autoreactive T cells past the BBB and into particular sites of the CNS. Using a mouse model of MS, experimental autoimmune encephalomyelitis (EAE), we recently defined the mechanism of the pathogenesis in which regional neural stimulations modulate the status of the blood vessel endothelium to allow the invasion of autoreactive T cells into specific sites of the CNS via the fifth lumbar cord. This gate for autoreactive T cells can be artificially manipulated by removing gravity forces on the hind legs or by electric pulses to the soleus muscles, quadriceps, and triceps of mice, resulting in an accumulation of autoreactive T cells in the intended regions via the activation of regional neurons. Gating blood vessels by regional neural stimulations, a phenomenon we call the gateway theory, has potential therapeutic value not only in preventing autoimmunity, but also in augmenting the effects of cancer immunotherapies.

Keywords: inflammation, cytokines, autoimmune diseases, inflammatory diseases, multiple sclerosis, gateway theory, neural activation, blood-brain barrier

INTRODUCTION

The immune system is a sophisticated protective mechanism that coordinates many types of bone-marrow derived hematopoietic cells including T cells, B cells, dendritic cells, and macrophages among others that have evolved to combat infectious agents and cancerous cells in the body. Careful regulation is required to control the immune system, because uncontrollable immune reactions, or chronic inflammation, are harmful and considered the pathogenesis of many diseases. It has been long recognized yet not well elucidated that neural activation directly influences the immune system. For example, mentally ill stresses in mice promote tumor progression, while good stresses, or eustress, which are induced by an enriched housing environment with increased space, physical activity, and social interactions, suppress it (Cao et al., 2010; Feng et al., 2012; Hassan et al., 2013). In human patients with autoimmune diseases, it has been suggested that psychological stresses including depression and anxiety are associated with disease progression and relapse (Mitsonis et al., 2009; Srivastava and Boyer, 2010). Whereas systemic modulation of the immune system by the nervous system through the secretion of corticosteroid is relatively well characterized, the regional interplay between these two biological systems is just beginning to be elucidated. Here we discuss the regional neuro-immune interactions during chronic inflammations including our recent findings.

INFLAMMATION UNDERLIES MANY TYPES OF CHRONIC DISEASES

Traditionally, inflammation has been defined as pathophysiological symptoms with dolor, calor, rubor, and tumor (Latin for pain, heat, redness, and swelling, respectively). We now know that these symptoms are the consequences of the local accumulation and activation of immune cells that produce soluble factors such as cytokines and lipid mediators. Therefore, it is not an oversimplification to define inflammation as a biological mechanism that locally recruits various immune cells followed by the disruption of local homeostasis. Inflammation, or the accumulation of immune cells, basically acts as a protective mechanism against infectious agents including viruses and bacteria. In fact, mice genetically lacking T lymphocytes, which secrete various cytokines to orchestrate the immune reactions (CD4+ helper T cells) and exert cytotoxic activities that kill unnecessary or undesirable cells, such as infected cells as well as cancer cells (CD8+ killer T cells), are unable to control pathogen invasion via inflammation induction.

At the same time, inflammation has to resolve immediately after these incidences come to an end, since chronically persistent inflammation has a rather adverse effect. Autoimmune diseases such as rheumatoid arthritis (RA) and multiple sclerosis (MS) are good examples of diseases that involve chronic inflammation. Signs of inflammation (i.e., local accumulation of immune cells followed by dysregulation of local homeostasis) are evident in the joints and the central nervous system (CNS) of RA and MS patients, respectively. We have also found the similar phenomena in the target organs of animal models for these diseases. In addition, accumulating evidence indicates that chronic inflammation underlies the pathogenesis of many other types of disorders including neurodegenerative diseases, metabolic syndromes, and even psychiatric diseases (Hamdani et al., 2012; Tabas and Glass, 2013). Thus, understanding the molecular mechanisms that convert protective acute inflammation into harmful chronic inflammation and how chronic inflammation persists is essential to the development of novel therapeutic interventions for many diseases and disorders.

THE INFLAMMATION AMPLIFIER PROVIDES A MOLECULAR MECHANISM FOR CHRONIC INFLAMMATION

ESTABLISHMENT OF A RHEUMATOID ARTHRITIS MODEL, F759 MICE

Interleukin (IL)-6 is a well-studied cytokine that promotes inflammation. In fact, IL-6 is found upregulated in the serum and affected areas of human diseases and disorders such as synovial fluids in the case of RA, while genome-wide association studies (GWAS) have revealed that the IL-6 gene is genetically associated with a wide range of diseases including autoimmunity, neurodegenerative diseases, and cancer (http://geneticassociationdb.nih.gov/). Therefore, the establishment of an IL-6-dependent disease model has been desired for understanding the pathogenesis of various inflammatory diseases. IL-6 signals emanating from IL-6 receptor complexes, gp130 and IL-6R, involve the activation of STAT3, the central transcription factor for the many biological effects of IL-6. SOCS3 is a target gene of IL-6 and known to negatively regulate the signal transduction of IL-6 by binding to the receptor subunit gp130 and Jak kinases (Kamimura et al., 2003; Murakami et al., 2004). Given that IL-6 is abundant in patients with inflammatory disorders, we hypothesized that persistent activation of IL-6/gp130 signaling might induce inflammatory diseases. We therefore generated a knock-in mouse with a point mutation at the binding site of SOCS3 in gp130, thereby enhancing the IL-6 signal pathway (Ohtani et al., 2000). As expected, this mouse strain, called F759 mice, develops RA-like joint diseases spontaneously (Atsumi et al., 2002).

DISCOVERY OF THE INFLAMMATION AMPLIFIER

Breeding experiments with various deficient mouse strains showed the joint disease in F759 mice mainly relies on CD4+ T cells, IL-6, and IL-17, which is a recently reported helper T-cell-derived cytokine involved in autoimmunity and activation of the transcription factor NF-κB (Sawa et al., 2006; Ogura et al., 2008). Indeed, the number of an IL-17-secreting CD4+ T cell subtype (Th17 cells) and the serum levels of IL-17 were increased in F759 mice. Furthermore, systemic expressions of IL-17 or IL-6 in F759 mice accelerated the disease onset and, interestingly, induced the production of IL-6 itself, suggesting a positive feedback loop (Ogura et al., 2008). Moreover, IL-17 expression in F759 mice induced an excessive level of IL-6 and chemokines. *In vitro* experiments using fibroblasts confirmed that IL-6 is a target of the simultaneous treatment of IL-17 and IL-6, but not of either cytokine alone (Ogura et al., 2008). DNA microarray analysis revealed that many chemokines are also targets of this synergism. Since chemokines recruit immune cells to promote inflammation via the dysregulation of local homeostasis, we named this synergistic mechanism the inflammation amplifier (formerly, IL-6 amplifier) (**Figure 1**) (Murakami and Hirano, 2012). Activation of the inflammation amplifier in endothelial cells is induced by the simultaneous activation of NF-κB and STAT3 followed by chemokine expressions. We expected that NF-κB and STAT3 stimulants, whether they are proinflammatory or anti-inflammatory cytokines, should enhance the expression of the chemokines. However, anti-inflammatory cytokines might indirectly suppress the activation of the inflammation amplifier by inhibiting activated helper T cells, which express various NF-κB and STAT3 stimulants including IL-17, IL-6, and TNFα. Moreover, as discussed in detail below, the inflammation amplifier, which can be regulated by neural inputs such as norepinephrine (NE), enhances the production of chemokines via NF-κB activation (**Figure 1**) (Arima et al., 2012).

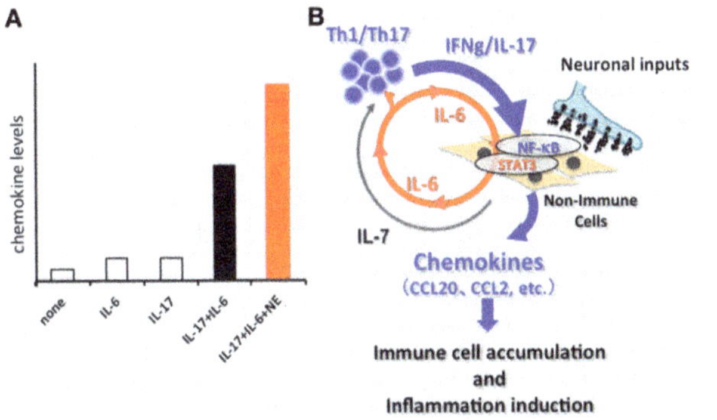

FIGURE 1 | The inflammation amplifier. (A) Image of the activation of the inflammation amplifier in the presence and absence of NE. A combination of IL-17 and IL-6 causes a synergistic effect on the induction of inflammation-amplifier target chemokines such as CCL20 in non-immune cells including fibroblasts, endothelial cells, and certain synovial cells. NE further enhances the chemokine production. Other neurotransmitters can also influence activation of the inflammation amplifier. See Arima et al. (2012) for the original data. **(B)** The synergistic effect seen in **(A)** requires the concomitant activation of two transcriptions factors, NF-kB and STAT3. In the case of autoimmune diseases, Th-17 derived IL-17 induces an initially low amount of IL-6 from non-immune cells via NF-κB activation. Secreted IL-6 together with IL-17 forms a positive feedback loop to produce excessive expression of the target genes including many inflammatory chemokines such as CCL20, CCL2, etc. Consequently, various immune cells are recruited at the region around the target cells via chemokine expression, and inflammation takes place. Persistent activation of the inflammation amplifier, as is the case in F759 mice, drives chronic inflammation. IL-7, a target of the amplifier and derived from non-immune cells, fuels the proliferation, and survival of Th17 cells. The activation of the inflammation amplifier can be modulated by regional neural activation.

THE INFLAMMATION AMPLIFIER IS ASSOCIATED WITH VARIOUS HUMAN DISEASES AND DISORDERS

Mice deficient in gp130 or STAT3 in fibroblasts and/or endothelial cells (i.e., inflammation amplifier-defective non-immune cells) are highly resistant to animal disease models including RA, MS, and allogeneic graft rejection, demonstrating that the inflammation amplifier is critical for multiple chronic inflammatory diseases *in vivo* (Ogura et al., 2008; Murakami et al., 2011; Arima et al., 2012; Lee et al., 2012). To explore the molecular mechanisms underlying the inflammation amplifier, we recently conducted genome-wide functional screening and identified around 1700 candidates that positively regulate it.

Interestingly, genes associated with human diseases including not only autoimmunity, but also metabolic syndromes, neurodegenerative diseases, and other inflammatory diseases including allergies and atopic dermatitis were significantly enriched in the candidate genes (Murakami et al., 2013). Based on these findings, we propose that de novo mutations, expression alterations, or epigenetic changes of these genes in non-immune cells during acute inflammation can cause dysregulation of the amplifier like that observed in F759 mice (i.e., a point-mutation of gp130), turning acute inflammation into a pathogenic chronic version.

NEURO-IMMUNE INTERACTIONS MEDIATE IMMUNE HOMEOSTASIS AND PATHOGENESIS

AUTOREACTIVE CD4+ T CELLS ENTER THE CNS FROM THE FIFTH LUMBAR CORD

MS is a chronic inflammatory disease in the CNS that, according to a recent genome-wide association study, involves CD4+ T cells (International Multiple Sclerosis Genetics et al., 2011). An animal model of MS, experimental autoimmune encephalomyelitis (EAE), is widely used to study the pathogenesis of MS, and autoreactive CD4+ T cells, in particular Th17 cells, have been demonstrated to be essential for the disease induction (Komiyama et al., 2006). In these experiments, mice or rats were immunized with CNS antigens such as myelin oligodendrocyte glycoprotein (MOG) or a proteolipid protein, resulting in the generation of autoreactive CD4+ T cells that target the CNS and the development of MS-like symptoms including progressive paralysis, particularly in the lower body. EAE can also be induced by a passive transfer method that is performed via the intravenous transfer of these autoreactive CD4+ T cells into naïve recipient animals. Indeed, the passive transfer method is suitable to track the behavior of the disease-causing CD4+ T cells without affecting the immune system systemically by adjuvant treatment. We have shown using the transfer method-induced EAE that the inflammation amplifier is critically involved in EAE development, because the disease symptoms were significantly ameliorated in amplifier-deficient mice such as type-1 collagen cre/gp130flox mice (Ogura et al., 2008; Arima et al., 2012). These results challenge traditional theories, because the blood-brain barrier (BBB) should block the migration of the pathogenic CD4+ T cells into the CNS. We thus sought the initial site where autoreactive CD4+ T cells invade the CNS during the development of EAE. A clinical symptom of typical EAE constantly begins with a loss of tonicity in the tail tip, suggesting immune attacks at a particular site in the lower body despite the uniform presence of the autoantigens in the CNS. Whole-mount sections of adult mice at a preclinical stage of EAE revealed that MOG-reactive CD4+ T cells preferentially entered the CNS from the dorsal vessels of the fifth lumbar (L5) cord (Arima et al., 2012).

DORSAL VESSELS OF THE L5 CORD EXPRESS VARIOUS CHEMOKINES VIA ACTIVATION OF THE INFLAMMATION AMPLIFIER, EVEN AT STEADY STATE

This accumulation of CD4+ T cells is dependent on the inflammation amplifier, as expected. In addition, the treatment of mice with antibodies against CCL20, a chemokine potently recruiting Th17 and a target gene of the inflammation amplifier, suppressed the CD4+ T cell accumulation at the L5 dorsal vessels, suggesting that amplifier-mediated CCL20 overproduction causes the recruitment of pathogenic Th17 at the L5 cord (Arima et al., 2012). In fact, not only CCL20, but also various chemokines were upregulated at L5 dorsal vessels during EAE as compared to dorsal vessels from the other spinal levels. Unexpectedly, the upregulation of chemokines at L5 vessels was observed even under steady state (i.e., the natural condition). Given that a certain number of immune cells are present in the CNS, probably for the purpose of immune surveillance, and that the CNS-resident microglia is of bone-marrow origin, the increase of chemokines at the L5 cord may function as a gate for their precursors from the periphery to the CNS, although further studies are needed to confirm this conclusion.

REGIONAL NEURAL ACTIVATION INDUCED BY GRAVITY PLAYS A ROLE IN CHEMOKINE EXPRESSION AT THE L5 GATE

Why the L5 is the location of the gate was answered by investigating a neuro-immune interaction. It is known that sensory neurons in the dorsal root ganglion (DRG) beside the L5 cord are connected to the soleus muscles, the main anti-gravity muscles (Ohira et al., 2004). We considered whether constant stimulation of the soleus muscles by a gravity force might mediate entry of the MOG-specific Th17 cells at the L5 cord. Indeed, when mice were tail-suspended so that the hind limbs were released from the gravity stimuli (**Figure 2**), MOG-specific Th17 cells no longer accumulated at the L5 cord. Instead, these Th17

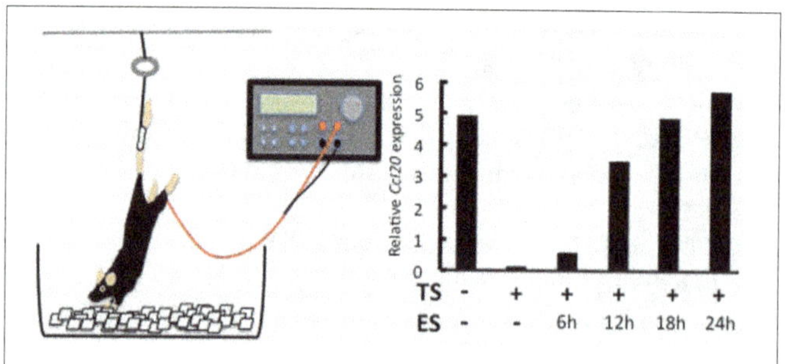

FIGURE 2 | Effects of regional neural activation on the invasion of Th17 cells into the CNS. Tail suspension and electric stimulation of the soleus muscles **(left)**. Tail suspension (TS) reduces CCL20 expression in the L5 dorsal vessel. Electric stimulations (ES) to the soleus muscles of TS mice restore the chemokine expression in a time-dependent manner **(right)**. See Arima et al. (2012) for the original data.

cells accumulated at cervical cords as if a new gate was opened by a gravitational burden on the fore limb muscles (Arima et al., 2012). Consistently, the tail suspension suppressed CCL20 mRNA expression in the L5 dorsal blood vessels and decreased the expression of the neural activation marker c-fos in the L5 DRG. Moreover, artificial electric stimulations to the soleus muscles of the tail-suspended mice restored CCL20 expression (**Figure 2**) and Th17 accumulation at the L5 cord, as well as c-fos levels in the L5 DRG (Arima et al., 2012). These results strongly suggest that neural inputs from the soleus muscles in response to the gravity force play a role in activating the inflammation amplifier and lead to the expression of various chemokines including Th17-attracting CCL20 in L5 dorsal blood vessels.

A SENSORY-SYMPATHETIC INTERACTION IS CRITICAL FOR THE L5 ENTRY OF THE AUTOREACTIVE T CELLS

What mechanisms do afferent sensory neurons from the soleus muscles use to regulate the status of blood vessels at L5? Although a precise neural network remains elusive, we have shown sympathetic nerves to be involved. Blood flow speeds at L5 dorsal vessels become slower when mice are tail suspended, while electronic stimulation of the soleus muscles increases the flow speed. These results clearly suggest that autonomic nerves including sympathetic neurons are involved in the response to the tail suspension. In addition, blood flow speeds in blood vessels other than the L5 region, such as the femoral vessels, brain surface vessels, and the portal vein, are not affected by tail suspension (Arima et al., 2012). Furthermore, treatment with atenolol, a β1 adrenergic receptor antagonist, or prazosin, an α1 adrenergic receptor antagonist, significantly inhibits CCL20 mRNA expression, NF-κB mRNA expression, and MOG-reactive Th17 accumulation at L5 vessels and also suppresses clinical signs of EAE (Arima et al., 2012). Consistent with these *in vivo* results, the addition of NE, which is a neurotransmitter from sympathetic neurons, to a culture of endothelial cells enhances chemokine expressions mediated by the activation of the inflammation amplifier (**Figure 1A**). Thus, anti-gravity responses of the soleus muscles lead to sympathetic nerve stimulation, creating a gateway for immune cells to pass through the CNS via L5 dorsal vessels (Arima et al., 2012). Based on these findings, we concluded that MOG-reactive, disease-causing Th17 cells make use of the L5 gateway to infiltrate the CNS and induce local inflammation by producing cytokines like IL-17 and IL-6, which further induces chemokines via the inflammation amplifier in parenchymal non-immune cells and results in chronic inflammation in the CNS (**Figure 3**). Thus, the neural response triggered by the gravity force creates a gate for immune cells to invade the CNS, although we also hypothesize that the clearance and/or apoptosis of immune cells in the CNS may contribute to the feed-forward mechanism of continued neuroinflammation (Goldmann et al., 2006). Our findings also imply that various types of neural activity affect the disease status differently. Indeed, we found and are currently studying the mechanism for how certain physical or mental stresses cause the deterioration or relapse of EAE in mice, which will shed new light on the molecular mechanism of the relapse and remission of MS.

THE GATEWAY THEORY

Neuronal innervation occurs throughout the body and appropriately controls all organs. One potential strategy to therapeutically manage neuro-immune interactions is to find and stimulate the appropriate peripheral neurons connected to the organs to be treated. To test this theory, we selectively stimulated sensory neurons via electric stimulations of different muscles and observed local chemokine expressions in the vessels of spinal cords as a

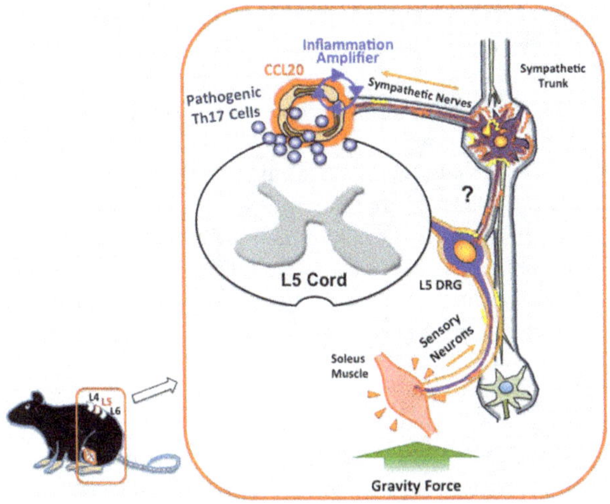

FIGURE 3 | Gateway for autoreactive T cells into the CNS. Continuous stimulation of the soleus muscles by gravity leads to the constant activation of L5 DRG sensory neurons, followed by the activation of sympathetic neurons at the L5 region via unidentified circuits (?). NE, a neurotransmitter from sympathetic neurons, augments the inflammation amplifier at the dorsal vessels of L5, causing an elevation of CCL20 and subsequent Th17 infiltration into the CNS.

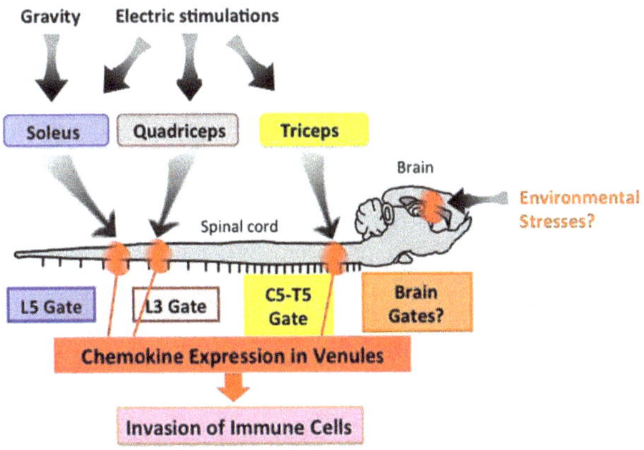

FIGURE 4 | The gateway theory. Electric pulses to the upper arm, thigh, and soleus muscles induce activation of the inflammation amplifier (chemokine upregulation), thereby opening a gate in the dorsal vessels of the fifth cervical to fifth thoracic (C5-T5), third lumbar (L3), and fifth lumbar (L5) cords, respectively. Environmental stresses such as those from social interactions and mental stresses might create a specific gate in the brain. This effect is potentially an attractive target for manipulating immune cell migration *in vivo*.

marker of the inflammatory response. Thigh muscles including the quadriceps are known to be regulated by L3 DRG neurons. Interestingly, electronic stimulation of these muscles followed by L3 DRG activation led to an increased expression of CCL20 in the L3 cord dorsal vessels of mice (Arima et al., 2012). In a similar fashion, chemokine levels in the fifth cervical to fifth thoracic cord vessels were upregulated by stimulations of the epitrochlearis/triceps brachii and upper arm muscles, are controlled by neurons located at the corresponding areas (**Figure 4**) (Arima et al., 2012). Based on these results, we propose "the gateway theory," which describes blood vessels that act as gates for immune cell infiltration into organs and is dependent on regional neural stimulations. The theory is supported by empirical evidence that shows stresses from environments can affect the disease status and trigger relapse in MS patients. Experimentally, we have found that certain environmental stresses influence the disease progression in EAE mice by creating gates for autoreactive helper T cells to enter the CNS (manuscript in preparation). We hypothesize that these stresses create gates at certain CNS vessels via neural control of the inflammation amplifier to modify the disease status at specific vessels (**Figure 4**).

FUTURE DIRECTIONS

Investigations on whether the gateway theory can be more generally applied to tissues beyond the CNS are currently ongoing. If true, artificial manipulation of the gate should have significant clinical benefits, as closing it in normal cells would dampen autoimmune inflammation in a target organ without any systemic immune suppression, while opening it in tumors could enhance cancer immunotherapy. The precise molecular mechanisms for gating still need to be studied, however, to confirm this possibility.

REFERENCES

Arima, Y., Harada, M., Kamimura, D., Park, J. H., Kawano, F., Yull, F. E., et al. (2012). Regional neural activation defines a gateway for autoreactive T cells to cross the blood-brain barrier. *Cell* 148, 447–457. doi: 10.1016/j.cell.2012.01.022

Atsumi, T., Ishihara, K., Kamimura, D., Ikushima, H., Ohtani, T., Hirota, S., et al. (2002). A point mutation of Tyr-759 in interleukin 6 family cytokine receptor subunit gp130 causes autoimmune arthritis. *J. Exp. Med.* 196, 979–990. doi: 10.1084/jem.20020619

Cao, L., Liu, X., Lin, E. J., Wang, C., Choi, E. Y., Riban, V., et al. (2010). Environmental and genetic activation of a brain-adipocyte BDNF/leptin axis causes cancer remission and inhibition. *Cell* 142, 52–64. doi: 10.1016/j.cell.2010.05.029

Feng, Z., Liu, L., Zhang, C., Zheng, T., Wang, J., Lin, M., et al. (2012). Chronic restraint stress attenuates p53 function and promotes tumorigenesis. *Proc. Natl. Acad. Sci. U.S.A.* 109, 7013–7018. doi: 10.1073/pnas.1203930109

Goldmann, J., Kwidzinski, E., Brandt, C., Mahlo, J., Richter, D., and Bechmann, I. (2006). T cells traffic from brain to cervical lymph nodes via the cribroid plate and the nasal mucosa. *J. Leukoc. Biol.* 80, 797–801. doi: 10.1189/jlb.0306176

Hamdani, N., Tamouza, R., and Leboyer, M. (2012). Immuno- inflammatory markers of bipolar disorder: a review of evidence. *Front. Biosci.* 4, 2170–2182. doi: 10.2741/534

Hassan, S., Karpova, Y., Baiz, D., Yancey, D., Pullikuth, A., Flores, A., et al. (2013). Behavioral stress accelerates prostate cancer development in mice. *J. Clin. Invest.* 123, 874–886. doi: 10.1172/JCI63324

International Multiple Sclerosis Genetics, C., Wellcome Trust Case Control, C., Sawcer, S., Hellenthal, G., Pirinen, M., Spencer, C. C., et al. (2011). Genetic risk and a primary role for cell-mediated immune mechanisms in multiple sclerosis. *Nature* 476, 214–219. doi: 10.1038/nature10251

Kamimura, D., Ishihara, K., and Hirano, T. (2003). IL-6 signal transduction and its physiological roles: the signal orchestration model. *Rev. Physiol. Biochem. Pharmacol.* 149, 1–38. doi: 10.1007/s10254-003-0012-2

Komiyama, Y., Nakae, S., Matsuki, T., Nambu, A., Ishigame, H., Kakuta, S., et al. (2006). IL-17 plays an important role in the development of experimental autoimmune encephalomyelitis. *J. Immunol.* 177, 566–573.

Lee, J., Nakagiri, T., Oto, T., Harada, M., Morii, E., Shintani, Y., et al. (2012). IL-6 amplifier, NF-kappaB-triggered positive feedback for IL-6 signaling, in grafts is involved in allogeneic rejection responses. *J. Immunol.* 189, 1928–1936. doi: 10.4049/jimmunol.1103613

Mitsonis, C. I., Potagas, C., Zervas, I., and Sfagos, K. (2009). The effects of stressful life events on the course of multiple sclerosis: a review. *Int. J. Neurosci.* 119, 315–335. doi: 10.1080/00207450802480192

Murakami, M., Harada, M., Kamimura, D., Ogura, H., Okuyama, Y., Kumai, N., et al. (2013). Disease-association analysis of the IL-6-amplifier, an inflammation-related feedback loop. *Cell Rep.* 3, 946–959. doi: 10.1016/j.celrep.2013.01.028

Murakami, M., and Hirano, T. (2012). The pathological and physiological roles of IL-6 amplifier activation. *Int. J. Biol. Sci.* 8, 1267–1280. doi: 10.7150/ijbs.4828

Murakami, M., Kamimura, D., and Hirano, T. (2004). New IL-6 (gp130) family cytokine members, CLC/NNT1/BSF3 and IL-27. *Growth Factors* 22, 75–77. doi: 10.1080/08977190410001715181

Murakami, M., Okuyama, Y., Ogura, H., Asano, S., Arima, Y., Tsuruoka, M., et al. (2011). Local microbleeding facilitates IL-6- and IL-17-dependent arthritis in the absence of tissue antigen recognition by activated T cells. *J. Exp. Med.* 208, 103–114. doi: 10.1084/jem.20100900

Ogura, H., Murakami, M., Okuyama, Y., Tsuruoka, M., Kitabayashi, C., Kanamoto, M., et al. (2008). Interleukin-17 promotes autoimmunity by triggering a positive-feedback loop via interleukin-6 induction. *Immunity* 29, 628–636. doi: 10.1016/j.immuni.2008.07.018

Ohira, Y., Kawano, F., Stevens, J. L., Wang, X. D., and Ishihara, A. (2004). Load-dependent regulation of neuromuscular system. *J. Gravit. Physiol.* 11, P127–P128.

Ohtani, T., Ishihara, K., Atsumi, T., Nishida, K., Kaneko, Y., Miyata, T., et al. (2000). Dissection of signaling cascades through gp130 *in vivo*: reciprocal roles for STAT3- and SHP2-mediated signals in immune responses. *Immunity* 12, 95–105. doi: 10.1016/S1074-7613(00)80162-4

Sawa, S., Kamimura, D., Jin, G. H., Morikawa, H., Kamon, H., Nishihara, M., et al. (2006). Autoimmune arthritis associated with mutated interleukin (IL)-6 receptor gp130 is driven by STAT3/IL-7-dependent homeostatic proliferation of CD4+ T cells. *J. Exp. Med.* 203, 1459–1470. doi: 10.1084/jem.20052187

Srivastava, S., and Boyer, J. L. (2010). Psychological stress is associated with relapse in type 1 autoimmune hepatitis. *Liver Int.* 30, 1439–1447. doi: 10.1111/j.1478-3231.2010.02333.x

Tabas, I., and Glass, C. K. (2013). Anti-inflammatory therapy in chronic disease: challenges and opportunities. *Science* 339, 166–172. doi: 10.1126/science.1230720

Fetal cholinergic anti-inflammatory pathway and necrotizing enterocolitis: the brain-gut connection begins *in utero*

L. Garzoni[1,2], C. Faure[1,2] and M.G. Frasch[1,3]*

[1] *CHU Sainte Justine Research Center, Montreal, QC, Canada*
[2] *Division of Gastroenterology, Hepatology and Nutrition, CHU Sainte-Justine, Montreal, QC, Canada*
[3] *Department of Obstetrics and Gynaecology, University of Montreal, Montreal, QC, Canada*

Edited by:
Beatriz Gomez-Gonzalez, Universidad Autonoma Metropolitana, Mexico

Reviewed by:
Lisa Goehler, University of Virginia, USA
Gianluca Matteoli, KU Leuven, Belgium

****Correspondence:***
M.G. Frasch, CHU Sainte-Justine Research Center, 3175 Côte Sainte Catherine, Montreal, QC H3T 1C5, Canada
e-mail: mg.frasch@umontreal.ca

Necrotizing enterocolitis (NEC) is an acute neonatal inflammatory disease that affects the intestine and may result in necrosis, systemic sepsis and multisystem organ failure. NEC affects 5–10% of all infants with birth weight ≤ 1500 g or gestational age less than 30 weeks. Chorioamnionitis (CA) is the main manifestation of pathological inflammation in the fetus and is strong associated with NEC. CA affects 20% of full-term pregnancies and upto 60% of preterm pregnancies and, notably, is often an occult finding. Intrauterine exposure to inflammatory stimuli may switch innate immunity cells such as macrophages to a reactive phenotype ("priming"). Confronted with renewed inflammatory stimuli during labour or postnatally, such sensitized cells can sustain a chronic or exaggerated production of proinflammatory cytokines associated with NEC (two-hit hypothesis). Via the cholinergic anti-inflammatory pathway, a neurally mediated innate anti-inflammatory mechanism, higher levels of vagal activity are associated with lower systemic levels of proinflammatory cytokines. This effect is mediated by the α7 subunit nicotinic acetylcholine receptor (α7nAChR) on macrophages. The gut is the most extensive organ innervated by the vagus nerve; it is also the primary site of innate immunity in the newborn. Here we review the mechanisms of possible neuroimmunological brain-gut interactions involved in the induction and control of antenatal intestinal inflammatory response and priming. We propose a neuroimmunological framework to (1) study the long-term effects of perinatal intestinal response to infection and (2) to uncover new targets for preventive and therapeutic intervention.

Keywords: necrotizing enterocolitis, chorioamnionitis, preterm birth, inflammation, neuroimmunology, vagus nerve, intestines, prevention

INTRODUCTION

In this review we summarize the emerging understanding of the mechanisms of necrotizing enterocolitis (NEC; **Table 1**) of the neonate and the clinical significance of the cholinergic anti-inflammatory pathway (CAP) as a neuroimmunological mechanism to prevent NEC. We propose how this emerging understanding of neuroimmunological basis for the NEC etiology may lead to new avenues of clinical research that could result in low cost widely available treatment strategies of NEC across the world. Overall, this review provides a comprehensive, up-to-date review of the literature about the role of CAP in the pathogenesis of NEC as a neuroimmunological modulation system and the emerging therapeutic strategies.

THE BURDEN OF NEC

NEC is an acute neonatal inflammatory disease that affects the intestine and may result in necrosis, systemic sepsis and multisystem organ failure. The incidence varies from 0.3 to 2.4 infants per 1000 live births, with nearly 90% of cases occurring in infants born at less than 36 weeks' gestation. NEC affects 5–10% of all infants with birth weight ≤ 1500 g or gestational age less than 30 weeks, and 2–5% of all preterm neonates (Lin and Stoll, 2006). NEC accounts for up to 8% of all admissions to the neonatal intensive care unit. Moreover, with the increased survival of very preterm infants with birth weights ≤ 800 g, the incidence of NEC has increased, despite surfactant replacement therapy (Lin et al., 2008). NEC is the leading cause of death and long-term disability from gastrointestinal disease in preterm infants. Overall mortality ranges from 10–50%, approaching 100% in infants with the most severe form of the disease, which is characterized by full-thickness destruction of the intestine leading to intestinal perforation, peritonitis, bacterial invasion, sepsis and multiorgan failure.

A NEC diagnosis in the very low birth weight infant poses a significant burden to the individual family and the neonatal community, as well as a serious financial burden to society as a whole. NEC is not only one of the most serious clinical problems in neonates, but also one of the most challenging to treat.

Table 1 | Abbreviations.

CAP	Cholinergic anti-inflammatory pathway
CNS	Central nervous system
ENS	Enteric nervous system
LPS	Lipopolysaccharide
α7nAChR	α7 subunit nicotinic acetylcholine receptor
NEC	Necrotizing enterocolitis
TNF-α	Tumor necrosis factor alpha

Because the etiology and underlying mechanisms are unknown, treatment is symptomatic. Minor cases and early stages are managed with antibiotics and cessation of oral feeding; advanced cases, marked by intestinal necrosis, may require intestinal resection.

Despite several decades of research on the pathogenesis of NEC (Hunter et al., 2008), the overall mortality rate remains high and our overall understanding of its causes remains low. Clearly, a more complete understanding of the causes of NEC is required to design more effective and widely affordable preventive strategies aimed at reducing the incidence of NEC as well as therapies (Bisquera et al., 2002; Ganapathy et al., 2012).

CHORIOAMNIONITIS: PATHOLOGICAL FETAL INFLAMMATION IS A RISK FACTOR

The events leading to NEC are complex and multifactorial, including preterm birth, complicated early neonatal trajectory, adverse intrauterine environment and poor perinatal transition. The most important ones are preterm birth and a history of enteral feeding (Lin and Stoll, 2006). Chorioamnionitis is the main manifestation of pathological inflammation in the fetus and affects 20% of term pregnancies and up to 60% of preterm pregnancies and is commonly an occult finding (Lahra and Jeffery, 2004; Gotsch et al., 2007). Chorioamnionitis is histologically defined by the presence of polymorphonuclear infiltrates in the placenta and its membranes. Even silent, asymptomatic inflammation may inhibit placental angiogenesis and thus modulate the course of the pregnancy (Garnier et al., 2008). Thus, a significant number of fetuses are exposed to various degrees of inflammation, which impacts on their intestinal development. Chorioamnionitis associated with maternal infection has been strongly implicated in fetal intracerebral hemorrhage (Andrews et al., 2006, 2008; Aziz et al., 2009). However, an increased incidence of NEC has also been reported in neonates of mothers presenting with chorioamnionitis, in several independent studies (Andrews et al., 2006; Aziz et al., 2009; Been et al., 2009) as well as a recent meta-analysis (Been et al., 2013), where clinical chorioamnionitis (OR 1.24; 95%, CI 1.02–1.52) and histological chorioamnionitis with fetal involvement (CI 3.29; 95%, OR 1.87–5.78) were significantly associated with NEC. However, the association of histological chorioamnionitis with NEC was not statistically significant. The role of prenatal infection in the development of NEC is most significant in very preterm infants (24–26 weeks' gestational age) (Aziz et al., 2009), but is also apparent in preterm births < 32 weeks (Andrews et al., 2006; Been et al., 2009) and in full-term births (Martinez-Tallo et al., 1997).

TIGHT JUNCTIONS: INTESTINAL PERMEABILITY AND INTEGRITY

After birth, the intestinal lumen is subject to external environmental influences, including bacterial colonization of the gastrointestinal tract (Gronlund et al., 1999). Cells that cover the intestinal surface must form a barrier to protect the "*milieu intérieur*" from the external world and prevent unrestricted exchange of materials. The intestinal epithelial barrier needs to allow the passage of water and nutrients but prevent microbial contamination and the invasion of interstitial tissues by foreign antigens (**Figure 1**) (Turner, 2009). Tight junctions, essential to the paracellular pathway, are the primary determinants of barrier function. Tight junctions are situated at the apical pole of epithelial cells, and comprise over 50 associated proteins. The first group includes claudins (a family of at least 24 members) and occludin. These proteins span the plasma membrane and are attached to a second group of proteins including zonula occludens (ZO) -1, -2 and -3, which link them to actin and myosin in the cytoskeleton (Turner, 2009).

The properties of tight junctions differ from one tissue to another, as evidenced by the 1000-fold variation in electrical resistance between different epithelia. Barrier properties are not fixed: they can be modulated and regulated on a short- or long-term basis. Short-term regulation is achieved by deformation of the cytoskeleton: myosin light chain phosphorylation permits interaction with actin and contraction of the actin filaments in the perijunctional ring. Contraction of the actin filaments favours the passage of macromolecules by opening the pores. Myosin light chain kinase-1 (MLCK-1) controls the phosphorylation/dephosphorylation of the myosin light chains in the villus enterocytes and surface colonocytes (Clayburgh et al., 2004). Further downstream, during alterations of the tight junction permeability, the transmembrane protein occludin is subject to endocytosis (Schwarz et al., 2007; Turner, 2009). Long-term regulation of intestinal permeability depends on the synthesis and trafficking of claudin-2, a molecule that is overexpressed in intestinal cells of animal models of colitis and in human ulcerative colitis specimens (Heller et al., 2005).

It has been suggested that abnormalities in intestinal permeability may be key to the facilitation of intestinal inflammation leading to NEC (Petrosyan et al., 2009). Intestinal barrier integrity and its appropriate regulation are essential to the prevention of antigen diffusion and bacterial contamination into the lamina propria and interstitial tissue. McElroy et al. (2012) however, have recently suggested an alternate "bottom up" hypothesis whereby NEC may be caused by injury to the Paneth cells located in the crypts of Lieberkühn (McElroy et al., 2012).

INTESTINAL PERMEABILITY IS INFLUENCED BY PATHOGENS AND INFLAMMATION

Intestinal barrier dysfunction in newborns may be triggered by exogenous agents. Such enteric pathogens trigger local inflammatory responses through specific receptors (e.g., toll-like receptor 4 (TLR4) for lipopolysaccharide (LPS) recognition) or by proinflammatory cytokines (e.g., tumour necrosis factor alpha

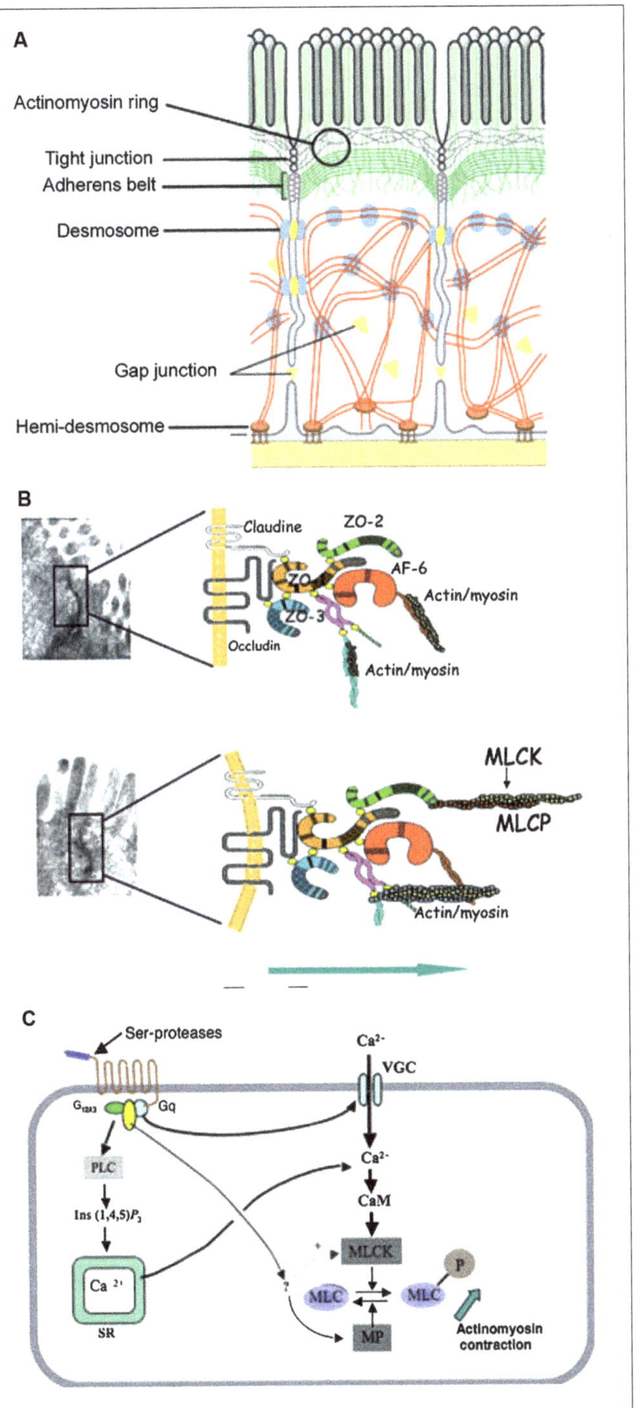

FIGURE 1 | Structures and factors controlling paracellular permeability. Tight junctions are luminal structures that filter the passage of ions and macromolecules **(A)**. The intercellular structural proteins, claudins and occludins, are anchored to the cytoskeleton actinomyosin apical ring through intermediary proteins (ZO-1, -2, -3, AF6). The phosphorylation of myosin light chain causing contraction is associated with opening of tight junctions and junction protein deformations that favour macromolecule passage and bacterial translocation **(B)**. The phosphorylation/dephosphorylation of myosin light chain is controlled by myosin light chain kinase (MLCK) and myosin phosphatase (MP). PAR-2 activation increases MLCK activity through external and internal calcium (Ca++) mobilization and calmodulin binding **(C)**. (With permission from John Wiley and Sons) (Bueno and Fioramonti, 2008).

(TNF-α) (Clayburgh et al., 2005), interferon-γ (Wang et al., 2005), interleukin (IL) 1-β (Al-Sadi et al., 2008) and high-mobility group box 1 (HMGB1) protein (Sappington et al., 2002; Liu et al., 2006; Raman et al., 2006). TNF-α-induced barrier loss is associated with increased transcription and translation of MLCK (Clayburgh et al., 2005). In vivo, intestinal epithelial MLCK is induced by TNF-α. In the rat model of sepsis, an intraperitoneal injection of LPS demonstrably resulted in a rapid rise of TNF-α in the colonic mucosa followed by an increase in myosin light chain phosphorylation and colonic permeability (Moriez et al., 2005). Interestingly, studies in the fetal rat model of NEC have also shown that prenatal bacterial LPS exposure alters the development and permeability of intestinal epithelium (Giannone et al., 2006) and increases ileal injury (Giannone et al., 2009). Similarly, in fetal sheep, preterm intra-amniotic LPS exposure induces abnormal expression of ZO-1 in the ileum (Wolfs et al., 2009).

ENS CONTROLS EPITHELIAL BARRIER FUNCTION

The enteric nervous system (ENS) is defined as the arrangement of neurons and supporting cells throughout the gastrointestinal tract, from the esophagus to the anus (Goyal and Hirano, 1996). The ENS is organized in ganglia that contain neurons, glial cells and interstitial cells. Each enteric ganglion contains many different neuron types (Furness, 2000). The ENS consists of some one hundred million neurons, or about one-tenth of the number of neurons of the spinal cord. Glial cells in the ENS have similar properties to those in the central nervous system (CNS) (Gershon et al., 1993). The numbers and types of neurotransmitters expressed by enteric neurons are comparable to those found in the CNS. The ENS is capable of autonomy with elicitation of reflexes (complete reflex circuitry in the intestinal wall comprises intrinsic sensory neurons, interneurons and intrinsic motor neurons) after total extrinsic denervation of the gut (Furness et al., 1995). However, the ENS is under physiological influence of the sympathetic and vagus nerves. The ENS controls intestinal motility, modulates visceral sensation and plays a role in the regulation of the intestinal blood supply and the secretion of digestive hormones (Costa and Brookes, 1994; Kunze and Furness, 1999; Boeckxstaens, 2002). It also plays a major role in water and electrolyte transport. As a consequence, intestinal permeability is under neural control (Keita and Soderholm, 2010). The ENS should thus be considered, along with the microflora, immune system and fibroblasts, as a major player in the maintenance of intestinal homeostasis and integrity. The ENS has the ability to fine-tune intestinal barrier function via the release of mediators such as acetylcholine that enhance—via muscarinic receptors—(Cameron and Perdue, 2007) and vasoactive intestinal peptide (VIP) that constrict (Neunlist et al., 2003) intestinal permeability over short-term or long-term periods (Neunlist et al., 2012). Similarly, the ENS can modulate the proliferation and differentiation of the intestinal epithelial barrier via the secretion of distinct neuromediators such as VIP (Neunlist et al., 2012). VIP exerts antiproliferative effects, while mediators such as acetylcholine, glucagon-like peptide 2 (GLP-2) or substance P stimulate intestinal epithelial cell proliferation (Neunlist et al., 2012).

NEC: IMMATURE IMMUNE RESPONSE

Local intestinal immune response is normally tightly controlled (Su et al., 2009).

The premature gastrointestinal tract has increased permeability, low levels of protective mucus and secretory immunoglobuline A, higher risk of bacterial overgrowth caused by dysmotility due to ENS immaturity and decreased regenerative capabilities (Neu, 2007). Uncontrolled intestinal inflammation may result from immaturity of the innate immune system of the developing gut (Lin and Stoll, 2006; Lin et al., 2008). Immature regulation could lead to an exaggerated inflammatory response, leading to greater injury and increased intestinal barrier damage. Alternatively, immature regulation could result in minimal immune response due to insufficient inflammatory signalling, thus contributing to bacterial overgrowth and invasion of interstitial tissue. The uncontrolled intestinal inflammation observed in NEC may also depend on dysregulation of intestinal permeability in relation to localized immune response (Turner, 2009). In most individuals and specifically in healthy full-term newborns, a localized break in the intestinal barrier induces a localized immune response that is finely tuned and controlled to avoid over-inflammation and a subsequent increase of intestinal permeability. This normal immunoregulatory response is the result of a delicate balance between pro-inflammatory (TNF-α, IL-1β) and anti-inflammatory (IL-10) processes. If even small anomalies occurred in any of the components of the system (tight junction dysregulation, immune regulatory response), the inflammatory response would be amplified and would result in intestinal injury. Such anomalies may occur secondary to immaturity in preterm babies.

Furthermore immunomodulatory nutrients such as glutamine, arginine, nucleotides, omega-3 polyunsaturated fatty acids and lactoferrin are provided with enteral nutrition and prevent diseases such as NEC. Difficulties with enteral feeding in the first weeks of life predispose premature infants to sepsis and NEC (Neu et al., 2013).

DEVELOPMENT AND MONITORING OF THE AUTONOMIC NERVOUS SYSTEM ACTIVITY

The autonomic nervous system (ANS) plays a predominant role in complex coordinated control of multiple vitally important physiological subsystems in the organism and is part of the neuroimmunological response to pathogens via CAP (Fairchild et al., 2011). Since ANS development and activity are reflected in the heart rate patterns, an appropriate analysis of the fetal heart rate variability (fHRV) may provide information regarding the individual fetal development (Hoyer et al., 2013; Van Leeuwen et al., 1999). fHRV is a non-invasively obtainable marker of changes in vagal (parasympathetic) and sympathetic activity (Frank et al., 2006). Increase in fHRV is associated with fetal growth in general and with the increase in neural integration in particular (Van Leeuwen et al., 2013). Understanding of the dynamics of fHRV in human and ovine fetuses during physiologic (e.g., sleep states) and pathophysiologic (e.g., asphyxia) conditions has evolved over the past two decades (Karin et al., 1993; Frank et al., 2006; Shapiro et al., 2013). Fetal heart rate (FHR) and fHRV are regulated by a complex interplay of the parasympathetic and sympathetic nervous systems accounting for the baseline FHR as well as short-term and long-term variability and nonlinear properties (Frasch et al., 2009; Gieraltowski et al., 2013). Nonlinear properties of fHRV in late gestation fetuses are present and a higher vagal tone is associated with more efficient regulation of homeostasis (Groome et al., 1999).

CAP CONTROLS IMMUNE HOMEOSTASIS

CAP has been implicated in the regulation of the inflammatory reflex in adult organisms including humans (Tracey, 2002, 2007, 2009; Cailotto et al., 2012; Olofsson et al., 2012). CAP is a neural mechanism that influences the magnitude of the innate immune response and maintains homeostasis. As part of CAP, increased vagal activity inhibits the release of proinflammatory cytokines (**Figures 2,3**). Vagal nerve stimulation decreases LPS-induced systemic TNF-α release in adult rats (Borovikova et al., 2000). Suppression of proinflammatory cytokine expression via agonistic action on the α7 subunit nicotinic acetylcholine receptor (α7nAChR) was confirmed in innate immune cells such as macrophages (reviewed in Tracey, 2007) (**Figures 2,3**). Systemically via CAP, this is mediated via the spleen: Adrenergic nerve fibres in the spleen activate acetylcholine-producing T-lymphocytes, thereby inhibiting systemic cytokine production (Huston et al., 2007; Rosas-Ballina et al., 2011; Olofsson et al., 2012).

Vagal nerve activity in basal conditions provides inhibitory input that dampens innate immune response (Haensel et al., 2008; Thayer and Fischer, 2009). The CAP influences the magnitude of the innate immune response and maintains homeostasis (Tracey, 2009). Depressed vagal nerve activity is associated with an exaggerated proinflammatory response and increased morbidity and mortality in various contexts such as acute or stable coronary heart disease, metabolic syndrome or impaired glucose tolerance and kidney failure (Haensel et al., 2008; Thayer and Fischer, 2009). The inhibitory role of CAP on innate immune function can be thought of as analogous to the inhibitory role of the vagus nerve on the resting heart rate (Tracey, 2009).

Under resting conditions, the inflammatory reflex helps establish the set point for the magnitude of the innate immune response to molecules arising from infection, injury or ischemia. Vagus nerve output maintains homeostasis by limiting proinflammatory response to the healthy, protective and non-toxic range (**Figure 4**). However, when vagal activity is absent or diminished, the set point increases; exposure to pathogens then results in an exaggerated proinflammatory response and eventual tissue damage as demonstrated in different experiments with murine models (Ghia et al., 2006, 2007a,b, 2008).

Numerous factors can experimentally or clinically impair the CAP, each resulting in an exaggerated innate immune response. For instance, in animal models with vagotomy or deficient in α7nAChR, the magnitude of the proinflammatory cytokine response and the extent of tissue damage increase during infection, haemorrhagic shock and stroke (Guarini et al., 2003; van Westerloo et al., 2005; Ghia et al., 2008; Ottani et al., 2009; Tracey, 2009). The observation that vagal nerve activity influences circulating TNF-α amounts and the shock response to endotoxemia has widespread implications. It is a previously

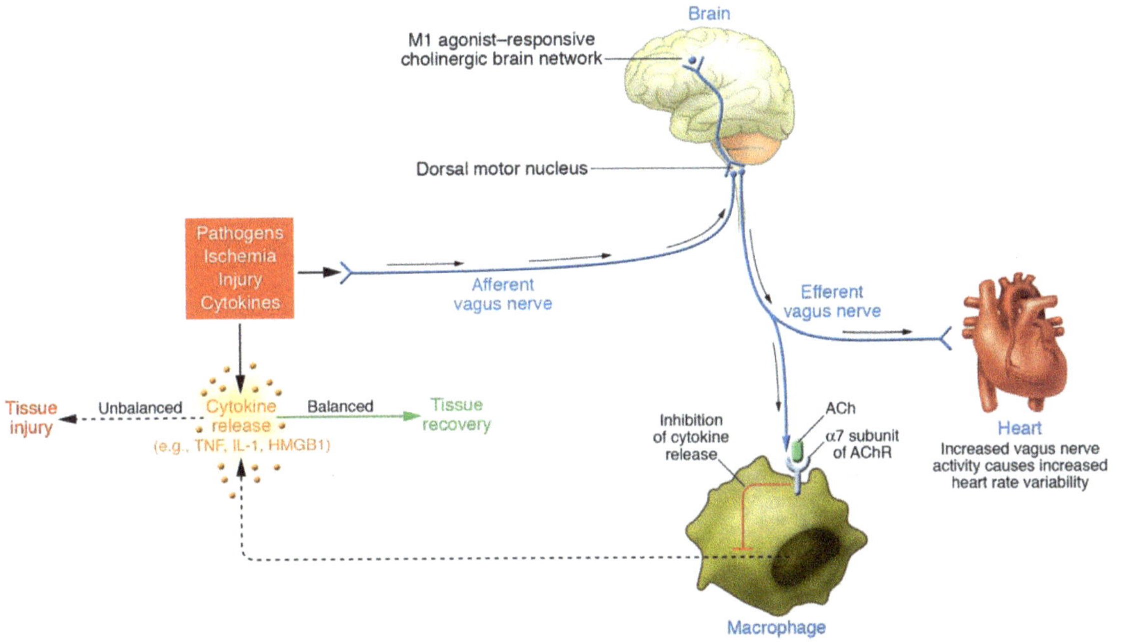

FIGURE 2 | Wiring of the cholinergic anti-inflammatory pathway (CAP), which balances cytokine production. Pathogens as well as ischemia and other forms of injury activate cytokine production, which normally restores health. If the cytokine response is excessive, however, then these same mediators can cause disease. Efferent signals from the vagus nerve inhibit cytokine production via pathways dependent on the *α7 subunit* of the acetylcholine receptor (*AChR*) on macrophages and other cells. Efferent vagus nerve activity also increases instantaneous heart rate variability (HRV). A cholinergic brain network that is responsive to M1 agonists can increase the activity of CAP and also increase instantaneous HRV. Afferent signals carried in the vagus nerve can activate an efferent response that inhibits cytokine release, termed the *inflammatory reflex* (With permission from American Society for Clinical Investigation) (Tracey, 2007).

unrecognized, direct and rapid endogenous mechanism that can suppress the lethal effects of biological toxins. The CAP has much shorter response times than humoral anti-inflammatory pathways. Electrical stimulation of the vagus nerve or administration of α7nAChR agonists reduces the magnitude of proinflammatory cytokine production by 50–75% but does not eliminate cytokine activity (Borovikova et al., 2000; Tracey, 2009). Activation of CAP has not been observed to cause immunosuppression because maximal suppression only reduces proinflammatory cytokine levels from the toxic to the healthy range (**Figure 4**). This concept has been studied as a potential treatment for a range of inflammatory diseases, including infection (reviewed in Tracey, 2009). The role of CAP in the perinatal inflammatory response and the priming of subsequent innate immune response require elucidation.

Adult clinical data indicate that loss of inhibition from the CAP unleashes innate immunity, produces higher levels of proinflammatory mediators, and exacerbates damage to the organism (Lindgren et al., 1993; Lanza et al., 2006; Thayer and Sternberg, 2006; Marsland et al., 2007; Sloan et al., 2007; Tateishi et al., 2007; Haensel et al., 2008; Holman and Ng, 2008; von Kanel et al., 2008) and exacerbation of tissue damage. Studies are needed to explore the impact of CAP activity on chorioamnionitis (Shapiro et al., 2013). Such studies could lead to the development of novel prognostic markers to better identify fetuses at risk of NEC. We hypothesize that increased CAP activity would inhibit the activation of intestinal innate immune cells such as macrophages and thus suppress the inflammatory response to bacterial infection. Effectively, pathological inflammation and intestinal permeability as a *locus minoris resistentiae* of incipient NEC would be decreased or normalized.

VAGAL NERVE STIMULATION AND THE GUT INFLAMMATION

As vagal nerve stimulation stimulates CAP activity without causing immunosuppression (Borovikova et al., 2000), it has been shown to improve intestinal inflammation in murine models of experimental colitis (Ghia et al., 2006, 2007a,b, 2008) and postoperative ileus (The et al., 2007; van Bree et al., 2012). The role of intestinal macrophages seems pivotal (The et al., 2007; Costantini et al., 2010a; Rosas-Ballina et al., 2011; van Bree et al., 2012). In a murine model of dextran sodium sulphate-induced colitis, Ghia et al. demonstrated an increased inflammatory response in the colonic mucosa of the vagotomy group as compared to control animals. They showed the protective effect of vagal activity in acute colitis (Ghia et al., 2006) and in acute relapses within a background of chronic inflammation (Ghia et al., 2007b).

In a murine model of postoperative ileus, the anti-inflammatory effect of intracerebroventricular injection of semapimod was abolished in the presence of vagotomy (The et al., 2011). Vagal nerve stimulation also modulates intestinal permeability and integrity. In a murine model of intestinal injury caused by severe burns, vagal nerve stimulation performed before injury improved intestinal barrier integrity through an efferent signalling pathway and was associated with improved tight junction

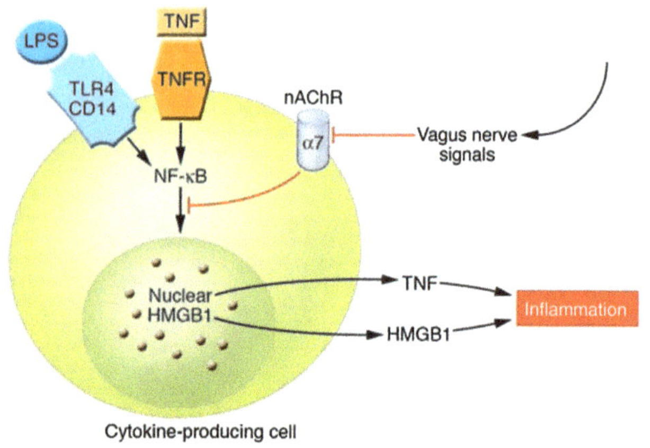

FIGURE 3 | Cholinergic signals derived from vagus nerve stimulation inhibit the release of TNF-α, IL-1, HMGB1, and other cytokines by transducing a cellular signal that inhibits the nuclear activity of NF-κB. TNFR stands for TNF receptor (Wang et al., 2004; Tracey, 2007). The cytokine producing cell can be a macrophage, among others. The nAChR family are ligand-gated ion channels that mediate diverse physiological functions and were originally identified in the nervous system. They consist of different subtypes formed by the specific assembly of five polypeptide subunits including α1-10, β1-4, γ, δ, and ϵ. The subunits fall into two groups: neuronal nicotinic receptors (consisting of α2–10 and β2–4) and muscle nicotinic receptors (consisting of α1, β1, γ, δ, and ϵ). Functional neuronal nAChR subtypes are either homomeric (consisting of 5 identical α-subunits, as in α7- or α9 nAChR) or heteromeric (consisting of combinations of the α- and β-subunits, such as $\alpha3\beta2$nAChR) (Yeboah et al., 2008). Remarkably, it is specifically the α7nAChR that is required for CAP's effects on peripheral innate immune cells (**Figures 2,3**) (With permission from American Society for Clinical Investigation) (Tracey, 2007).

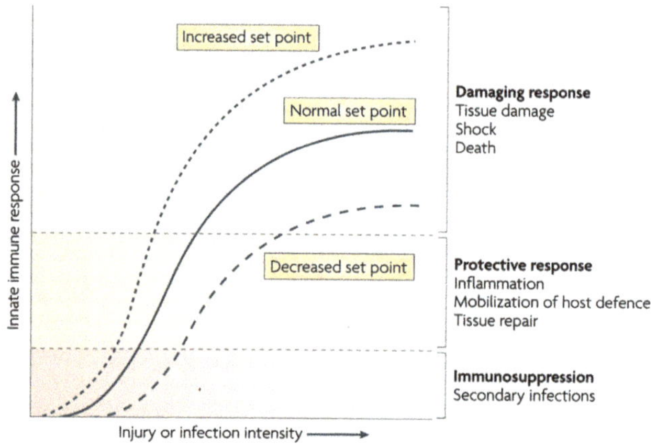

FIGURE 4 | The set point function of the immune response is defined by the magnitude of innate immune responses relative to the infection or injury stimulus. Increasing the set point or shifting the curve to the left increases the chance that tissue damage will occur from the response to infection or injury. Decreasing the set point or shifting the curve to the right reduces the probability that tissue damage will occur. CAP is the neural circuit that provides acute compensatory input to adjust the magnitude of the immune response relative to the set point (With permission from Nature Publishing Group) (Tracey, 2009).

protein expression (Costantini et al., 2010b). In the same model, stimulating the vagus nerve at the time of injury promoted enteric glial cell activation. Either method could prevent intestinal barrier injury (Costantini et al., 2010a). Activation of enteric glial cells has been reported in a rat model of burn-induced stress and gut injury (Costantini et al., 2010a).

The optimal choice of vagal nerve stimulation parameters in order to activate the CAP for therapeutic purposes remains challenging. Although the literature provides a spectrum of possibilities, further studies are needed. Huston et al., 2007 demonstrated improved survival in murine polymicrobial sepsis with transcutaneous vagal nerve stimulation (Huston et al., 2007), suggesting that this mode might be an effective therapy for sepsis generally and NEC specifically. Pharmacologically, cholinergic neuronal circuitry can be stimulated peripherally using α7nAChR agonists to act on macrophages; or centrally using intracerebroventricular injections of semapimod (The et al., 2011), muscarinic receptor agonist McN-A-343 (Pavlov et al., 2006), or an acetylcholinesterase inhibitor (galantamine) (Pavlov et al., 2009). Importantly, enteral feeding of lipid-rich nutrition may also be used to activate the CAP pathway (Luyer et al., 2005).

SIGNIFICANCE AND NOVELTY

Intrauterine infection leads to macrophage activation in LPS-induced chorioamnionitis in fetal sheep and in a rat model of postnatal sepsis. Intrauterine infection may prime innate immune cells for subsequent exacerbated response and increase intestinal permeability. However, the effects of CAP on this process have not been elucidated. The existence of CAP in adult mammals, including humans, is by now well established. CAP may play an important role in fetal and perinatal development by serving as a neuroimmunological network for "internal surveillance" linking the CNS and the vagus nerve to modulate systemic and intestinal inflammation. The presence of such a brain-gut network and its significance for perinatal health have not yet been fully studied. Further research on the physiology and pathophysiology of fetal and perinatal neuroimmunological interactions may open new avenues for diagnosis of fetuses at risk of intestinal injury, such that appropriate preventive or therapeutic interventions may be taken. Specifically, fetal CAP activation is likely to suppress the adverse effects of macrophage activation thus decreasing antenatal and perinatal intestinal injury. New pharmacologic targets or validated non-invasive methods of vagus nerve stimulation for manipulating the inflammatory response in compromised fetuses may emerge to improve perinatal and postnatal outcome.

ACKNOWLEDGMENTS

The authors are grateful to Danielle Buch, medical writer/editor at the Applied Clinical Research Unit of the CHU Sainte-Justine Research Centre, for a quick revision of the manuscript.

FUNDING SUPPORT ACKNOWLEDGMENT

L. Garzoni: Swiss National Science Foundation (SNSF). M.G. Frasch: Canadian Institutes of Health Research (CIHR), Fonds de Recherche Santé Québec (FRSQ) and Molly Towell Perinatal Research Foundation.

REFERENCES

Al-Sadi, R., Ye, D., Dokladny, K., and Ma, T. Y. (2008). Mechanism of IL- 1beta-induced increase in intestinal epithelial tight junction permeabil- ity. *J. Immunol.* 180,5653–5661.

Andrews, W. W., Cliver, S. P., Biasini, F., Peralta-Carcelen, A. M., Rector, R., Alriksson-Schmidt, A. I., et al. (2008). Early preterm birth: association between in utero exposure to acute inflammation and severe neurodevelopmental disability at 6 years of age. *Am. J. Obstet. Gynecol.* 198, 466. e1–466.e11. doi:10.1016/j.ajog. 2007.12.031

Andrews, W. W., Goldenberg, R. L., Faye-Petersen, O., Cliver, S., Goepfert, A. R., and Hauth, J. C. (2006). The alabama preterm birth study: polymorphonuclear and mononuclear cell placental infiltrations, other markers of inflammation, and outcomes in 23- to 32-week preterm newborn infants. *Am. J. Obstet. Gynecol.* 195, 803–808. doi: 10.1016/j.ajog.2006. 06.083

Aziz, N., Cheng, Y. W., and Caughey, A. B. (2009). Neonatal outcomes in the setting of preterm premature rup- ture of membranes complicated by chorioamnionitis. *J. Matern. Fetal Neonatal. Med.* 22,780–784. doi:10. 1080/14767050902922581

Been, J. V., Lievense, S., Zimmermann, L. J., Kramer, B. W., and Wolfs, T. G. (2013). Chorioamnionitis as a risk factor for necrotizing ente- rocolitis: a systematic review and meta-analysis. *J. Pediatr.* 162, 236- 242.e2. doi: 10.1016/j.jpeds.2012. 07.012

Been, J. V., Rours, I. G., Kornelisse, R. F., Lima Passos, V., Kramer, B. W., Schneider, T. A., et al. (2009). Histologic chorioamnioni- tis, fetal involvement, and antenatal steroids: effects on neona- tal outcome in preterm infants. *Am. J. Obstet. Gynecol.* 201, 587, e581–e588. doi:10.1016/j.ajog.2009. 06.025

Bisquera, J. A., Cooper, T. R., and Berseth, C. L. (2002). Impact of necrotizing enterocolitis on length of stay and hospital charges in very low birth weight infants. *Pediatrics* 109, 423–428. doi: 10.1542/peds. 109.3.423

Boeckxstaens, G. E. (2002). Under- standing and controlling the enteric nervous system. *Best Pract. Res. Clin. Gastroenterol.* 16, 1013–1023. doi: 10.1053/bega.2002.0336

Borovikova, L. V., Ivanova, S., Zhang, M., Yang, H., Botchkina, G. I., Watkins, L. R., et al. (2000). Vagus nerve stimulation attenuates the systemic inflammatory response to endotoxin. *Nature* 405, 458–462. doi: 10.1038/35013070

Bueno, L., and Fioramonti, J. (2008). Protease-activated receptor 2 and gut permeability: a review. *Neuro- gastroenterol. Motil.* 20, 580–587. doi: 10.1111/j.1365-2982.2008. 01139.x

Cailotto, C., Costes, L. M., Van Der Vliet, J., Sh, V. a. N. B., Jj, V. a. N. H., Buijs, R. M., and Boeckxs- taens, G. E. (2012). Neuroanatomi- cal evidence demonstrating the exis- tence of the vagal anti-inflammatory reflex in the intestine. *Neurogas- troenterol. Motil.* 24,e191–e193. doi: 10.1111/j.1365-2982.2011.01824.x

Cameron, H. L., and Perdue, M. H. (2007). Muscarinic acetyl- choline receptor activation increases transcellular transport of macro- molecules across mouse and human intestinal epithelium in vitro. *Neu- rogastroenterol. Motil.* 19, 47–56. doi: 10.1111/j.1365-2982.2006. 00845.x

Clayburgh, D. R., Barrett, T. A., Tang, Y., Meddings, J. B., Van Eldik, L. J., Watterson, D. M., et al. (2005). Epithelial myosin light chain kinase-dependent barrier dysfunc- tion mediates T cell activation- induced diarrhea in vivo. *J. Clin. Invest.* 115, 2702–2715. doi: 10. 1172/jci24970

Clayburgh, D. R., Rosen, S., Witkowski, E. D., Wang, F., Blair, S., Dudek, S., et al. (2004). A differentiation- dependent splice variant of myosin light chain kinase, MLCK1, reg- ulates epithelial tight junction permeability. *J. Biol. Chem.* 279, 55506–55513. doi: 10.1074/jbc. m408822200

Costa, M., and Brookes, S. J. (1994). The enteric nervous system. *Am. J. Gastroenterol.* 89, S129–S137.

Costantini, T. W., Bansal, V., Krzyza- niak, M. J., Putnam, J. G., Peterson, C. Y., Loomis, W. H., et al. (2010a). Vagal nerve stimula- tion protects against burn-induced intestinal injury through activation of enteric glia cells. *Am. J. Phys- iol. Gastrointest. Liver Physiol.* 299, G1308–G1318. doi: 10.1152/ajpgi. 00156.2010

Costantini, T. W., Bansal, V., Peterson, C. Y., Loomis, W. H., Putnam, J. G., Rankin, F., et al. (2010b). Efferent vagal nerve stimulation attenuates gut barrier injury after burn: modu- lation of intestinal occludin expres- sion. *J. Trauma.* 68, 1349–1354; dis- cussion 1354–1346. doi: 10.1097/ta. 0b013e3181dccea0

Fairchild, K. D., Srinivasan, V., Moor- man, J. R., Gaykema, R. P., and Goehler, L. E. (2011). Pathogen- induced heart rate changes associ- ated with cholinergic nervous sys- tem activation. *Am. J. Physiol. Regul. Integr. Comp. Physiol.* 300, R330– R339. doi: 10.1152/ajpregu.00487. 2010

Frank, B., Frasch, M. G., Schneider, U., Roedel, M., Schwab, M., and Hoyer, D. (2006). Complexity of heart rate fluctuations in near-term sheep and human fetuses during sleep. *Biomed. Tech. (Berl)* 51, 233–236. doi: 10. 1515/bmt.2006.044

Furness, J. B. (2000). Types of neu- rons in the enteric nervous system. *J. Auton. Nerv. Syst.* 81,87–96. doi: 10.1016/s0165-1838(00)00127-2

Furness, J. B., Johnson, P. J., Pompolo, S., and Bornstein, J. C. (1995). Evi- dence that enteric motility reflexes can be initiated through entirely intrinsic mechanisms in the guinea- pig small intestine. *Neurogastroen- terol. Motil.* 7, 89–96. doi:10.1111/j. 1365-2982.1995.tb00213.x

Ganapathy, V., Hay, J. W., and Kim, J. H. (2012). Costs of necrotizing enterocolitis and cost-effectiveness of exclusively human milk-based prod- ucts in feeding extremely premature infants. *Breastfeed. Med.* 7, 29–37. doi:10.1089/bfm.2011.0002

Garnier, Y., Kadyrov, M., Gantert, M., Einig, A., Rath, W., and Huppertz, B. (2008). Proliferative responses in the placenta after endotoxin exposure in preterm fetal sheep. *Eur. J. Obstet. Gynecol. Reprod. Biol.* 138, 152–157. doi: 10.1016/j.ejogrb.2007.08.016

Gershon, M. D., Chalazonitis, A., and Rothman, T. P. (1993). From neu- ral crest to bowel: development of the enteric nervous system. *J. Neuro- biol.* 24, 199–214. doi: 10.1002/neu. 480240207

Ghia, J. E., Blennerhassett, P., and Collins, S. M. (2007a). Vagus nerve integrity and experimental colitis. *Am. J. Physiol. Gastrointest. Liver Physiol.* 293, G560–G567. doi: 10. 1152/ajpgi.00098.2007

Ghia, J. E., Blennerhassett, P., and Collins, S. M. (2008). Impaired parasympathetic function increases susceptibility to inflammatory bowel disease in a mouse model of depression. *J. Clin. Invest.* 118, 2209–2218. doi: 10.1172/jci32849

Ghia, J. E., Blennerhassett, P., El- Sharkawy, R. T., and Collins, S. M. (2007b). The protective effect of the vagus nerve in a murine model of chronic relapsing colitis. *Am. J. Physiol. Gastrointest. Liver Physiol.* 293,G711–G718. doi: 10.1152/ajpgi. 00240.2007

Ghia, J. E., Blennerhassett, P., Kumar- Ondiveeran, H., Verdu, E. F., and Collins, S. M. (2006). The vagus nerve: a tonic inhibitory influence associated with inflam- matory bowel disease in a murine model. *Gastroenterology* 131, 1122–1130. doi: 10.1053/j.gastro.2006. 08.016

Giannone, P. J., Nankervis, C. A., Richter, J. M., Schanbacher, B. L., and Reber, K. M. (2009). Prena- tal lipopolysaccharide increases postnatal intestinal injury in a rat model of necrotizing enterocoli- tis. *J. Pediatr. Gastroenterol. Nutr.* 48, 276–282. doi: 10.1097/mpg. 0b013e31818936b8

Giannone, P. J., Schanbacher, B. L., Bauer, J. A., and Reber, K. M. (2006). Effects of prenatal lipopolysaccharide exposure on epithelial development and function in newborn rat intestine. *J. Pediatr. Gastroenterol. Nutr.* 43, 284–290. doi: 10.1097/01.mpg. 0000232572.56397.d6

Gieraltowski, J., Hoyer, D., Tetschke, F., Nowack, S., Schneider, U., and Zebrowski, J. (2013). Development of multiscale complexity and multifractality of fetal heart rate variabil- ity. *Auton. Neurosci.* doi: 10.1016/j. autneu.2013.01.009. [Epub ahead of print].

Gotsch, F., Romero, R., Kusanovic, J. P., Mazaki-Tovi, S., Pineles, B. L., Erez, O., et al. (2007). The fetal inflam- matory response syndrome. *Clin. Obstet. Gynecol.* 50,652–683.

Goyal, R. K., and Hirano, I. (1996). The enteric nervous system. *N. Engl. J. Med.* 334, 1106–1115. doi: 10. 1056/NEJM199604253341707

Gronlund, M. M., Lehtonen, O. P., Eerola, E., and Kero, P. (1999). Fecal microflora in healthy infants born by different methods of deliv- ery: permanent changes in intestinal flora after cesarean delivery. *J. Pedi- atr. Gastroenterol. Nutr.* 28, 19–25. doi: 10.1097/00005176-199901000- 00007

Groome, L. J., Loizou, P. C., Holland, S. B., Smith, L. A., and Hoff, C. (1999). High vagal tone is associated with more efficient reg- ulation of homeostasis in low-risk human fetuses. *Dev. Psychobiol.* 35, 25–34. doi: 10.1002/(sici)1098-2302(199907)35:1<25::aid-dev4>3.0.co;2-q

Guarini, S., Altavilla, D., Cainazzo, M. M., Giuliani, D., Bigiani, A., Marini, H., et al. (2003). Efferent vagal fibre stimulation blunts nuclear factor- kappaB activation and protects against hypovolemic hemorrhagic shock. *Circulation* 107, 1189–1194. doi: 10.1161/01.cir.0000050627. 90734.ed

Haensel, A., Mills, P. J., Nelesen, R. A., Ziegler, M. G., and Dimsdale, J.E. (2008). The relationship between heart rate variability and inflam- matory markers in cardiovascu- lar diseases. *Psychoneuroendocrinol- ogy* 33, 1305–1312. doi: 10.1016/j. psyneuen.2008.08.007

Heller, F., Florian, P., Bojarski, C., Richter, J., Christ, M., Hillenbrand, B., et al. (2005). Interleukin-13 is the key effector Th2 cytokine in ulcera- tive colitis that affects epithelial tight junctions, apoptosis, and cell resti- tution. *Gastroenterology* 129, 550–564. doi: 10.1016/j.gastro.2005.05.002

Holman, A. J., and Ng, E. (2008). Heart rate variability predicts anti-tumor necrosis factor therapy response for inflammatory arthritis. *Auton. Neu- rosci.* 143, 58–67. doi: 10.1016/j. autneu.2008.05.005

(2013). Fetal develop- ment of complex autonomic con- trol evaluated from multiscale heart rate patterns. *Am. J. Physiol. Regul. Integr. Comp. Physiol.* 304, R383– R392. doi: 10.1152/ajpregu.00120. 2012

Hunter, C. J., Upperman, J. S., Ford, H. R., and Camerini, V. (2008). Understanding the susceptibility of the premature infant to necrotizing enterocolitis (NEC). [Review]. *Pedi- atr. Res.* 63, 117–123. doi: 10.1203/PDR.0b013e31815ed64c

Huston, J. M., Gallowitsch-Puerta, M., Ochani, M., Ochani, K., Yuan, R., Rosas-Ballina, M., et al. (2007). Transcutaneous vagus nerve stimulation reduces serum high mobility group box 1 levels and improves survival in murine sepsis. *Crit. Care Med.* 35, 2762–2768. doi: 10.1097/01.ccm.0000288102. 15975.ba

Karin, J., Hirsch, M., and Akselrod, S. (1993). An estimate of fetal autonomic state by spectral analy- sis of fetal heart rate fluctuations. *Pediatr. Res.* 34, 134–138. doi: 10. 1203/00006450-199308000-00005

Keita, A. V., and Soderholm, J. D. (2010). The intestinal barrier and its regulation by neuroimmune fac- tors. *Neurogastroenterol. Motil.* 22, 718–733. doi: 10.1111/j.1365-2982.2010.01498.x

Kunze, W. A., and Furness, J. B. (1999). The enteric nervous system and regulation of intestinal motility. *Annu. Rev. Physiol.* 61, 117–142. doi: 10. 1146/annurev.physiol.61.1.117

Lahra, M. M., and Jeffery, H. E. (2004). A fetal response to chorioamnioni- tis is associated with early sur- vival after preterm birth. *Am. J. Obstet. Gynecol.* 190, 147–151. doi: 10.1016/j.ajog.2003.07.012

Lanza, G. A., Sgueglia, G. A., Cianflone, D., Rebuzzi, A. G., Angeloni, G., Ses- tito, A., et al. (2006). Relation of heart rate variability to serum lev- els of C-reactive protein in patients with unstable angina pectoris. *Am. J. Cardiol.* 97, 1702–1706. doi: 10. 1016/j.amjcard.2006.01.029

Lin, P. W., Nasr, T. R., and Stoll, B. J. (2008). Necrotizing enterocolitis: recent scientific advances in patho- physiology and prevention. *Semin. Perinatol.* 32, 70–82. doi: 10.1053/j. semperi.2008.01.004

Lin, P. W., and Stoll, B. J. (2006). Necrotising enterocolitis. *Lancet* 368,1271–1283.

Lindgren, S., Stewenius, J., Sjolund, K., Lilja, B., and Sundkvist, G. (1993). Autonomic vagal nerve dysfunction in patients with ulcerative colitis. *Scand. J. Gastroenterol.* 28, 638–642. doi: 10.3109/00365529309096103

Liu, S., Stolz, D. B., Sappington, P. L., Macias, C. A., Killeen, M. E., Ten- hunen, J. J., et al. (2006). HMGB1 is secreted by immunostimulated enterocytes and contributes to cytomix-induced hyperpermeabil- ity of Caco-2 monolayers. *Am. J. Physiol. Cell Physiol.* 290, C990– C999. doi: 10.1152/ajpcell.00308. 2005

Luyer, M. D., Greve, J. W., Had- foune, M., Jacobs, J. A., Dejong, C. H., and Buurman, W. A. (2005). Nutritional stimulation of cholecys- tokinin receptors inhibits inflam- mation via the vagus nerve. *J. Exp. Med.* 202, 1023–1029. doi: 10. 1084/jem.20042397

Marsland, A. L., Gianaros, P. J., Prather, A., Jennings, J. R., Neumann, S. A., and Manuck, S. B. (2007). Stim- ulated production of proinflam- matory cytokines covaries inversely with heart rate variability. *Psycho- som. Med.* 69, 709–716. doi: 10. 1097/psy.0b013e3181576118

Martinez-Tallo, E., Claure, N., and Bancalari, E. (1997). Necrotizing enterocolitis in full-term or near-term infants: risk factors. *Biol. Neonate* 71, 292–298. doi: 10. 1159/000244428

McElroy, S. J., Underwood, M. A., and Sherman, M. P. (2012). Paneth cells and necrotizing enterocolitis: a novel hypothesis for disease patho- genesis. *Neonatology* 103, 10–20. doi: 10.1159/000342340

Moriez, R., Salvador-Cartier, C., Theodorou, V., Fioramonti, J., Eutamene, H., and Bueno, L. (2005). Myosin light chain kinase is involved in lipopolysaccharide- induced disruption of colonic epithelial barrier and bacterial translocation in rats. *Am. J. Pathol.* 167, 1071–1079. doi: 10. 1016/s0002-9440(10)61196-0

Neu, J. (2007). Gastrointestinal devel- opment and meeting the nutritional needs of premature infants. *Am. J. Clin. Nutr.* 85,629S–634S.

Neu, J., Mihatsch, W. A., Zegarra, J., Supapannachart, S., Ding, Z. Y., and Murguia-Peniche, T. (2013). Intesti- nal mucosal defense system, Part Consensus recommendations for immunonutrients. *J. Pediatr.* 162, S56–S63. doi: 10.1016/j.jpeds.2012. 11.054

Neunlist, M., Toumi, F., Oreschkova, T., Denis, M., Leborgne, J., Laboisse, C. L., et al. (2003). Human ENS regu- lates the intestinal epithelial barrier permeability and a tight junction- associated protein ZO-1 via VIPer- gic pathways. *Am. J. Physiol. Gas- trointest. Liver Physiol.* 285, G1028– G1036.

Neunlist, M., Van Landeghem, L., Mahe, M. M., Derkinderen, P., Bru- ley Des Varannes, S. B., and Rolli- Derkinderen, M. (2012). The diges- tive neuronal-glial-epithelial unit: a new actor in gut health and disease. *Nat. Rev. Gastroenterol. Hepatol.* 10, 90–100. doi: 10.1038/nrgastro.2012. 221

Olofsson, P. S., Rosas-Ballina, M., Levine, Y. A., and Tracey, K. J. (2012). Rethinking inflammation: neural circuits in the regulation of immunity. *Immunol. Rev.* 248, 188– 204. doi: 10.1111/j.1600-065x.2012. 01138.x

Ottani, A., Giuliani, D., Mioni, C., Galantucci, M., Minutoli, L., Bitto, A., et al. (2009). Vagus nerve mediates the protective effects of melanocortins against cerebral and systemic damage after ischemic stroke. *J. Cereb. Blood Flow. Metab.* 29, 512–523. doi: 10.1038/jcbfm.2008.140

Pavlov, V. A., Ochani, M., Gallowitsch- Puerta, M., Ochani, K., Huston, J. M., Czura, C. J., et al. (2006). Cen- tral muscarinic cholinergic regula- tion of the systemic inflammatory response during endotoxemia. *Proc. Natl. Acad. Sci. U S A* 103, 5219– 5223. doi: 10.1073/pnas.0600506103

Pavlov, V. A., Parrish, W. R., Rosas-Ballina, M., Ochani, M., Puerta, M., Ochani, K., et al. (2009). Brain acetylcholinesterase activity controls systemic cytokine levels through the cholinergic anti- inflammatory pathway. *Brain Behav. Immun.* 23, 41–45. doi: 10.1016/j. bbi.2008.06.011

Petrosyan, M., Guner, Y. S., Williams, M., Grishin, A., and Ford, H. R. (2009). Current concepts regard- ing the pathogenesis of necrotizing enterocolitis. *Pediatr. Surg. Int.* 25, 309–318. doi: 10.1007/s00383-009-2344-8

Raman, K. G., Sappington, P. L., Yang, R., Levy, R. M., Prince, J. M., Liu, S., et al. (2006). The role of RAGE in the pathogenesis of intestinal bar- rier dysfunction after hemorrhagic shock. *Am. J. Physiol. Gastrointest. Liver Physiol.* 291, G556–G565. doi: 10.1152/ajpgi.00055.2006

Rosas-Ballina, M., Olofsson, P. S., Ochani, M., Valdes-Ferrer, S. I.,Levine, Y. A., Reardon, C., et al. (2011). Acetylcholine-synthesizing T cells relay neural signals in a vagus nerve circuit. *Science* 334, 98–101. doi: 10.1126/science.1209985

Sappington, P. L., Yang, R., Yang, H.,Tracey, K. J., Delude, R. L., and Fink, M. P. (2002). HMGB1 B box increases the permeability of Caco-2 enterocytic monolayers and impairs intestinal barrier function in mice. *Gastroenterology* 123, 790–802. doi: 10.1053/gast.2002.35391

Schwarz, B. T., Wang, F., Shen, L., Clayburgh, D. R., Su, L., Wang, Y., et al. (2007). LIGHT signals directly to intestinal epithelia to cause bar- rier dysfunction via cytoskeletal and endocytic mechanisms. *Gastroen- terology* 132, 2383–2394. doi: 10. 1053/j.gastro.2007.02.052

Shapiro, G., Fraser, W. D., Frasch,M. G., and Seguin, J. R. (2013). Psychosocial stress in pregnancy and preterm birth: associations and mechanisms. *J. Perinat. Med.* doi: 10.1515/jpm-2012-0295

Sloan, R. P., Mccreath, H., Tracey, K. J., Sidney, S., Liu, K., and Seeman,T. (2007). RR interval variabilityis inversely related to inflammatory markers: the CARDIA study. *Mol. Med.* 13, 178–184.

Su, L., Shen, L., Clayburgh, D. R., Nalle, S. C., Sullivan, E. A., Meddings, J. B., et al. (2009). Targeted epithelial tight junction dysfunction causes immune activation and contributes to development of experimental col- itis. *Gastroenterology* 136, 551–563. doi:10.1053/j.gastro.2008.10.081

Tateishi, Y., Oda, S., Nakamura, M., Watanabe, K., Kuwaki, T., Moriguchi, T., et al. (2007). Depressed heart rate variability is associated with high IL-6 blood level and decline in the blood pressure in septic patients. *Shock* 28, 549–553. doi: 10.1097/shk. 0b013e318063e8d1

Thayer, J. F., and Fischer, J. E. (2009). Heart rate variability, overnight uri- nary norepinephrine and C-reactive protein: evidence for the choliner- gic anti-inflammatory pathway in healthy human adults. *J. Intern. Med.* 265, 439–447. doi: 10.1111/j. 1365-2796.2008.02023.x

Thayer, J. F., and Sternberg, E. (2006). Beyond heart rate variability: vagal regulation of allostatic systems. *Ann. NY Acad. Sci.* 1088, 361–372. doi: 10. 1196/annals.1366.014

The, F. O., Boeckxstaens, G. E., Snoek, S. A., Cash, J. L., Bennink, R., Larosa, G. J., et al. (2007). Activation of the cholinergic anti- inflammatory pathway ameliorates postoperative ileus in mice. *Gas- troenterology* 133, 1219–1228. doi: 10.1053/j.gastro.2007.07.022

The, F., Cailotto, C., Van Der Vliet, J., De Jonge, W. J., Bennink, R. J., Buijs, R. M., et al. (2011). Central activation of the cholinergic anti-inflammatory pathway reducessurgical inflammation in experi- mental post-operative ileus. *Br. J. Pharmacol* 163, 1007–1016. doi: 10. 1111/j.1476-5381.2011.01296.x

Tracey, K. J. (2002). The inflammatory reflex. *Nature* 420, 853–859. doi: 10. 1038/nature01321

Tracey, K. J. (2007). Physiology and immunology of the cholinergic antiinflammatory pathway. *J. Clin. Invest.* 117, 289–296. doi: 10. 1172/jci30555

Tracey, K. J. (2009). Reflex control of immunity. *Nat. Rev. Immunol.* 9, 418–428. doi:10.1038/nri2566

Turner, J. R. (2009). Intestinal mucosal barrier function in health and dis- ease. *Nat. Rev. Immunol.* 9, 799–809. doi: 10.1038/nri2653 van Bree, S. H., Nemethova, A., Cailotto, C., Gomez-Pinilla, P. J., Matteoli, G., and Boeckxstaens, G. E. (2012). New therapeutic strategies for postoperative ileus. *Nat. Rev. Gastroenterol. Hepatol.* 9, 675–683. doi: 10.1038/nrgastro.2012.134

Hatzmann, W. (1999). Fetal heart rate variability and complexity in the course of pregnancy. *Early Hum. Dev.* 54, 259–269. doi: 10. 1016/s0378-3782(98)00102-9

van Westerloo, D. J., Giebelen, I. A., Florquin, S., Daalhuisen, J., Bruno, M. J., De Vos, A. F., et al. (2005). The cholinergic anti-inflammatory pathway regulates the host response during septic peritonitis. *J. Infect. Dis.* 191, 2138–2148. doi: 10.1086/ 430323

von Kanel, R., Nelesen, R. A., Mills, P. J., Ziegler, M. G., and Dimsdale, J. E. (2008). Relationship between heart rate variability, interleukin-6, and soluble tissue factor in healthy subjects. *Brain Behav. Immun.* 22, 461–468. doi: 10.1016/j. bbi.2007. 09.009

Wang, F., Graham, W. V., Wang, Y., Witkowski, E. D., Schwarz, B. T., and Turner, J. R. (2005). Interferon-gamma and tumor necrosis factor-alpha synergize to induce intestinal epithelial bar- rier dysfunction by up-regulating myosin light chain kinase expres- sion. *Am. J. Pathol.* 166, 409– 419. doi: 10.1016/ s0002-9440(10) 62264-x

Wang, H., Liao, H., Ochani, M., Justiniani, M., Lin, X., Yang, L., et al. (2004). Cholinergic agonists inhibit HMGB1 release and improve survival in experimental sepsis. *Nat. Med.* 10, 1216–1221. doi: 10. 1038/nm1124

Wolfs, T. G., Buurman, W. A., Zoer,B., Moonen, R. M., Derikx, J. P., Thuijls, G., et al. (2009). Endotoxin induced chorioamnionitis prevents intestinal development during ges- tation in fetal sheep. *PLoS One*4:e5837. doi: 10.1371/journal.pone. 0005837

Yeboah, M. M., Xue, X., Javdan, M.,Susin, M., and Metz, C. N. (2008). Nicotinic acetylcholine receptor expression and regulation in the rat kidney after ischemia-reperfusion injury. *Am. J. Physiol. Renal. Physiol.* 295, F654–F661. doi: 10. 1152/ajprenal.90255.2008

17

Programming of neuroendocrine self in the thymus and its defect in the development of neuroendocrine autoimmunity

Vincent Geenen[1]*, Gwennaëlle Bodart[1], Séverine Henry[1], Hélène Michaux[1], Olivier Dardenne[1], Chantal Charlet-Renard[1], Henri Martens[1] and Didier Hober[2]

[1] *Department of Biomedical and Preclinical Sciences, Center of Immunoendocrinology, GIGA Research Institute, Fund of Scientific Research, University of Liege, Liege-Sart Tilman, Belgium*

[2] *Laboratory of Virology EA3610, University of Lille 2 and CHRU Lille, Lille, France*

Edited by:
Jaleel A. Miyan, The University of Manchester, UK

Reviewed by:
Francisco Gaytán, University of Cordoba, Spain
Saheem Ahmad, Loyola University Medical Center, Loyola University of Chicago, USA

****Correspondence:***
Vincent Geenen, Center of Immunology, GIGA I3 Research, CHU-B34, B-4000 Liege-Sart Tilman, Belgium
e-mail: vgeenen@ulg.ac.be

For centuries after its first description by Galen, the thymus was considered as only a vestigial endocrine organ until the discovery in 1961 by Jacques FAP Miller of its essential role in the development of T (thymo-dependent) lymphocytes. A unique thymus first appeared in cartilaginous fishes some 500 million years ago, at the same time or shortly after the emergence of the adaptive (acquired) immune system. The thymus may be compared to a small brain or a computer highly specialized in the orchestration of central immunological self-tolerance. This was a necessity for the survival of species, given the potent evolutionary pressure imposed by the high risk of autotoxicity inherent in the stochastic generation of the diversity of immune cell receptors that characterize the adaptive immune response. A new paradigm of "neuroendocrine self-peptides" has been proposed, together with the definition of "neuroendocrine self." Neuroendocrine self-peptides are secreted by thymic epithelial cells (TECs) not according to the classic model of neuroendocrine signaling, but are processed for presentation by, or in association with, the thymic major histocompatibility complex (MHC) proteins. The autoimmune regulator (AIRE) gene/protein controls the transcription of neuroendocrine genes in TECs. The presentation of self-peptides in the thymus is responsible for the clonal deletion of self-reactive T cells, which emerge during the random recombination of gene segments that encode variable parts of the T cell receptor for the antigen (TCR). At the same time, self-antigen presentation in the thymus generates regulatory T (Treg) cells that can inhibit, in the periphery, those self-reactive T cells that escaped negative selection in the thymus. Several arguments indicate that the origin of autoimmunity directed against neuroendocrine glands results primarily from a defect in the intrathymic programming of self-tolerance to neuroendocrine functions. This defect may be genetic or acquired, for example during an enteroviral infection. This novel knowledge of normal and pathologic functions of the thymus constitutes a solid basis for the development of a novel type of tolerogenic/negative self-vaccination against type 1 diabetes (T1D).

Keywords: thymus, self-tolerance, autoimmunity, type 1 diabetes, neuroendocrine self-peptides, oxytocin, insulin-like growth factor 2, AIRE

INTRODUCTION

Galen (129–210 AC), who, with Hippocrates, is recognized as one of the fathers of Western medicine, first observed, behind the sternum and before the cardiac area, an organ that he named "thymus" because of its resemblance to the leaf of the thyme plant *Thymus vulgaris.* Galen also suspected that the thymus was the seat of courage and affection because of its close vicinity to the heart; in Ancient Greece, the word "thumos or thymos (θυμός)" indicated a physical association between breath and blood, and referred to one of Plato's three constituent parts of human psyche.

The function of the thymus remained unknown for many centuries and it was considered only as a vestigial organ that had become redundant both during phylogeny and ontogeny after puberty. Then, at the beginning of the 20th century, Hammar (Sweden) published a series of important studies describing hyperplasia of the thymus in various endocrine diseases including acromegaly and Graves' disease, and after castration (Hammar, 1921). A few years later, Hans Selye reported that massive thymus atrophy is observed soon after administration of glucocorticoids (Selye, 1941), and this dramatic decrease in thymus size soon became a hallmark of the general adaptation and stress syndrome. At that time, the thymus was thought to be an endocrine gland but, despite the identification of several thymic "hormones," the model of endocrine signaling failed to characterize the molecular dialogue between thymic epithelial cells (TECs) and immature thymic T cells (thymocytes). The hypothesis that the thymus had an endocrine nature then progressively faded, after Miller demonstrated the immunological function of the thymus (Miller, 1961). In this seminal paper, Miller postulated that lymphocytes leaving the thymus are specially selected in an epithelial environment. To the best of our knowledge, Burnet and Mackay published in *The Lancet* the first hypothesis connecting autoimmune diseases with histological abnormalities in the lympho-epithelial structure of the thymus (Burnet and Mackay, 1963). Immunological tolerance was first shown to be induced by thymic epithelial grafts in birds (Ohki et al., 1987), and the prominent role of the thymus in the induction of central tolerance was established by investigating the fate of developing thymocytes in response to superantigens (Kappler et al., 1987) or in T cell receptor (TCR) transgenic mice bearing a receptor for a HY-derived antigen (Kisielow et al., 1988). The identification of thymus-derived regulatory T cells (tTreg) (Sakagushi et al., 1995) completed our essential knowledge about the physiological function of the thymus, *i.e.*, the generation of a diverse repertoire of TCRs that are self-tolerant and competent against non-self. The central role of thymus-dependent central self-tolerance has now become a cornerstone of immune physiology (Mathis and Benoist, 2004; Kyewski and Klein, 2006).

THYMUS ORGANOGENESIS

Epithelial cells of the thymic cortex (cTECs, including thymic "nurse" cells) and medulla (mTECs) constitute around 85% of the thymus parenchyme. Other cells of the thymic stroma—dendritic cells (DCs) and macrophages—derive from the bone marrow. TECs arise from the endoderm of the 3rd pharyngeal pouch that, at around day 9 of embryonic development in the mouse (E9.0), contains thymic common epithelial progenitors (Blackburn and Manley, 2004; Anderson et al., 2007). Further development of this primitive epithelial rudiment between E9.5 and E12.5 depends on mesenchyme derived from the cephalic neural crest, the role of which extends beyond the early stages of thymus organogenesis (Foster et al., 2008).

Some human diseases and animal models involve a defect in thymus development, which leads to primary immune deficiencies. Di George's syndrome associates congenital absence or hypoplasia of the thymus and parathyroid glands together with defects in the heart and truncal vessels. This syndrome results partly from a migration failure of the cephalic neural crest. More recently, transgenic mouse models have revealed some of the molecular mechanisms involved in thymus development. Thus, *Hoxa3*$^{-/-}$ mice present thymic aplasia, parathyroid hypoplasia, that are often accompanied by defects of the heart and the great truncal vessels (Manley and Capecchi, 1995). In mice, the "nude" phenotype results from mutations in the *nude* gene locus on chromosome 11 that encodes the transcription factor winged-helix nude (*whn*) or forkhead box N1 (*Foxn1*) (Nehls et al., 1994). *Foxn1* is a master regulator gene of the TEC differentiation programme; it controls lineage progression in cTECs and mTECs, and regulates a series of genes implicated in TEC function, although is not essential for medullary sublineage divergence (Nowell et al., 2011). Importantly, the genetic mechanisms responsible for murine thymus organogenesis are conserved in humans (Farley et al., 2013) and this is important with regard to current attempts to regenerate the thymus in aging, as well as in many other clinical conditions associated with compromised immune function (Holländer et al., 2010). Indeed, contrary to earlier dogma, the thymus is functional until an advanced age, and thymopoiesis plays a central role in immune reconstitution after intensive chemotherapy or anti-retroviral treatment (Douek et al., 1998).

OVERVIEW OF T CELL DIFFERENTIATION IN THE THYMUS

The T cell immune system may be regarded as a 6th sensory organ that responds to different kinds of danger signals that are not detected by nerve cells. From the fetal liver, and later from the bone marrow, T lymphocyte progenitors migrate through the boundary between cortex and medulla into the thymic epithelial rudiment in response to chemoattractant factors (Wilkinson et al., 1999). They undergo many mitotic divisions in the outer cortex, and then differentiate after presentation of peptides by major histocompatibility complex (MHC) proteins expressed by thymic antigen-presenting cells (essentially cTECs, mTECs, DCs, and macrophages). The stochastic rearrangement of related β– then α-chains generates an enormous diversity of TCRs, many of which can bind self-antigen/MHC complexes with high affinity and are subsequently deleted (negative selection). Clonal deletion of thymocytes can occur both in the cortex and in the medulla (McCaughtry et al., 2008), but is most effective in the medulla.

Self-antigen presentation by thymic MHC proteins determines the whole process of T cell differentiation, which includes three alternative and exclusive fates for developing thymocytes: (1) Negative selection of self-reactive T cells generated during the random generation of TCR diversity due to the activity of the two recombination-activating enzymes RAG-1 and RAG-2; (2) Generation of self-specific tTreg cells; and (3) Positive selection of CD4+ and CD8+ effector and self-tolerant T cells. The first two events establish the establishment of the central arm of self-tolerance, while the avidity-affinity of the TCR—self-antigen—MHC interaction determines T cell negative or positive selection (Ashton-Rickardt et al., 1994). A remaining question is how the same MHC—self-peptide complexes can mediate either negative selection of self-reactive T cells or generation of self-specific tTreg cells (Klein et al., 2009; Stritesky et al., 2012). Another crucial question concerns the precise biochemical nature of self-peptides that are presented in the thymus, in particular during fetal life.

NEUROHYPOPHYSIAL FAMILY-RELATED PEPTIDES AND RECEPTORS IN THE THYMUS NETWORK

At the beginning of the 20th century, English scientists reported the galactogogue activity of thymus and corpus luteum extracts after their injection into the goat (Ott and Scott, 1910). At that time, oxytocin (OT) had not yet been identified as the specific factor of galactokinesis, which would be established in the late 50's by Vincent du Vigneaud and his team. In 1986, human thymus extracts were shown to possess potent uterine oxytocic activity, and OT was identified as the dominant member of the neurohypophysial family synthesized by TECs and thymic nurse cells in humans and different animal species (Geenen et al., 1986). Thymic T cells also express the OT receptor (OTR) and the V1b (or V3) vasopressin (AVP) receptor, which transduce nanomolar concentrations of OT and, accordingly to the rules of signaling induced by OTR and V1b, these receptors transduce low concentrations of OT and AVP via the phosphoinositide pathway in mitogenic signals for freshly isolated thymocytes (reviewed in Martens et al., 1996a,b). Together, these data showed the existence of a functional signaling within the thymus mediated by OT synthesized by TECs acting on functional OTR and V1b receptors expressed by developing T cells. Further molecular characterization of the neurohypophysial receptors present in the murine thymus showed that *Otr* is transcribed by all thymic T cell subsets, while *V1b* is expressed only in double positive CD4+8+ and single positive CD8+ T cells (Hansenne et al., 2005). Because intrathymic OT concentrations are in agreement with the high affinity Kd (10^{-9}–10^{-10} M) of neurohypophysial receptors expressed by pre-T cells, the physico-chemical conditions are conducive to a functional signaling within the thymus network, which is not the case for the blood-borne OT and AVP, due to their low plasma concentration (10^{-11}–10^{-12} M).

Despite the strong evidence for the presence of neurohypophysial ligands and receptors in the thymus network, no secretion of OT or neurophysin could be detected in primary cultures of freshly isolated human TECs. Moreover, in the murine thymus, OT is not located in secretory granules but is diffuse in cytosol, in vesicles of the endoplasmic reticulum, and associated with keratin filaments (Wiemann and Ehret, 1993). This posed a fundamental problem, since the neuropeptide OT had been the basis for the development of the neurosecretion model by the Sharrer's in the 40's. However, in 1990, Funder proposed a model of cell-to-cell cryptocrine (hidden secretion) signaling to characterize the direct membrane-to-membrane exchange of information between large epithelial nursing cells (like TECs in the thymus and Sertoli cells in the testis) and immature elements that migrate and differentiate at their contact (respectively, thymocytes and spermatocytes).

We thus proposed that, in the thymus, OT mediates a cryptocrine signaling between TECs and pre-T cells (Geenen et al., 1991). The observation of numerous points of focal adhesion between OT+ TECs and immature T cells (Wiemann and Ehret, 1993) prompted us to investigate the hypothesis that thymic OT could stimulate the activation of focal adhesion kinases (FAKs) in thymocytes. Among the proteins phosphorylated by OT in murine pre-T cells, two were precipitated with an anti-FAK mAb: one was identified as the $p125^{FAK}$, while the other was a coprecipitating 130-kD protein (most probably $p130^{Cas}$). In pre-T cells, OT also phosphorylates paxillin, a 68-kD protein located at focal adhesion sites and associated with $p125^{FAK}$ (Martens et al., 1998). Together, these data establish the existence of a functional OT-mediated cryptocrine signaling in the thymus network. The OT-mediated promotion of focal adhesion may contribute to the establishment of immunological "synapses" between TECs and immature T cells, which is fundamental for the completion of the T cell differentiation programme.

A PARADIGM SHIFT: FROM THYMIC NEUROPEPTIDES TO "NEUROENDOCRINE SELF-PEPTIDES"

As discussed above, self-antigen presentation by thymic MHC proteins is the essential mechanism that determines the whole process of T cell differentiation. Because OT and its associated neurophysin are self-peptides synthesized in TECs, we hypothesized a processing of the thymic OT precursor that would be related to antigen presentation rather than classical neurosecretion. If true, such a processing would fit with the model of cryptocrine signaling, which implicates a membrane targeting of the ligand. Following affinity-chromatography with a mAb against the monomorphic part of human MHC class I molecules, we identified, in human TEC plasma membrane, a 55-kD protein that was labeled by both anti-MHC class I mAb and a specific anti-neurophysin antiserum. Because this antiserum does not cross-react either with MHC class I proteins, or with β2-microglobulin, this 55-kD membrane protein could represent a hybrid protein including a neurophysin domain (10 kD) and a MHC class I heavy chain-related domain (45 kD). The formation of this hybrid could reside at the post-transcriptional level (such as a trans-splicing event) or at the post-translational level (such as ATP-dependent ubiquitinylation). The MHC class I domain could be implicated in the membrane targeting of the hybrid, whereas the neurophysin domain would bind OT for final presentation to pre-T cells. According to this explanation, the neurophysin part of the OT precursor could fulfill the same function in the thymus and in the hypothalamo-neurohypophysial axis: binding of the peptide OT and transport to the external limit of TECs or magnocellular neurons, respectively. The tyrosine residue in position 2 of OT plays an important role in its binding to neurophysin (Griffin et al., 1973) and, interestingly, the tyrosine residue in the same position plays a crucial role in the binding of antigens to some MHC class I alleles for their presentation (Maryanski et al., 1991).

The antigenic behavior of thymic OT is also supported by another type of experiment. The recognition of OT by specific mAbs at the outer surface of TEC plasma membrane induces a marked increase in the secretion of interleukin 6 (IL-6) and leukemia inhibitory factor (LIF) in the supernatant of human TEC primary cultures (Martens et al., 1996a,b). Given the nature of the specific epitopes recognized by anti-OT mAbs, it was concluded that OT is fully processed at the level of the TEC plasma membrane. The absence of any effect of anti-AVP mAbs further supports the conclusion that thymic OT behaves as the self-peptide of the neurohypophysial family.

Because OT is a cyclic nonapeptide, and since antigen presentation mostly concerns linear sequences, the hypothesis of a similar processing was investigated with the linear neurotensin (NT). Primary cultures of human TECs contain around 5 ng of NT/10^6 cells, of which 5% is associated with TEC plasma membranes. Again, no NT was detected in the supernatant of human TEC cultures. High performance liquid chromatography analysis of NT present in human TEC revealed a major peak of NT corresponding to intact NT_{1-13}. Using the same affinity column prepared with an anti-MHC class I mAb, NT, and NT-related peptides were retained on the column and were eluted together with MHC class I proteins (Vanneste et al., 1997). The C-terminal sequence of NT includes tyrosine, isoleucine, and leucine residues that all can be used to anchor most of MHC class I alleles. Thus, NT and NT-derived C-terminal fragments could be natural ligands for MHC class I alleles.

At this point and in association with the characterization of the thymic peptides related to different neuroendocrine families (Geenen et al., 1998), the biochemical nature and properties of the *"neuroendocrine self"* could be defined according to the following features:

1. Neuroendocrine self-peptides are the dominant members of neuroendocrine gene/protein families that are expressed in TECs of many species and usually correspond to sequences that have been highly conserved during the evolution of a given family.
2. A hierarchy characterizes their expression profile. In the neurohypophysial family, OT is the dominant peptide expressed in TECs from different species. In the tachykinin family, neurokinin A (NKA)—but not substance P—is the peptide generated from the processing in TECs of the preprotachykinin A gene product (Ericsson et al., 1990). In the insulin family, all members are expressed in the thymus network: IGF-2 (cTECs and mTECs) > IGF-1 (cTECs, mTECs, and macrophages) >> Insulin (rare subsets of mTECs). This hierarchical pattern is important, because the strength of immunological tolerance to a protein/peptide is proportional to its concentration in the thymus (Ashton-Rickardt et al., 1994). Blocking thymic IGF-mediated signaling at the level of IGF ligands (in particular IGF-2) or IGF receptors interferes with the early stages of T cell differentiation, while one mAb to proinsulin did not exert any significant effect (Kecha et al., 2000).
3. The autoimmune regulator gene/protein (AIRE) controls the degree of intrathymic transcription of the genes encoding neuroendocrine self-peptides (Anderson et al., 2002).
4. In the thymus, neuroendocrine precursors are not processed according to the model of neurosecretion but undergo antigenic processing for presentation by—or in association with—MHC proteins. This processing differs between thymic antigen-presenting cells (APCs) and professional APCs (DCs, B cells, and macrophages) in the periphery. For some neuroendocrine self-peptides (OT and NT), such differences imply that their presentation in the thymus is not tightly restricted by MHC alleles as much as presentation of nonself antigens and autoantigens by dedicated APCs in the periphery.
5. For some precursors of neuroendocrine self-peptide precursors, their transcription in TECs precedes their orthotopic expression in peripheral neuroendocrine glands/cells (Hansenne et al., 2005).

Therefore, depending on their behavior either as the source of neuroendocrine self-peptides or cryptocrine signals, the thymic repertoire of neuroendocrine precursors recapitulates at the molecular level the dual role of the thymus in T cell negative and positive selection.

INTEGRATED COEVOLUTION OF THE NEUROENDOCRINE AND IMMUNE SYSTEMS (FIGURE 1)

Throughout evolution, the neuroendocrine and innate immune systems have evolved in parallel, and coexist in all animal species without any apparent aggression of the innate immune system toward neuroendocrine glands. Indeed, Toll-like receptors, which are the essential mediators of innate response, do not react against normal or undamaged self. Some anticipatory immune responses are present even in jawless vertebrates (agnathans), mediated by

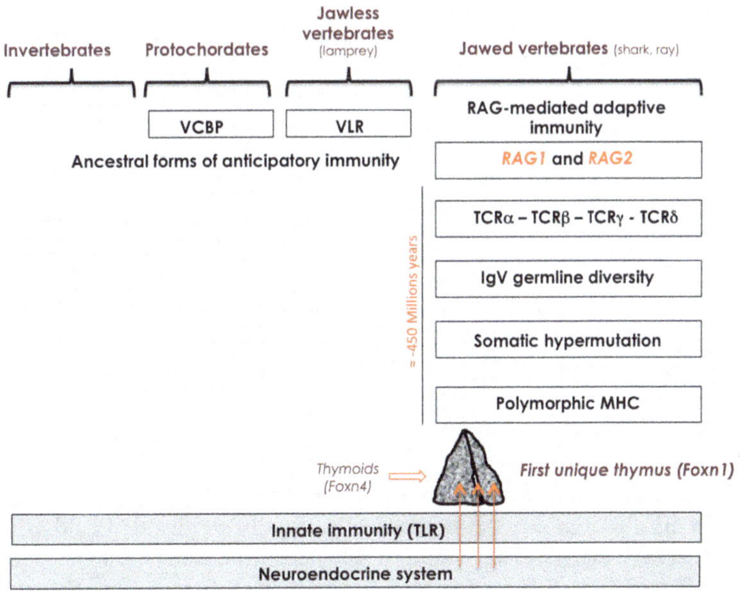

FIGURE 1 | Integrated evolution of the immune and neuroendocrine systems. Neuroendocrine principles are evolutionarily ancient and did not evolve extensively except by gene duplication and differential RNA splicing. A high risk of inherent autoimmunity toward the neuroendocrine tissues resulted from the appearance of RAG-dependent adaptive immunity in jawed cartilaginous fishes. Preceded by ancestor thymoids in lamprey larvae, the first unique thymus emerged in jawed vertebrates, and the intrathymic presentation of neuroendocrine self-peptides (arrows) may be viewed *a posteriori* as a very efficient and economical way to instruct the adaptive T cell system in tolerating neuroendocrine functions as early as during thymus-dependent cell differentiation. VCBP, variable region-containing chitin-binding protein; VLR, variable lymphocyte receptor.

diverse variable lymphocyte receptors (VLRs), with 4–12 leucine-rich repeat modules assembled by some gene conversion process. Some 500 million years ago, the emergence of transposon-like genes coding for recombination-activating enzymes RAG-1 and RAG-2 in cartilaginous fishes (sharks and rays, mainly) initiated the development of adaptive immunity (Agrawal et al., 1998; Boehm and Bleul, 2007; Hirano et al., 2011). The appearance of these two genes in the genome of gnathostomes (probably via horizontal transmission), and the subsequent appearance of the combinatorial immune system has been sometimes described as the "Big Bang" of immunology. Gene recombination in somatic lymphoid cells is responsible for the stochastic generation of diverse immune receptors for antigen, B-cell receptors (BCRs, $\pm 5 \times 10^{13}$ combinations) and T-cell receptors (TCRs, $\pm 10^{18}$ combinations). This extreme diversity of antigen receptors was directly associated with a high inherent risk of autoxicity that threatened survival of both species and individuals. This evolutionary pressure was so strong that, in accordance with Paul Ehrlich's concept of *horror autotoxicus*, novel structures, and mechanisms appeared with the specific role of protecting self against potential autoimmune attacks and orchestrating immunological self-tolerance. The first unique thymus also appeared in jawed cartilaginous fishes, concomitantly or very shortly after the emergence of adaptive immunity. The thymus did not abruptly appear but, as elegantly demonstrated by Bajoghli et al. (2011), was preceded by thymus-like lymphoepithelial structures in the gill baskets of lamprey larvae. These "thymoids" express the gene encoding forkhead box N4 (*Foxn4*), the ortholog of *Foxn1*, the transcription factor responsible for the differentiation of TECs in higher vertebrates as discussed above. *Foxn1* thus stands at a crucial place in the emergence of thymus epithelium that is essential for the control of T cell differentiation and self-tolerance programming (Boehm, 2011). The same study also provided strong evidence for a functional analogy between VLR assembly in thymoids and TCR recombination in the thymus, opening the hypothesis of autoimmune-like phenomena in jawless vertebrates.

The hierarchic organization of the thymic repertoire of neuroendocrine self-peptides is also very significant from an evolutionary point of view. Because major neuroendocrine principles had been established before the emergence of the anticipatory adaptive immune response, they had to be protected from the risk of autoimmunity inherent to this immune lottery. OT is a hypothalamic nonapeptide that is closely implicated at different steps of the reproductive process, from social affiliation and bonding to control of parturition and lactation. Thus, OT is fundamental for the preservation of animal and human species. Through its dominant expression in TECs, OT is much more tolerated than AVP, its hypothalamo-neurohypophysial homolog, which mainly controls water homeostasis and vascular tone. Interestingly, rare cases of autoimmune hypothalamitis with AVP deficiency and diabetes insipidus have been repeatedly observed (de Bellis et al., 2004), but no autoimmunity against OT has ever been reported. Similarly in the insulin family, insulin is the primary autoantigen of type 1 diabetes (T1D) while there is no report of autoimmunity against IGF-2, a growth factor fundamental for fetus development and individual ontogeny. However, because of their close homology, however, thymic neuroendocrine self-peptides promote immunological cross-tolerance to their whole family, and tolerance to insulin is indeed lower in *Igf2*$^{-/-}$ than in wild-type mice (Hansenne et al., 2006). Despite IGF-2 ubiquitous expression in extrathymic tissues, the deletion of *Igf2* in murine *Foxn1*+ TECs is also associated with a significant decrease in immunological tolerance to IGF-2 and to insulin (unpublished observations).

A DEFECT OF CENTRAL SELF-TOLERANCE AS THE PRIMARY EVENT DRIVING DEVELOPMENT OF AUTOIMMUNITY (FIGURE 2)

The evidence that T cells are programmed to recognize and tolerate the whole insulin family during their differentiation in the thymus prompted us to investigate the hypothesis of a defect in this education process as a potential source of self-reactive T cells directed specifically against insulin-secreting β cells of the pancreas. In other words, instead of considering autoimmune T1D as pathology of the pancreas, should we now consider the thymus as the primary defective organ? Already in 1973, Burnet theorized that the pathogenesis of autoimmune diseases first depends on a failure of self-tolerance and the appearance of "forbidden" self-reactive immune clones in the peripheral repertoire (Burnet, 1973), and even before the development of transgenic mice, a number of studies had provided elegant data supporting this hypothesis. Neonatal thymectomy prevents the emergence of autoimmune diabetes in an animal model of human T1D, the bio-breeding (BB) rat (Like et al., 1982). This benefit of neonatal thymectomy may now be explained by the removal of a defective thymus responsible for the continuous release and peripheral enrichment of the peripheral T cell repertoire with "forbidden" intolerant self-reactive T cells. Conversely, transplantation of thymus from diabetes-resistant (BBDR) to diabetes-prone BB (BBDR) rats prevents autoimmune diabetes in the latter (Georgiou and Bellgrau, 1989). Grafts of pure TECs from NOD mouse embryos to newborn C57BL/6 athymic nude mice also induce CD4 and CD8 T cell-mediated insulitis and sialitis (Thomas-Vaslin et al., 1997). Central tolerance and intrathymic apoptosis of self-reactive T cells were suspected to be defective in the NOD thymus (Kishimoto and Sprent, 2001; Zucchelli et al., 2005). However, a very careful recent study has established that thymic negative selection is functional in NOD mice (Mingueneau et al., 2012).

Transcription of all insulin-related genes has been investigated in the thymus of BBDR and BBDP rats. *Ins* and *Igf1* transcripts were detected in all BBDP and BBDR thymi whereas *Igf2* transcripts were also detected in all BBDR thymi but in only in 4 of 15 BBDP thymi. Such a defect of *Igf2* transcription in BBDP thymus could contribute both to their lymphopenia (including CD8+ T and RT6+ Treg cells) and to the absence of central tolerance to islet β cells (Kecha-Kamoun et al., 2001). In humans, *INS* transcripts are measured at a lower level in the thymus from fetuses with short class I variable number of tandem repeat (VNTR) alleles, the second genetic trait (*IDDM2*) of T1D susceptibility (Pugliese et al., 1997; Vafiadis et al., 1997). A number of other genetic loci associated with susceptibility to T1D could certainly determine disturbances in the

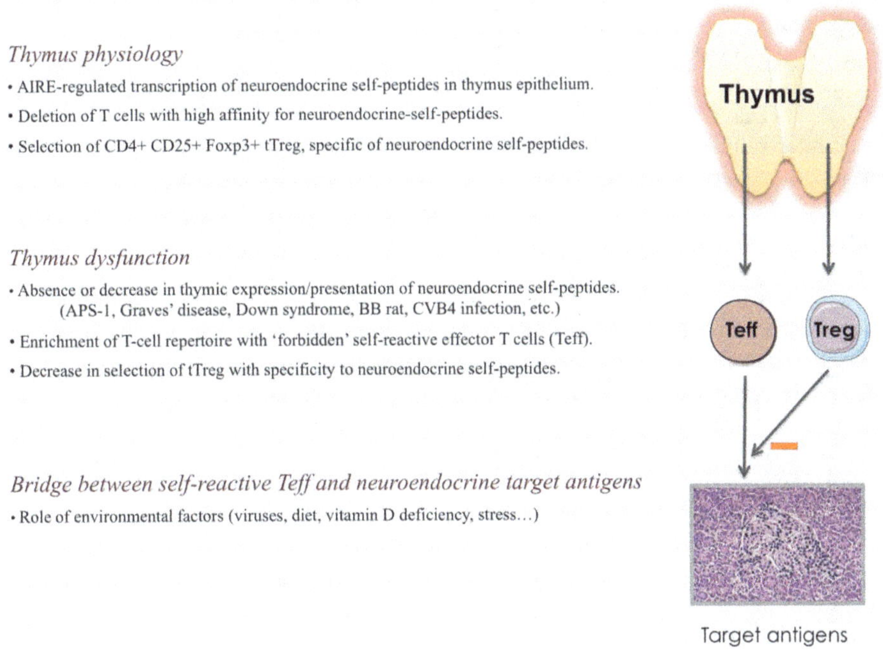

FIGURE 2 | Physiology of the thymus and the primary role of a thymus dysfunction in the development of autoimmune endocrine diseases. Throughout life, the thymus generates naïve T cells that are self-tolerant and competent against nonself-antigens, as well as self-specific thymus-dependent regulatory T (tTreg) cells. Under AIRE control, thymus epithelium (and mTECs particularly) transcribes genes encoding neuroendocrine self-peptides, as well as other tissue-restricted antigens. The absence or decrease in the intrathymic presentation of neuroendocrine self-peptides conducts to a continuous enrichment of the peripheral T cell repertoire with "forbidden" self-reactive T cells (Teff) bearing a TCR directed against neuroendocrine self-antigens, while thymic generation of specific tTreg cells is severely impaired. This thymus defect results in the absence of central self-tolerance to neuroendocrine tissues/cells, which is a condition necessary but not sufficient to initiate an autoimmune endocrine disease. Environmental factors also intervene in the promotion of a molecular bridge between self-reactive Teff and target neuroendocrine antigens.

thymus-dependent programming of central self-tolerance toward islet β cells.

In mice, where two genes code for (pro)insulin (*Ins1* and *Ins2*), *Ins2* is predominantly transcribed in rare subsets of mTECs while *Ins1* is dominantly expressed in murine islet β cells, which leads to a higher immunological tolerance to *Ins2*. This difference in the topography of *Ins2* and *Ins1* expression explains why breeding of *Ins2*$^{-/-}$ mice onto the NOD background markedly accelerates insulitis and diabetes onset (Thebault-Baumont et al., 2003), while the incidence of insulitis and autoimmune diabetes is considerably reduced in *Ins1*$^{-/-}$ congenic NOD mice (Moriyama et al., 2003). Susceptibility to autoimmune diabetes is also correlated with the level of *Ins2* transcription in the murine thymus (Chentoufi and Polychronakos, 2002). The role of thymic insulin in mediating central tolerance to islet β cells was demonstrated by the very rapid onset of autoimmune diabetes after a thymus-specific *Ins1* and *Ins2* deletion resulting from the crossing of *Ins1*$^{-/-}$ mice with others presenting a specific *Ins2* deletion in *Aire*-expressing mTECs (Fan et al., 2009). Of note, *Ins2* transcription in mTEC clones is not regulated by glucose (Levi and Polychronakos, 2009) and is increased about 20-fold by anti-lymphotoxin β mAb (Palumbo et al., 2006). *Ins* transcription in mTECs uses a start site different than in pancreatic islet β cells (Villasenor et al., 2008). In addition to Aire, the insulin transactivator MafA also induces *Ins* transcription in the thymus; targeted *Mafa* disruption reduces *Ins2* expression in the thymus and induces anti-islet autoantibodies (Noso et al., 2010).

The identification of the autoimmune regulator (*AIRE*) gene, a member of the zinc-finger gene family, led to an extremely important advancement in our knowledge of the central role played by a thymus dysfunction in the pathogenesis of organ-specific autoimmune diseases (The Finnish-German APECED Consortium, 1997). *AIRE* mutations are responsible for a rare recessive congenital syndrome called autoimmune polyglandular syndrome type 1 (APS-1) or Autoimmune Poly-Endocrinopathy, Candidiasis, Ectodermal Dystrophy (APECED) syndrome. *AIRE* encodes a protein with structural characteristics of a transcription factor: its transcription is maximal in thymus epithelium, and *Aire*$^{-/-}$ mice develop several autoimmune processes associated with a marked decrease in the intrathymic expression of numerous neuroendocrine self-peptides (Anderson et al., 2002). It also appears that both VNTR alleles (*IDDM2*) and the level of *AIRE* transcription in the thymus determine the concentration of *INS* transcripts in the human thymus (Sabater et al., 2005). The two plant homeodomains (PHDs) are critical regions for Aire function (Peterson et al., 2008); PHD2 strongly influences the ability of Aire to control the mTEC transcriptome and is therefore crucial for effective central tolerance induction (Yang et al., 2013). RANK signals from CD4+CD3− lymphoid tissue inducer (LTi) cells regulate the development and differentiation of *Aire*-expressing mTECs (Rossi et al., 2007). Very recently, a mutual interdependence between Aire and microRNAs (miRs) was evidenced in the thymus since the profile of miR expression is severely affected in isolated murine and human mTECs from *Aire*$^{-/-}$ mice and since, in turn, *Aire* expression is downregulated in mTECs of Dicer null mutant mice (Macedo et al., 2012; Ucar et al., 2013).

An additional level of protection against autoimmunity is also provided by peripheral mechanisms of immunological tolerance that inactivate self-reactive T lymphocytes that have escaped the thymic censorship. Interestingly, extrathymic *Aire*-expressing cells were very recently identified as distinct bone marrow-derived tolerogenic cells that anergize effector self-reactive CD4+ T cells in secondary lymphoid organs (Gardner et al., 2008, 2013). These data further demonstrate that the Aire gene/protein is an essential shield against autoimmunity (Metzger and Anderson, 2011).

For several years, we have been investigating a novel hypothesis according which an infection by the enterovirus Coxsackie B4 (CVB4) could induce a thymus dysfunction and an impairment of central tolerance to the insulin protein/gene family. CVB4 can directly infect the epithelial and lymphoid compartments of the human and murine thymus, and promote a severe thymus dysfunction with massive pre-T cell depletion and a marked-up regulation of MHC class I expression by TECs and by double positive CD4+CD8+ immature thymic T cells (Brilot et al., 2002, 2004). CVB4 infection of murine fetal thymic organ cultures also interferes with T cell differentiation (Brilot et al., 2008). Outbred mice can be infected with CVB4 following oral inoculation, which results in systemic spreading of viral RNA and a prolonged detection of CVB4 RNA in thymus, spleen, and blood up to 70 days after inoculation (Jaïdane et al., 2006). Moreover, CVB4 infection of a murine mTEC line induces a dramatic decrease in *Igf2* mRNA and IGF-2 protein in this cell line, while *Igf1* transcripts were relatively unaffected. In this mTEC line, *Ins2* transcripts could not be detected (Jaïdane et al., 2012). Together, our data strongly suggest that CVB4 infection of the thymus could disrupt central self-tolerance to the insulin family, and could also enhance CVB4 virulence through induction of central tolerance to this virus.

With regard to autoimmune thyroiditis, which is the most frequent autoimmune endocrine disease, all major thyroid-specific antigens, i.e., thyroperoxydase, thyroglobulin, and thyrotropin receptor (TSHR), are also transcribed in human TECs in normal conditions (Paschke and Geenen, 1995; Sospedra et al., 1998). As first reported by Hammar, thymic hyperplasia is commonly observed in Graves' disease (Murakami et al., 1996), and homozygotes for an SNP allele predisposing to Graves' disease have significantly lower intrathymic *TSHR* transcripts than carriers of the protective allele (Colobran et al., 2011).

With regard to autoimmunity directed against peripheral nonendocrine organs, a defect in α-myosin expression in TECs was recently shown to exert a central role in the pathogenesis of autoimmune myocarditis in mice and humans (Lv et al., 2011; Lv and Lipes, 2012). Also, a defect in Aire-mediated central tolerance to myelin protein zero promotes the development of an autoimmune Th1 effector response toward peripheral nerves (Su et al., 2012).

THE CONCEPT OF "NEGATIVE/TOLEROGENIC SELF-VACCINATION"

Although *Ins2* is expressed at low levels in rare mTECs, thymic (pro)insulin has an essential role in protecting islet β cells against diabetogenic autoimmunity. However, insulin *per se* does not exert any significant tolerogenic properties that could be exploited to reprogram immunological tolerance to islet β cells. With the exception of two studies (Fourlanos et al., 2011; Roep et al., 2013), all the clinical trials based on insulin administration by different ways failed to preserve the residual β cell mass once the autoimmune attack has induced patent T1D. On the contrary, the potent immunogenic properties of insulin were revealed in different studies (Blanas et al., 1996; Liu et al., 2002), and this immunogenicity could be related to the very low level of insulin gene transcription in the thymus. Other studies have also evidenced the risk of hypersensitivity or anaphylaxis following administration of an autoantigen (Pedotti et al., 2001).

Nevertheless, the development of peptide-based therapeutic vaccines remains an attractive approach because of the specificity of immune suppression or regulation directed to specific pathogenic self-reactive T cells. In this context, infusion of a strongly active insulin mimetope was recently shown to convert naïve T cells into Foxp3+ Treg cells *in vivo* and to prevent autoimmune diabetes in NOD mice (Daniel et al., 2011). We proposed that IGF-2 could be a safer and more valuable basis for developing a specific "negative/tolerogenic self-vaccination," on the basis that *Igf2* transcription is defective in the thymus of BBDP rats (Kecha-Kamoun et al., 2001) and that IGF-2 mediates significant cross-tolerance to insulin (Hansenne et al., 2006). The concept of negative self-vaccination implies both the competition between IGF-2 and insulin-derived epitopes for presentation by DQ2 and DQ8 alleles, as well as a tolerogenic response—including recruitment of Treg cells–induced by MHC-presentation of IGF-2 self-peptides (Geenen et al., 2004, 2010).

CONCLUSION

Our studies have established that the thymus is not a classical neuroendocrine gland, but an obligatory intersection between the adaptive immune and neuroendocrine systems (Geenen, 2010). Moreover, they have elucidated how thymic epithelium is responsible for the programming of immunological central self-tolerance toward neuroendocrine functions through presentation of neuroendocrine self-peptides. They have also helped to resolve three major questions concerning the pathogenesis of autoimmune endocrine disorders: Why are the neuroendocrine glands so frequently tackled by an autoimmune process? What is the origin of the pathogenic effector self-reactive T cells? And what explains the tissue/cell-specificity of the autoimmune processes? There is no doubt that this novel knowledge will soon be exploited for the development of innovative strategies to prevent and cure a variety of organ-specific devastating autoimmune diseases such as T1D.

ACKNOWLEDGMENTS

Vincent Geenen is Research Director and Gwennaëlle Bodart is Research Assistant of the Belgian Fund for Scientific Research of Belgium (F.S.R.-NFSR). We are extremely grateful to Pr Gareth

Leng (University of Edinburgh) for his critical reading of this manuscript. These studies are or have been supported by F.S.R.-NFSR and the Fund for Research in Industry and Agronomy (FRIA, Belgium), by the Fund Leon Fredericq for biomedical research at the University Hospital of Liege, by the Special Research Fund of the University of Liege, by the Fund A. Rahier for research in diabetes, by Wallonia (Tolediab, ThymUp and Raparray conventions), by the European Federation for the Study of Diabetes (EFSD, Düsseldorf), by the Juvenile Diabetes Research Foundation (JDRF, New York), and by the European Commission (Eurothymaide PF6 Integrated Project, contract LHSB-CT-2003-503410, www.eurothymaide.org).

REFERENCES

Agrawal, A., Eastman, Q. M., and Schatz, D. G. (1998). Transposition mediated by RAG1 and RAG2 and its implications for the evolution of the immune system. *Nature* 394, 744–751. doi:10.1038/29457

Anderson, G., Lane, P. J. L., and Jenkinson, E. J. (2007). Generating intrathymic microenvironments to establish T-cell tolerance. *Nat. Rev. Immunol.* 7, 954–962. doi: 10.1038/nri2187

Anderson, M. S., Venanzi, E. S., Klein, L., Chen, Z., Berzin, S. P., Turley, S. J., et al. (2002). Projection of an immunological self shadow within the thymus by the aire protein. *Science* 298, 1395–1401. doi:10.1126/science.1075958

Ashton-Rickardt, P., Bandeira, A., Delaney, J. R., Van Kaer, L., Pircher, H. P., Zinkernagel, R. M., et al. (1994). Evidence for a differential avidity model of T cell selection in the thymus. *Cell* 76, 651–663. doi: 10.1016/0092-8674(94)90505-3

Bajoghli, B., Guo, P., Aghaallaei, N., Hirano, M., Strohmeier, C., McCurley, N., et al. (2011). A thymus candidate in lam- preys. *Nature* 470, 90–94. doi: 10.1038/nature09655

Blackburn, C. C., and Manley, N. R. (2004). Developing a new paradigm for thymus organogenesis. *Nat. Rev. Immunol.* 4, 278–289. doi: 10.1038/nri1331

Blanas, E., Carbone, F. R., Allison, J., Miller, J. F. A. P., and Heath, W. R. (1996). Induction of autoim- mune diabetes by oral admin- istration of autoantigen. *Science* 274, 1707–1709. doi: 10.1126/sci- ence.274.5293.1707

Boehm, T. (2011). Design principles of adaptive immune systems. *Nat. Rev. Immunol.* 11, 307–317. doi: 10.1038/nri2944

Boehm, T., and Bleul, C. (2007). The evolutionary history of lymphoid organs. *Nat. Immunol.* 8, 131–135. doi: 10.1038/ni1435

Brilot, F., Chehadeh, W., Charlet- Renard, C., Martens, H., Geenen, V., and Hober, D. (2002). Persistent infection of human thymic epithe- lial cells by coxsackievirus B4. *J. Virol.* 76, 5260–5265. doi: 10.1128/JVI.76.10.5260-5265.2002

Brilot, F., Geenen, V., Hober, D., and Stoddart, C. (2004). Coxsackievirus B4 infection of human fetal thymus cells. *J. Virol.* 78, 9854–9861. doi: 10.1128/JVI.78.18.9854-9861.2004

Brilot, F., Jaïdane, H., Geenen, V., and Hober, D. (2008). Coxsackievirus B4 infection of murine foetal thymus organ cultures. *J. Med. Virol.* 80, 659–666. doi: 10.1002/jmv.21016

Burnet, F. M. (1973). A reassessment of the forbidden clone hypothesis of autoimmune diseases. *Aust. J. Exp. Biol. Med. Sci.* 50, 1–9. doi: 10.1038/icb.1972.1

Burnet, F. M., and Mackay, I. R. (1963). Lymphoepithelial structures and autoimmune disease. *Lancet* 2, 1030–1033.

Chentoufi, A. A., and Polychronakos, C. (2002). Insulin expression lev- els in the thymus modulate insulin- specific autoreactive T-cell toler- ance. *Diabetes* 51, 1383–1390. doi: 10.2337/diabetes.51.5.1383

Colobran, R., del Pilar Armengol, M., Faner, R., Gärtner, M., Tykocinski, L. O., Lucas, A., et al. (2011). Association of an SNP with intrathymic transcription of TSHR and Graves' disease: a role for defective tolerance. *Hum. Mol. Genet.* 20, 3415–3423. doi: 10.1093/hmg/ddr247

Daniel, C., Weigmann, B., Bronson, R., and von Boehmer, H. (2011). Prevention of type 1 diabetes in mice by tolerogenic vaccination with a strong insulin mimetope. *J. Exp. Med.* 208, 1501–1510. doi: 10.1084/jem.20110574

de Bellis, A., Bizzarro, A., and Bellastella, A. (2004). "Autoimmune central diabetes insipidus," in *Immunoendocrinology in Health and Disease*, eds V. Geenen and G. P. Chrousos (New York, NY: Marcel Dekker), 461–490.

Douek, D. C., MacFarland, R. D., Keiser, P. H., Gage, E. A., Massey, J. M., Haynes, B. F., et al. (1998). Changes in thymic function with age and during the treatment of HIV infection. *Nature* 396, 690–695. doi: 10.1038/25374

Ericsson, A., Geenen, V., Robert, F., Legros, J. J., Vrindts-Gevaert, Y., Franchimont, P., et al. (1990). Expression of preprotachykinin A and neuropeptide-Y messenger RNA in the thymus. *Mol. Endocrinol.* 4, 1211–1218. doi: 10.1210/mend-4-8-1211

Fan, Y., Rudert, W. A., Grupillo, M., He, J., Sisino, G., and Trucco, M. (2009). Thymus specific deletion of insulin induces autoimmune dia- betes. *EMBO J.* 28, 2812–2824. doi: 10.1038/emboj.2009.212

Farley, A. M., Morris, L. X., Vroegindeweij, E., Depreter, M. L., Vaidya, H., Stenhouse, F. H., et al. (2013). Dynamics of thymus organogenesis and colonization in early human development. *Development* 140, 2015–2026. doi: 10.1242/dev.087320

Foster, K., Sheridan, J., Veiga- Fernandes, H., Roderick, K., Pachnis, V., Adams, R., et al. (2008). Contribution of neural crest-derived cells in the embryonic and adult thymus. *J. Immunol.* 180, 3183–3189.

Fourlanos, S., Perry, C., Gellert, S. A., Martinuzzi, E., Mallone, R., Butler, J., et al. (2011). Evidence that nasal insulin induces immune tolerance to insulin in adults with autoimmune diabetes. *Diabetes* 60, 1237–1245. doi: 10.2337/db10-1360

Funder, J. W. (1990). Paracrine, cryptocrine, acrocrine. *Mol. Cell. Endocrinol.* 70, C21–C24. doi: 10.1016/0303-7207(90)90052-A

Gardner, J. M., Devos, J. J., Friedman, R. S., Wong, D. J., Ta, Y. X., Zhou, X., et al. (2008). Deletional tolerance mediated by extrathymic Aire-expressing cells. *Science* 321, 843–847. doi: 10.1126/science.1159407

Gardner, J. M., Metzger, T. C., McMahon, E. J., Au-Yeung, B. B., Krawisz, A. K., Lu, W., et al. (2013). Extrathymic Aire-expressing cells are a distinct bone marrow- derived population that induce functional activation of CD4+ T cells. *Immunity* 39, 560–572. doi: 10.1016/j.immuni.2013.08.005

Geenen, V. (2010). The thymus as an obligatory intersection between the immune and neuroendocrine systems: phar- macological implications. *Curr. Opin. Pharmacol.* 10, 406–407. doi: 10.1016/j.coph.2010.05.011

Geenen, V., Kecha, O., and Martens, H. (1998). Thymic expression of neuroendocrine self-peptide pre- cursors: role in T cell survival and self-tolerance. *J. Neuroendocrinol.* 10, 811–822. doi: 10.1046/j.1365-2826.1998.00269.x

Geenen, V., Legros, J. J., Franchimont, P., Baudrihaye, M., Defresne, M. P., and Boniver, J. (1986). The neuroendocrine thymus: coexistence of oxytocin and neurophysin in the human thy- mus. *Science* 232, 508–511. doi: 10.1126/science.3961493

Geenen, V., Louis, C., Martens, H., and The Belgian Diabetes Registry. (2004). An insulin-like growth fac- tor 2-derived self antigen inducing a regulatory cytokine profile after presentation to peripheral blood mononuclear cells form DQ8+ type 1 diabetic adolescents: pre- liminary design of a thymus-based tolerogenic self-vaccination. *Ann. N.Y. Acad. Sci.* 1037, 59–64. doi: 10.1196/annals.1337.008

Geenen, V., Mottet, M., Dardenne, O., Kermani, H., Martens, H., Francois, J. M., et al. (2010). Thymic self-antigens for the design of a negative/tolerogenic self- vaccination against type 1 diabetes. *Curr. Opin. Pharmacol.* 10, 461–472. doi: 10.1016/j.coph.2010.04.005

Geenen, V., Robert, F., Martens, H., Benhida, A., De Giovanni, G., Defresne, M. P., et al. (1991). At the cutting edge. Biosynthesis and paracrine/cryptocrine actions of 'self' neurohypophysial-related peptides in the thymus. *Mol. Cell. Endocrinol.* 76, C27–C31. doi: 10.1016/0303-7207(91)90277-Y

Georgiou, H. M., and Bellgrau, D. (1989). Thymus transplantation and disease prevention in the diabetes-prone Bio-Breeding rat. *J. Immunol.* 142, 3400–3405.

Griffin, G. H., Alazard, R., and Cohen, P. (1973). Complex formation between bovine neurophysin I and oxytocin, vasopressin and tripeptide analogs of their NH_2- terminal region. *J. Biol. Chem.* 248, 7975–7978.

Hammar, J. A. (1921). The new views as to the morphology of the thy- mus gland and their bearing on the problem of the function of the thy- mus. *Endocrinology* 5, 543–573. doi: 10.1210/endo-5-5-543

Hansenne, I., Charlet-Renard, C., Greimers, R., and Geenen, V. (2006). Dendritic cell differentia- tion and tolerance to insulin-related peptides in *Igf2*-deficient mice. *J. Immunol.* 176, 4651–4657.

Hansenne, I., Rasier, G., Péqueux, C., Brilot, F., Renard, Ch., Breton, C. et al. (2005). Ontogenesis and func- tional aspects of oxytocin and vaso- pressin gene expression in the thy- mus network. *J. Neuroimmunol.* 158, 67–75. doi: 10.1016/j.jneuroim. 2004.08.007

Hirano, M., Das, S., Guo, P., and Cooper, M. D. (2011). The evo- lution of adaptive immunity in vertebrates. *Adv. Immunol.* 109, 125–157. doi: 10.1016/B978-0-12-387664-5.00004-2

Holländer, G. A., Krenger, W., and Blazar, B. R. (2010). Emerging strategies to boost thymic function. *Curr. Opin. Pharmacol.* 10, 443–453. doi: 10.1016/j.coph.2010.04.008

Jaïdane, H., Caloone, D., Lobert, P. E., Sane, F., Dardenne, O., Naquet, P., et al. (2012). Persistent infec- tion of thymic epithelial cells with coxsackievirus B4 results in decreased expression of type 2 insulin-like growth factor. *J. Virol.* 86, 11151–11162. doi: 10.1128/JVI.00726-12

Jaïdane, H., Gharbi, J., Lobert, P. E., Lucas, B., Hiar, R., M'Hadheb, M. B., et al. (2006). Prolonged viral RNA detection in blood and lym- phoid tissues from coxsackievirus B4-E2 orally-inoculated mice. *Microbiol. Immunol.* 50, 971–974.

Kappler, J. W., Roehm, N., and Marrack, P. (1987). T cell toler- ance by clonal elimination in the thymus. *Cell* 49, 273–280. doi: 10.1016/0092-8674(87)90568-X

Kecha, O., Brilot, F., Martens, H., Franchimont, N., Renard, C., Greimers, R., et al. (2000). Involvement of insulin-like growth factors in early T cell develop- ment: a study using fetal thymic organ cultures. *Endocrinology* 141, 1209–1217. doi: 10.1210/en.141. 3.1209

Kecha-Kamoun, O., Achour, I., Martens, H., Collette, J., Lefèbvre, P. J., Greiner, D. L., et al. (2001). Thymic expression of insulin- related genes in an animal model of type 1 diabetes. *Diabetes Metab. Res. Rev.* 17, 146–152. doi: 10.1002/dmrr.182

Kishimoto, H., and Sprent, J. (2001). A defect in central tolerance in NOD mice. *Nat. Immunol.* 2, 1025–1031. doi: 10.1038/ni726

Kisielow, P., Bluethmann, H., Staerz, D., Steinmetz, M., and von Boehmer, H. (1988). Tolerance in T cell receptor transgenic mice: dele- tion of nonmature CD4+8+ thy- mocytes. *Nature* 333, 742–746. doi: 10.1038/333742a0

Klein, L., Hinterberger, M., Wirnsberger, G., and Kyewski, B. (2009). Antigen presentation in the thymus for positive selection and central tolerance induction. *Nat. Rev. Immunol.* 9, 833–844. doi: 10.1038/nri2669

Kyewski, B., and Klein, L. (2006). A central tole for central tolerance. *Annu. Rev. Immunol.* 24, 571–606. doi: 10.1146/annurev.immunol.23. 021704.115601

Levi, D., and Polychronakos, C. (2009). Regulation of insulin gene expression by cytokines and cell-cell interactions in mouse medullary thymic epithelial cells. *Diabetologia* 52, 2151–2158. doi: 10.1007/s00125-009-1448-y

Like, A. A., Kislaukis, E., Williams, R. M., and Rossini, A. A. (1982). Neonatal thymectomy prevents spontaneous diabetes mellitus in the BB:W rat. *Science* 216, 644–646. doi: 10.1126/science.7041259

Liu, E., Moriyama, H., Abiru, N., Miao, D., Yu, L., Taylor, R. M., et al. (2002). Anti-peptide autoantibodies and fatal anaphylaxis in NOD mice in response to insulin self-peptides. *J. Clin. Invest.* 110, 1021–1027. doi: 10.1172/JCI215488

Lv, H., Havari, E., Pinto, S., Gottumukkala, R. V., Cornivelli, L., Raddassi, K., et al. (2011). Impaired thymic tolerance to a- myosin directs autoimmunity to the heart in mice and humans. *J. Clin. Invest.* 121, 1561–1573. doi: 10.1172/JCI44583

Lv, H. J., and Lipes, M. A. (2012). Role of impaired central tolerance to a-myosin in inflamma- tory heart disease. *Trends Cardiovasc. Med.* 22, 113–117. doi: 10.1016/j.tcm.2012.07.005

Macedo, C., Evangelista, A. F., Marques, M. M., Octavillio-Silva, S., Donadi, E. A., Sakamoto-Hojo, E. T., et al. (2012). Autoimmune regulator (Aire) controls the expression of microRNAs in medullary thymic epithelial cells. *Immunobiology* 218, 554–560. doi: 10.1016/j.imbio.2012. 06.013

Manley, N. R., and Capecchi, M. R. (1995). The role of Hoxa-3 in mouse thymus and thyroid development. *Development* 121, 1989–2003.

Martens, H., Kecha, O., Charlet Renard, C., Defresne, M. P., and Geenen, V. (1998). Neurohypophysial peptides stim- ulate the phosphorylation of pre-T cells focal adhesion kinases. *Neuroendocrinology* 67, 282–289. doi: 10.1159/000054324

Martens, H., Malgrange, B., Robert, F., Charlet, C., De Groote, D., Heymann, D., et al. (1996a). Cytokine production by human thymic epithelial cells: control by the immune recognition of the neurohypophysial self- antigen. *Regul. Pept.* 67, 39–45. doi: 10.1016/S0167-0115(96)00105-X

Martens, H., Goxe, B., and Geenen, (1996b). The thymic repertoire of neuroendocrine self-antigens: physiological implications in T-cell life and death. *Immunol. Today* 17, 312–317. doi: 10.1016/0167-5699(96)10023-2

Maryanski, J. L., Romero, P., Van Pel, A., Boon, T., Salemme, F. R., Cerrottini, J. C., et al. (1991). The identification of tyrosine as a common key residue in unrelated H-2K^d restricted anti- genic peptides. *Int. Immunol.* 3, 1035–1042. doi: 10.1093/intimm/3. 10.1035

Mathis, D., and Benoist, C. (2004). Back to central tolerance. *Immunity* 20, 509–516. doi: 10.1016/S1074-7613(04)00111-6

McCaughtry, T. M., Baldwin, T. A., Wilken, M. S., and Hogquist, K. A. (2008). Clonal deletion of thy- mocytes can occur in the cortex with no involvement of the medulla. *J. Exp. Med.* 205, 2575–2584. doi: 10.1084/jem.20080866

Metzger, T. C., and Anderson, M. S. (2011). Control of central and peripheral tolerance by Aire. *Immunol. Rev.* 241, 89–103. doi: 10.1111/j.1600-065X.2011.01008.x

Miller, J. F. A. P. (1961). Immunological function of the thymus. *Lancet* 2, 748–749. doi: 10.1016/S0140-6736(61)90693-6

Mingueneau, M., Jiand, W., Feuerer, M., Mathis, D., and Benoist, C. (2012). Thymic negative selec- tion is functional in NOD mice. *J. Exp. Med.* 209, 623–637. doi: 10.1084/jem.20112593

Moriyama, H., Abiru, N., Paronen, J., Sikora, K., Liu, E., Miao, D., et al. (2003). Evidence for a primary islet autoantigen (pre- proinsulin 1) for insulitis and diabetes in the nonobese dia- betic mouse. *Proc. Natl. Acad. Sci. U.S.A.* 100, 10376–10381. doi: 10.1073/pnas.1834450100

Murakami, M., Hosoi, Y., Negishi, T., Kamiya, Y., Miyashita, K., Yamada, M., et al. (1996). Thymic hyper- plasia in patients with Graves' dis- ease. Identification of thyrotropin receptors in human thymus. *J. Clin. Invest.* 98, 2228–2234. doi: 10.1172/ JCI119032

Nehls, M., Pfeifer, D., Schorpp, M., Hedrich, H., and Boehm, T. (1994). New member of the winged-helix protein family disrupted in mouse and rat nude mutations. *Nature* 372, 103–106. doi: 10.1038/372103a0

Noso, S., Kataoka, K., Kawabata, Y., Babaya, N., Hiromine, Y., Yamaji, K., et al. (2010). Insulin transacti- vator MafA regulates intrathymic expression of insulin and affects susceptibility to type 1 diabetes. *Diabetes* 59, 2579–2587. doi: 10.2337/db10-0476

Nowell, C. S., Bredenkamp, N., Tetélin, S., Jin, X., Tischner, C., Vaidya, H., et al. (2011). Foxn1 regulates lineage progression in cortical and medullary thymic epithe- lial cells but is dispensable for medullary sublineage divergence. *PLoS Genet.* 7:e1002348. doi: 10.1371/journal.pgen.1002348

Ohki, H., Martin, C., Corbel, C., Coltey, M., and Le Douarin, N. M. (1987). Tolerance induced by thymic epithelial grafts in birds. *Science* 237, 1032–1035. doi: 10.1126/science.3616623

Ott, I., and Scott, J. C. (1910). The galactogogue action of the thy- mus and corpus luteum. *Proc. Soc. Exp. Biol. Med.* 8, 49–53. doi: 10.3181/00379727-8-28

Palumbo, M. O., Levi, D., Chentoufi, A. A., and Polychronakos, C. (2006). Isolation and character- isation of proinsulin-producing medullary thymic epithelial cells clones. *Diabetes* 55, 2595–2601. doi: 10.2337/db05-1651

Paschke, R., and Geenen, V. (1995). Messenger RNA expression for a TSH receptor variant in the thymus of a two-year old child. *J. Mol. Med.* 73, 577–580. doi: 10.1007/BF00195143

Pedotti, R., Mitchell, D., Wedemeyer, ., Karpuj, M., Chabas, D., Hattab, E. M., et al. (2001). An unex- pected version of horror autotox- icus: anaphylactic shock to a self- peptide. *Nat. Immunol.* 2, 216–222. doi: 10.1038/85266

Peterson, P., Org, T., and Rebane, A. (2008). Transcriptional regula- tion by AIRE: molecular mech- anisms of central tolerance. *Nat. Rev. Immunol.* 8, 948–957. doi: 10.1038/nri2450

Pugliese, A., Zeller, M., Fernandez, A. Jr., Zalcberg, L. J., Barnett, R. J., Ricordi, C., et al. (1997). The insulin gene is transcribed in the human thymus and transcription levels cor- relate with allelic variation at the *INS* VNTR-*IDDM2* susceptibility locus for type 1 diabetes. *Nat. Genet.* 15, 293–297. doi: 10.1038/ ng0397-293

Roep, B. O., Solvason, N., Gottlieb, P. A., Abreu, J. R., Harrison, L. C., Eisenbarth, G. S., et al. (2013). Plasmid-encoding proinsulin pre- serves C-peptide while specifically reducing proinsulin-specific CD8+ T cells in type 1 diabetes. *Sci. Transl. Med.* 5, 191ra82. doi: 10.1126/sci- translmed.3006103

Rossi, S. W., Kim, M. Y., Leibbrandt, A., Parnell, S. M., Jenkinson, W. E., Glanville, S. H., et al. (2007). RANK signals from CD4(+)3(-) inducer cells regulate develop- ment of Aire-expressing epithelial cells in the thymic medulla. *J. Exp. Med.* 204, 1267–1272. doi: 10.1084/jem.20062497

Sabater, L., Ferrer-Francesch, X., Transcription of a broad range of self-antigens in human thymus sug- gests a role for central mecha- nisms in tolerance toward periph- eral antigens. *J. Immunol.* 161, 5918–5929.

Stritesky, G. L., Jameson, S. C., and Hogquist, K. A. (2012). Selection of self-reactive T cells in the thymus. *Annu. Rev. Immunol.* 30, 95–114. doi: 10.1146/annurev-immunol- 020711-075035

Su, M. A., Davini, D., Cheng, P., Giang, K., Fan, U., DeVoss, J. J., et al. (2012). Defective autoim- mune regulator-dependent central tolerance to myelin protein zero is linked to autoimmune periph- eral neuropathy. *J. Immunol.* 188, 4906–4912. doi: 10.4049/jimmunol. 1200493

The bault-Baumont, K., Dubois- Laforgue, D., Krief,P.,Briand,J. P., Halbout, P.,Vallon- Geoffroy, K., etal.(2003).Acceleration of type 1 diabetes mellitusin proinsulin 2-deficient NOD mice. J. Clin. Invest. 111, 851–857.doi: 10.1172/ JCI16584

The Finnish-German Consortium. (1997). Anautoimmunedisease, APECED, caused by mutations in a novel gene featuring two PHD- type zinc-finger domains. Nat. Genet. 17,399–403.doi:10.1038/ ng1297-399

Thomas-Vaslin, V., Damotte, D., Coltey, M., LeDouarin, N.M., Coutinho,A.,andSalaün,J.(1997). Abnormal Tcellselectionon NOD thymic epithelium is sufficient to induce autoimmune mani-festations in C57/BL/6 athymic nude mice. Proc. Natl. Acad. Sci.U.S.A. 94, 4598–4603.doi: 10.1073/ pnas.94.9.4598

Ucar, O., Tykocinski, L.-O., Dooley, J., Liston, A.,and Kyewski, B. (2013). An evolutionary conserved mutual interdependence between Aire and microRNAs in promis-cuous gene expression. Eur.J. Immunol. 43,1769–1778.doi: 10.1002/ eji.201343343

Vafiadis, P., Bennett, S. T., Todd, J. A., Nadeau, J., Grabs, R., Goodyer, C. G., et al. (1997). Insulin expression in human thymus is modulated by *INS* VNTR alleles at the *IDDM2* locus.*Nat.Genet.* 15,289–292.doi: 10.1038/ng0397-289

Vanneste, Y., Ntodou Thome, A., Vandersmissen, E., Charlet, C., Franchimont,D.,Martens, H.,et al. (1997). Identification of neurotensin-related peptides in human thymic epithelial cell membranes and relationship with major his to compatibility complex class I molecules. J. Neuroimmunol. 76, 161–166. doi:10.1016/S0165-5728 (97)00052-0

Villasenor, J., Besse, W., Benoist, C., and Mathis, D. (2008). Ectopic expression of peripheral-tissue antigens in the thymic epithe- lium: probabilistic, monoallelic, misinitiated. *Proc. Natl. Acad. Sci. U.S.A.* 105, 15854–15859. doi: 10.1073/pnas.0808069105

Wiemann, M., and Ehret, G. (1993). Subcellular localization of immunoreactive oxytocin within thymic epithelial cells of the male mouse. *Cell Tissue Res.* 273, 79–87. doi: 10.1007/BF00304614

Wilkinson, B., Owen, J. J. T., and Jenkinson, E. J. (1999). Factors reg- ulating stem cell recruitment to the fetal thymus. *J. Immunol.* 162, 3873–3881.

Yang, S., Bansal, K., Lopes, J., Benoist, C., and Mathis, D. (2013). Aire's plant homeodomain (PHD)-2 is critical for induction of immunological tolerance. *Proc. Natl. Acad. Sci. U.S.A. 110, 1833–1838. doi : 10.1073/ pnas. 1222023110*

Zucchelli, S., Holler, P.,Yamagata, T.,Roy, M., Benoist, C., and Mathis,D.(2005). Defective central tolerance induction in NOD mice: genomics and genetics. Immunity 22, 385–396.doi: 10.1016/j. immuni. 2005.01.015

18

Pericytes: brain-immune interface modulators

Gabriela Hurtado-Alvarado, Adrian M. Cabañas-Morales and Beatriz Gómez-Gónzalez*

Area of Neurosciences, Department of Biology of Reproduction, Unidad Iztapalapa, Universidad Autónoma Metropolitana, Mexico City, Mexico

Edited by:
Sidney A. Simon, Duke University, USA

Reviewed by:
Patrizia Casaccia, University of Medicine and Dentistry, USA
Antonio Pereira, Federal University of Rio Grande do Norte, Brazil

****Correspondence:***
Beatriz Gómez-Gónzalez, Area of Neurosciences, Department Biology of Reproduction, Unidad Iztapalapa, Universidad Autónoma Metropolitana, Avenida San Rafael Atlixco No. 186, Colonia Vicentina, Iztapalapa, Mexico City 09340, Mexico
e-mail: bgomezglez@gmail.com; bgomez@xanum.uam.mx

The premise that the central nervous system is immune-privileged arose from the fact that direct contact between immune and nervous cells is hindered by the blood–brain barrier. However, the blood–brain barrier also comprises the interface between the immune and nervous systems by secreting chemo-attractant molecules and by modulating immune cell entry into the brain. The majority of published studies on the blood–brain barrier focus on endothelial cells (ECs), which are a critical component, but not the only one; other cellular components include astroglia, microglia, and pericytes. Pericytes are poorly studied in comparison with astrocytes or ECs; they are mesenchymal cells that can modify their ultrastructure and gene expression in response to changes in the central nervous system microenvironment. Pericytes have a unique synergistic relationship with brain ECs in the regulation of capillary permeability through secretion of cytokines, chemokines, nitric oxide, matrix metalloproteinases, and by means of capillary contraction. Those pericyte manifestations are related to changes in blood–brain barrier permeability by an increase in endocytosis-mediated transport and by tight junction disruption. In addition, recent reports demonstrate that pericytes control the migration of leukocytes in response to inflammatory mediators by up-regulating the expression of adhesion molecules and releasing chemo-attractants; however, under physiological conditions they appear to be immune-suppressors. Better understanding of the immune properties of pericytes and their participation in the effects of brain infections, neurodegenerative diseases, and sleep loss will be achieved by analyzing pericyte ultrastructure, capillary coverage, and protein expression. That knowledge may provide a mechanism by which pericytes participate in the maintenance of the proper function of the brain-immune interface.

Keywords: pericytes, blood–brain barrier, immune response, inflammation, cytokines, REM sleep loss, brain endothelial cell, tight junction disruption

INTRODUCTION

The brain must respond to blood-borne signals but has no direct access to them (Persidsky et al., 2006; Saper, 2010). Likewise, the immune system does not contact directly the brain *milieu*; they interact through the brain-immune interface, the blood–brain barrier. The interface is comprised by endothelial cells (ECs), astrocytes, microglia, pericytes, and extracellular matrix components (basal lamina and glycocalyx; Risau, 1991; Ballabh et al., 2004; Ueno, 2007; Gómez-González et al., 2012). ECs limit blood-borne macromolecules or cells from crossing into the brain through junction complexes that fasten together adjacent cell membranes. In addition, transcellular trafficking of molecules is limited by the minimal expression of endocytosis and the presence of specialized carrier systems (Zlokovic, 2008; Abbott et al., 2010). Although ECs provide the physical and chemical barrier function *per se*, all elements are crucial for the development and maintenance of the blood–brain barrier, allowing it to be the interface between peripheral systems and the brain (Zlokovic, 2008).

Pericytes have been increasingly implicated in the regulation of local blood-flow in brain regions with increased synaptic activity, a phenomenon known as neurovascular coupling (reviewed in Hamilton et al., 2010); furthermore, they have also been involved in the regulation of the blood–brain barrier permeability to circulating molecules (Armulik et al., 2010). Better understanding of the immune properties of pericytes and their participation in the changes observed during brain infections and neurodegenerative diseases will provide a mechanism by which pericytes participate in the maintenance of the proper function of the brain-immune interface, the blood–brain barrier. Here we present recent evidence depicting the new roles of pericytes in regulating blood–brain barrier function under normal and pathological conditions and hypothesize its potential role in the regulation of the blood–brain barrier after chronic sleep loss.

PERICYTES AS BLOOD–BRAIN BARRIER COMPONENTS

Pericytes are smooth muscle-derived cells that play a crucial role in keeping brain homeostasis given their presence at the blood–brain barrier and particularly their active role in what is known as the neurovascular unit (Zlokovic, 2008; Gómez-González et al., 2012). Rouget (1874), for the first time, described a population of branched cells with contractile properties that surrounded ECs. Fifty years later, these mesenchymal cells were renamed "pericytes" by Zimmerman in concordance with their anatomical location: abluminal to ECs and luminal to parenchymal cells (Kim et al., 2006; Sá-Pereira et al., 2012). Anatomically, pericytes have projections that wrap around capillaries and are embedded within the basal lamina. The diversity in pericyte marker expression may be related to vessel size or embryonic origin; the main markers are α-smooth muscle actin (αSMA), desmin, the regulator of G-protein signaling 5 (RGS-5), neuron-glial antigen 2 (NG2), platelet-derived growth factor receptor (PDGFRα and PDGFRβ), and amino-peptidase-N (CD13; Ozerdem et al., 2002; Bergers and Song, 2005). These proteins show different expression patterns under physiological and pathological states (see **Table 1**). Furthermore, pericytes express numerous macrophage markers, namely CD4, CD11b, CD146, and proteins related to immune function such as the fragment crystallizable receptor (FcR) and the major histocompatibility complex (MHC) classes I and II (Bergers and Song, 2005; Kamouchi et al., 2011). Differences in the expression of those markers are based on the local environmental influences on pericytes. For example, it has been reported that CD146 is expressed during embryonic development but not in all freshly isolated pericytes in adulthood. Also, RGS-5 protein expresses during embryonic development, but decreases after birth and is absent in pericytes of the normal adult central nervous system (Dore-Duffy, 2008; Sá-Pereira et al., 2012).

Although pericyte identification is rather difficult owing to the lack of one specific marker (Özen et al., 2012), its ultrastructure was described (Nag, 2003; Sá-Pereira et al., 2012). Two classes of pericytes exist in the brain: granular and agranular; this classification arises from the presence or absence of lysosome-like granules in the cytoplasm (Farrell et al., 1987). In humans, less than 5% of the pericyte population is agranular (Farrell et al., 1987; Nag, 2003). Both, granular and agranular pericytes exhibit an oval cell body and a prominent round nucleus that is different from the elongated nucleus of ECs. Each pericyte may cover 100 μm of capillary length with up to 90 ramifications 300–800 nm wide (Nag, 2003; Sá-Pereira et al., 2012). Pericyte distribution is intermittent along the walls of arterioles, venules and, particularly, in capillaries (Dore-Duffy, 2003). They are crucial for the development and maintenance of the main nervous system barriers, namely, blood–spinal cord barrier, blood–retinal barrier, blood–nerve barrier and blood–brain barrier. In fact, pericyte coverage of brain ECs *in vitro* is approximately 80%, in the capillaries of the retina it is 90%, and in the microvessels of the spinal cord it is less than 60%. Pericyte coverage and

Table 1 | Pericyte markers in health and disease.

Pericyte marker/ location	Main function	Main physiological role	Health	Disease	Reference
PDGFRβ/cell surface protein	Tyrosine-protein kinase; Kinase receptor	Embryonic development, proliferation, chemotaxis, host-virus interaction	+	+/– Fibrosis Tumor Blood–brain barrier disruption	Song et al. (2005), Armulik et al. (2010), Dore-Duffy and Cleary (2011)
αSMA/Filament protein	Contractility	Regulation of blood flow and motility	–	++ Fibrosis Tumor Blood–brain barrier disruption	Song et al. (2005), Dore-Duffy and Cleary (2011)
NG2/cell surface protein	Cell adhesion protein	Vasculo-genesis	+	+ Fibrosis Tumor Blood–brain barrier disruption	Ozerdem et al. (2002), Dore-Duffy and Cleary (2011)
RGS-5/intracellular protein	GTPase-activating protein	Cell motility	+	++ Fibrosis Tumor Blood–brain barrier disruption	Song et al. (2005), Dore-Duffy and Cleary (2011)
Desmin/filament protein	Contractility	Regulation of blood flow and motility	+	+ Fibrosis Tumor Blood–brain barrier disruption	Dore-Duffy and Cleary (2011), Kamouchi et al. (2011)
CD13/cell surface protein	Ectopeptidase	Pericyte differentiation	+	++ Fibrosis Tumor Blood–brain barrier disruption	Armulik et al. (2010), Kamouchi et al. (2011)

Symbols are as follow: (+) Indicates that the marker is present; (–) indicates that the marker is absent; (+/–) indicates a decrease in marker expression and; (++) indicates that the marker is over expressed.

number is related to the permeability of the biological-barriers, higher coverage correlates with lower permeability (Winkler et al., 2012). Specifically, it has been shown that pericytes contribute to regulate capillary structure and diameter (Peppiatt et al., 2006; Armulik et al., 2010; Bell et al., 2010; Daneman et al., 2010). Pericytes express junctional complexes that include gap junctions, tight junctions (Tjs), and focal adhesions with ECs (Zlokovic, 2008). These associations lead to the maintenance of low permeability of the cerebral endothelium (Lai and Kuo, 2005; Nakagawa et al., 2007). Brain pericytes promote a reduction in vesicular transport, (Daneman et al., 2010), and promote endothelial Tj protein expression (Zonula occludens, ZO-1, claudin-5, occludin; **Figure 1**; Armulik et al., 2005, 2010; Daneman et al., 2010). In addition, the morphological pattern of pericyte projections around brain capillaries is linked to their function and intimately correlates with brain health state (normal, angiogenic, or injured; Dore-Duffy and Cleary, 2011). The classic wrapping pattern consists of broad processes with a large continuous surface in the external wall of brain microvessels (Dore-Duffy, 2003; Nag, 2003; Dore-Duffy and Cleary, 2011). Under normal conditions, the wrapping pattern predominates, but in pathological conditions detachment and migrating patterns can be observed with the formation of finger-like projections followed by retraction of projections (**Figure 1**; Dore-Duffy and Cleary, 2011). Different morphological patterns in pericyte processes may appear in response to changes in the microenvironment. For example, the migrating pattern is associated to up-regulation of cell surface proteases in aversive conditions, and also with early stages of angiogenesis, in contrast with the wrapping pattern that predominates in normal capillaries (Dore-Duffy, 2003; Sá-Pereira et al., 2012).

Morphological changes in pericytes vary as a function of exposure to soluble molecules released by blood–brain barrier components such as ECs, neurons, microglia or astrocytes; pericytes can differentiate into fibroblasts, smooth muscle cells or macrophages, depending on the stimulus received (**Figure 1**). The molecules released to the basal lamina that can promote pericyte morphological changes include neurotransmitters, neurohormones and inflammatory mediators (Özen et al., 2012). To illustrate this, it has been shown that adenosine and adenosine triphosphate (ATP) released by neurons and glial cells may modify pericyte status by activating purinergic receptors; in addition, rat brain pericytes express ecto-nucleotidase 1 and 2 (Ceruti et al., 2011; Lecca et al., 2012). After immune challenges such as lipopolysaccharide (LPS) administration, hippocampal brain pericytes present increased ecto-nucleotidase expression and function and also morphological changes (Kittel et al., 2007). Activation of purinergic receptor P2X7 initiates an inflammatory response by inducing interleukin (IL) 1β secretion from ECs, astrocytes, microglia, and also pericytes (Derks and Beaman, 2004; Lecca et al., 2012).

Pericyte versatility is, for the most part, unexplored, but several studies suggest that pericytes may play potential roles in brain repair through contractile, migratory, pro-angiogenic and phagocytic functions but they can also promote brain impairment by uncontrolled immune response (Dore-Duffy et al., 2000; Dore-Duffy et al., 2006; Özen et al., 2012; Sá-Pereira et al., 2012).

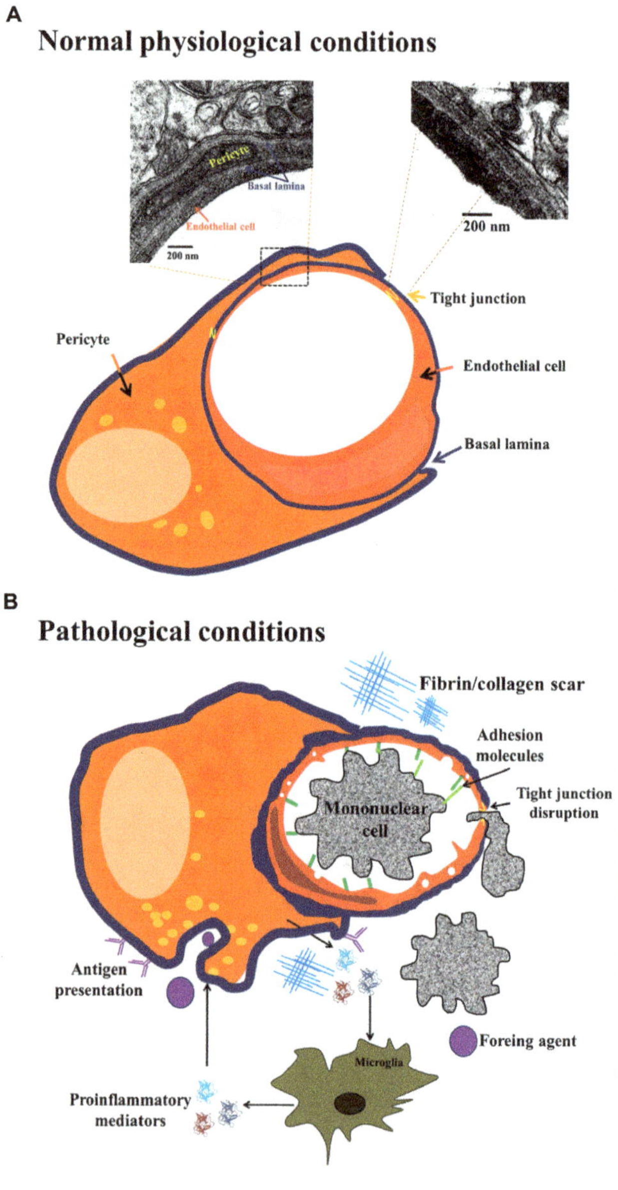

FIGURE 1 | Brain pericyte phenotype in normal and pathological conditions. Under normal physiological conditions **(A)** brain pericytes exhibit tight junctions (Tjs) with endothelial cells (ECs), and are embedded in the basal lamina. Under pathological conditions, such as injury, infection or neurodegeneration **(B)**, pericytes present a migrating phenotype with up-regulation of ICAM expression, pro-inflammatory cytokine release with ensuing recruitment of peripheral mononuclear cells. Additionally, under pathological conditions, the continuity of basal lamina is lost and the existence of fibrin scars contributes to blood–brain barrier impairment.

IMMUNE PROPERTIES OF BRAIN PERICYTES

Mesodermal or neural crest origins of pericytes are generally accepted. Pericytes are considered as "brain macrophages". In fact, for some authors, they represent the first line of defense in the central nervous system due to their antigen presentation properties and because they are directly associated with the microvasculature, in contrast to microglia (**Figure 1**; Balabanov et al., 1999; Guillemin and Brew, 2004). Thomas (1999) reported pericytes leaving the basal lamina and migrating to the perivascular space where they are indistinguishable from perivascular macrophages and reactive microglia (Guillemin and Brew, 2004). Pericyte de-differentiation into cells presenting antigens may initiate a local pro-inflammatory response. Immune response in the brain induces monocyte and lymphocyte recruitment; this process is mediated by the increased expression of adhesion molecules (e.g., intracellular adhesion molecule 1, ICAM-1) in the luminal region of ECs that correlates with decreases in the number of Tjs (**Figure 1**; Guillemin and Brew, 2004). In addition, pericytes are able to produce chemo-attractants and promote transmigration to the brain of circulating immune cells, starting an inflammatory process. Pericytes may also release inflammatory mediators, such as IL-1β, IL-6, tumor necrosis factor (TNF) α, reactive oxygen species, nitric oxide (NO), and matrix metalloproteinases (MMP-2 and MMP-9), all of which contribute to pericyte detachment and blood–brain barrier disruption (Kovac et al., 2011).

These immunoactive properties of pericytes suggest mechanisms by which they can act as an integral part of the blood–brain barrier during brain inflammatory processes. A pro-inflammatory component is the hallmark of several brain diseases. Vascular damage associated to pericyte deficiency may precede neurodegeneration in brain infections, Alzheimer's or Parkinson's disease, diabetes (Özen et al., 2012), and perhaps in less-explored phenomena that exhibit considerable cognitive impairments, such as sleep loss.

PERICYTES AND BRAIN INFECTIONS

The blood–brain barrier provides a shield against foreign agents that initiate inflammatory responses (Al-Ghananeem et al., 2013). The structural variability and the nature of biotic/abiotic inflammatory agents that may promote neuropathology are reflected in the mechanisms used to access the brain. These mechanisms include receptor-mediated endocytosis, unspecific transport by pinocytotic vesicles, paracellular diffusion, transmigration through infected leukocytes, and crossing after blood–brain barrier breakdown (Alcendor et al., 2012; Nakagawa et al., 2012; Pulzova et al., 2012).

The inflammatory response to a foreign agent may cause irreversible brain damage by continuous exposure to pathogen-derived toxic molecules and immune mediators (Kumar et al., 2009; Hirooka and Kaji, 2012). Factors that promote a pro-inflammatory state in the brain include abiotic agents such as heavy metal ions or viruses, and biotic factors such as bacteria, fungi, and parasites (Gasque et al., 1998; Liou and Hsu, 1998; Alvarez and Teale, 2007; Hirooka and Kaji, 2012; Nakagawa et al., 2012). There is scant knowledge of pericyte function and structure under inflammatory response induced by foreign agents.

Heavy metal ions, such as methyl-mercury, cadmium and inorganic mercury induce a potent inflammatory response in the brain. These metal ions have high affinity to sulfhydryl groups favoring the formation of a methionine-like complex that easily crosses the blood–brain barrier. The methionine-like complex enters the brain by the large neutral amino acid transporter (LAT-1); once inside, the heavy metal ions induce cytokine and growth factor release by blood–brain barrier components. Heavy metal ions associate with the fibroblast growth factor type 2 (FGF-2); this union may cause cell damage because FGF-2 is unable to repair endothelial damage; therefore, heavy metal ions promote less auto-regulatory signaling inhibition of EC proliferation (Hirooka and Kaji, 2012).

In the case of viral and bacterial infections, such as congenital human cytomegalovirus (HCMV), human immunodeficiency virus type 1 (HIV-1), Japanese encephalitis (JE) virus and bacterial meningitis, the main transport routes through the blood–brain barrier include endocytosis of blood-circulating vesicles, microvessel wall degradation, and indirect crossing via previous blood–brain barrier disruption. When infectious agents are detected, pericytes begin an inflammatory response through increased expression of pro-inflammatory cytokines, such as IL-1β, IL-6, and TNF-α (Liou and Hsu, 1998; Alcendor et al., 2012; Nakagawa et al., 2012). In HIV-1 infection, pericytes express the chemokine receptors CXCR4 and CCR5 that are used by infected cells to contribute to the formation of viral reservoirs in the brain (Nakagawa et al., 2012). It is known that 80% of cultured pericytes infected by HCMV generate an inflammatory response; in fact, only 72 h after infection, a huge rise in IL-1β, a medium increase in IL-6, and a minimal increase in TNF-α concentration are observed. However, later on those pro-inflammatory cytokine profiles are reversed by the compensatory effect of anti-inflammatory cytokines (Alcendor et al., 2012). In contrast, bacterial meningitis infection increases expression of receptors C5a and C3a in brain pericytes. These complement molecules are powerful chemo-attractants to recruit polimorfonuclear cells and macrophages to the inflammation site causing cell activation (Gasque et al., 1998). On the other hand, it has been reported that *Taenia solium* infiltrates cause brain inflammation by pericyte release of pro-inflammatory cytokines and MMP-2 and MMP-9, which are associated to blood–brain barrier disruption. Blood–brain barrier breakdown allows infiltration of antigen-presenting cells and specialized immune cells (B cells and T cells), exacerbating the inflammatory condition (Alvarez and Teale, 2007).

These studies illustrate that although each pathogen exhibits a characteristic pathway, the same inflammatory mediators participate in the orchestration of the brain immune response (**Figure 2**). It is known that rises in pro-inflammatory cytokines, particularly IL-1 β, IL-6, and TNF-α, disrupt Tjs by down-regulating occludin and ZO-1 expression (Liou and Hsu, 1998; Alcendor et al., 2012; Nakagawa et al., 2012). Pro-inflammatory cytokines alter Tj integrity by promoting an increase in prostaglandin-E (PGE) receptors in pericytes, which leads to MMP overproduction and release, causing pericyte uncoupling with ECs (Alvarez and Teale, 2007). In fact, ECs are the unique brain cell type that expresses PGE-2 synthase (Yamagata et al., 2001); PGE-2 is produced in response to immune challenges (e.g., IL-1 or LPS administration; Cao et al., 1997; Laflamme et al., 1999) suggesting a relevant role of perivascular cells (astrocytes, interneurons and particularly pericytes) in the response to low doses of immune stimulators (Schiltz and Sawchenko, 2002). Interestingly, perivascular cell response is different for each type of molecule; e.g., pericytes elicit cyclooxygenases in brain ECs in response to low doses of IL-1, but with low doses of LPS perivascular cells

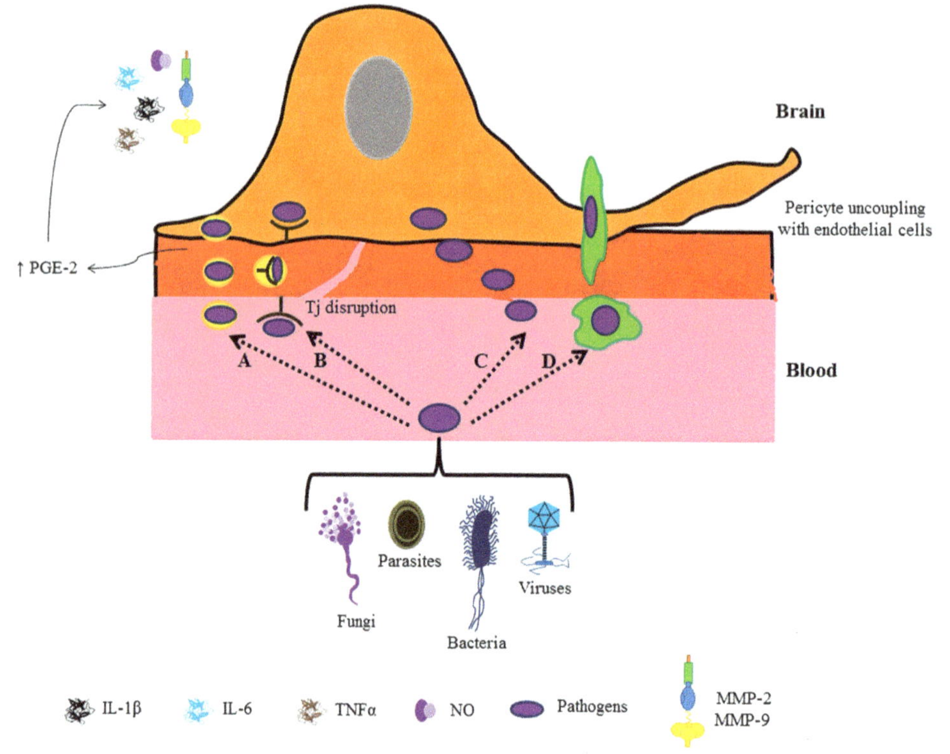

FIGURE 2 | Pathogen entry to the brain. The cartoon depicts different routes for pathogen entry to the brain: caveolae **(A)**, receptor-mediated transport **(B)**, paracellular diffusion **(C)**, and transmigration through infected leukocytes **(D)**. In all cases a pericyte-mediated immune response followed by blood–brain barrier breakdown is observed.

apparently have an inhibitory effect on cyclooxygenase production (Schiltz and Sawchenko, 2002). Some neuro-infections are associated with neurodegenerative diseases, for example, the bacteria *Borrelia burgdorferi* in Alzheimer's disease (Miklossy et al., 2004). So, is the pathogenic action on pericytes a promoter of neurodegenerative disease? Undoubtedly, pericyte function has an important role in the progression of brain pathologies. Although several studies provide relevant information on the immune role of pericytes in the protection of the brain against an infectious threat, the molecular and cellular mechanisms involved in blood–brain barrier disruption are poorly understood.

ROLE OF PERICYTES IN NEURODEGENERATIVE DISORDERS

Similar to infectious processes, during neurodegenerative and cerebrovascular diseases inflammatory phenomena occur, which are characterized by increased release of pro-inflammatory cytokines (IL-1β, IL-6, and TNF-α), subsequent hyperthermia, and mononuclear cell infiltration (Bleys and Cowen, 2001). In both, neurodegenerative and cerebrovascular diseases, pericyte detachment of ECs and differentiation into fibroblasts or phagocytes correlates with an increase in vesicle number in ECs, Tj disruption and immune cell recruitment (Özen et al., 2012). Additionally, fibrosis-like pathophysiological changes are described (**Figure 3**); pericyte-derived fibrin and collagen form scars, which are involved in cell death by neurotoxicity (Armulik et al., 2010; Fernández et al., 2013). Deposits of extracellular matrix components and organ failure are common after prolonged exposure to pro-inflammatory cytokines, suggesting that the first step leading to cell death relates to the immune response (Lin et al., 2008; Armulik et al., 2010). Furthermore, cytokine production is accompanied by oxidative stress; both, inflammatory mediators and oxidative stress are directly involved in increased blood–brain barrier permeability through the same signaling pathways.

Recent studies revealed the role of NO released by microglia and pericytes in neurodegenerative diseases and neuro-immune interactions; it was shown that amyloid β deposits in Alzheimer's disease promote pericyte constriction despite NO over-production. The role of NO in blood–brain barrier disruption is also related to its high ability to form free radicals such as peroxynitrite (ONOO-•), which may induce cell death (Hamilton et al., 2010; Kovac et al., 2011). In addition, it has been reported that amyloid β deposits promote over-production of reactive oxygen species in pericytes, endothelial, and glial cells (Veszelka et al., 2013). Blood–brain barrier disruption promotes lymphocyte recruitment in neurodegenerative diseases and stroke; hence, after cerebral ischemia, polymorphonuclear leukocytes impede reperfusion leading to generation of free radicals, and promoting pericyte constriction. Indeed, pericyte detachment from the vessel wall occurs following ischemia and reperfusion (Takahashi et al., 1997). Recently, Tigges et al. (2013) reported an increase in fibronectin and collagen I deposits in animal models of Alzheimer's disease, these deposits are related to pericyte

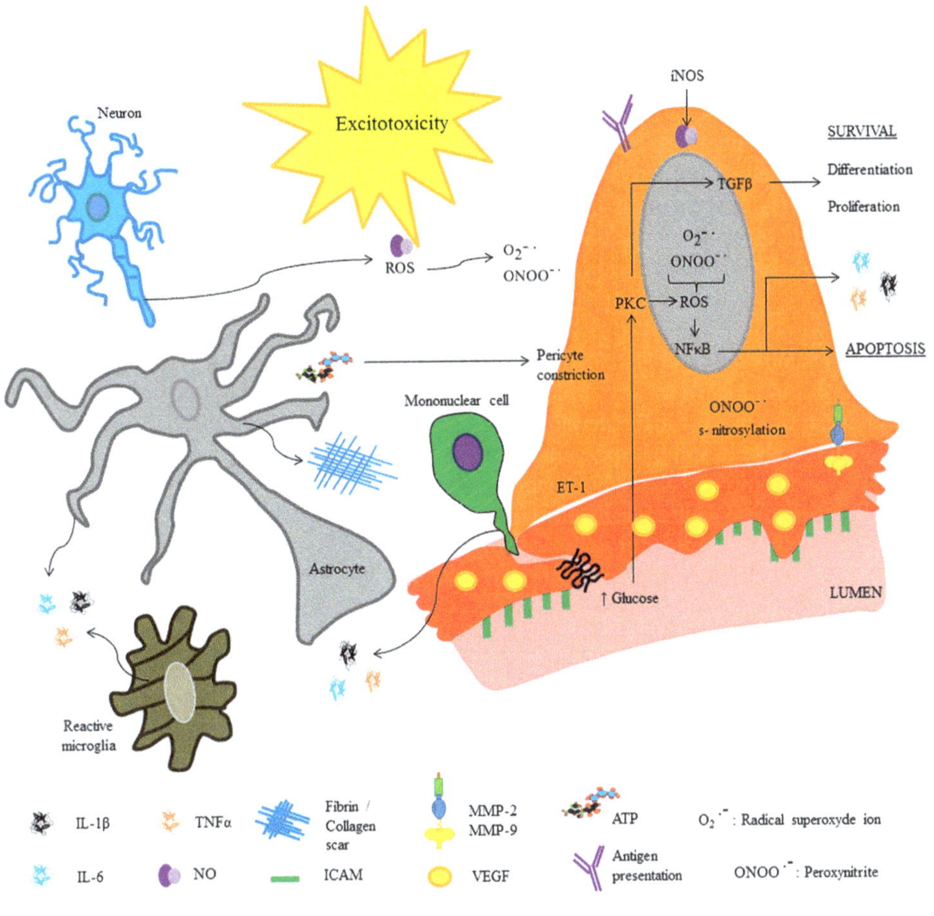

FIGURE 3 | Molecular inflammatory changes in brain pericytes in pathophysiological conditions. The cartoon depicts molecules released by pericytes under altered physiological conditions (e.g., neurodegeneration, infections or brain injury). Excitotoxicity may occur secondary to blood–brain barrier disruption.

differentiation and migration. Tigges et al. (2013) showed that under normal conditions, brain pericytes express high levels of α5 integrin and lower levels of α1, α2, and α6 integrins. This expression pattern has a crucial role in the attachment of pericytes to the vessel wall; in fact, an *in vivo* study shows that TNF-α promotes pericyte proliferation and detachment as well as a switch in integrin expression pattern, with predominance of α2 integrin (Tigges et al., 2013). Interestingly, Tigges et al. (2013) also found that α2 integrin expression strongly correlated with brain vessel remodeling in experimental autoimmune encephalomyelitis. Similarly, in Alzheimer's disease it is reported that fibrin deposition and increased extravascular immunoglobulin G (IgG) correlate with a reduction in pericyte coverage of ECs (Sengillo et al., 2013).

Fibrin deposits are a signal of fibroblast activity and probably represent an index of de-differentiation from pericytes to fibroblasts. Transforming growth factor-β (TGF-β) is the most potent known growth inhibitor for ECs, fibroblasts, neurons, and lymphoid cells. TGF-β inhibits proliferation of T-lymphocytes by down-regulating pro-inflammatory cytokines, e.g., IL-2-mediated proliferative signals (Dohgu et al., 2005). Under diabetic conditions, pericytes release TGF-β, which increases fibronectin levels (Shimizu et al., 2013). Shimizu et al. (2013) suggest that advanced glycation end-products (AGEs) induce blood–brain barrier disruption in diabetic conditions by stimulation of autocrine TGF-β signaling in pericytes, and up-regulation of vascular endothelial growth factor (VEGF) and MMP-2. Both, VEGF and MMP-2 modify trans-endothelial electric resistance (TEER) leading to Tj disruption and increased vesicular transport (Thanabalasundaram et al., 2011). Pericyte deficiency reported in diabetes is attributed to raises in glucose concentration, and production of reactive oxygen species through the NFκB pathway (Hamilton et al., 2010). Interestingly, in diabetic animal models, pericytes are highly immunosuppressive; under early hyperglycemic conditions retinal-derived pericytes inhibit T cell proliferation and protect ECs from inflammation-induced apoptosis (Tu et al., 2011). In addition, it is known that pericytes are especially susceptible to oxidative stress; for example, high glucose levels cause oxidative stress and apoptosis (Shah et al., 2013). In addition to the reactive oxygen species effect, the production of large amounts of NO by inducible-nitric oxide synthase (iNOS) can lead to changes in cerebral blood-flow, nitrosative stress, and subsequent cell death of pericytes, ECs and neurons through toxicity caused by excitatory amino acids and massive entry of toxic molecules to the brain (Kischer, 1992; Li et al., 1997; Tu et al., 2011; Baloyannis and Baloyannis, 2012). A decrease in pericyte capillary coverage and cell number has been reported in hyperglycemia, early diabetes retinopathy, brain tumors, and Alzheimer's disease. Therefore, brain microvascular alterations seem to reciprocally interact with underlying neurodegeneration in inducing cognitive impairments (Pimentel-Coelho and Rivest, 2012). The role of pericytes in the genesis of neurodegenerative diseases and in brain regeneration is poorly studied; however, pericytes undoubtedly, cause alterations in brain physiology.

PERICYTES AND SLEEP LOSS: AN IMMUNOLOGICAL PERSPECTIVE

Sleep loss is a common problem in modern society (Mills et al., 2007; Yehuda et al., 2009) and a risk factor for the development of obesity, metabolic syndrome, diabetes, and neurodegenerative diseases (Tasali et al., 2009; van Leeuwen et al., 2009; Reynolds et al., 2012). Similar to infections and neurodegenerative diseases, sleep loss has an important pro-inflammatory component (Mills et al., 2007; Zager et al., 2007). Specific sleep function is yet unclear; but it has been proposed that sleep is associated with changes in parameters of host defense (Benca and Quintas, 1997). Sleep is divided into two distinct stages namely; slow wave sleep and rapid eye movement (REM) sleep (Siegel, 2010). Particularly, REM sleep has an important role in biological processes; REM sleep loss decreases neurogenesis in the hippocampus (Guzman-Marin et al., 2008; Mueller et al., 2008), alters the brain neurochemical content (Mohammed et al., 2011), and impairs learning and memory in both rodents and humans (Meerlo et al., 2008). Prolonged wakefulness promotes an increase of inflammatory mediators such as adenosine and NO (Kalinchuk et al., 2011; Cespuglio et al., 2012; Raymond et al., 2012), and increases plasma levels of IL-1β, IL-6, IL-17A, TNF-α (Yehuda et al., 2009), and endothelin-1 (ET-1; Mills et al., 2007). These changes may act directly on the blood–brain barrier components; for example, IL-1, IL-17, and ET-1 disrupt the blood–brain barrier (Banks et al., 1995; Blamire et al., 2000; Didier et al., 2003; Huppert et al., 2010). REM sleep deprivation also increases body temperature (Jaiswal and Mallick, 2009), which also disrupts the blood–brain barrier (Kiyatkin and Sharma, 2009).

Our research group recently found that chronic REM sleep restriction induces a generalized blood–brain barrier breakdown, and subsequent sleep opportunity is capable of restoring blood–brain barrier integrity. In addition, we studied EC ultrastructure and observed alterations in vesicle trafficking (Gómez-González et al., 2013). It is highly likely that pericyte dysfunction may contribute to increases in blood–brain barrier permeability secondary to sleep loss because ultrastructural changes in ECs are similar to those reported in pericyte-deficient mice, e.g., increased caveolae density, and endothelial derangement (Armulik et al., 2010). Chronic exposure to pro-inflammatory cytokines, NO and other inflammatory mediators released during sleep restriction may directly induce pericyte detachment from the vessel wall and subsequent differentiation into migratory and phagocytic phenotypes, mediating blood–brain barrier disruption. It is likely that the synthesis of antioxidants and anti-inflammatory molecules during sleep recovery may restore normal blood–brain barrier permeability through neutralization of free radicals (**Figure 4**).

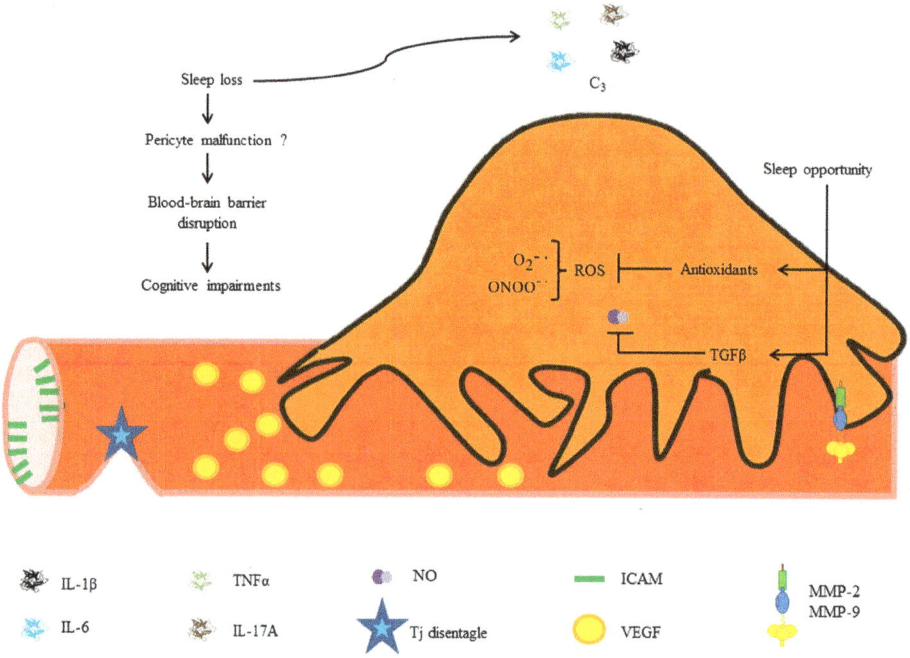

FIGURE 4 | Hypothetical roles of pericytes in REM sleep loss-induced blood–brain barrier disruption. Increased cytokine and chemokine concentrations during sleep loss may disrupt the blood–brain barrier. Brief periods of sleep opportunity may reestablish the blood–brain barrier integrity through synthesis of antioxidants and anti-inflammatory cytokines (e.g., TGF-β).

CONCLUSION

Classically, pericytes have been considered a cell population involved mainly in microvessel contractility. New research on pericyte contribution to optimal blood–brain barrier function and neural pathogenesis shows that they have a substantial influence on the neuro-immune response. The immunoactive properties of pericytes suggest mechanisms by which they could act as an integral component of the blood–brain barrier during inflammatory processes, such as during brain infections, neurodegenerative diseases or sleep loss. Future studies are needed to elucidate pericyte role under inflammatory conditions. Knowledge on pericyte contribution to disease pathogenesis will allow more specific treatment of brain pathologies and perhaps the development of better diagnostic markers. The field study of pericytes is generating frontier knowledge and may be exploited as an example of neuro-integration. Certainly, pericytes are crucial cells in optimal brain function, but their deficit results from molecular interactions between all brain cells.

ACKNOWLEDGMENTS

The authors express their gratitude to Dr. Edith Monroy for the correction of the English language. Supported by Grant 14412025 from CONACyT to B Gómez-González.

REFERENCES

Abbott, N. J., Patabendige, A. A. K., Dolman, D. E. M., Yusof, S. R., and Begley, D. J. (2010). Structure and function of the blood-brain barrier. *Neurobiol. Dis.* 37, 13–25. doi: 10.1016/j.nbd.2009.07.030

Alcendor, D. J., Charest, A. M., Zhu, W. Q., Vigil, H. E., and Knobel, S. M. (2012). Infection and upregulation of proinflammatory cytokines in human brain vascular pericytes by human cytomegalovirus. *J. Neuroinflammation* 9, 95. doi: 10.1186/1742-2094-9-95

Al-Ghananeem, A. M., Smith, M., Coronel, M. L., and Tran, H. (2013). Advances in brain targeting and drug delivery of anti-HIV therapeutic agents. *Expert Opin. Drug Deliv.* 10, 973–985. doi: 10.1517/17425247.2013.781999

Alvarez, J. I., and Teale, J. M. (2007). Evidence for differential changes of junctional complex proteins in murine neurocysticercosis dependent upon CNS vasculature. *Brain Res.* 1169, 98–111. doi: 10.1016/j.brainres.2007.07.010

Armulik, A., Abramsson, A., and Betsholtz, C. (2005). Endothelial/pericyte interactions. *Circ. Res.* 97, 512–523. doi: 10.1161/01.RES.0000182903.16652.d7

Armulik, A., Genové, G., Mäe, M., Nisancioglu, M. H., Wallgard, E., Niaudet, C., et al. (2010). Pericytes regulate the blood-brain barrier. *Nature* 25, 557–561 doi: 10.1038/nature09522

Balabanov, R., Beaumont, T., and Dore-Duffy, P. (1999). Role of central nervous system microvascular pericytes in activation of antigen-primed splenic T-lymphocytes. *J. Neurosci. Res.* 1, 578–587. doi: 10.1002/(SICI)1097-4547(19990301)55:5<578::AID-JNR5>3.0.CO;2-E

Ballabh, P., Braun, A., and Nedergaad, M. (2004). The blood-brain barrier: an overview. Structure, regulation, and clinical implications. *Neurobiol. Dis.* 16, 1–13. doi: 10.1016/j.nbd.2003.12.016

Baloyannis, S. J., and Baloyannis, I. S. (2012). The vascular factor in Alzheimer's disease: a study in Golgi technique and electron microscopy. *J. Neurol. Sci.* 15, 117–121. doi: 10.1016/j.jns.2012.07.010

Banks, W. A., Kastin, A. J., and Broadwell, R. D. (1995). Passage of cytokines across the blood-brain barrier. *Neuroimmunomodulation* 2, 241–248. doi: 10.1159/000097202

Bell, R. D., Winkler, E. A., Sagare, A. P., Singh, I., LaRue, B., Deane, R., et al. (2010). Pericytes control key neurovascular functions and neural phenotype in the adult brain and during brain aging. *Neuron* 68, 409–427. doi: 10.1016/j.neuron.2010.09.043

Benca, R. M., and Quintas, J. (1997). Sleep and host defenses: a review. *Sleep* 20, 1027–1037.

Bergers, G., and Song, S. (2005). The role of pericytes in blood-vessels formation and maintenance. *Neuro Oncol.* 7, 452–464. doi: 10.1215/S1152851705000232

Blamire, A. M., Anthony, D. C., Rajagopalan, B., Sibson, N. R., Perry, V. H., and Styles, P. (2000). Interleukin-1 beta -induced changes in blood-brain barrier permeability, apparent diffusion coefficient, and cerebral blood volume in the rat brain: a magnetic resonance study. *J. Neurosci.* 1, 8153–8159.

Bleys, R., and Cowen, T. (2001). Innervation of cerebral blood vessels: morphology, plasticity, age-related, and Alzheimer's disease-related neurodegeneration. *Microsc. Res. Tech.* 53, 106–118. doi: 10.1002/jemt.1075

Cao, C., Matsumura, K., Yamagata, K., and Watanabe, Y. (1997). Involvement of cyclooxygenase-2 in LPS-induced fever and regulation of its mRNA by LPS in the rat brain. *Am. J. Physiol.* 272, R1712–R1725.

Ceruti, S., Colombo, L., Magni, G., Viganò, F., Boccazzi, M., Deli, M. A., et al. (2011). Oxygen-glucose deprivation increases the enzymatic activity and the microvescicle-mediated release of ectonucleotidases in the cells composing the blood–brain barrier. *Neurochem. Int.* 59, 259–271. doi: 10.1016/j.neuint.2011.05.013

Cespuglio, R., Amrouni, D., Meiller, A., Buguet, A., and Gautier-Sauvigné, S. (2012). Nitric oxide in the regulation of the sleep-wake states. *Sleep Med. Rev.* 16, 265–279. doi: 10.1016/j.smrv.2012.01.006

Daneman, R., Zhou, L., Kebede, A. A., and Barres, B. A. (2010). Pericytes are required for blood–brain barrier integrity during embryogenesis. *Nature* 468, 562–566. doi: 10.1038/nature09513

Derks, R., and Beaman, K. (2004). Regeneration and tolerance factor modulates the effect of adenosine triphosphate-induced interleukin 1 beta secretion in human macrophages. *Hum. Immunol.* 65, 676–682. doi: 10.1016/j.humimm.2004.04.006

Didier, N., Romero, I. A., Créminon, C., Wijkhuisen, A., Grassi, J., and Mabondzo, A. (2003). Secretion of interleukin-1beta by astrocytes mediates endothelin-1 and tumour necrosis factor-alpha effects on human brain microvascular endothelial cell permeability. *J. Neurochem.* 86, 246–254. doi: 10.1046/j.1471-4159.2003.01829.x

Dohgu, S., Takata, F., Yamauchi, A., Nakagawa, S., Egawa, T., Naito, M., et al. (2005). Brain pericytes contribute to the induction and up-regulation of blood–brain barrier functions through transforming growth factor-β production. *Brain Res.* 1038, 208–215. doi: 10.1016/j.brainres.2005.01.027

Dore-Duffy, P. (2003). Isolation and characterization of cerebral microvascular pericytes. *Methods Mol. Med.* 89, 375–382. doi: 10.1385/1-59259-419-0:375

Dore-Duffy, P. (2008). Pericytes: pluripotent cells of the blood brain barrier. *Curr. Pharm. Des.* 14, 1581–1593. doi: 10.2174/138161208784705469

Dore-Duffy, P., and Cleary, K. (2011). "Morphology and properties of pericytes," in *Methods in molecular biology,* Vol. 686, *The Blood-Brain and Other Neural Barriers, Reviews, and Protocols,* ed. S. Nag (Philadelphia: Springer Science+Business Media, LLC), 49–68.

Dore-Duffy, P., Katychev, A., Wang, X., and Van Buren, E. (2006). CNS microvascular pericytes exhibit multipotential stem cell activity. *J. Cereb. Blood Flow Metab.* 26, 613–624. doi: 10.1038/sj.jcbfm.9600272

Dore-Duffy, P., Owen, C., Balavanov, R., Murphy, S., Beamount, T., and Rafols, J. A. (2000). Pericyte migration from the vascular wall in response to traumatic brain injury. *Microvasc. Res.* 60, 55–69. doi: 10.1006/mvre.2000.2244

Farrell, C. R., Stewart, P. A., Farrell, C. L., and Del Maestro, R. F. (1987). Pericytes in human cerebral microvasculature. *Anat. Rec.* 218, 466–469. doi: 10.1002/ar.1092180416

Fernández, K. F., Potas, J. R., Hilpert, D., Blazej, K., Radke, J., Huck, J., et al. (2013). Early loss of pericytes and perivascular stromal cell-induced scar formation after stroke. *J. Cereb. Blood Flow Metab.* 33, 428–439. doi: 10.1038/jcbfm.2012.187

Gasque, P., Singhrao, S. K., Neal, J. W., Wang, P., Sayah, S., Fontaine, M., et al. (1998). The receptor for complement anaphylatoxin C3a is expressed by myeloid cells and nonmyeloid cells in inflamed human central nervous system: analysis in multiple sclerosis and bacterial meningitis. *J. Immunol.* 160, 3543–3554.

Gómez-González, B., Hurtado-Alvarado, G., Esqueda-León, E., Santana-Miranda, R., Rojas-Zamorano, J. A., and Velazquéz-Moctezuma, J. (2013). REM sleep loss and recovery regulates blood-brain barrier function. *Curr. Neurovasc. Res.* 10, 197–207. doi: 10.2174/15672026113109990002

Gómez-González, B., Hurtado-Alvarado, G., and Velazquéz-Moctezuma, J. (2012). "Local and temporal regulation of the blood-brain barrier during normal and altered physiological states", in *The Blood-Brain Barrier New Research,* eds P. A. Montenegro and S. M. Juárez (New York: Nova Science Publishers, Inc.), 1–42.

Guillemin, G. J., and Brew, B. J. (2004). Microglia, macrophages, perivascular macrophages, and pericytes: a review of function and identification. *J. Leukoc. Biol.* 75, 388–397. doi: 10.1189/jlb.0303114

Guzman-Marin, R., Suntsova, N., Bashir, T., Nienhuis, R., Szymusiak, R., and McGinty, D. (2008). Rapid eye movement sleep deprivation contributes to reduction of neurogenesis in the hippocampal dentate gyrus of the adult rat. *Sleep* 31, 167–175.

Hamilton, N. B., Attwell, D., and Hall, C. N. (2010). Pericyte-mediated regulation of capillary diameter: a component of neurovascular coupling in health and disease. *Front. Neuroenergetics* 2:5. doi: 10.3389/fnene.2010.00005

Hirooka, T., and Kaji, T. (2012). The cytotoxicity of methylmercury in human microvascular endothelial cells and pericytes in culture. *Biol. Pharm. Bull.* 35, 1201–1205. doi: 10.1248/bpb.b12-00394

Huppert, J., Closhen, D., Croxford, A., White, R., Kulig, P., Pietrowski, E., et al. (2010). Cellular mechanisms of IL-17-induced blood-brain barrier disruption. *FASEB J.* 24, 1023–1034. doi: 10.1096/fj.09–141978

Jaiswal, M. K., and Mallick, B. N. (2009). Prazosin modulates rapid eye movement sleep deprivation-induced changes in body temperature in rats. *J. Sleep Res.* 18, 349–356. doi: 10.1111/j.1365-2869.2008.00731.x

Kalinchuk, A. V., McCarley, R. W., Porkka-Heiskanen, T., and Basheer, R. (2011). The time course of adenosine, nitric oxide (NO) and inducible NO synthase changes in the brain with sleep loss and their role in the non-rapid eye movement sleep homeostatic cascade. *J. Neurochem.* 116, 260–272. doi: 10.1111/j.1471-4159.2010.07100.x

Kamouchi, M., Ago, T., and Kitazono, T. (2011). Brain pericytes: emerging concepts and functional roles in brain homeostasis. *Cell. Mol. Neurobiol.* 31, 175–193. doi: 10.1007/s10571-010-9605-x

Kim, J. A., Tran, N. D., Li, Z., Yang, F., Zhou, W., and Fisher, M. J. (2006). Brain endothelial hemostasis regulation by pericytes. *J. Cereb. Blood Flow Metab.* 26, 209–217. doi: 10.1038/sj.jcbfm.9600181

Kischer, C. W. (1992). The microvessels in hypertrophic scars, keloids and related lesions: a review. *J. Submicrosc. Cytol. Pathol.* 24, 281–296.

Kittel, A., Sperlagh, B., Pelletier, J., Sevigny, J., and Kirley, T. L. (2007). Transient changes in the localization and activity of ectonucleotidases in rat hippocampus following lipopolysaccharide treatment. *Int. J. Dev. Neurosci.* 25, 275–282. doi: 10.1016/j.ijdevneu.2007.05.007

Kiyatkin, E. A., and Sharma, H. S. (2009). Permeability of the blood-brain barrier depends on brain temperature. *Neuroscience* 161, 926–939. doi: 10.1016/j.neuroscience.2009.04.004

Kovac, A., Erickson, E. A., and Banks, W. A. (2011). Brain microvascular pericytes are immunoactive in culture: cytokine, chemokine, nitric oxide, and LRP-1 expression in response to lipopolysaccharide. *J. Neuroinflammation* 8, 139. doi: 10.1186/1742-2094-8–139

Kumar, P., Shen, Q., Pivetti, C. D., Lee, E. S., Wu, M. H., and Yuan, S. Y. (2009). Molecular mechanisms of endothelial hyperpermeability: implications in inflammation. *Expert Rev. Mol. Med.* 11, e19. doi: 10.1017/S14623994090 01112

Lai, C. H., and Kuo, K. H. (2005). The critical component to establish in vitro BBB model: pericyte. *Brain Res. Rev.* 50, 258–265. doi: 10.1016/j.brainresrev.2005. 07.004

Laflamme, N., Lacroix, S., and Rivest, S. (1999). An essential role of interleukin-1beta in mediating NF-kappaB activity and COX-2 transcription in cells of the blood-brain barrier in response to a systemic and localized inflammation but not during endotoxemia. *J. Neurosci.* 19, 10923–10930.

Lecca, D., Ceruti, S., Fumagalli, M., and Abbracchio, M. P. (2012). Purinergic trophic signalling in glial cells: functional effects and modulation of cell proliferation, differentiation, and death. *Purinergic Signal.* 8, 539–557. doi: 10.1007/s11302-012-9310-y

Li, W., Yanoff, M., Liu, X., and Ye, X. (1997). Retinal capillary pericyte apoptosis in early human diabetic retinopathy. *Chin. Med. J.* 110, 659–663.

Lin, S. L., Kisseleva, T., Brenner, D. A., and Duffield, J. S. (2008). Pericytes and perivascular fibroblasts are the primary source of collagen-producing cells in obstructive fibrosis of the kidney. *Am. J. Pathol.* 173, 1617–1627. doi: 10.2353/ajpath.2008.080433

Liou, M. L., and Hsu, C. Y. (1998). Japanese encephalitis virus is transported across the cerebral blood vessels by endocytosis in mouse brain. *Cell Tissue Res.* 293, 389–394. doi: 10.1007/s004410051130

Meerlo, P., Sgoifo, A., and Suchecki, D. (2008). Restricted and disrupted sleep: effects on autonomic function, neuroendocrine stress systems and stress responsivity. *Sleep Med. Rev.* 12, 197–210. doi: 10.1016/j.smrv.2007. 07.007

Miklossy, J., Khalili, K., Gern, L., Ericson, R. L., Darekar, P., Bolle, L., et al. (2004). *Borrelia burgdorferi* persists in the brain in chronic lyme neuroborreliosis and may be associated with Alzheimer disease. *J. Alzheimers Dis.* 6, 639–649.

Mills, P. J., von Känel, R., Norman., Natarajan, L., Ziegler, M. G., and Dimsdale, J. E. (2007). Inflammation and sleep in healthy individuals. *Sleep* 30, 729–735.

Mohammed, H. S., Aboul Ezz, H. S., Khadrawy, Y. A., and Noor, N. A. (2011). Neurochemical and electrophysiological changes induced by paradoxical sleep deprivation in rats. *Behav. Brain Res.* 225, 39–46. doi: 10.1016/j.bbr.2011. 06.018

Mueller, A. D., Pollock, M. S., Lieblich, S. E., Epp, J. R., Galea, L. A., and Mistlberger, R. E. (2008). Sleep deprivation can inhibit adult hippocampal neurogenesis independent of adrenal stress hormones. *Am. J. Physiol. Regul. Integr. Comp. Physiol.* 294, R1693–R1703. doi: 10.1152/ajpregu.00858.2007

Nag, S. (2003). Morphology and molecular properties of cellular components of normal cerebral vessels. *Methods Mol. Med.* 89, 3–36.

Nakagawa, S., Castro, V., and Toborek, M. (2012). Infection of human pericytes by HIV-1 disrupts the integrity of the blood–brain barrier. *J. Cell. Mol. Med.* 16, 2950–2957. doi: 10.1111/j.1582-4934.2012.01622.x

Nakagawa, S., Deli, M. A., Nakao, S., Honda, M., Hayashi, K., Nakaoke, R., et al. (2007). Pericytes from brain microvessels strengthen the barrier integrity in primary cultures of rat brain endothelial cells. *Cell. Mol. Neurobiol.* 27, 687–694. doi: 10.1007/s10571-007-9195-4

Özen, I., Boix, J., and Paul, G. (2012). Perivascular mesenchymal stem cells in the adult human brain: a future target for neuroregeneration? *Clin. Transl. Med.* 1, 30. doi: 10.1186/2001-1326-1-30

Ozerdem, U., Monosov, E., and Stallcup, W. B. (2002). NG2 proteoglycan expression by pericytes in pathological microvasculature. *Microvasc. Res.* 63, 129–134. doi: 10.1006/mvre.2001.2376

Peppiatt, C. M., Howarth, C., Mobbs, P., and Attwell, D. (2006). Bidirectional control of CNS capillary diameter by pericytes. *Nature* 12, 700–704. doi: 10.1038/nature05193

Persidsky, Y., Ramirez, S. H., and Haorah, J. (2006). Blood–brain barrier: structural components and function under physiologic and pathologic conditions. *J. Neuroimmune Pharmacol.* 1, 223–236. doi: 10.1007/s11481-006-9025-3

Pimentel-Coelho, P. M., and Rivest, S. (2012). The early contribution of cerebrovascular factors to the pathogenesis of Alzheimer's disease. *J. Neurosci.* 35, 1917–1937. doi: 10.1111/j.1460-9568.2012.08126.x

Pulzova, L., Mlynarcik, P., Bencurova, E., and Bhine, M. (2012). "It takes to tango: protein-protein interaction in the translocation of pathogens across a blood-brain barrier," in *The Blood-Brain Barrier New Research,* ed. P. A. Montenegro and S. M. Juárez (New York: Nova Science Publishers, Inc), 79–115.

Raymond, C., Donia, A., Anne, M., Alain, B., and Sabine, G. (2012). Nitric oxide in the regulation of the sleep-wake states. *Sleep Med. Rev.* 16, 265–279. doi: 10.1016/j.smrv.2012.01.006

Reynolds, A. C., Dorrian, J., Liu, P. Y., Van Dongen, H. A., and Wittert, G. A. (2012). Impact of five nights of sleep restriction on glucose metabolism, leptin and testosterone in young adult men. *PLoS ONE* 7:e41218. doi: 10.1371/journal.pone.0041218

Risau, W. (1991). Induction of blood-brain barrier endothelial cell differentiation. *Ann. N. Y. Acad. Sci.* 633, 405–419. doi: 10.1111/j.1749-6632.1991.tb15630.x

Rouget, C. (1874). Note sur le developpement de la tunique contractile des vaisseaux. *C. R. Acad. Sci.* 59, 559–562.

Saper, C. B. (2010). The dance of the perivascular and endothelial cells: mechanisms of brain response to immune signaling. *Neuron* 65, 4–6. doi: 10.1016/j.neuron.2009.12.029

Sá-Pereira, I., Brites, D., and Brito, M. A. (2012). Neurovascular unit: a focus on pericytes. *Mol. Neurobiol.* 45, 327–347. doi: 10.1007/s12035-012-8244-2

Schiltz, J. C., and Sawchenko, P. E. (2002). Distinct brain vascular cell types manifest inducible cyclooxygenase expression as a function of the strength and nature of immune insults. *J. Neurosci.* 22, 5606–5618.

Sengillo, J. D., Winkler, E. A., Walker, C. T., Sullivan, J. S., Johnson, M., and Zlokovic, B. V. (2013). Deficiency in mural vascular cells coincides with blood-brain barrier disruption in Alzheimer's disease. *Brain Pathol.* 23, 303–310. doi: 10.1111/bpa.12004

Shah, G. N., Price, T. O., Banks, W. A., Morofuji, Y., Kovac, A., Ercal, N., et al. (2013). Pharmacological inhibition of mitochondrial carbonic anhydrases protects mouse cerebral pericytes from high glucose-induced oxidative stress and apoptosis. *J. Pharmacol. Exp. Ther.* 344, 637–645. doi: 10.1124/jpet.112.201400

Shimizu, F., Sano, Y., Tominaga, O., Maeda, T., Abe, M. A., and Kanda, T. (2013). Advanced glycation end-products disrupt the blood-brain barrier by stimulating the release of transforming growth factor-β by pericytes and vascular endothelial growth factor and matrix metalloproteinase-2 by endothelial cells in vitro. *Neurobiol. Aging* 4, 1902–1912. doi: 10.1016/j.neurobiolaging.2013.01.012

Siegel, J. M. (2010). Do all animals sleep? *Trends Neurosci.* 31, 208–213. doi: 10.1016/j.tins.2008.02.001

Song, S., Ewald, A. J., Stallcup, W., Werb, Z., and Bergers, G. (2005). PDGFRbeta+ perivascular progenitor cells in tumours regulate pericyte differentiation and vascular survival. *Nat. Cell Biol.* 7, 870–879. doi: 10.1038/ncb1288

Takahashi, A., Park, H. K., Melgar, M. A., Alcocer, L., Pinto, J., Lenzi, T., et al. (1997). Cerebral cortex blood flow and vascular smooth muscle contractility in a rat model of ischemia: a correlative laser Doppler flowmetric and scanning electron microscopic study. *Acta Neuropathol.* 93, 354–368. doi: 10.1007/s004010050627

Tasali, E., Leproult, R., and Spiegel, K. (2009). Reduced sleep duration or quality: relationships with insulin resistance and type 2 diabetes. *Prog. Cardiovasc. Dis.* 51, 381–391. doi: 10.1016/j.pcad.2008.10.002

Thanabalasundaram, G., Schneidewind, J., Pieper, C., and Galla, H. J. (2011). The impact of pericytes on the blood-brain barrier integrity depends critically on the pericyte differentiation stage. *Int. J. Biochem. Cell Biol.* 43, 1284–1293. doi: 10.1016/j.biocel.2011.05.002

Thomas, W. E. (1999). Brain macrophages: on the role of pericytes and perivascular cells. *Brain Res. Rev.* 31, 42–57. doi: 10.1016/S0165-0173(99)00024-7

Tigges, U., Boroujerdi, A., Welser-Alves, J. V., and Milner, R. (2013). TNF-alpha promotes cerebral pericyte remodeling in vitro, via a switch from alpha1 to alpha2 integrins. *J. Neuroinflammation* 1, 331–310.

Tu, Z., Li, Y., Smith, D. S., Sheibani, N., Huang, S., Kern, T., et al. (2011). Retinal pericytes inhibit activated T cell proliferation. *Invest. Ophthalmol. Vis. Sci.* 52, 9005–9010. doi: 10.1167/iovs.11–8008

Ueno, M. (2007). Molecular anatomy of the brain endothelial barrier: an overview of the distributional features. *Curr. Med. Chem.* 14, 1199–1206. doi: 10.2174/092986707780597943

van Leeuwen, W. M. A., Lehto, M., Karisola, P., Lindholm, H., and Luukkonen, R. (2009). Sleep Restriction increases the risk of developing Cardiovascular diseases by augmenting proinflammatory responses through IL-17 and CRP. *PLoS ONE* 4:e4589. doi: 10.1371/journal.pone.0004589

Veszelka, S., Tóth, A. E., Walter, F. R., Datki, Z., Mózes, E., Fülöp, L., et al. (2013). Docosahexaenoic acid reduces amyloid-B induced toxicity in cells of the neurovascular unit. *J. Alzheimers Dis.* 36, 487–501. doi: 10.3233/JAD-120163

Winkler, E. A., Sengillo, J. D., Bell, R. D., Wang, J., and Zlokovic, B. V. (2012). Blood-spinal cord barrier pericyte reductions contribute to increased capillary permeability. *J. Cereb. Blood Flow Metab.* 32, 1841–1852. doi: 10.1038/jcbfm.2012.113

Yamagata, K., Matsumura, K., Inoue, W., Shiraki, T., Suzuki, K., Yasuda, S., et al. (2001). Coexpression of microsomal-type prostaglandin E synthase with cyclooxygenase-2 in brain endothelial cells of rats during endotoxin-induced fever. *J. Neurosci.* 21, 2669–2677.

Yehuda, S., Sredni, B., Carasso, R. L., and Kenigsbuch-Sredni, D. (2009). REM sleep deprivation in rats results in inflammation and interleukin-17 elevation. *J. Interferon Cytokine Res.* 29, 393–398. doi: 10.1089/jir.2008.0080

Zager, A., Andersen, M. L., Ruiz, F. S., Antunes, I. B., and Tufik, S. (2007). Effects of acute and chronic sleep loss on immune modulation of rats. *Am. J. Physiol. Regul. Integr. Comp. Physiol.* 293, R504–R509. doi: 10.1152/ajpregu.00105.2007

Zlokovic, B. V. (2008). The blood–brain barrier in health and chronic neurodegenerative disorders. *Neuron* 57, 178–201. doi: 10.1016/j.neuron.2008.01.003

Conflict of Interest Statement: The authors declare that the research was conducted in the absence of any commercial or financial relationships that could be construed as a potential conflict of interest.

19

Brain immune interactions and air pollution: macrophage inhibitory factor (MIF), prion cellular protein (PrP^C), interleukin-6 (IL-6), interleukin 1 receptor antagonist (IL-1Ra), and interleukin-2 (IL-2) in cerebrospinal fluid and MIF in serum differentiate urban children exposed to severe vs. low air pollution

Lilian Calderón-Garcidueñas **[1,2]***, ***Janet V. Cross*** **[3]**, ***Maricela Franco-Lira*** **[2]**, ***Mariana Aragón-Flores*** **[2]**, ***Michael Kavanaugh*** **[1]**, ***Ricardo Torres-Jardón*** **[4]**, ***Chih-kai Chao*** **[1]**, ***Charles Thompson*** **[1]**, ***Jing Chang*** **[5]**, ***Hongtu Zhu*** **[5]** ***and Amedeo D'Angiulli*** **[6]**

[1] *Department of Biomedical Sciences, The Center for Structural and Functional Neurosciences, The University of Montana, Missoula, MT, USA*
[2] *Hospital Central Militar, Secretaria de la Defensa Nacional, Mexico City, Mexico*
[3] *Department of Pathology, School of Medicine, University of Virginia, Charlottesville, VA, USA*
[4] *Centro de Ciencias de la Atmósfera, Universidad Nacional Autónoma de México, Mexico City, Mexico*
[5] *Department of Biostatistics, Gillings School of Global Public Health, University of North Carolina, Chapel Hill, NC, USA*
[6] *Department of Neuroscience, Carleton University, Ottawa, ON, Canada*

Edited by:
Adam Denes, University of Manchester, UK

Reviewed by:
Zsuzsanna Környei, Institute of Experimental Medicine of the Hungarian Academy of Sciences, Hungary
Muhammad Sajjad, University of Bonn, Germany
Jesus M. Pradillo, University Complutense of Madrid, Technical University of Madrid, Spain

****Correspondence:***
Lilian Calderón-Garcidueñas, The Center for Structural and Functional Neurosciences, The University of Montana, 32 Campus Drive, Skaggs Building 287, Missoula, MT 59812, USA
e-mail: lilian.calderon-garciduenas@umontana.edu

Mexico City Metropolitan Area children chronically exposed to high concentrations of air pollutants exhibit an early brain imbalance in genes involved in oxidative stress, inflammation, innate and adaptive immune responses along with accumulation of misfolded proteins observed in the early stages of Alzheimer and Parkinson's diseases. A complex modulation of serum cytokines and chemokines influences children's brain structural and gray/white matter volumetric responses to air pollution. The search for biomarkers associating systemic and CNS inflammation to brain growth and cognitive deficits in the short term and neurodegeneration in the long-term is our principal aim. We explored and compared a profile of cytokines, chemokines (Multiplexing LASER Bead Technology) and Cellular prion protein (PrP^C) in normal cerebro-spinal-fluid (CSF) of urban children with high vs. low air pollution exposures. PrP^C and macrophage inhibitory factor (MIF) were also measured in serum. Samples from 139 children ages 11.91 ± 4.2 years were measured. Highly exposed children exhibited significant increases in CSF MIF ($p = 0.002$), IL6 ($p = 0.006$), IL1ra ($p = 0.014$), IL-2 ($p = 0.04$), and PrP^C ($p = 0.039$) vs. controls. MIF serum concentrations were higher in exposed children ($p = 0.009$). Our results suggest CSF as a MIF, IL6, IL1Ra, IL-2, and PrP^C compartment that can possibly differentiate air pollution exposures in children. MIF, a key neuro-immune mediator, is a potential biomarker bridge to identify children with CNS inflammation. Fine tuning of immune-to-brain communication is crucial to neural networks appropriate functioning, thus the short and long term effects of systemic inflammation and dysregulated neural immune responses are of deep concern for millions of exposed children. Defining the linkage and the health consequences of the brain / immune system interactions in the developing brain chronically exposed to air pollutants ought to be of pressing importance for public health.

Keywords: Alzheimer, air pollution, children, innate immunity, neurodegeneration, neuroinflammation, particulate matter, prion cellular protein

INTRODUCTION

Air pollution is a significant health problem in megacities around the world (Molina and Molina, 2004; Chen and Kan, 2008; Bloom, 2011). In the first 50 years of this century (Bloom, 2011), the projected world population will have a further increase of 2–4.5 billion making the issue of deteriorating environments and their health impact critical.

Mexico City Metropolitan Area (MCMA) children with no known risk factors for neurological or cognitive disorders exhibit significant deficits in a combination of fluid and crystallized cognition tasks vs. low air pollution exposed children (Calderón-Garcidueñas et al., 2008a). Brain structural and volumetric changes are seen in both MCMA children and young animal facility dogs (Calderón-Garcidueñas et al., 2008a, 2011a, 2012a). The canine frontal white matter lesions are characterized by vascular sub-cortical pathology associated with neuroinflammation, gliosis, and ultrafine particulate matter deposition (Calderón-Garcidueñas et al., 2008a). Young MCMA residents exhibit the neuropathological hallmarks of Alzheimer and Parkinson's diseases i.e., amyloid beta42 (Aβ42) plaques, tau hyperphosphorylation with pre-tangles and α-synuclein accumulation (Calderón-Garcidueñas et al., 2012b).

The complex modulation of cytokines and chemokines that influence children's central nervous system (CNS) structural and volumetric responses to air pollution obligate the search for biomarkers associating systemic and CNS inflammation to brain growth and cognitive deficits in the short term and neurodegeneration in the long-term (Calderón-Garcidueñas et al., 2008a,b, 2011a,b, 2012b). A good candidate biomarker, macrophage migration inhibitory factor (MIF) is a cytokine expressed in the CNS and involved in innate and adaptive immune responses (Bernhagen et al., 1993; Bacher et al., 2010; Edwards et al., 2010; Moon et al., 2012; Savaskan et al., 2012; Bucala, 2013; Cox et al., 2013; Freiria-Oliveira et al., 2013; Turtzo et al., 2013). MIF participates in the induction of neural stem/progenitor cells (Ohta et al., 2012), the protection of mice female brains after experimental stroke (Turtzo et al., 2013), the mediation of the antidepressant action of exercise (Moon et al., 2012), and of key importance for this work, MIF plays a key role in neuroinflammatory responses (Savaskan et al., 2012; Cox et al., 2013).

In clinical practice and in the experimental setting, MIF has been used as a marker of neurological worsening in progressive neurodegenerative processes including multiple sclerosis and autoimmune-mediated neuroinflammation (Hagman et al., 2011; Cox et al., 2013), as a key neuro-immune mediator linking depressive symptoms with inflammation and HPA dysregulation (Edwards et al., 2010), and as a predictor of lack of response to antidepressants (Cattaneo et al., 2013). Moreover, in the scenario of air pollution and the early hallmarks of Alzheimer's disease (AD) in Mexico City children (Calderón-Garcidueñas et al., 2008a, 2012a), two key issues are of utmost interest to us: the increased concentrations of MIF in the cerebro-spinal-fluid (CSF) of AD patients and the capacity of MIF to enhance the ability of the tau/Aβ42 ratio to discriminate cognitively normal vs. mildly demented patients (Lee et al., 2008; Bacher et al., 2010; Craig-Schapiro et al., 2011). In addition MIF promotes the production of several inflammatory mediators including IL-6, TNF α, and IFN γ (Popp et al., 2009). Given the wide spectrum of serum and CSF responses to pathological processes including neuroinflammation and neurodegenerative diseases such as AD and Parkinson's disease (PD) (Dziedzic, 2006; Helmy et al., 2012; Yan et al., 2012; Giralt et al., 2013; Martinez et al., 2013; Mooijaart et al., 2013; Smolen et al., 2013), we have selected a 41 cytokine/chemokine panel and MIF to explore the CSF responses to high air pollution residency.

Cellular prion protein (PrP^C) is a conserved GPI-anchored membrane protein located on the surface of neurons, at both pre and post-synaptic sites, with a high abundance in the hippocampus, frontal cortex and stratium (Stellato et al., 2011; Ding et al., 2013; Watt et al., 2013). The PRNP gene located in chromosome 20 likely plays key roles in neuronal development, synaptic plasticity, myelin sheath maintenance, cell adhesion, CNS development, and neuroprotection via inhibition of the mitochondrial apoptotic pathway (Mitsios et al., 2007; Altmeppen et al., 2012; Bradford and Mabbott, 2012; Kaiser et al., 2012; Ding et al., 2013).

We are particularly interested in the critical role PrP^C may play in the integrity of the CNS under a neuroinflammatory insult, precisely the key marker of air pollution exposure in urban children (Bremer et al., 2010; Popko, 2010; Gourdain et al., 2012; Scalabrino and Veber, 2012). The role of PrP^C in cellular immunity (Tsutsui et al., 2008), cognitive functioning (Breitling et al., 2012), oxidative stress, and the impact of prion proteins upon the toxic effect of environmental neurotoxic metals (Choi et al., 2007; Oh et al., 2012) are at the core of our research.

The primary aim of this study was to measure the concentrations of PrP^C and selected inflammatory mediators in normal CSF from cohorts of children with high exposures to urban air pollution vs. low pollution control children. Concurrently, we also explored serum MIF and PrP^C in clinically healthy children representing cohorts with high and low air pollution exposures.

Our results identify CSF as a MIF, IL6, IL-1Ra, IL-2, and PrP^C compartment that differentiates children with high vs. low air pollution exposures. The MIF increases in CSF and serum compartments in highly vs. low exposed children strongly suggest MIF could be a serum biomarker bridge to identify children at risk for brain inflammation. Short and long term effects of dysregulated neural immune responses and systemic inflammation are of pressing importance for public health.

PROCEDURE

STUDY AREAS

Children's cohorts were selected from the MCMA and several small cities in Mexico, characterized by clean environments with concentrations of the six criteria air pollutants (ozone, particulate matter, sulfur dioxide, nitrogen oxides, carbon monoxide and lead) below the current US EPA standards.

PARTICIPANTS

This research was approved by the research ethics committee of the Hospital Central Militar in Mexico City. Children gave active assent and their parents gave written informed consent to participation in the study. This work includes data from 139 children 74F, 65M (*Meanage* = 11.91 years, *SD* = 4.2), carefully selected to represent comparable populations from a larger longitudinal cohort research program. There were two groups of children included in this study: Group 1 (*n*: 28, *Meanage* = 10.46 years, *SD* = 4.2, low pollution 8F/6M; high pollution 6F/8M) corresponded to children admitted to the hospital from either MCMA or a low polluted city with a work up diagnosis of acute lymphoblastic leukemia entering a clinical protocol, which included a spinal tap. Only cases with a normal CSF were included in this study. None of the selected CSF samples belonged to children with previous oncological and/or hematological treatments. Group 2 (*n*: 111, 44 controls (24F/20M), 67 MCMA (33F/34M), *Meanage* = 13.37 years, *SD* = 4.2) were clinically healthy children from MCMA and control cities and their serum samples were taken as part of their pediatric examination during a longitudinal follow-up. Inclusion criteria for all participating children were: negative smoking history and environmental tobacco exposure, lifelong residency in MCMA or a control city, residency within 5 miles of the city monitoring stations, full term birth, and unremarkable clinical histories prior to the hospital admission (for the children CSF donors). Low and high pollution exposed children were matched by age, gender, and socioeconomic status.

CSF SAMPLES

Spinal tap was performed in the supine position from lumbar levels using a standard 22 spinal needle. CSF was collected dripping in free air in1 ml aliquot into Nalge Nunc polypropylene CryoTubes. Lumbar puncture samples were collected during non-traumatic, non-complicated procedures. CSF pleocytosis was defined as CSF white blood cell (WBC) counts of >7 cells per mm^3. CSF samples were used for the laboratory procedures without dilution steps.

PERIPHERAL BLOOD ANALYSIS

Blood was collected from an antecubital vein using a 21-G needle. After centrifugation at 3000 rpm for 10 min, aliquots of 1.5 ml serum were transferred to CryoTubes and samples were frozen at −20°C and then transferred to −80°C and stored until further analysis. Blood samples were also collected for a complete blood count (CBC) with differential. Serum samples were processed for Multiplexing LASER Bead Technology (Eve Technologies, Calgary, Canada) that included 41 cytokines and chemokines: EGF, Eotaxin, FGF-2, Flt-3L, Fractalkine, G-CSF, GM-CSF, GRO, IFNα2, IFNγ, IL-1α, IL-1β, IL-1ra, IL-2, IL-3, IL-4, IL-5, IL-6, IL-7, IL-8, IL-9, IL-10, IL-12 (p40), IL-12 (p70), IL-13, IL-15, IL-17a, IP-10, MCP-1, MCP-3, MDC, MIP-1α, MIP-1β, PDGF-AA, PDGF-AB/BB, RANTES, sCD40L, TGFα, TNFα, TNFβ, and VEGF. An ELISA was done for the quantification of PrPc in serum and CSF, BetaPrion®Human EIA (AJ RoboScreen GmbH, Leipzig, Germany). Macrophage inhibitory factor (MIF) was done using an ELISA procedure from R&D (Minneapolis, MN 55413, USA). Serum samples were run without dilution steps.

DATA ANALYSIS

First, we calculated the summary statistics (mean ± standard deviation) of all relevant variables including age, inflammatory mediators and PrPc results. In the 28 CSF samples, we worked with 42 variables and established with independent samples *t*-tests which variables were statistically significant between children with high exposures to air pollutants (Mexico City) and children residing in low pollution cities (Controls). Spearman correlations were run between the CSF target inflammatory mediators and PrPc. In the 111 serum samples, we worked with 2 variables and established with independent samples *t*-tests which variables were statistically significant between Mexico City and control children. Significance was assumed at $p < 0.05$ and data expressed as mean values ± SD. All the statistical analyses described above were performed on statistical software "R" (http://www.r-project.org/).

RESULTS

CSF DATA

CSF samples were clear, colorless, with a normal opening pressure, a mean WBC count of 2.1 ± 1 cells per mm^3 and no RBC. Glucose was 55.9 ± 6.7 mg/100 ml in controls and 54.8 ± 11.7 mg/100ml in Mexico City children ($p = 0.3$). **Table 1** shows the results of the 42 variables included in the analysis. Six variables

Table 1 | Cerebro-spinal- fluid inflammatory mediators in Control vs. Mexico City children (values are shown in pg/ml).

Variables	Mean (controls)	*SD* (controls)	Mean (Mexico City)	*SD* (Mexico City)	*p*-value
EGF	1.627	2.258	2.416	2.665	0.396
FGF2	11.972	20.495	13.294	12.858	0.838
TGFalpha	2.810	1.637	1.800	1.667	0.111
GCSF	8.389	3.668	10.602	12.673	0.526
FIT.3L	23.429	18.261	35.249	34.856	0.261
GM.CSF	4.327	2.253	2.907	1.500	0.060
Fractalkine	41.711	18.529	218.851	422.998	0.127
IFNα2	4.931	2.468	5.349	2.989	0.683
IFNγ	0.278	0.148	1.296	2.006	0.070
GRO	8.057	13.421	19.084	22.972	0.125
IL10	0.259	0.258	2.593	4.966	0.091
MCP3	3.574	3.358	3.594	5.018	0.990
IL12p40	2.030	1.131	2.526	1.564	0.335
MDC	16.996	6.852	20.768	11.320	0.285
IL12	0.473	0.939	0.637	0.516	0.571
PDGF.AA	4.351	4.690	3.210	3.483	0.467
IL13	0.516	0.229	0.477	0.255	0.673
PDGF-BB	0.963	1.494	0.635	1.301	0.535
IL15	2.920	2.491	5.237	5.317	0.144
sCD40l	2.391	5.617	1.334	1.547	0.507
IL17a	5.165	18.595	0.225	0.021	0.338
IL1ra	0.475	0.579	1.915	1.954	0.014
IL1a	0.323	0.365	0.905	1.329	0.122
IL9	0.996	1.229	0.952	0.861	0.913
IL1beta	0.231	0.043	0.642	1.389	0.272
IL2	0.218	0.042	0.530	0.532	0.040
IL3	0.220	0	0.709	1.929	0.343
IL4	2.099	0.890	2.788	1.627	0.167
IL5	0.534	0.385	3.769	12.514	0.334
IL6	1.161	0.650	21.26	38.5	0.006
IL7	0.251	0.080	0.429	0.445	0.147
IL8	17.306	26.099	26.341	37.853	0.459
IP10	207.479	492.590	296.127	519.441	0.641
MCP1	1061.199	1159.217	1521.123	2698.525	0.553
MIP1α	1.130	1.846	6.497	9.129	0.041
MIP1β	6.776	3.065	7.049	3.761	0.832
RANTES	2.121	1.720	8.667	13.963	0.093
TNFα	0.368	0.224	1.441	3.0208	0.191
TNFβ	0.471	0.843	0.987	2.384	0.442
VEGF	4.542	4.494	24.503	43.563	0.099
PrPc	4.396	3.228	8.036	5.506	0.039
MIF	66.918	24.454	329.930	264.342	0.002

were statistically significant, including: MIF, PrP^C, IL-6, IL1Ra, IL-2, and MIP1α (this is not an effect of the number of multiple comparisons, i.e., inflation of Type I error, because the binomial probability that 6 comparisons out of 42 would turn out to be significant by chance is less than 0.0001). Relevant Spearman correlations between CSF PrP^C and target inflammatory mediators are seen in **Table 2**. We found significant correlations between PrP^C and IL-15 ($p = 0.025$) and RANTES ($p = 0.04$), MIF and IL-6 ($p < 0.000$) and IL-6 with IL-15 and RANTES ($p = 0.03$).

SERUM DATA

MIF and PrP^C results in serum are seen in **Table 3**. MIF was significantly higher ($p = 0.009$) in Mexico City children, while PrP^C showed no differences between cohorts.

DISCUSSION

Cerebro-spinal-fluid concentrations of Macrophage migration inhibitory factor MIF, IL-6, IL-1Ra, IL-2, Macrophage Inflammatory Protein 1-α [MIP1α,Chemokine (C-C Motif) Ligand 3] and PrP^C differentiate children with high vs. low air pollution exposures and suggest a complex interplay of a network of multipotent cytokines and normal cellular proteins with known neuromodulatory actions participating in neuroinflammatory responses associated with exposures to air pollutants. Our data also suggests that MIF in serum is a potential biomarker bridge to identify children with CNS inflammation.

IL-6, IL-1Ra, IL-2, and MIF are important players in the pathogenesis of neuroinflammation and the systemic inflammation associated with chronic exposures to high concentrations of air pollutants, while the increased CSF concentrations of PrP^C could potentially represent a neuroprotective response against oxidative stress (Griffiths et al., 2007; Carnini et al., 2010).

IL-6 is a pleiotropic cytokine with key roles in inflammatory responses and in directing T cell differentiation in adaptive immunity. The elevation of IL-6 in the CSF of highly exposed children and its significant correlation with other potent chemokines and cytokines regulating and coordinating innate and adaptive immune responses is important in the developing CNS.

IL-6 has been implicated in systemic and brain neoangiogenesis (Gertz et al., 2012). In traumatic brain injury the presence of low concentrations of IL-6 [IL-6 knock-out (KO) mice] is associated with poor behavior performance, and impacts the expression of IL1β, another powerful pro-inflammatory cytokine (Ley et al., 2011). Neuroprotective associations of specific IL-6 SNP (i.e., the G-allele of the SNP rs1800795) on hippocampal volumes (Baune et al., 2012), the protection of midbrain dopaminergic neurons by IL-6 in the model of 1-methyl-4-phenyl-1,2,3,6-tetrahydropyridine (MPTP) (Spittau et al., 2012), and the significant attenuation of IL-6 concentrations and lower gray volume in old rhesus macaques by a caloric-restricted diet (Willette et al., 2010) support a complex interaction between IL-6, other inflammatory mediators and protective brain responses. The role of IL-6 in long-term potentiation (LTP) and learning is well known (Del Rey et al., 2013). The increased expression of IL-6 is causally related to an increase in synaptic strength since it was abrogated when LTP was interfered by blockade of NMDA-glutamate receptors (Del Rey et al., 2013).

Detrimental effects on the other hand, are described between high concentrations of IL-6, reduced hippocampal volumes and major depressive disorders (Frodl et al., 2012) and in chronic systemic inflammatory conditions with increased risk of stroke (Drake et al., 2011). In advanced HIV infection, CSF concentrations of IL-6 show elevations in patients on suppressive combination antiretroviral therapy regardless of cognitive status, implying the persistence of intra-thecal inflammation even in the absence of clinical manifestations (Kamat et al., 2012).

Of utmost importance for this work and the higher concentrations of CSF IL-6 in Mexico City children is the fact we are seeing the hallmarks of Alzheimer i.e., hyperphosphorilated tau and Aβ42 amyloid plaques in 44 and 51%, respectively, of highly exposed Mexico City teens vs. 0% in low pollution control children. In the literature involving elderly individuals, the associations between IL-6 and dementia are controversial (Papassotiropoulos et al., 2001; Jellinger, 2010; Helmy et al., 2012). Galimberti et al., reported the highest CSF IL-6 concentrations in AD patients with mild cognitive deterioration, suggesting to the authors a key role of IL-6 in the initial phases of neurodegeneration (Galimberti et al., 2008). Combarros et al., suggested that dysregulation of IL-6 in some elderly people contributes to the development of AD (Combarros et al., 2009). Oxidative damage and neuroinflammation are crucial players in neurodegenerative diseases (Nunomura et al., 2001, 2006, 2012a,b), and both are present in the context of air pollution exposures (Calderón-Garcidueñas et al., 2012a). Moreover, under experimental conditions, exposures to different components of air pollutants

Table 3 | Serum MIF and PrP^C in Control v Mexico City children.

Variable	Controls	Mexico City	*p*-value
MIF	425.1 ± 188	711.1 ± 488.7	0.009
PrP^C	1.671 ± 0.96	1.647 ± 1.465	0.21

Values are shown in pg/ml.

Table 2 | Speaman correlations in CSF target inflammatory mediators and PrP^C Control v Mexico City children.

Mediator	PrP^C *r*/*p*-value	MIF *r*/*p*-value	IL-6 *r*/*p*-value	IL-15 *r*/*p*-value	RANTES *r*/*p*
PrP^C	1000	0.307 /0.113	0.236/0.302	0.424/0.025	0.406/0.044
MIF	0.307/0.113	1000	0.773/0.000	0.233/0.232	0.236/0.256
IL-6	0.236/0.302	0.773/0.000	1000	0.467/0.033	0.476/0.034
IL-15	0.424/0.025	0.233/0.232	0.467/0.033	1000	0.692/0.000
RANTES	0.406/0.044	0.236/0.256	0.476/0.034	0.692/0.000	1000

cause oxidative stress, neuroinflammation and neurodegeneration (Calderón-Garcidueñas et al., 2003, 2008a, 2012a,b; Levesque et al., 2011, 2013). Thus, the CSF and brain inflammatory imbalance observed in highly exposed children could represent an early physiological reaction to chronic environmental stress contributing later to the establishment of neurodegenerative processes with childhood clinical manifestations (Calderón-Garcidueñas et al., 2008b, 2011b, 2012b, 2013). Of critical importance are the portals of entry of air pollutants in the urban setting: (i) the nasal pathway through the olfactory, trigeminal nerves and accessory posterolateral nerve, (ii) the red blood cells and monocytes transporting ultrafine PM and then delivering the particles to distant organs including the brain, (iii) the direct access of PM organic and inorganic components to the systemic circulation through the alveolar-capillary interphase, (iv) the gastrointestinal and vagal pathways (Calderón-Garcidueñas et al., 2007; Block and Calderón-Garcidueñas, 2009; Dhuria et al., 2010; Bleier et al., 2012; Lucchini et al., 2012).

Thus, the association between IL-6 serum increases and deficits in verbal memory (Grassi-Oliveira et al., 2011) obligates us to explore the cognitive consequences of an inflammatory imbalance and cognitive impairment in highly exposed cohorts (Aung et al., 2011; Tsai et al., 2012; Uski et al., 2012; Wittkopp et al., 2013).

Intrathecal inflammation in these children is counterbalanced by the increased production of interleukin 1 receptor antagonist (IL-1Ra), a natural endogenous antagonist of IL-1, critical for a variety of brain effects (Arend, 2002; Gadek-Michalska and Bugajski, 2010; Akash et al., 2013; Peters et al., 2013). IL-1RA exhibits low uptake in the normal brain, with rapid metabolism, a short biological half-life (4–6 h), and excretion via the kidneys (Cawthorne et al., 2011). IL-1Ra higher CSF concentrations in highly exposed children, is a key observation since we have previously described a significant frontal up-regulation of IL-1β in Mexico City children (Calderón-Garcidueñas et al., 2008a). IL-1Ra has clear neuroprotective effects in experimental perinatal inflammation and hypoxic-ischemic injuries (Girard et al., 2012), reduces ischemic brain damage and inflammation in co-morbid rats (Pradillo et al., 2012), prevents postoperative cognitive decline and neuroinflammation in older rats (Barrientos et al., 2012), and plays a key anti-inflammatory role in AD (Rubio-Perez and Morillas-Ruiz, 2012). Interestingly, experimental endotoxemia in healthy male volunteers produces significant transient increases in IL-1Ra and decreases in mood, likely reflecting a compensatory strategy or a greater social cognitive processing as a function of sickness (Kullmann et al., 2013). We interpreted the CSF IL-1Ra increases as a neuroprotective response in Mexico City children.

On the other hand, the increases in CSF IL-2 are in keeping with the critical role of this pro-inflammatory cytokine in both effector T-cell development and FoxP3(+) CD4(+) Treg-cell homeostasis (Shameli et al., 2013). Of utmost interest in the context of air pollution is the role of IL-2 in regulating inflammation in an organ-specific manner through the migration and retention of CD4(+) T-cells (both Th1 and Th2) (Ju et al., 2012). Since IL-2 is also required for regulating the Th2 cytokine response during T-cell activation and participates in multifactorial autoimmune responses (Wang et al., 2009; Baine et al., 2013), the issue of autoimmunity to CNS components warrants full investigation in exposed children especially those with extensive white matter hyperintense lesions (Calderón-Garcidueñas et al., 2008b, 2012b).

Macrophage Inflammatory Protein 1-α [Chemokine (C-C Motif) Ligand 3/CCR3] CSF increases in Mexico City children relate to its well known role in inflammatory responses, angiogenesis and tissue remodeling through binding with receptors to other chemokines (i.e., CCR1, CCR4, CCR5) (Gaspar et al., 2013).

MIF is a newly arrived player in the air pollution scenario, is an active participant in innate and acquired immunity (Savaskan et al., 2012), its association with the production of several inflammatory mediators including IL-6, TNF-α, and IFN-γ, and the identification of CSF MIF as a biomarker in AD and mild cognitive impairment patients (MCI) (Popp et al., 2009; Craig-Schapiro et al., 2011) has a great impact in air pollution-related brain effects.

The role of MIF as a neuro-immune mediator linking inflammation with depressive symptoms and HPA dysregulation (Anisman and Hayley, 2012; Savaskan et al., 2012), and its concomitant increases in CSF and serum makes MIF a potential biomarker to identify children with systemic and CNS inflammation. A facet of MIF of importance for us is the potentiation with autoimmune-mediated neuroinflammation (Cox et al., 2013). Cox et al. demonstrated that MIF is essential for microglial activation and the production of IL-6, IL-1β, TNF-α, and inducible NO synthase in an experimental autoimmune encephalomyelitis model. Cox et al., work is important to us because the target cytokines described in their paper are up-regulated in brain tissues of highly exposed children, and the same cytokines exhibit higher serum concentrations when compared with low pollution exposed children (Calderón-Garcidueñas et al., 2008a,b, 2009, 2011a, 2012a,b).

The CSF increases of the normal cellular isoform of the prion protein (PrP^C) in exposed children deserve to be discussed under three important headings:

1. The PrP^C neuroprotective role related primarily to its antioxidant properties, its capacity as a radical scavenger, its key role in signal transduction and cell survival, neuronal zinc regulation, and its functional importance in the protection against oxidative stress and metal toxicity (Brown et al., 1997; Kuwahara et al., 1999; Viles et al., 1999; Milhavet and Lehmann, 2002; Hu et al., 2007; Westergard et al., 2007; Carnini et al., 2010; Martins et al., 2010; Bertuchi et al., 2012; Alfaidy et al., 2013; Watt et al., 2013).
2. The PrP^C role in animal behavior suggesting that the absence of the prion protein could result in altered neural processing (Massimino et al., 2013).
3. The associations of PrP^C with neuropathology apart from the conventional prion diseases (Jiménez-Huete et al., 1998; Ferrer et al., 2001; Voigtländer et al., 2001; Checler and Vincent, 2002; Aguzzi and Haass, 2003; Rezaie et al., 2005; Schwarze-Eicker et al., 2005; Ramljak et al., 2008). Of interest to us are the controversial issues in the literature linking Aβ oligomers and

PrP^C (Laurén et al., 2009; Nygaard and Strittmatter, 2009; Gunther and Striitmatter, 2010; Kessels et al., 2010; Barry et al., 2011; Saijo et al., 2011; Larson et al., 2012; Um et al., 2012; Chen et al., 2013; Kudo et al., 2013; Whitehouse et al., 2013; Younan et al., 2013). A few specific examples to make the point: Kudo et al. showed that Prnp (-/-) mice are resistant to the neurotoxic effect of oligomeric Aβ *in vivo* and *in vitro* (Kudo et al., 2013). Chen et al. have shown PrP^C overexpression down-regulated tau protein and PrP^C lacking the Aβ oligomer binding site was incapable of rescuing the level of tau reduction. These authors demonstrated that PrP^C down-regulated tau via Fyn pathway and the effect can be regulated by Aβ oligomers (Chen et al., 2013). Whitehouse et al. measured PrP^C in the frontal cortex of 24 sporadic AD brains vs. 24 age-matched controls and found a significant decreased of PrP^C in AD brains. Interestingly, PrP^C significantly inversely correlated with BACE1 activity, Aβ load, soluble Aβ, and insoluble Aβ and with the stage of disease, as indicated by Braak tangle stage (Whitehouse et al., 2013). The authors concluded that brain PrP^C level may be important in influencing the onset and progression of sporadic AD (Whitehouse et al., 2013).

Why are all these papers relevant to our work? We recently published a paper (Calderón-Garcidueñas et al., 2012a) showing a 15 fold frontal down-regulation of mRNA PrP^C in Mexico City residents (18 ± 8.7 years) vs. low air pollution age matched controls. In the same work, we showed frontal tau hyperphosphorylation and Aβ diffuse plaques in the exposed kids, but none in low air pollution controls. Thus, the regional frontal PrP^C down-regulation shown by microarray analysis is of deep concern given the age of the autopsy subjects (on average 8 years older) than our CSF children in this study. PrP^C might have significant longitudinal variations in mRNA expression by brain region (Rezaie et al., 2005; Velayos et al., 2009), age, gender, and other factors in the setting of air pollution. Moreover, because the CSF is produced and reabsorbed throughout the entire CSF-Interstitial fluid (IF) functional unit (Chikly and Quaghebeur, 2013), our results highlight the need to define PrP^C changes both directly in different regions of the brain and in the CSF in low vs. high pollution exposed children and young adults. Furthermore, since PrP^C likely plays a key protective role against sporadic AD (Whitehouse et al., 2010; Griffiths et al., 2012) we will expect age-related decreases in specific regional brain areas inversely related to the development of AD hallmarks in highly exposed individuals.

The second reason for concern is the impact of PrP^C in cognition. Gimbel et al. showed that AD transgenic mice with intact PrP^C expression exhibit deficits in spatial learning and memory, while mice lacking PrP^C, but containing Aβ plaque derived from APPswe/PSen1DeltaE9 transgenes, show no detectable impairment of spatial learning and memory (Gimbel et al., 2010). Thus, deletion of PrP^C expression dissociates Aβ accumulation from behavioral impairment in AD mice, with the cognitive deficits selectively requiring PrP^C (Gimbel et al., 2010). Interestingly, Schmidt et al. (2013) showed no association between CSF PrP^C and cognitive status in 114 AD patients, while Breitling et al. reported in a 5 years follow-up study of 1322 elderly Germans (aged 65+ years at baseline), an inverse association between serum PrPc and cognitive functioning (Breitling et al., 2012). In our study, CSF PrP^C was significantly higher in exposed vs. low pollution children, while serum PrP^C concentrations showed no differences.

The significant correlations of PrP^C with RANTES and IL-15 deserve a comment. Regulated upon Activation, Normal T-cell Expressed and Secreted (RANTES) is a proinflammatory chemokine produced by neurons and capable of upregulating neurotrophic factors and extending cell survival after ischemic stroke (Tokami et al., 2013), while IL-15 instructs the generation of a distinct memory T-lymphocyte subset, intermediate between naive and central memory cells (Cieri et al., 2013). These findings highlight the complex link between normal brain proteins, powerful chemokines, and immune driven cytokines.

It has been clear for a number of years that neuroinflammation has critical implications for cognition, behavior, altered brain growth and neurodegeneration. Brain dysbalances in inflammatory mediators and alterations of essential proteins with key roles in CNS development and neuroprotection will inevitably have detrimental consequences for young brains. We already described some of these consequences in Mexico City youth: differences in white matter volumes involving right parietal and bilateral temporal areas and cognitive deficits consistent with impairment of the targeted lobes, olfaction deficits, auditory and vestibular nuclei accumulating α synuclein and/or β amyloid and significant involvement of the medial superior olive neurons, critically involved in brainstem auditory evoked potentials. Elevation of indices of neuroinflammation and oxidative stress, and AD and PD associated pathology completing the grim picture (Calderón-Garcidueñas et al., 2003, 2008a,b, 2010, 2011a,b, 2012a,b, 2013; Calderón-Garcidueñas and Torres-Jardón, 2012).

At the core of our observations lies the complex dynamic interaction in different compartments of cytokines, chemokines and brain proteins responding to the constant state of inflammation and oxidative stress resulting from unhealthy environmental exposures. The short term consequences are having an impact in the performance of children in school and in their violent behavior (Calderón-Garcidueñas and Torres-Jardón, 2012), while the longer effects are already seen in neuropathological studies of children with accidental deaths (Calderón-Garcidueñas et al., 2008b, 2012b, 2013). There is no doubt of the close linkage between the brain and the immune system particularly in the developing brain (Bilbo and Schwarz, 2012). Brisk responses are at hand both systemically and in the brain upon endogenous and exogenous environmental signals, however, the developing brain is delicately sensitive to chronic stimuli and the end result could be a pathological process with deleterious outcomes for the individual.

LOOKING FORWARD AND LIMITATIONS

Despite controversy regarding the mechanistic pathways involved in the CNS damage associated with exposure to air pollutants, we agree that oxidative stress, endothelial dysfunction vascular damage and neuroinflammation are at the core of the pathology, and the same factors play a key role in neurodegenerative diseases (Qin et al., 2007; Rivest, 2009; Levesque et al., 2011; Castellani and Perry, 2012; de la Torre, 2012; Nunomura et al., 2012a,b; Calderón-Garcidueñas et al., 2013). We are looking forward to bridging the gap between early neuroinflammation and its neurodegenerative consequences, an issue of importance in childhood and adolescence when cognitive performance is critical.

There is a need for looking into the CSF early responses to air pollution because we can connect with the knowledge available for elderly populations, i.e., the progression of Alzheimer core biomarkers [Aβ(1-42), total tau and phosphorylated tau] and inflammatory markers useful in the clinical practice to evaluate patients with mild cognitive impairment and their course to AD. This is critical, given that implementation of early preventive pathways (Castellani and Perry, 2012) in the developing brain could ameliorate or drastically modified the pathology in later years.

Our results are potentially limited by the fact our CSF normal samples were taken from a population of children with a hematological workup for a neoplastic process, albeit no CNS involvement, while our serum samples were from clinically healthy children. As pediatricians we are totally aware of the ethical issues in taking CSF samples from healthy children, so the readily available normal CSF samples destined to be discarded are a good initial source of exploratory samples. Nevertheless, the robust CSF increase in the described inflammatory mediators in highly exposed children warrants extensive investigations using available normal CSF samples in Mexico and around the world. Two issues are important here: the selection of multiplex platforms and knowledge of their ability to accurately and sensitively detect cytokines in CSF and blood (serum/plasma) (Malekzadeh et al., 2012). The second one, the use of standardized operating procedures for the recollection of CSF samples, a key point if we want to decrease the variability attributed to different preanalytical procedures between laboratories (del Campo et al., 2012).

SUMMARY

We have quantified CSF responses for a selected panel de inflammatory mediators and PrP^C in two groups of children with contrasting air pollution lifetime exposures. Our results identify MIF, IL6, IL1Ra, IL-2, and PrP^C as potential CSF biomarkers differentiating the high vs. low air pollution exposed children, supporting the previous evidence of an ongoing neuroinflammatory process in Mexico City children. Serum MIF was identified as a robust biomarker in Mexico City children.

Fine tuning of immune-to-brain communication is crucial to neural networks appropriate functioning, thus the short and long term effects of systemic inflammation and dysregulated neural immune responses are of deep concern for millions of highly exposed children.

A large body of work on PrP^c, IL-6, MIF, IL-2, and the IL-1 family already exists, thus expanding this knowledge in the scenario of air pollution pediatric effects could greatly facilitate our understanding of the downstream mechanisms of the complex interaction of cytokines/chemokines/ PrP^c immune responses in the developing brain and the resulting short and long term brain effects.

The role of PrP^c in highly exposed children is an issue worth investigating further as the field moves forward, since we believe knowledge on PrP^c responses in a developing brain will shed light on neuroprotective mechanisms against the onset of Alzheimer disease.

Although the two objectives of this study were accomplished: (i) To evaluate the concentrations of PrP^C and selected inflammatory mediators in normal CSF from cohorts of children with high vs. low pollution controls and (ii) To explore serum PrP^C and MIF in clinically healthy children representing cohorts with high and low air pollution exposures, our immediate goal will be to assess whether the identified biomarkers will be useful in the identification of children at higher risk for cognitive deficits, behavioral disorders, and structural and volumetric brain alterations.

Our ultimate goal is that following the identification of children at the highest risk for detrimental brain effects, we protect them through multidimensional interventions yielding both impact and reach. The prospective of our efforts is readily apparent.

Defining the linkage and the health consequences of the brain/immune system interactions in the developing brain chronically exposed to air pollutants ought to be of pressing importance for public health.

AUTHOR CONTRIBUTIONS

Lilian Calderón-Garcidueñas planned and directed the study, wrote the manuscript, performed all experiments and supported the study from personal funds. Janet V. Cross planned the study, performed the MIF determinations and wrote the manuscript. Amedeo D'Angiulli wrote, edited and formatted the manuscript and performed part of the statistic analysis. Maricela Franco-Lira and Mariana Aragón-Flores obtained patient consent and ethical approvals, got the samples and wrote the manuscript. Michael Kavanaugh wrote the manuscript. Chih-kai Chao and Charles Thompson performed the PrP^C and wrote the manuscript. Ricardo Torres-Jardón wrote the manuscript and Jing Chang and Hongtu Zhu performed the statistical analysis. All authors approved the final draft of the manuscript for publication.

ACKNOWLEDGMENTS

This work was supported in part by the UM-CHPBS Endowment Fund Program, NIMHD grant # S21-MD000236 and a AUCC LACREG grant to Drs. Calderón and D'Angiulli. We thank Dennis Templeton, MD PhD, Chair, Department of Pathology, School of Medicine, University of Virginia, Charlottesville, VA for his generous support of this research while Dr. Lilian Calderón-Garcidueñas was a U Virginia visiting professor. We also thank Lara Ferreira-Azevedo, 5th year Pharmacy visiting student from Brazil for her technical assistance.

REFERENCES

Aguzzi, A., and Haass, C. (2003). Games played by rogue proteins in prion disorders and Alzheimer's disease. *Science* 302, 814–818. doi: 10.1126/science.1087348

Akash, M. S., Rehman, K., and Chen,S. (2013). IL-1Ra and its deliv- ery strategies: inserting the associa- tion in perspective. *Pharm. Res.* doi: 10.1007/s11095-013-1118-0. [Epub ahead of print].

Alfaidy, N., Chauvet, S., Donadio- Andrei, S., Salomon, A., Saoudi, Y., Richaud, P., et al. (2013). Prion protein expression and functional importance in developmental angiogenesis: role in oxidative stress and copper homeostasis. *Antioxid. Redox Signal.* 18, 400–411. doi: 10.1089/ars.2012.4637

Altmeppen, H. C., Puig, B., Dohler, F., Thurm, D. K., Falker, C., Krasemann, S., et al. (2012). Proteolytic processing of the prion protein in health and disease. *Am. J. Neurodegener. Dis.* 1, 15–31.

Anisman, H., and Hayley, S. (2012). Inflammatory factors contribute to depression and its comorbid conditions. *Sci. Signal.* 5:pe45. doi: 10.1126/scisignal.2003579

Arend, W. P. (2002). The balance between IL-1 and IL-1Ra in disease. *Cytokine Growth Factor Rev.* 13, 323–340. doi: 10.1016/S1359-6101(02)00020-5

Aung, H. H., Lame, M. W., Gohil, K., He, G., Denison, M. S., Rutledge, J. C., et al. (2011). Comparative gene responses to collected ambi- ent particles *in vitro*: endothelial responses. *Physiol. Genomics* 43, 917–929. doi: 10.1152/physiolge- nomics.00051.2011

Bacher, M., Deuster, O., Aljabari, B.,Egensperger, R., Neff, F., Jessen, F., et al. (2010). The role of macrophage migration inhibitory factor in Alzheimer's disease. *Mol. Med.* 16, 116–121. doi: 10.2119/molmed.2009.00123

Baine, I., Basu, S., Ames, R., Sellers, R. S., and Macian, F. (2013). Helios induces epigenetic silencing of IL2 gene expression in regulatory T cells. *J. Immunol.* 190, 1008–1016. doi: 10.4049/jimmunol.1200792

Barrientos, R. M., Hein, A. M., Frank, M. G., Watkins, L. R., and Maier, S. F. (2012). Intracisternal interleukin-1 receptor antag- onist prevents postoperative cognitive decline and neuroin- flammatory response in aged rats. *J. Neurosci.* 32, 14641–14648. doi: 10.1523/JNEUROSCI.2173-12.2012

Barry, A. E., Klyubin, I., McDonald, J. M., Mably, A. J., Farrell, M. A., Scott, M., et al. (2011). Alzheimer's disease brain-derived amyloid- β-mediated inhibition of LTP *in vivo* is prevented by immuno- targeting cellular prion protein. *J. Neurosci.* 31, 7259–7263. doi: 10.1523/JNEUROSCI.6500-10.2011

Baune, B. T., Konrad, C., Grotegerd, D., Suslow, T., Birosova, E., Ohrmann, P., et al. (2012). Interleukin-6 gene (IL6): a possible role of brain mor- phology in the healthy adult brain. *J. Neuroinflammation* 9:125. doi: 10.1186/1742-2094-9-125

Bernhagen, J., Calandra, T., Mitchell, R. A., Martin, S. B., Tracey, K. J., Voelter, W., et al. (1993). MIF is a pituitary-derived cytokine that potentiates lethal endotoxemia. *Nature* 365, 756–759. doi: 10.1038/ 365756a0

Bertuchi, F. R., Bourgeon, D. M., Landemberger, M. C., Martins, V. R., and Cerchiaro, G. (2012). PrPC displays an essential protective role from oxidative stress in an astrocyte cell line derived from PrPC knock- out mice. *Biochim. Biophys. Res. Commun.* 418, 27–32. doi: 10.1016/ j.bbrc.2011.12.098

Bilbo, S. D., and Schwarz, J. M. (2012). The immune system and developmental programming of brain and behavior. *Front. Neuroendocrinol.* 33, 267–286. doi: 10.1016/j.yfrne.2012.08.006

Bleier, B. S., Feldman, R., Sadow, P. M., Wu, A., Ting, J., and Metson, R. (2012). The acces- sory posterolateral nerve: an immunohistological analysis. *Am. J. Rhinol. Allergy* 26, 271–273. doi: 10.2500/ajra.2012.26.3804

Block, M., and Calderón-Garcidueñas, L. (2009). Air Pollution: mechanisms of neuroinflammation and CNS disease. *Trends Neurosci.* 32, 506–516. doi: 10.1016/j.tins.2009. 05.009

Bloom, D. E. (2011). 7 Billion and counting. *Science* 333, 562–569. doi: 10.1126/science.1209290

Bradford, B. M., and Mabbott, N. A. (2012). Prion disease and the innate immune system. *Viruses* 4, 3389–3419. doi: 10.3390/v4123389

Breitling, L. P., Muller, H., Stegmaier, C., Kliegel, M., and Brenner, H. (2012). Association of prion pro- tein with cognitive functioning in humans. *Exp. Gerontol.* 47, 919–24. doi: 10.1016/j.exger.2012. 08.001

Bremer, J., Baumann, F., Tiberi, C., Wessig, C., Fischer, H., Schwarz, P., et al. (2010). Axonal prion protein is required for peripheral myelin maintenance. *Nat. Neurosci.* 13, 310–318. doi: 10.1038/nn.2483

Brown, D. R., Schmidt, B., and Kretzschmar, H. A. (1997). Effects of oxidative stress on prion protein expression in PC12 cells. *Int. J. Dev. Neurosci.* 15, 961–972. doi: 10.1016/S0736-5748(97)00042-7

Bucala, R. (2013). MIF, MIF alleles, and prospects for therapeutic inter- vention in autoimmunity. *J. Clin. Immunol.* 33(Suppl. 1), S72–S78. doi: 10.1007/s10875-012-9781-1

Calderón-Garcidueñas, L., Engle, R., Mora-Tiscareño, A., Styner, M., Gomez-Garza, G., Zhu, H., et al. (2011a). Exposure to severe urban pollution influences cognitive outcomes, brain volume and systemic inflammation in clinically healthy children. *Brain Cognition* 77, 345–355. doi: 10.1016/j.bandc.2011.09.006

Calderón-Garcidueñas, L., D'Angiulli, A., Kulesza, R. J., Torres-Jardón, R., Romero, L., Keefe, S., et al. (2011b). Air pollution is associ- ated with brainstem auditory nuclei pathology and delayed brainstem auditory evoked potentials. *Int. J. Dev. Neurosci.* 29, 365–375. doi: 10.1016/j.ijdevneu.2011.03.007

Calderón-Garcidueñas, L., Franco- Lira, M., Henríquez-Roldán, C., González-Maciel, A., Reynoso- Robles, R., Villarreal-Calderon, R., et al. (2010). Urban air pol- lution: influences on olfactory function and pathology in exposed children and young adults. *Exp. Toxicol. Pathol.* 62, 91–102. doi: 10.1016/j.etp.2009.02.117

Calderón-Garcidueñas, L., FrancoLira, M., Mora Tiscareño, A., Medina-Cortina, H., Torres-Jardón, R., and Kavanaugh, M. (2013). Early Alzheimer's and Parkinson's disease pathology in urban children: friend versus foe responses- it is time to face the evidence. *Biomed. Res. Int.* doi: 10.1155/2013/ 161687

Calderón-Garcidueñas, L., Franco Lira, M., Torres-Jardón, R., Henriquez Roldán, C., Valencia-Salazar, G., González-Maciel, A., et al. (2007). Pediatric and systemic effects of chronic air pollution exposure: nose, lung, heart, and brain pathol- ogy. *Toxicol. Pathol.* 35, 154–162. doi: 10.1080/01926230601059985

Calderón-Garcidueñas, L., Kavanaugh, M., Block, M. L., D'Angiulli, A., Delgado-Chávez, R., Torres- Jardón, R., et al. (2012a). Neuroinflammation, hyperphos- phorilated tau, diffuse amyloid plaques and down- regulation of the cellular prion protein in air pollution exposed children and adults. *J. Alzheimers Dis.* 28, 93–107.

Calderón-Garcidueñas, L., Mora Tiscareño, A., Styner, M., Gómez-Garza, G., Zhu, H., Torres- Jardón, R., et al. (2012b). White matter hyperintensities, systemic inflammation, brain growth and cognitive functions in chil- dren exposed to air pollution. *J. Alzheimers Dis.* 31, 183–91. Calderón-Garcidueñas, L., Macías Parra, M., Hoffmann, H. J., Valencia-Salazar, G., Henríquez-Roldán, C., Monte, O. C., et al. (2009). Immunotoxicity and envi- ronment: immunodysregulation and systemic inflammation in children. *Toxicol. Pathol.* 37, 161–169. doi: 10.1177/0192623308329340

Calderón-Garcidueñas, L., Maronpot, R. R., Torres Jardón, R., Henriquez Roldán, C., Schoonhoven, R., Acuña-Ayala, H., et al. (2003). DNA damage in nasal and brain tissues of canines exposed to air pollutants is associated with evidence of chronic brain inflam- mation and neurodegeneration. *Toxicol. Pathol.* 31, 524–538. doi: 10.1080/01926230390226645

Calderón-Garcidueñas, L., Solt, A. C., Henríquez-Roldán, C., Torres Jardón, R., Nuse, B., Herritt, L., et al. (2008a). Long-term air pollution exposure is associated with neuroinflammation, an altered innate immune response, disrup- tion of the blood-brain-barrier, ultrafine particulate deposition, and accumulation of amyloid beta-42 and alpha-synuclein in children and young adults. *Toxicol. Pathol.* 36, 289–310.

Calderón-Garcidueñas, L., Mora Tiscareño, A., Gómez Garza, G., Broadway, J., Chapman, S., Valencia-Salazar, G., et al. (2008b). Air pollution, cognitive deficits and brain abnormalities: a pilot study with children and dogs. *Brain Cogn.* 68, 117–127. doi: 10.1016/j.bandc.2008.04.008

Calderón-Garcidueñas, L., and Torres Jardón, R. (2012). Air pollution, socioeconomic status and children's cognition in megacities: the Mexico City scenario. *Front. Psychol.* 3:217. doi: 10.3389/fpsyg.2012.00217

Carnini, A., Casha, S., Yong, V. W., Hurlbert, R. J., and Braun, J. E. (2010). Reduction of PrPC in human cerebrospinal fluid after spinal cord injury. *Prion* 4, 80–86. doi: 10.4161/pri.4.2.11756

Castellani, R. J., and Perry, G. (2012). Pathogenesis and disease modifying therapy in Alzheimer's disease: the flat line of progress. *Arch. Med. Res.* 43, 694–698. doi: 10.1016/j.arcmed.2012.09.009

Cattaneo, A., Gennarelli, M., Uher, R., Breen, G., Farmer, A., Aitchison, K. J., et al. (2013). Candidate genes expression profile aasociated with antidepressants response in the GENDEP study: dif- ferentiating between baseline predictors and longitudinal targets. *Neuropsychopharmacology* 38, 377–385. doi: 10.1038/npp. 2012.191

Cawthorne, C., Prenant, C., Smigova, A., Julvan, P., Maroy, R., Herholz, K., et al. (2011). Biodistribution, pharmacokinetics and metabolism of interleukin-1 receptor antago- nist (IL-1RA) using [^{18}F] IL1RA and PET imaging in rats. *Br. J. Pharmacol.* 162, 659–672. doi: 10.1111/j.1476-5381.2010.01068.x

Checler, F., and Vincent, B. (2002). Alzheimer's and prion diseases: distinct pathologies, common proteolytic denominators. *Trends Neurosci.* 25, 616–620. doi: 10.1016/ S0166-2236(02)02263-4

10.1021/cn400085q Chikly, B., and Quaghebeur, J. (2013). Reassessing cerebrospinal fluid (CSF) hydrodynamics: a literature review presenting a novel hypothesis for CSF physiology. *J. Bodyw. Mov. Ther.* 17, 344–354. doi: 10.1016/j.jbmt.2013.02.002

Choi, C. J., Anantharam, V., Saetveit, N. J., Houk, R. S., Kanthasamy, A., and Kanthasamy, A. G. (2007). Normal cellular prion protein pro- tects against manganese-induced oxidative stress and apoptotic cell death. *Toxicol. Sci.* 98, 495–509. doi: 10.1093/toxsci/kfm099

Cieri, N., Camisa, B., Cocchiarella, F., Forcato, M., Oliveira, G., Provasi, E., et al. (2013). IL-7 and IL-15 instruct the generation of human memory stem T cells from naive precursors. *Blood* 121, 573–584. doi: 10.1182/blood-2012-05-431718

Combarros, O., van Duijn, C. M., Hammond, N., Belbin, O., Arias Vásquez, A., Cortina-Borja, M., et al. (2009). Replication by the epistasis project of the interaction between the genes for IL-6 and IL-10 in the risk of Alzheimer's disease. *J. Neuroinflammation* 6:22. doi: 10.1186/1742-2094-6-22

Cox, G. M., Kithcart, A. P., Pitt, D., Guan, Z., Alexander, J., Williams, J. L., et al. (2013). Macrophage migration inhibitory factor potentiates autoimmune-mediated neu- roinflammation. *J. Immunol.* 191, 1043–1054. doi: 10.4049/jimmunol. 1200485

Craig-Schapiro, R., Kuhn, M., Xiong, C., Pickering, E. H., Liu, J., Misko, T. P., et al. (2011). Multiplex immunoassay panel identifies novel CSF biomarkers for Alzheimer's disease diagnosis and progno- sis. *PLoS ONE* 6:e18850. doi: 10.1371/journal.pone.0018850

de la Torre, J. C. (2012). A turning point for Alzheimer's disease? *Biofactors* 38, 78–83. doi: 10.1002/biof.200

del Campo, M., Mollenhauer, B., Bertolotto, A., Engelborghs, S., Hampel, H., Simonsen, A. H., et al. (2012). Recommendations to standardize preanalytical con- founding factors in Alzheimer's and Parkinson's disease cerebrospinal fluid biomarkers: an update. *Biomark. Med.* 6, 419–430. doi: 10.2217/bmm.12.46

Del Rey, A., Balschun, D., Wetzel, W., Randolf, A., and Besedovsky, H. O. (2013). A cytokine network involv- ing brain-borne IL-1β, IL-1Ra, IL- 18, IL-6 and TNF-α operates during long-term potentiation and learn- ing. *Brain Behav. Immun.* 33, 15–23. doi: 10.1016/j.bbi.2013.05.011

Dhuria, S. V., Hanson, L. R., and Frey, W. H. 2nd. (2010). Intranasal delivery to the central nervous sys- tem: mechanisms and experimen- tal considerations. *J. Pharm. Sci.* 99, 1654–1673. doi: 10.1002/jps.21924

Ding, T., Zhou, X., Kouadir, M., Shi, F., Yang, Y., Liu, J., et al. (2013). Cellular prion protein participates in the regulation of inflammatory response and apoptosis in BV2 microglia during infection with Mycobacterium bovis. *J. Mol. Neurosci.* 51, 118–126. doi: 10.1007/ s12031-013-9962-2

Drake, C., Boutin, H., Jones, M. S., Denes, A., McColl, B. W., Selvarajah, J. R., et al. (2011). Brain inflammation is induced by co-morbidities and risk fac- tors for stroke. *Brain Behav. Immun.* 25, 1113–1122. doi: 10.1016/j.bbi.2011.02.008

Dziedzic, T. (2006). Systemic inflam- matory markers and risk of dementia. *Am. J. Alzheimers Dis. Other Demen.* 21, 258–262. doi: 10.1177/1533317506289260

Edwards, K. M., Bosch, J. A., Engeland, C. G., Cacioppo, J. T., and Marucha, P. T. (2010). Elevated macrophage migration inhibitory factor (MIF) is associated with depressive symptoms, blunted cortisol reac- tivity to acute stress, and lowered morning cortisol. *Brain Behav. Immun.* 24, 1202–1208. doi: 10.1016/j.bbi.2010.03.011

Ferrer, I., Blanco, R., Carmona, M., Puig, B., Ribera, R., Rey, M. J., et al. (2001). Prion protein expression in senile plaques in Alzheimer's disease. *Acta Neuropathol.* 101, 49–56.

Freiria-Oliveira, A. H., Blanch, G. T., Li, H., Colombari, E., Colombari, D. S., and Sumners, C. (2013). Macrophage inhibitory factor in the nucleus of solitary tract decreases blood pressure in SHRs. *Cardiovasc. Res.* 97, 153–160. doi: 10.1093/cvr/cvs297

Frodl, T., Carballedo, A., Hughes, M. M., Saleh, K., Fagan, A., Skokauskas, N., et al. (2012). Reduced expression of glucocorticoid-inducible genes GILZ and SGK-1: high IL6 levels are associated with reduced hippocam- pal volumes in major depressive dis- order. *Transl. Psychiatry* 2:e88. doi: 10.1038/tp.2012.14

Gadek-Michalska, A., and Bugajski, J. (2010). Interleukin-1 (IL-1) in stress-induced activation of limbic- hypothalamic-pituitary adrenal axis. *Pharmacol. Rep.* 62, 969–982.

Galimberti, D., Venturelli, E., Fenoglio, C., Guidi, I., Villa, C., Bergamaschini, L., et al. (2008). Intratechal levels of IL6, IL11 and LIF in Alzheimer's disease and frontotemporal lobar degenera- tion. *J. Neurol.* 255, 539–544. doi: 10.1007/s00415-008-0737-6

Gaspar, K., Kukova, G., Bunemann, E., Buhren, B. A., Sonkolv, E., Szollosi, A. G., et al. (2013). The chemokine receptor CCR3 par- ticipates in tissue remodeling during atopic skin inflammation. *J. Dermatol. Sci.* 71, 12–21. doi: 10.1016/j.jdermsci.2013.04.011

Gertz, K., Kronenberg, G., Kälin, R. E., Baldinger, T., Werner, C., Balkaya, M., et al. (2012). Essential role of interleukin-6 in post-stroke angio- genesis. *Brain* 135, 1964–1980. doi: 10.1093/brain/aws075

Gimbel, D. A., Nygaard, H. B., Coffey, E. E., Gunther, E. C., Laurén, J., Gimbel, Z. A., et al. (2010). Memory impairment in transgenic Alzheimer mice requires cellular prion protein. *J. Neurosci.* 30, 6367–6374. doi: 10.1523/JNEUROSCI.0395-10.2010

Giralt, M., Ramos, R., Quintana, A., Ferrer, B., Erta, M., Castro-Freire, M., et al. (2013). Induction of atypi- cal EAE mediated by transgenic pro- duction of IL6 in astrocytes in the absence of systemic IL6. *Glia* 61, 587–600. doi: 10.1002/glia.22457

Girard, S., Sébire, H., Brochu, M. E., Briota, S., Sarret, P., and Sébire, G. (2012). Postnatal administration of IL-1Ra exerts neuroprotec- tive effects following perinatal inflammation and/or hypoxic- ischemic injuries. *Brain Behav. Immun.* 26, 1331–1339. doi: 10.1016/j.bbi.2012.09.001

Gourdain, P., Ballerini, C., Nicot, A. B., and Carnaud, C. (2012). Exacerbation of experimental autoimmune encephalomyeli- tis in prion protein PrPc-null mice: evidence for a critical role of the central nervous system. *J. Neuroinflammation* 9:25. doi: 10.1186/1742-2094-9-25

Grassi-Oliveira, R., Bauer, M. E., Pezzi, J. C., Teixeira, A. L., and Brietzke, E. (2011). Interleukin-6 and verbal memory in recurrent major depres- sive disorder. *Neuro Endocrinol. Lett.* 32, 540–544.

Griffiths, H. H., Whitehouse, I. J., and Hooper, N. M. (2012). Regulation of amyloid-β production by the prion protein. *Prion* 6, 217–222. doi: 10.4161/pri.18988

Griffiths, M., Neal, J. W., and Gasque, P. (2007). Innate immunity and protective neuroinflammation: new emphasis on the role of neu- roimmune regulatory proteins. *Int. Rev. Neurobiol.* 82, 29–55. doi: 10.1016/S0074-7742(07)82002-2

Gunther, E. C., and Striitmatter, S. M. (2010). Beta-amyloid oligomers and cellular prion protein in Alzheimer's disease. *J. Mol. Med.* 88, 331–338. doi: 10.1007/s00109-009-0568-7

Hagman, S., Raunio, M., Rossi, M., Dastidar, P., and Elovaara, I. (2011). Disease-associated inflam- matory biomarker profiles in blood in different subtypes of multiple sclerosis: prospective clinical and MRI follow-up Study. *J. Neuroimmunol.* 234, 141–147. doi: 10.1016/j.jneuroim.2011.02.009

Helmy, A. A., Naseer, M. M., Shafie, S. E., and Nada, M. A. (2012). Role of interleukin 6 and alpha-globulins in differentiating Alzheimer and vas- cular dementias. *Neurodegener. Dis.* 9, 81–86. doi: 10.1159/000329568

Hu, W., Rosenberg, R. N., and Stüve, (2007). Prion proteins: a bio- logical role beyond prion diseases. *Acta Neurol. Scand.* 116, 75–82. doi: 10.1111/j.1600-0404.2007.00868.x Jellinger, A. K. (2010). Intrathecal levels of IL6 in Alzheimer's dis- ease. *J. Neurol.* 257, 142. doi: 10.1007/s00415-009-5312-2

Jiménez-Huete, A., Lievens, P. M., Vidal, R., Piccardo, P., Ghetti, B., Tagliavini, F., et al. (1998). Endogenous proteolytic cleavage of normal and disease-associated iso- forms of the human prion protein in neural and non-neural tissues. *Am. J. Pathol.* 153, 1561–1572. doi: 10.1016/S0002-9440(10)65744-6

Ju, S. T., Sharma, R., Gaskin, F., and Fu, S. M. (2012). IL-2 controls trafficking receptor gene expression and Th2 response for skin and lung inflammation. *Clin. Immunol.* 145, 82–88. doi: 10.1016/j.clim.2012.07.015

Kaiser, D. M., Acharya, M., Leighton, L. A., Wang, H., Daude, N., Wohlgemuth, S., et al. (2012). Amyloid beta precursor pro- tein and prion protein have a conserved interaction affecting cell adhesion and CNS develop- ment. *PLoS ONE* 7:e51305. doi: 10.1371/journal.pone.0051305

Kamat, A., Lyons, J. L., Misra, V., Uno, H., Morgello, S., Singer, E. J., et al. (2012). Monocyte acti- vation markers in cerebrospinal fluid associated with impaired neurocognitive testing in advanced HIV infection. *J. Acquir. Immune Defic. Syndr.* 60, 234–243. doi: 10.1097/QAI.0b013e318256f3bc

Kessels, H. W., Nguyen, L. N., Nabavi, S., and Malinow, R. (2010). The prion protein as a receptor for amyloid-beta. *Nature* 466, E3–E4. doi: 10.1038/nature09217

Kudo, W., Petersen, R. B., and Lee, H. G. (2013). Cellular prion pro- tein and Alzheimer disease: link to oligomeric amyloid-β and neuronal cell death. *Prion* 7, 114–116. doi: 10.4161/pri.22848

Kullmann, J. S., Grigoleit, J. S., Wolf, O. T., Engler, H., Oberbeck, R., Elsenbruch, S., et al. (2013). Experimental human endotoxemia enhances brain activity during social cognition. *Soc. Cogn. Affect. Neurosci.* doi: 10.1093/scan/nst049. [Epub ahead of print].

Lee, K. S., Chung, J. H., Lee, K. H., Shin, M. J., Oh, B. H., and Hong, C. H. (2008). Bioplex analysis of plasma cytokines in Alzheimer's dis- ease and mild cognitive impair- ment. *Immunol. Lett.* 121, 105–109. doi:10.1016/j.imlet.2008.09.004

Levesque, S., Surace, M. J., McDonald, J., and Block, M. L. (2011). Air pollution and the brain: subchronic diesel exhaust exposure causes neu- roinflammation and elevates early markers of neurodegenerative dis- ease. *J. Neuroinflammation* 8:105. doi:10.1186/1742-2094-8-105

Levesque, S., Taetzsch, T., Lull, M. E., Johnson, J. A., McGraw, C., and Block, M. L. (2013). The role of MAC1 in diesel exhaust particle- induced microglial activation and loss of dopaminergic neuron func- tion. *J. Neurochem.* 125, 756–765. doi:10.1111/jnc.12231

Ley, E. J., Clond, M. A., Singer, M. B., and Salim, A. (2011). IL6 defi- ciency affects function after trau- matic brain injury. *J. Surg. Res.* 170, 253–256. doi: 10.1016/j.jss. 2011.03.006

Lucchini, R. G., Dorman, D. C., Elder, A., and Veronesi, B. (2012). Neurological impacts from inhalation of pollutants and the nose-brain connection. *Neurotoxicology* 33, 838–841. doi: 10.1016/j.neuro.2011.12.001

Malekzadeh, A., de Groot, V., Beckerman, H., van Oosten, B. W., Blankenstein, M. A., and Teunissen, C. (2012). Challenges in multiplex and monoplex platforms for the discovery of inflammatory profiles in neurodegenerative dis- eases. *Methods* 56, 508–513. doi: 10.1016/j.ymeth.2012.03.017

Martinez, A. N., Mehra, S., and Kaushal, D. (2013). Role of Interleukin-6 (IL6) in innate immunity to Mycobacterium tuber- culosis infection. *J. Infect. Dis.* 207, 1253–1261. doi: 10.1093/infdis/ jit037

Martins, V. R., Beraldo, F. H., Hajj, G. N., Lopes, M. H., Lee, K. S., Prado, M. A., et al. (2010). Prion protein: orchestrating neurotrophic activities. *Curr. Issues Mol. Biol.* 12, 63–86.

Massimino, M. L., Redaelli, M., Bertoli, A., Sorgato, M. C., and Mucignat-Caretta, C. (2013). Altered behavioral aspects of aged mice lacking the cellular prion protein. *Physiol. Behav.* 119C, 86–91. doi: 10.1016/j.physbeh.2013.06.006

Milhavet, O., and Lehmann, S. (2002). Oxidative stress and the prion protein in transmissible spongi- form encephalopathies. *Brain Res. Brain Res. Rev.* 38, 328–339. doi: 10.1016/S0165-0173(01)00150-3

Mitsios, N., Saka, M., Krupinski, J., Pennucci, R., Sanfeliu, C., Turu, M. M., et al. (2007). Cellular prion protein is increased in the plasma and peri-infarcted brain tissue after acute stroke. *J. Neurosci. Res.* 85, 602–611. doi: 10.1002/jnr.21142

Molina, L. T., and Molina, M. J. (2004). Improving air quality in megaci- ties: Mexico City case study. *Ann. N.Y. Acad. Sci.* 1023, 142–158. doi: 10.1196/annals.1319.006

Mooijaart, S. P., Sattar, N., Trompet, S., Lucke, J., Stott, D. J., Ford, I., et al. (2013). Circulating interleukin-6 concentration and cognitive decline in old age: the PROSPER study. *J. Intern. Med.* 274, 77–85. doi: 10.1111/joim.12052

Moon, H. Y., Kim, S. H., Yang, Y. ., Song, P., Yu, H. S., Park, H. G., et al. (2012). Macrophage migration inhibitory factor medi- ates the antidepressant actions of voluntary exercise. *Proc. Natl. Acad. Sci. U.S.A.* 109, 13094–13099. doi: 10.1073/pnas.1205535109

Nunomura, A., Castellani, R. J., Lee, H. G., Moreira, P. I., Zhu, X., Perry, G., et al. (2006). Neuropathology in Alzheimer's disease: awakening from a hundred-year old dream. *Sci. Aging Knowledge Environ.* 2006, pe10. doi: 10.1126/sageke.2006.8.pe10

Nunomura, A., Perry, G., Aliev, G., Hirai, K., Takeda, A., Balraj, E. K., et al. (2001). Oxidative damage is the earliest event in Alzheimer's dis- ease. *J. Neuropathol. Exp. Neurol.* 60, 759–767.

Nunomura, A., Tamaoki, T., Motohashi, N., Nakamura, M., McKeel, D. W. Jr., Tabaton, M., et al. (2012a). The earliest stage of cognitive impairment in tran- sition from normal aging to Alzheimer's disease is marked by prominent RNA oxidation in vulnerable neurons. *J. Neuropathol. Exp. Neurol.* 71, 233–241. doi: 10.1097/NEN.0b013e318248e614

Nunomura, A., Moreira, P. I., Castellani, R. J., Lee, H. G., Zhu, X., Smith, M. A., et al. (2012b). Oxidative damage to RNA in aging and neurodegenerative disorders. *Neurotox. Res.* 22, 231–248. doi: 10.1007/s12640-012-9331-x

Nygaard, H. B., and Strittmatter, S. M. (2009). Cellular protein mediates the toxicity of beta- amyloid oligomers: implications for Alzheimer disease. *Arch. Neurol.* 66, 1325–1328. doi: 10.1001/ archneurol.2009.223

Oh, J. M., Choi, E. K., Carp, R. I., and Kim, Y. S. (2012). Oxidative stress impairs autophagic flux in prion protein-deficient hippocam- pal cells. *Autophagy* 8, 1448–1461. doi: 10.4161/auto.21164

Ohta, S., Misawa, A., Fukaya, R., Inoue, S., Kanemura, Y., Okano, H., et al. (2012). Macrophage migra- tion inhibitory factor (MIF) pro- motes cell survival and prolifera- tion of neural stem/progenitor cells. *J. Cell Sci.* 125, 3210–3220. doi: 10.1242/jcs.102210

Papassotiropoulos, A., Hock, C., and Nitsch, R. M. (2001). Genetics of Interleukin 6: impli- cations for Alzheimer's disease. *Neurobiol. Aging* 22, 863–871. doi: 10.1016/S0197-4580(01)00294-9

Peters, V. A., Joesting, J. J., and Freund, G. G. (2013). IL-1 receptor 2 (IL-1R2) and its role in immune regula- tion. *Brain Behav. Immun.* 32, 1–8. doi: 10.1016/j.bbi.2012.11.006

Popko, B. (2010). Myelin mainte- nance: axonal support required. *Nat. Neurosci.* 13, 275–277. doi: 10.1038/nn0310-275

Popp, J., Bacher, M., Kölsch, H., Noelker, C., Deuster, O., Dodel, R., et al. (2009). Macrophage inhibitory factor in mild cognitive impair- ment and Alzheimer's disease. *J. Psychiatr. Res.* 43, 749–753. doi: 10.1016/j.jpsychires.2008.10.006

Pradillo, J. M., Denes, A., Greenhalgh, A. D., Boutin, H., Drake, C., McColl, B. W., et al. (2012). Delayed administration of interleukin-1 receptor antagonist reduces ischemic brain damage and inflam- mation in comorbid rats. *J. Cereb. Blood Flow Metab.* 32, 1810–1819. doi: 10.1038/jcbfm.2012.101

Qin, L., Wu, X., Block, M. L., Liu, Y., Breese, G. R., Hong, J. S., et al. (2007). Systemic LPS causes chronic neuroinflammation and progres- sive neurodegeneration. *Glia* 55, 453–462. doi:10.1002/glia.20467

Ramljak, S., Asif, A. R., Armstrong, V. W., Wrede, A., Groschup, M. H., Buschmann, A., et al. (2008). Physiological role of the cellular prion protein (PrPc): protein profil- ing study in two cell culture systems. *J. Proteome Res.* 7, 2681–2695. doi: 10.1021/pr7007187

Rezaie, P., Pontikis, C. C., Hudson, L., Caims, N. J., and Lantos, P. L. (2005). Expression of cellular prion protein in the frontal and occipital lobe in Alzheimer's disease, diffuse Lewy body disease, and in normal brain: an immunohistochemical study. *J. Histochem. Cytochem.* 53, 929–940. doi: 10.1369/jhc.4A6551. 2005

Rivest, S. (2009). Regulation of innate immune responses in the brain. *Nat. Rev. Immunol.* 9, 429–439. doi: 10.1038/nri2565

Rubio-Perez, J. M., and Morillas-Ruiz, J. M. (2012). A review: inflam- matory process in Alzheimer's disease, role of cytokines. *ScientificWorldJournal* 2012:756357. doi: 10.1100/2012/756357

Saijo, E., Scheff, S. W., and Telling, G. C. (2011). Unaltered prion pro- tein expression in Alzheimer dis- ease patients. *Prion* 5, 109–116. doi: 10.4161/pri.5.2.16355

Savaskan, N. E., Fingerle-Rowson, G., Buchfelder, M., and Eyüpoglu, I. Y. (2012). Brain miffed by macrophage inhibitory factor. *Int. J. Cell Biol.* 2012:139573. doi: 10.1155/2012/ 139573

Scalabrino, G., and Veber, D. (2012). Normal prions as a new target of cobalamin (vitamin B12) in rat cen- tral nervous system. *Clin. Chem. Lab. Med.* 51, 601–606. doi: 10.1515/ cclm-2012-0474

Schmidt, C., Artjomova, S., Hoeschel, M., and Zerr, I. (2013). CSF prion protein concentration and cogni- tion in patients with Alzheimer dis- ease. *Prion* 7, 229–234. doi: 10.4161/ pri.23904

Schwarze-Eicker, K., Keyvani, K., Görtz, N., Westaway, D., Sachser, N., and Paulus, W. (2005). Prion protein (PrPc) promotes beta amyloid plaque formation. *Neurobiol. Aging* 26, 1177–1182. doi: 10.1016/j. neurobiolaging.2004.10.004

Shameli, A., Yamanouchi, J., Tsai, ., Yang, Y., Clemente-Casares, X., Moore, A., et al. (2013). IL-2 promotes the function of memory- like autoregulatory CD8+T cells but suppresses their develop- ment via FoxP3+ Treg cells. *Eur. J. Immunol.* 43, 394–403. doi: 10.1002/eji.201242845

Smolen, J. S., Schoels, M. M., Nishmoto, N., Breedveld, F. C., Burmester, G. R., Dougados, M., et al. (2013). Consensus state- ment on blocking the effects of interleukin-6 and in particular by interleukin-6 receptor inhibi- tion in rheumatoid arthritis and other inflammatory conditions. *Ann. Rheum. Dis.* 72, 482–492. doi: 10.1136/annrheumdis-2012- 202469

Spittau, B., Zhou, X., Ming, M., and Krieglstein, K. (2012). IL6 protects MN9D cells and mid- brain dopaminergic neurons from MPP+-induced neurodegener- ation. *Neuromolecular Med.* 14, 317–327. doi: 10.1007/s12017-012- 8189-7

Stellato, F., Spevacek, A., Proux, O., Minicozzi, V., Millhauser, G., and Morante, S. (2011). Zinc modulates copper coordination mode in prion protein octa- repeats subdomains. *Eur. Biophys. J.* 40, 1259–1270. doi: 10.1007/s00249-011-0713-4

Tokami, H., Ago, T., Sugimori, H., Kuroda, J., Awano, H., Suzuki, K., et al. (2013). RANTES has a potential to play a neuroprotective role in an autocrine/paracrine manner after ischemic stroke. *Brain Res.* 1517, 122–132. doi: 10.1016/j.brainres.2013.04.022

Tsai, D. H., Amvai, N., Marques-Vidal, P., Wang, J. L., Riediker, M., Mooser, V., et al. (2012). Effects of particu- late matter on inflammatory mark- ers in the general adult popula- tion. *Part. Fibre Toxicol.* 9, 24. doi: 10.1186/1743-8977-9-24

Turtzo, L. C., Li, J., Persky, R., Benashski, S., Weston, G., Bucala, R., et al. (2013). Deletion of macrophage migration inhibitory factor worsens stroke outcome in female mice. *Neurobiol. Dis.* 54, 421–431. doi: 10.1016/j.nbd.2013. 01.016

Um, J. W., Nygaard, H. B., Heiss, J. K., Kostylev, M. A., Stagi, M., Vortmeyer, A., et al. (2012). Alzheimer amyloid-beta oligomer bound to postsynaptic prion protein activates Fyn to impair neu- rons. *Nat. Neurosci.* 15, 1227–1235. doi: 10.1038/nn.3178

Uski, O. J., Happo, M. S., Jalava, P. I., Brunner, T., Kelz, J., Obemberger, I., et al. (2012). Acute systemic and lung inflammation in C57Bl/6J mice after intratracheal aspira- tion of particulate matter from small-scale biomass combustion appliances based on old and mod- ern technologies. *Inhal. Toxicol.* 24, 952–965. doi: 10.3109/08958378. 2012.742172

Velayos, J. L., Irujo, A., Cuadrado- Tejedor, M., Paternain, B., Moleres, F. J., and Ferrer, V. (2009). The cel- lular prion protein and its role in Alzheimer disease. *Prion* 3, 110–117. doi: 10.4161/pri.3.2.9135

Viles, J. H., Cohen, F. E., Prusiner, S. B., Goodin, D. B., Wright, P. E., and Dyson, H. J. (1999). Copper binding to the prion protein: struc- tural implications of four identical cooperative binding sites. *Proc. Natl. Acad. Sci. U.S.A.* 96, 2042–2047. doi: 10.1073/pnas.96.5.2042

Voigtländer, T., Klöppel, S., Birner, P., Jarius, C., Flicker, H., Verghese-Nikolakaki, S., et al. (2001). Marked increase of neuronal prion protein immunoreactivity in Alzheimer's disease and human prion diseases. *Acta Neuropathol.* 101, 417–423.

Wang, J., Wicker, L. S., and Santamaria, P. (2009). IL-2 and its high- affinity receptor: genetic control of immunoregulation and autoimmu- nity. *Semin. Immunol.* 21, 363–371. doi: 10.1016/j.smim.2009.04.004

Watt, N. T., Griffiths, H. H., and Hooper, N. M. (2013). Neuronal zinc regulation and the prion protein. *Prion* 7, 203–208. doi: 10.4161/pri.24503

Westergard, L., Christensen, H. M., and Harris, D. A. (2007). The cellular prion protein (PrP^{C}): its physiological func- tion and role in disease. *Biochim. Biophys. Acta* 1772, 629–644. doi: 10.1016/j.bbadis.2007.02.011

Whitehouse, I. J., Jackson, C., Turner, A. J., and Hooper, N. M. (2010). Prion protein is reduced in aging and in speoradic but not in famil- ial Alzheimer's disease. *J. Alzheimers Dis.* 22, 1023–1031.

Whitehouse, I. J., Miners, J. S., Glennon, E. B., Kehoe, P. G., Love, S., Kellet, K. A., et al. (2013). Prion protein is decreased in Alzheimer's brain and inversely correlates with BACE1 activ- ity, amyloid-β levels and Braak stage. *PLoS ONE* 8:e59554 doi: 10.1371/journal.pone.0059554

Willette, A. A., Bendlin, B. B., McLaren, D. G., Canu, E., Kastman, E. K., Kosmatka, K. J., et al. (2010). Age-related changes in neural volume and microstructure asso- ciated with interleukin-6 are ameliorated by a calorie-restricted diet in old rhesus monkeys. *Neuroimage* 51, 987–994. doi: 10.1016/j.neuroimage.2010.03.015

Wittkopp, S., Staimer, N., Tjoa, T., Gillen, D., Daher, N., Shafer, M., et al. (2013). Mitochondrial genetic background modifies the relationship between traffic- related air pollution exposure and systemic biomarkers of inflam- mation. *PLoS ONE* 8:e64444. doi: 10.1371/journal.pone.0064444

Yan, J., Liu, J., Lin, C. Y., Anzgene, A. N., Csurhes, P. A., Pender, M. P., et al. (2012). Interleukin-6 gene promoter-572 C allele may play a role in rate of disease progres- sion in multiple sclerosis. *Int. J. Mol. Sci.* 13, 13667–13679. doi: 10.3390/ijms131013667

Younan, N. D., Sarell, C. J., Davies, P., Brown, D. R., and Viles, J. H. (2013). The cellular prion pro- tein traps Alzheimer's Aβ in an oligomeric form and disassem- bles amyloid fibers. *FASEB J.* 27, 1847–1858. doi: 10.1096/fj.12-222588

Permissions

All chapters in this book were first published in BBTGFNI, by Frontiers; hereby published with permission under the Creative Commons Attribution License or equivalent. Every chapter published in this book has been scrutinized by our experts. Their significance has been extensively debated. The topics covered herein carry significant findings which will fuel the growth of the discipline. They may even be implemented as practical applications or may be referred to as a beginning point for another development.

The contributors of this book come from diverse backgrounds, making this book a truly international effort. This book will bring forth new frontiers with its revolutionizing research information and detailed analysis of the nascent developments around the world.

We would like to thank all the contributing authors for lending their expertise to make the book truly unique.

They have played a crucial role in the development of this book. Without their invaluable contributions this book wouldn't have been possible. They have made vital efforts to compile up to date information on the varied aspects of this subject to make this book a valuable addition to the collection of many professionals and students.

This book was conceptualized with the vision of imparting up-to-date information and advanced data in this field. To ensure the same, a matchless editorial board was set up. Every individual on the board went through rigorous rounds of assessment to prove their worth. After which they invested a large part of their time researching and compiling the most relevant data for our readers.

The editorial board has been involved in producing this book since its inception. They have spent rigorous hours researching and exploring the diverse topics which have resulted in the successful publishing of this book. They have passed on their knowledge of decades through this book. To expedite this challenging task, the publisher supported the team at every step. A small team of assistant editors was also appointed to further simplify the editing procedure and attain best results for the readers.

Apart from the editorial board, the designing team has also invested a significant amount of their time in understanding the subject and creating the most relevant covers. They scrutinized every image to scout for the most suitable representation of the subject and create an appropriate cover for the book.

The publishing team has been an ardent support to the editorial, designing and production team. Their endless efforts to recruit the best for this project, has resulted in the accomplishment of this book. They are a veteran in the field of academics and their pool of knowledge is as vast as their experience in printing. Their expertise and guidance has proved useful at every step. Their uncompromising quality standards have made this book an exceptional effort. Their encouragement from time to time has been an inspiration for everyone.

The publisher and the editorial board hope that this book will prove to be a valuable piece of knowledge for researchers, students, practitioners and scholars across the globe.

List of Contributors

Charity E. Onore, Milo Careaga and Paul Ashwood
The MIND Institute, University of California, Davis, CA, USA
Department of Medical Microbiology and Immunology, University of California, Davis, CA, USA

Brooke A. Babineau
Department of Pediatrics, University of California, San Francisco, CA, USA
Institute for Human Genetics, University of California, San Francisco, CA, USA

Jared J. Schwartzer and Robert F. Berman
The MIND Institute, University of California, Davis, CA, USA
Department of Neurological Surgery, University of California, Davis, CA, USA

Sonia Leon-Cabrera
Departamento de Biología de la Reproduccióny Clínicade Desórdenes de Sueño,Universidad Autónoma Metropolitana-Iztapalapa, D.F., México

Guillermo Robles-Díaz
Laboratorio de Hígado, Páncreas y Motilidad, Unidadde Medicina Experimental, Hospital General de México, D.F., México

Lourdes Solís-Lozano, Karina Suárez-Álvarez and Galileo Escobedo
Laboratorio de Hígado, Páncreas y Motilidad, Unidadde Medicina Experimental, Hospital General de México, D.F., México
Facultad de Medicina, Departamento de Medicina Experimental, Hospital General de México, Universidad Nacional Autónoma de México, D.F., México

Antonio González-Chávez
Servicio de Medicina Interna, Hospital General de México, D.F., México

Yadira L. Béjar
Servicio de Bancode Sangre, Hospital General de Méx-ico, D.F., México

Evan Papps and Bernhard T. Baune
Discipline of Psychiatry, School of Medicine, University of Adelaide, Adelaide, SA, Australia

Harris A. Eyre
Discipline of Psychiatry, School of Medicine, University of Adelaide, Adelaide, SA, Australia
School of Medicine and Dentistry, James Cook University, Townsville, QLD, Australia

J. Luis Quintanar and Irene Guzmán-Soto
Laboratory of Neurophy siology, Department of Physiology and Pharmacology, Centro de Ciencias Básicas, Universidad Autónoma de Aguascalientes, Aguascalientes, México

Daniel K. Goyal and Jaleel A. Miyan
Faculty of Life Sciences, The University of Manchester, Manchester, UK

Rafael Campos-Rodríguez, MaryCarmen Godínez-Victoria, Edgar Abarca-Rojano, Judith Pacheco-Yépez, Humberto Reyna-Garfias and Reyna Elizabeth Barbosa-Cabrera
Sección de Posgrado e Investigación, Escuela Superior de Medicina, Instituto Politécnico Nacional, Distrito Federal, México

Maria Elisa Drago-Serrano
Departamento de Sistemas Biológicos, Unidad Xochimilco, Universidad Autónoma Metropolitana, Distrito Federal, México

Lidia Garcia-Bonilla, Corinne Benakis, Jamie Moore, Costantino Iadecola and Josef Anrather
Brain and Mind Research Institute, Weill Cornell Medical College, New York, NY, USA

Helen B. Stolp
Department of Perinatal Imaging and Health, King's College London, London, UK
Department of Physiology, Anatomy and Genetics, University of Oxford, Oxford, UK

Shane A. Liddelow
Department of Neurobiology, Stanford University, Stanford, CA, USA
Department of Pharmacology and Therapeutics, University of Melbourne, Parkville, VIC, Australia

Katarzyna M. Dziegielewska and Norman R. Saunders
Department of Pharmacology and Therapeutics, University of Melbourne, Parkville, VIC, Australia

Inês Sá-Pereira
Department of Pharmacology, University of Oxford, Oxford, UK

Joanne I. Pennock
Translational Medicine, Faculty of Medical and Human Sciences, The University of Manchester, Manchester, UK

Bakri M. Assas
Translational Medicine, Faculty of Medical and Human Sciences, The University of Manchester, Manchester, UK
Department of Immunology, Faculty of Applied Sciences, King Abdulaziz University, Jeddah, SaudiArabia

Jaleel A. Miyan
Neurosciences, Faculty of Life Sciences,The University of Manchester, Manchester, UK

Nela Monasterio and Teresa Morales
Departamento de Neurobiología Celulary Molecular, Instituto de Neurobiología, Universidad Nacional Autónoma de México, Santiago de Querétaro, México

Edgar Vergara
Departamento de Biología, Facultad de Química, Universidad Nacional Autónoma de México, Ciudadde México, México

Brian M. Campbell, Erik Charych, Anna W. Lee and Thomas Möller
Neuroinflammation Disease Biology Unit, Lundbeck Research USA, Paramus, NJ, USA

Augusto J. Montiel-Castro
Centro Darwinde Pensamiento Evolucionista and Philosophy Department, Social Sciences and Humanities Division, Universidad Autonoma Metropolitana Iztapalapa, Mexico City, Mexico

Gabriela Bravo-Ruiseco and Gustavo Pacheco-López
Health Sciences Department, Biological and Health Sciences Division, Universidad Autonoma Metropolitana Lerma, Lerma, Mexico

Rina M. González-Cervantes
Health Sciences Department, Biological and Health Sciences Division, Universidad Autonoma Metropolitana Lerma, Lerma, Mexico
Biological Systems Department, Biological and Health Sciences Division, Universidad Autonoma Metropolitana Xochimilco, Mexico City, Mexico

Jesus M. Pradillo, Caroline Drake, Hannah Buggey, Nancy J. Rothwell and Stuart M. Allan
Faculty of Life Sciences, University of Manchester, Manchester, UK

Adam Denes
Faculty of Life Sciences, University of Manchester, Manchester, UK
Laboratory of Molecular Neuroendocrinology, Institute of Experimental Medicine, Budapest, Hungary

Marco A. Meraz-Ríos
Departamento de Biomedicina Molecular, Centro de Investigación y de Estudios Avanzados, Mexico City, Mexico

Danira Toral-Rios
Departamento de Fisiología Biofísica y Neurociencias, Centrode Investigación y de Estudios Avanzados, Mexico City, Mexico

Diana Franco-Bocanegra
Posgrado en Ciencias Biológicas, Universidad Nacional Autónoma de México, Mexico City, Mexico

Juana Villeda-Hernández
Departamento de Neuropatología Experimental, Instituto Nacional de Neurología y Neurocirugía, Mexico City, Mexico

Victoria Campos-Peña
Laboratorio Experimental de Enfermedades Neurodegenerativas, Instituto Nacional de Neurología y Neurocirugía Manuel Velasco Suárez, Mexico City, Mexico

Daisuke Kamimura, Moe Yamada, Masaya Harada, Lavannya Sabharwal, Jie Meng, Hidenori Bando, Hideki Ogura, Toru Atsumi, Yasunobu Arima and Masaaki Murakami
JST-CREST, WPI Immunology Frontier Research Center, Graduate School of Frontier Biosciences, Graduate School of Medicine, Osaka University, Suita, Osaka, Japan

L. Garzoni and C. Faure
CHU Sainte Justine Research Center, Montreal, QC, Canada
Division of Gastroenterology, Hepatology and Nutrition, CHU Sainte-Justine, Montreal, QC, Canada

M. G. Frasch
CHU Sainte Justine Research Center, Montreal, QC, Canada
Department of Obstetrics and Gynaecology, University of Montreal, Montreal, QC, Canada

Vincent Geenen, Gwennaëlle Bodart, Séverine Henry, Hélène Michaux, Olivier Dardenne, Chantal Charlet-Renard and Henri Martens
Department of Biomedical and Preclinical Sciences, Center of Immunoendocrinology, GIGA Research Institute, Fund of Scientific Research, University of Liege, Liege-Sart Tilman, Belgium

Didier Hober
Laboratory of Virology EA3610, University of Lille 2and CHRU Lille, Lille, France

Gabriela Hurtado-Alvarado, Adrian M. Cabañas-Morales and Beatriz Gómez-González
Area of Neurosciences, Department of Biology of Reproduction, Unidad Iztapalapa, Universidad Autónoma Metropolitana, Mexico City, Mexico

Michael Kavanaugh, Chih-kai Chao and Charles Thompson
Department of Biomedical Sciences, The Center for Structural and Functional Neurosciences, The University of Montana, Missoula, MT, USA

Maricela Franco-Lira and Mariana Aragón-Flores
Hospital Central Militar, Secretaria de la Defensa Nacional, Mexico City, Mexico

Lilian Calderón-Garcidueñas
Department of Biomedical Sciences, The Center for Structural and Functional Neurosciences, The University of Montana, Missoula, MT, USA
Hospital Central Militar, Secretaria de la Defensa Nacional, Mexico City, Mexico

Janet V. Cross
Department of Pathology, School of Medicine, University of Virginia, Charlottesville, VA, USA

Ricardo Torres-Jardón
Centro de Ciencias de la Atmósfera, Universidad Nacional Autónoma de México, Mexico City, Mexico

Jing Chang and Hongtu Zhu
Department of Biostatistics, Gillings School of Global Public Health, University of North Carolina, Chapel Hill, NC, USA

Amedeo D'Angiulli
Department of Neuroscience, Carleton University, Ottawa, ON, Canada

Index

A

Adolescence, 14, 37, 61, 228

Air Pollution, 222-223, 225-229, 232

Alzheimer's Disease, 5, 17, 37-39, 44, 122, 125, 131, 141-142, 144-147, 173-174, 183-187, 216-220, 229-232

Amyloid-B , 173, 185, 230, 232

Anaesthesia, 164-171

Anaphylatoxin, 176, 219

Anti-inflammatory Strategies, 173

Astrocytes, 16, 19, 21-23, 35, 37-38, 79, 86, 91, 97-98, 102, 104, 127, 130-131, 138, 143-144, 173-180, 183-186, 212, 214-215, 219, 230

Autism, 1-2, 6-9, 58-59, 61, 64-66, 97, 151, 158, 160, 163

Autism Spectrum Disorder, 8, 58-59, 64, 163

B

Blood-brain Barrier, 47, 53, 75, 82, 90, 92, 96-98, 100-109, 122, 124, 143, 175, 178, 188, 190, 192, 212-221

Bone Marrow, 2-3, 7, 37, 43, 51, 54, 99, 104, 107, 111-117, 128, 135, 144, 164-165, 167-171, 203

Brain Development, 96-99, 104-105

Brain-gut Axis, 67, 70, 162

C

C Fibers, 110-115

Cannabinoids, 74, 87, 90, 93, 95

Central Nervous System, 1, 16, 40, 43, 61, 67, 84, 86, 96, 98, 107-108, 115, 144, 147, 149, 151, 173, 183, 185, 188-189, 194-195, 212-214, 219, 223, 230

Cerebrospinal Fluid, 59, 96, 98, 106-108, 137, 143-146, 161, 176, 184, 186, 222, 229-230

Choroid Plexus, 21-22, 96-109

Cns Disease, 64, 127, 141, 146, 229

Corticosteroids, 71, 120, 128, 151, 181, 183

Craniotomy, 164-169

Cytokines, 1, 8, 14, 19, 23, 27, 32, 36, 40, 44, 47, 51, 53, 55, 59, 62, 66, 69, 74, 77, 82, 90, 94, 97, 100, 107, 113, 120, 124, 127, 136, 138, 143, 145, 150, 157, 164, 173, 179, 182, 185, 188, 191, 193, 196, 198, 200, 210, 212, 215, 222, 231

D

Dentate Gyrus, 21, 24, 32, 37, 40, 122, 220

Depression, 8, 16-27, 31, 35-41, 44, 63, 77-78, 80, 82, 91-92, 95, 130, 134, 136-138, 142-147, 151, 157, 161, 188, 199, 229

E

Encephalomyelitis, 44, 54, 56, 96, 107, 117, 123, 125, 133, 142-143, 146-147, 162, 188, 192, 217

Endotoxin, 2-3, 27, 38, 41, 78, 84, 90, 93-94, 114-115, 137, 141, 144, 167-168, 199, 201, 221

Epigenetics, 77, 93

Evolutionary Psychology, 149, 162

Experimental Stroke, 75, 84, 92, 164-165, 170-171

G

Gastrointestinal, 43, 45, 63, 66, 76, 117-118, 149, 160, 193, 195-196, 200, 226

Glucocorticoid, 16-17, 24, 35, 47, 73-74, 76, 119, 121, 139, 142, 159, 181, 230

Gut Microbiota, 24, 58, 66, 71, 149-151, 153-154, 157, 159-162

Gut-brain Axis, 110, 149-150, 157, 160-161

H

Heterogeneity, 39, 58, 61-62, 64, 108, 117, 144

Huntington's Disease, 132-133, 141-147

Hyperinsulinemia, 14

Hypothalamus, 15, 32, 42-43, 45, 48-49, 54, 63, 67-69, 73, 119-120, 123, 150

Hypothermia, 77, 79-81, 90, 92, 95

I

Immune System, 1, 17, 21, 23, 36-37, 41-53, 55-57, 60-61, 63, 65, 67, 69, 74, 76-78, 80, 82, 86, 88-92, 99, 104, 106-107, 120-123, 125, 133, 136, 141, 144, 149, 152, 163, 171-172, 177, 188, 190, 195, 202-, 205-206, 212, 222, 227-229

Innate Immunity, 8, 90-91, 93, 161, 163, 193, 197, 222, 230-231

Intestinal Mucosa, 67

Ischemic Tolerance, 77-78, 81, 85, 90, 92-95

K

Kynurenine, 38, 127-128, 130-148

L

Lactation, 119-126, 153, 155

Leptin, 10-15, 192, 220

Leuprolide Acetate, 50-52

Low-grade Inflammation, 10, 15

M

Macrophage, 1-5, 7-8, 14-17, 22, 31, 38, 40, 45, 51, 54, 59-60, 66, 100, 113-115, 117, 122-123, 128, 130, 134, 137, 140, 145, 175, 178, 185, 198, 213, 222-226, 229-232

Metabolic Disease, 10

Microglia, 1, 7-8, 16, 19-23, 27, 32, 34-41, 59, 64, 86, 97, 99-107, 109, 118, 127-135, 139-145, 147, 173-180, 182-187, 190, 212, 214-216, 219, 230

Micrornas, 40, 77-78, 89-95, 208, 210-211

Monocytes, 7-8, 22, 32, 36, 46-47, 51, 66, 81, 86, 93, 100, 105, 111-112, 114-117, 128, 131, 144-145, 170, 172, 178, 183, 185, 226

Mononuclear Cells, 15, 44, 47, 49-50, 53-54, 116, 122, 209, 214

Multiple Sclerosis, 5, 8, 37, 44, 52, 54, 56, 96, 100-101, 107-108, 121, 126, 133-135, 141-146, 188-190, 192, 219, 223, 230, 232

N

Neuro-immune, 7, 58, 63, 110, 124, 188, 190-191, 216, 219, 222-223, 226

Neurobiology, 16, 19, 58, 65-66, 96, 149-150, 162-163

Neurodegeneration, 39-40, 123, 132-134, 136, 145, 148, 173, 175-177, 183, 185-186, 214, 217, 219, 222, 227, 229, 231

Neuroimmune, 16-17, 19-20, 22, 24-28, 31-39, 74, 76, 110, 116, 119-120, 172, 185, 200, 220

Neuroimmunology, 110, 115, 183, 193

Neuroinflammation, 8, 16, 19-20, 24, 27, 33-34, 37-40, 58-59, 64, 90, 92, 94-96, 100, 107-108, 127, 132-133, 136-138, 140, 142-143, 145-148, 163-164, 172-173, 177, 183-187, 191, 219-223, 225-231

O

Oligodendrocytes, 21, 106, 109, 123, 175, 185-186

P

Parkinson's Disease, 44, 102, 107, 109, 132, 143-144, 146-148, 183, 215, 223, 229-230

Particulate Matter, 222-223, 232

Preconditioning, 77-81, 83, 85-95, 171

Prion Cellular Protein, 222

Progesterone, 119-125

Prolactin, 42-43, 56, 119-120, 122-126

Psychiatry, 8-9, 16-18, 36-41, 58, 64-66, 75, 109, 142-144, 146-147, 184-185, 230

Psychoneuroimmunology, 144, 149

R

Rapid Eye Movement, 218, 220

Restraint-stress, 67

S

Schizophrenia, 8, 16, 44, 58, 97, 131, 138-139, 141-147, 157, 160

Social Bonds, 149-150, 154, 157-159, 162

Spleen, 15, 43-45, 49-50, 54-57, 73, 112, 115, 121, 164-165, 168-170, 196, 208

T

Testis, 43, 45, 54, 56, 204

Tetrahydropyridine, 132, 141, 143-144, 225

Trachea, 116, 169

Type 2 Diabetes, 10, 41, 221

www.ingramcontent.com/pod-product-compliance
Lightning Source LLC
LaVergne TN
LVHW081039210926
848485LV00004B/1059